AND
THE BAND
PLAYED ON

ALSO BY RANDY SHILTS:

The Mayor of Castro Street:
The Life & Times of Harvey Milk

AND THE BAND PLAYED ON

POLITICS, PEOPLE, AND THE AIDS EPIDEMIC

RANDY SHILTS

St. Martin's Press

NEW YORK

Design by Claire Counihan

Shilts, Randy.
    And the band played on.

    1. AIDS (Disease)—Political aspects—United States.
2. AIDS (Disease)—Social aspects—United States.
I. Title.
RA644.A25S48   1987   362.1'969792'00973   87-16528
ISBN 0-312-00994-1

For Ann Neuenschwander

CONTENTS

PART VIII. THE BUTCHER'S BILL/1985

PART IX. EPILOGUE/AFTER

ACKNOWLEDGMENTS

I would not have been able to write this book if I had not been a reporter at the *San Francisco Chronicle,* the only daily newspaper in the United States that did not need a movie star to come down with AIDS before it considered the epidemic a legitimate news story deserving thorough coverage. Because of the *Chronicle*'s enlightened stance, I have had free rein to cover this epidemic since 1982; since 1983, I have spent virtually all my time reporting on AIDS. My reporting provided the core of this book. While this newspaper's commitment is a credit to all levels of *Chronicle* management, I particularly want to thank my city editor, Alan Mutter, who believed in the value of this story long before it was fashionable. I'm also grateful to the following *Chronicle* colleagues for their guidance and assistance: Katy Butler, David Perlman, Jerry Burns, Keith Power, and Kathy Finberg. The *Chronicle*'s library staff, especially Charlie Malarkey, also helped immensely.

My newspaper reporting would never have been transformed into a book if it were not for the faith of my editor at St. Martin's Press, Michael Denneny. He believed in this project when most in publishing doubted that the epidemic would ever prove serious enough to warrant a major book. I'm also grateful to the confidence of my agent, Fred Hill.

A number of other people helped me edit the manuscript. Without the constant encouragement, hand-holding, and insightful editing of Doris Ober, I could never have made it to the end of what became a very long tome. I'm also grateful to Katie Leishman and Rex Adkins for devoting their extraordinary editing talents to the manuscript.

The research phase of the book required much travel and would not have been tolerable without hosts such as Poul Birch Eriksen in Copenhagen, Mark Pinney in New York City, and Bob Canning and Steve Sansweet in Los Angeles. I'm also thankful to Frank Robinson, who kept voluminous files on the epidemic and generously shared them all with me. Among the other people who charitably opened their files to me were Tim Westmoreland, Dan Turner, David Nimmons, Jeff Richardson, Lawrence Schulman, Tom Murray of *The Sentinel,* Don Michaels of the *Washington Blade,* Terry Biern of the American Foundation for AIDS Research, and Jim Kepner of the AIDS History Project at the International Gay and Lesbian Archives in Los Angeles. Steve Unger and Fred Hoffman provided expert computer assistance. I would be remiss if I didn't acknowledge the help I got from the media relations staffs of San Francisco General Hospital, Pasteur Institute, National Cancer Institute, National Institute for Allergy and Infectious Diseases, and especially Chuck Fallis at the Centers for Disease Control. They made my job much easier.

I remain indebted to my brothers Reed Shilts, Russell Dennis Shilts III, and Gary Shilts for their support during the long writing process. I'm also blessed by some terrific friends who stuck by me during the insanity of this project: Janie Krohn, Bill Reiner, David Israels, Bill Cagle, Will Pretty, and Rich Shortell. Thanks also to the friends of Bill W. who sustained me with their experience, strength, and hope.

Ultimately, a reporter is only as good as his sources. The people to whom I remain most grateful are the hundreds who shared their time with me both during my newspaper reporting and during the book research. Many were scientists and doctors who carved large blocks of time out of hectic schedules. My deep background and off-the-record sources were also invaluable; you know who you are, and I thank you.

The people for whom I will always bear special reverence are those who were suffering from AIDS and who gave some of their last hours for interviews, sometimes while they were on their deathbeds laboring for breath. When I'd ask why they'd take the time for this, most hoped that something they said would save someone else from suffering. If there is an act that better defines heroism, I have not seen it.

DRAMATIS PERSONAE

DR. FRANCOISE BARRE, a researcher with the Pasteur Institute, the first to isolate the AIDS virus.

DR. BOB BIGGAR, a researcher with the Environmental Epidemiology branch of the National Cancer Institute.

FRANCES BORCHELT, a San Francisco grandmother.

DR. EDWARD BRANDT, Assistant Secretary for Health of the U.S. Department of Health and Human Services.

JOE BREWER, a gay psychotherapist in San Francisco's Castro Street neighborhood.

HARRY BRITT, the only openly gay member of San Francisco's board of supervisors, the local equivalent of a city council.

U.S. REPRESENTATIVE PHILIP BURTON, a staunch liberal who represented San Francisco in Congress.

U.S. REPRESENTATIVE SALA BURTON succeeded her husband in Congress.

MICHAEL CALLEN, a rock singer who organized the People With AIDS Coalition in New York City.

LU CHAIKIN, a lesbian psychotherapist in San Francisco's Castro Street neighborhood.

DR. JEAN-CLAUDE CHERMANN, part of the Pasteur Institute team that first isolated the AIDS virus.

DR. MARCUS CONANT, a dermatologist affiliated with the University of California at San Francisco.

DR. JAMES CURRAN, an epidemiologist and director of AIDS research efforts at the U.S. Centers for Disease Control in Atlanta.

WILLIAM DARROW, a sociologist and epidemiologist involved with AIDS research at the Centers for Disease Control.

DR. WALTER DOWDLE, director of the Center for Infectious Diseases.

DR. SELMA DRITZ, assistant director of the Bureau of Communicable Disease Control at the San Francisco Department of Public Health.

GAETAN DUGAS, a French-Canadian airline steward for Air Canada, one of the first North Americans diagnosed with AIDS.

DR. MYRON "MAX" ESSEX, a retrovirologist with Harvard University School of Public Health.

SANDRA FORD, a drug technician at the Centers for Disease Control.

DR. WILLIAM FOEGE, director of the Centers for Disease Control during the first years of the AIDS epidemic.

DR. DONALD FRANCIS, a retrovirologist who directed laboratory efforts for AIDS research at the Centers for Disease Control.

DR. ROBERT GALLO, a retrovirologist with the National Cancer Institute in Bethesda.

DR. MICHAEL GOTTLIEB, an immunologist with the University of California at Los Angeles.

ENRIQUE "KICO" GOVANTES, a gay San Francisco artist, lover of Bill Kraus.

DR. JAMES GROUNDWATER, a dermatologist who treated San Francisco's first reported AIDS case.

DR. MARY GUINAN, an epidemiologist involved with early AIDS research at the Centers for Disease Control.

MARGARET HECKLER, Secretary of the U.S. Department of Health and Human Services from early 1983 through the end of 1985.

KEN HORNE, the first reported AIDS case in San Francisco.

DR. HAROLD JAFFE, an epidemiologist with the AIDS program at the Centers for Disease Control.

CLEVE JONES, a San Francisco gay activist, organizer of the Kaposi's Sarcoma Research and Education Foundation.

LARRY KRAMER, novelist, playwright, and film producer, organizer of Gay Men's Health Crisis in New York City.

BILL KRAUS, prominent San Francisco gay leader, aide to U.S. Reps. Philip and Sala Burton.

MATTHEW KRIEGER, a San Francisco graphic designer, lover of Gary Walsh.

DR. MATHILDE KRIM, socially prominent cancer researcher, organized the AIDS Medical Foundation.

DR. DALE LAWRENCE, conducted early studies of AIDS in hemophiliacs and blood transfusion recipients for the Centers for Disease Control.

MICHAEL MALETTA, hair dresser who was one of San Francisco's early AIDS cases.

DR. JAMES MASON, director of the Centers for Disease Control since late 1983, served as acting Assistant Secretary for Health in 1985.

RODGER MCFARLANE, executive director of the Gay Men's Health Crisis in New York City.

DR. DONNA MILDVAN, AIDS researcher at Beth Israel Medical Center in Manhattan.

DR. LUC MONTAGNIER, head of the Pasteur Institute team that first isolated the AIDS virus.

JACK NAU, one of New York City's early AIDS cases, a former lover of Paul Popham.

ENNO POERSCH, a graphic designer drawn into AIDS organizing because of the death of his lover, Nick, in early 1981.

PAUL POPHAM, Wall Street businessman, president of Gay Men's Health Crisis.

DR. GRETHE RASK, Danish surgeon in Zaire, first westerner documented to have died of AIDS.

DR. WILLY ROZENBAUM, leading AIDS clinician in Paris.

DR. ARYE RUBINSTEIN, immunologist in the Bronx, among the first to detect AIDS in infants.

DR. DAVID SENCER, health commissioner of New York City.

DR. MERVYN SILVERMAN, director of the San Francisco Department of Public Health.

DR. PAUL VOLBERDING, director of the San Francisco General Hospital AIDS Clinic.

GARY WALSH, a San Francisco gay psychotherapist, early organizer of AIDS sufferers.

U.S. REPRESENTATIVE HENRY WAXMAN of Los Angeles, chair of House Subcommittee on Health and the Environment.

DR. JOEL WEISMAN, a prominent gay physician in Los Angeles, among the first to detect the AIDS epidemic.

RICK WELLIKOFF, a Brooklyn schoolteacher who was among the nation's first AIDS cases, close friend of Paul Popham.

TIM WESTMORELAND, counsel to the House Subcommittee on Health and the Environment.

DR. DAN WILLIAM, a prominent gay physician in New York City.

THE
BUREAUCRACY

In the government of the United States, health agencies are part of the **U.S. Department of Health and Human Services (HHS)**. Most of the key health and scientific research agencies fall under the umbrella of the **U.S. Public Health Service (PHS)**, which is directed by the Assistant Secretary for Health of the Department of Health and Human Services. The **National Institutes of Health (NIH)**, **Food and Drug Administration (FDA)**, and **Centers for Disease Control (CDC)** are among the agencies that comprise the PHS.

The **National Institutes of Health** is comprised of various separate institutes that conduct most of the government's laboratory research into health matters. The two largest institutes at the NIH are also the two that were most involved in AIDS research, the **National Cancer Institute (NCI)** and the **National Institute of Allergy and Infectious Diseases (NIAID)**.

The **Centers for Disease Control** is comprised of different centers that handle various public health problems. The largest is the **Center for Infectious Diseases**, under which AIDS research has been handled through most of the epidemic. The **Kaposi Sarcoma–Opportunistic Infections Task Force (KSOI Task Force)**, which changed its name to the **AIDS Task Force**, and later to the **AIDS Activities Office**, was part of the CID.

The **Kaposi's Sarcoma Research and Education Foundation (KS Foundation)** was organized in San Francisco in early 1982. In 1983, it split into the **National Kaposi's Sarcoma/AIDS Research and Education Foundation (National KS Foundation)**, which dissolved in 1984, and the **San Francisco Kaposi's Sarcoma/AIDS Research Foundation**. The latter group subsequently changed its name to the **San Francisco AIDS Foundation**.

The **AIDS Medical Foundation** was organized in New York City in 1983. In 1985, it merged with the **National AIDS Research Foundation** to become the **American Foundation for AIDS Research (AmFAR)**.

AND
THE BAND
PLAYED ON

PROLOGUE

By October 2, 1985, the morning Rock Hudson died, the word was familiar to almost every household in the Western world.

AIDS.

Acquired Immune Deficiency Syndrome had seemed a comfortably distant threat to most of those who had heard of it before, the misfortune of people who fit into rather distinct classes of outcasts and social pariahs. But suddenly, in the summer of 1985, when a movie star was diagnosed with the disease and the newspapers couldn't stop talking about it, the AIDS epidemic became palpable and the threat loomed everywhere.

Suddenly there were children with AIDS who wanted to go to school, laborers with AIDS who wanted to work, and researchers who wanted funding, and there was a threat to the nation's public health that could no longer be ignored. Most significantly, there were the first glimmers of awareness that the future would always contain this strange new word. AIDS would become a part of American culture and indelibly change the course of our lives.

The implications would not be fleshed out for another few years, but on that October day in 1985 the first awareness existed just the same. Rock Hudson riveted America's attention upon this deadly new threat for the first time, and his diagnosis became a demarcation that would separate the history of America before AIDS from the history that came after.

The timing of this awareness, however, reflected the unalterable tragedy at the heart of the AIDS epidemic: By the time America paid attention to the disease, it was too late to do anything about it. The virus was already pandemic in the nation, having spread to every corner of the North American continent. The tide of death that would later sweep America could, perhaps, be slowed, but it could not be stopped.

The AIDS epidemic, of course, did not arise full grown from the biological landscape; the problem had been festering throughout the decade. The death tolls of the late 1980s are not startling new developments but an unfolding of events predicted for many years. There had been a time when much of this suffering could have been prevented, but by 1985 that time had passed. Indeed, on the day the world learned that Rock Hudson was stricken, some 12,000 Americans were already dead or dying of AIDS and hundreds of thousands more were infected with the virus that caused the disease. But few had paid any attention to this; nobody, it seemed, had cared about them.

The bitter truth was that AIDS did not just happen to America—it was allowed to happen by an array of institutions, all of which failed to perform their appropriate tasks to safeguard the public health. This failure of the system leaves a legacy of unnecessary suffering that will haunt the Western world for decades to come.

There was no excuse, in this country and in this time, for the spread of a deadly new epidemic. For this was a time in which the United States boasted the world's most sophisticated medicine and the world's most extensive public health system, geared to eliminate such pestilence from our national life. When the virus appeared, the world's richest nation housed the most lavishly financed scientific research establishments— both inside the vast governmental health bureaucracy and in other institutions—to investigate new diseases and quickly bring them under control. And making sure that government researchers and public health agencies did their jobs were the world's most unfettered and aggressive media, the public's watchdogs. Beyond that, the group most affected by the epidemic, the gay community, had by then built a substantial political infrastructure, particularly in cities where the disease struck first and most virulently. Leaders were in place to monitor the gay community's health and survival interests.

But from 1980, when the first isolated gay men began falling ill from strange and exotic ailments, nearly five years passed before all these institutions—medicine, public health, the federal and private scientific research establishments, the mass media, and the gay community's leadership—mobilized the way they should in a time of threat. The story of these first five years of AIDS in America is a drama of national failure, played out against a backdrop of needless death.

People died while Reagan administration officials ignored pleas from government scientists and did not allocate adequate funding for AIDS research until the epidemic had already spread throughout the country.

People died while scientists did not at first devote appropriate attention to the epidemic because they perceived little prestige to be gained in studying a homosexual affliction. Even after this denial faded, people died while some scientists, most notably those in the employ of the United States government, competed rather than collaborated in international research efforts, and so diverted attention and energy away from the central struggle against the disease itself.

People died while public health authorities and the political leaders who guided them refused to take the tough measures necessary to curb the epidemic's spread, opting for political expediency over the public health.

And people died while gay community leaders played politics with the disease, putting political dogma ahead of the preservation of human life.

People died and nobody paid attention because the mass media did not like covering stories about homosexuals and was especially skittish about stories that involved gay sexuality. Newspapers and television largely avoided discussion of the disease until the death toll was too high to ignore and the casualties were no longer just the outcasts. Without the media to fulfill its role as public guardian, everyone else was left to deal—and not deal—with AIDS as they saw fit.

In those early years, the federal government viewed AIDS as a budget problem, local public health officials saw it as a political problem, gay leaders considered AIDS a public relations problem, and the news media regarded it as a homosexual problem that wouldn't interest anybody else. Consequently, few confronted AIDS for what it was, a profoundly threatening medical crisis.

Fighting against this institutional indifference were a handful of heroes from disparate callings. Isolated teams of scientists in research centers in America and Europe risked their reputations and often their jobs to pioneer early research on AIDS. There were doctors and nurses who went far beyond the call of duty to care for its victims. Some public health officials struggled valiantly to have the epidemic addressed in earnest. A handful of gay leaders withstood vilification to argue forcefully for a sane community response to the epidemic and to lobby for the funds that provided the first breakthroughs in research. And there were many victims of the epidemic who fought rejection, fear, isolation, and their own deadly prognoses to make people understand and to make people care.

Because of their efforts, the story of politics, people, and the AIDS epidemic is, ultimately, a tale of courage as well as cowardice, compassion as well as bigotry, inspiration as well as venality, and redemption as well as despair.

It is a tale that bears telling, so that it will never happen again, to any people, anywhere.

PART I

BEHOLD, A PALE HORSE

And I looked, and behold a pale horse:
and his name that sat on him
was Death, and Hell followed with
him. And power was given unto
them over the fourth part of the
earth, to kill with sword, and with
hunger, and with death, and with
the beasts of the earth.

—REVELATION 6:8

1 THE FEAST OF THE HEARTS

July 4, 1976
NEW YORK HARBOR

Tall sails scraped the deep purple night as rockets burst, flared, and flourished red, white, and blue over the stoic Statue of Liberty. The whole world was watching, it seemed; the whole world was there. Ships from fifty-five nations had poured sailors into Manhattan to join the throngs, counted in the millions, who watched the greatest pyrotechnic extravaganza ever mounted, all for America's 200th birthday party. Deep into the morning, bars all over the city were crammed with sailors. New York City had hosted the greatest party ever known, everybody agreed later. The guests had come from all over the world.

This was the part the epidemiologists would later note, when they stayed up late at night and the conversation drifted toward where it had started and when. They would remember that glorious night in New York Harbor, all those sailors, and recall: From all over the world they came to New York.

Christmas Eve, 1976
KINSHASA, ZAIRE

The hot African sky turned black and sultry; it wasn't like Christmas at all.

The unrelenting mugginess of the equatorial capital made Dr. Ib Bygbjerg even lonelier for Denmark. In the kitchen, Dr. Grethe Rask, determined to assuage her young colleague's homesickness, began preparing an approximation of the dinner with which Danes traditionally begin their Christmas observance, the celebration known through centuries of custom as the Feast of the Hearts.

The preparations brought back memories of the woman's childhood in Thisted, the ancient Jutland port nestled on the Lim Fiord not far from the North Sea. As the main course, Grethe Rask knew, there needed to be something that flies. In Jutland that would mean goose or duck; in Zaire, chicken would have to suffice. As she began preparing the fowl, Grethe again felt the familiar fatigue wash over her. She had spent the last two years haunted by weariness, and by now, she knew she couldn't fight it.

Grethe collapsed on her bed. She had been among the Danish doctors who came to replace the Belgian physicians who were no longer welcome in this new nation eager to forget its recent colonial incarnation as the Belgian Congo. Grethe had first gone there in 1964, returning to Europe for training in stomach surgery and tropical diseases. She had spent the last four years in Zaire but, despite all this time in Africa, she remained unmistakably from the Danish stock who proudly announce themselves as north of the fjord. To be north of the Lim Fiord was to be direct and decisive, independent and plainspoken. The Jutlanders born south of the stretch of water that divides the Danish peninsula tend toward weakness, as anyone north of the fjord might explain. Far from the kings in Copenhagen, these hardy northern people had nurtured their collective heritage for centuries. Grethe Rask from Thisted mirrored this.

It explained why she was here in Zaire, 5,000 miles from where she might forge a lucrative career as a surgeon in the sprawling modern hospitals of Copenhagen. Such a cosmopolitan career meant people looking over her shoulder, giving orders. Grethe preferred the work she had done at a primitive hospital in the remote village of Abumombazi in the north of Zaire. She alone was in charge there.

The hospital conditions in Abumombazi were not as deplorable as in other parts of the country. A prominent Zairian general came from the region. He had had the clout to attract a white doctor to the village, and there, with Belgian nuns, Grethe worked with what she could beg and borrow. This was Central Africa, after all, and even a favored clinic would never have such basics as sterile rubber gloves or disposable needles. You just used needles again and again until they wore out; once gloves had worn through, you risked dipping your hands in your patient's blood because that was what needed to be done. The lack of rudimentary supplies meant that a surgeon's work had risks that doctors in the developed world could not imagine, particularly because the undeveloped part, specifically Central Africa, seemed to sire new diseases with nightmarish regularity. Earlier that year, not far from Abumombazi, in a village along the Ebola River on the Zaire-Sudan border, a virulent outbreak of a horrifying new disease had demonstrated the dangers of primitive medicine and new viruses. A trader from the village of Enzara, suffering from fevers and profuse, uncontrollable bleeding, had come to the teaching hospital for nurses in Maridi. The man apparently had picked up the disease sexually. Within days, however, 40 percent of the student nurses in Maridi were stricken with the fever, transmitted by contact with the patient's infected blood either through standard care procedures or through accidental needle-sticks.

Frightened African health officials swallowed their pride and called the World Health Organization, who came with a staff from the American Centers for Disease Control. By the time the young American doctors arrived, thirty-nine nurses and two doctors were dead. The CDC doctors worked quickly, isolating all patients with fevers. Natives were infuriated when the Americans banned the traditional burials of the victims since the ritual bathing of the bodies was clearly spreading the disease further. Within weeks, however, the epidemic was under control. In the end, the Ebola Fever virus, as it came to be known, killed 53 percent of the people it infected, seizing 153 lives before it disappeared as suddenly and mysteriously as it had arisen. Sex and blood were two horribly efficient ways to spread a new virus, and years later, a tenuous relief would fill the voices of doctors who talked of how fortunate it was for humankind that this new killer had awakened in this most remote corner of the world and had been stamped out so quickly. A site just a bit closer to regional crossroads could have unleashed a horrible plague. With modern roads and jet travel, no corner of the earth was very remote anymore; never again could diseases linger undetected for centuries among a distant people without finding some route to fan out across the planet.

The battle between humans and disease was nowhere more bitterly fought than here in the fetid equatorial climate, where heat and humidity fuel the generation of new life forms. One historian has suggested that humans, who first evolved in Africa eons ago, migrated north to Asia and Europe simply to get to climates that were less hospitable to the deadly microbes the tropics so efficiently bred.

Here, on the frontiers of the world's harshest medical realities, Grethe Rask tended the sick. In her three years in Abumombazi, she had bullied and cajoled people for the resources to build her jungle hospital, and she was loved to the point of idolization by the local people. Then, she returned to the Danish Red Cross Hospital, the largest medical institution in the bustling city of Kinshasa, where she assumed the duties of chief surgeon. Here she met Ib Bygbjerg, who had returned from another rural outpost in the south. Bygbjerg's thick dark hair and small compact frame belied his Danish ancestry, the legacy, he figured, of some Spanish sailor who made his way to Denmark centuries ago. Grethe Rask had the features one would expect of a woman from Thisted, high cheekbones and blond hair worn short in a cut that some delicately called mannish.

To Bygbjerg's eye, on that Christmas Eve, there were troubling things to note about Grethe's appearance. She was thin, losing weight from a mysterious diarrhea. She had been suffering from the vague yet persistent malaise for two years now, since her time in the impoverished northern villages. In 1975, the problem had receded briefly after drug treatments, but for the past year, nothing had seemed to help. The surgeon's weight dropped further, draining and weakening her with each passing day.

Even more alarming was the disarray in the forty-six-year-old woman's lymphatic system, the glands that play the central role in the body's never-ending fight to make itself immune from disease. All of Grethe's lymph glands were swollen and had been for nearly two years. Normally, a lymph node might swell here or there to fight this or that infection, revealing a small lump on the neck, under an arm, or perhaps, in the groin. There didn't seem to be any reason for her glands to swell; there was no precise infection anywhere, much less anything that would cause such a universal enlargement of the lymph nodes all over her body.

And the fatigue. It was the most disconcerting aspect of the surgeon's malaise. Of course, in the best of times, this no-nonsense woman from north of the fjord did not grasp the concept of relaxation. Just that day, for example, she had not been scheduled to work, but she put in a full shift, anyway; she was always working, and in this part of the world nobody could argue because there was always so much to be done. But the weariness, Bygbjerg could tell, was not bred by overwork. Grethe had always been remarkably healthy, throughout her arduous career. No, the fatigue was something darker; it had become a constant companion that weighted her every move, mocking the doctor's industry like the ubiquitous cackling of the hyena on the savannah.

Though she was neither sentimental nor particularly Christian, Grethe Rask had wanted to cheer her young colleague; instead, she lay motionless, paralyzed again. Two hours later, Grethe stirred and began, halfheartedly, to finish dinner. Bygbjerg was surprised that she was so sick then that she could not muster the strength to stay awake for something as special as the Feast of the Hearts.

November 1977
HJARDEMAAL, DENMARK

A cold Arctic wind blistered over the barren heath outside a whitewashed cottage that sat alone, two miles from the nearest neighbors in the desolate region of Denmark north of the Lim Fiord. Sweeping west, from the North Sea over the sand dunes and low, bowed pines, the gusts made a whoosh-whooshing sound. Inside the little house, under a neat red-tiled roof, Grethe Rask gasped her short, sparse breaths from an oxygen bottle.

"I'd better go home to die," Grethe had told Ib Bygbjerg matter-of-factly.

The only thing her doctors could agree on was the woman's terminal prognosis. All else was mystery. Also newly returned from Africa, Bygbjerg pondered the compounding mysteries of Grethe's health. None of it made sense. In early 1977, it appeared that she might be getting better; at least the swelling in her lymph nodes had gone down, even as she became more fatigued. But she had continued working, finally taking a brief vacation in South Africa in early July.

Suddenly, she could not breathe. Terrified, Grethe flew to Copenhagen, sustained on the flight by bottled oxygen. For months now, the top medical specialists of Denmark had tested and studied the surgeon. None, however, could fathom why the woman should, for no apparent reason, be dying. There was also the curious array of health problems that suddenly appeared. Her mouth became covered with yeast infections. Staph infections spread in her blood. Serum tests showed that something had gone awry in her immune system; her body lacked T-cells, the quarterbacks in the body's defensive line against disease. But biopsies showed she was not suffering from a lymph cancer that might explain not only the T-cell deficiency but her body's apparent inability to stave off infection. The doctors could only gravely tell her that she was suffering from progressive lung disease of unknown cause. And, yes, in answer to her blunt questions, she would die.

Finally, tired of the poking and endless testing by the Copenhagen doctors, Grethe Rask retreated to her cottage near Thisted. A local doctor fitted out her bedroom with oxygen bottles. Grethe's longtime female companion, who was a nurse in a nearby hospital, tended her. Grethe lay in the lonely whitewashed farmhouse and remembered her years in Africa while the North Sea winds piled the first winter snows across Jutland.

In Copenhagen, Ib Bygbjerg, now at the State University Hospital, fretted continually about his friend. Certainly, there must be an answer to the mysteries of her medical charts. Maybe if they ran more tests. . . . It could be some common tropical culprit they had overlooked, he argued. She would be cured, and they would all chuckle over how easily the problem had been solved when they sipped wine and ate goose on the Feast of the Hearts. Bygbjerg pleaded with the doctors, and the doctors pleaded with Grethe Rask, and reluctantly the wan surgeon returned to the old *Rigshospitalet* in Copenhagen for one last chance.

Bygbjerg would never forgive himself for taking her away from the cottage north of the fjord. The virulent microbes that were haunting her body would not reveal themselves in the bombardment of tests she endured in those last days. On December 12, 1977, just twelve days before the Feast of the Hearts, Margrethe P. Rask died. She was forty-seven years old.

Later, Bygbjerg decided he would devote his life to studying tropical medicine. Before he died, he wanted to know what microscopic marauder had come from the African jungles to so ruthlessly rob the life of his best friend, a woman who had been so intensely devoted to helping others.

An autopsy revealed that Grethe Rask's lungs were filled with millions of organisms known as *Pneumocystis carinii;* they had caused a rare pneumonia that had slowly suffocated the woman. The diagnosis raised more questions than answers: Nobody died of *Pneumocystis.* Intrigued, Bygbjerg wanted to start doing research on the disease, but he was dissuaded by wizened professors, who steered him toward work in malaria. Don't study *Pneumocystis,* they told him; it was so rare that there would be no future in it.

PART II

BEFORE: 1980

All history resolves itself quite easily into the biography of
a few stout and earnest persons.

—RALPH WALDO EMERSON,
"Self-Reliance"

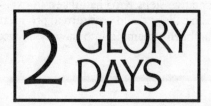

2 GLORY DAYS

June 29, 1980
SAN FRANCISCO

The sun melted the morning fog to reveal a vista so clear, so crystalline that you worried it might break if you stared too hard. The Transamerica Pyramid towered over the downtown skyline, and the bridges loped toward hills turning soft gold in the early summer heat. Rainbow flags fluttered in the gentle breezes.

Seven men were beginning their day. Bill Kraus, fresh from his latest political triumph in Washington, D.C., was impatient to get to the foot of Market Street to take his place at the head of the largest parade in San Francisco. There was much to celebrate.

In his apartment off Castro Street, in the heart of San Francisco's gay ghetto, Cleve Jones waited anxiously for his lover to get out of bed. This was parade day, Cleve kept repeating. No man, even the delightful muffin lolling lazily in the bed next to him, would make him late for this day of days. Cleve loved the sight of homosexuals, thousands strong. It was he who had led the gay mob that rioted at City Hall just a year ago, although he had now refashioned himself into the utterly respectable aide to one of California's most powerful politicians. He wasn't selling out, Cleve told friends impishly; he was just adding a new chapter to his legend. "Meet me at the parade," he called to his sleepy partner as he finally dashed for the door. "I can't be late."

A few blocks away, Dan William waited to meet David Ostrow. The two doctors were in town for a gathering of gay physicians at San Francisco State University. At home in New York City, gay parades drew only 30,000 or so; Dan William tried to imagine what a parade with hundreds of thousands of gays would look like. From what he had heard, David Ostrow was glad they didn't have parades like San Francisco's in Chicago; it would never play.

On California Street, airline steward Gaetan Dugas examined his face closely in the mirror. The scar, below his ear, was only slightly visible. His face would soon be unblemished again. He had come all the way from Toronto to enjoy this day, and for the moment he would put aside the troubling news the doctors had delivered just a few weeks before.

In the Mission District, the Gay Freedom Day Parade was the event twenty-two-year-old Kico Govantes had anticipated the entire five weeks he'd been in San Francisco. The tentative steps Kico had taken in exploring his homosexuality at a small Wisconsin college could now turn to proud strides. Maybe among the thousands who had been streaming into the city all week, Kico would find the lover he sought.

○

Before.

It was to be the word that would define the permanent demarcation in the lives of millions of Americans, particularly those citizens of the United States who were gay. There was life after the epidemic. And there were fond recollections of the times before.

Before and after. The epidemic would cleave lives in two, the way a great war or depression presents a commonly understood point of reference around which an entire society defines itself.

Before would encompass thousands of memories laden with nuance and nostalgia. Before meant innocence and excess, idealism and hubris. More than anything, this was the time before death. To be sure, Death was already elbowing its way through the crowds on that sunny morning, like a rude tourist angling for the lead spot in the parade. It was still an invisible presence, though, palpable only to twenty, or perhaps thirty, gay men who were suffering from a vague malaise. This handful ensured that the future and the past met on that single day.

People like Bill Kraus and Cleve Jones, Dan William and David Ostrow had lived through a recent past that had offered triumphs beyond their hopes; the future would present challenges beyond anything they could possibly fear. For them, and millions more, including many who considered themselves quite separate from such lives in San Francisco, this year would provide the last clear memories of the time before. Nothing would ever be the same again.

○

Bill Kraus looked up Market Street toward the Castro District, unable to find an end to the colorful crowd that had converged on downtown San Francisco for the Gay Freedom Day Parade. Bill ran his hands through his thick, curly brown hair and decided again that never was there a better place and time to be homosexual than here in this beautiful city on this splendid day when all gay people, no matter how diverse, became expressions of the same thought: We don't need to hide anymore.

Standing at the front of the parade, behind the banner announcing the gay and lesbian delegates to the 1980 Democratic National Convention, Bill Kraus retraced the steps that had brought him to this day and this parade. Primarily, he recalled the hiding and that nameless fear of being what he was, a homosexual. For years he had hidden the truth from others and, even worse, from himself. It was hard now to fathom the fear and self-hatred of those years without hope. The entire epoch seemed some kind of dream, a memory that had no real part in his waking life today.

At times, he wondered what he had been thinking all those years. Of what had he been so afraid? It wasn't just being Catholic. The edification of thirteen years of Cincinnati parochial schools dissipated within months of his arrival at Ohio State in 1968. There, he grew his hair long and answered the call of the Bob Dylan songs he played incessantly on his beat-up stereo. "The first one now will later be last," Dylan said. The times, they were a-changing. The message never rang true to him, not in the years of anti–Vietnam War marches or social activism, not until Bill had moved to Berkeley just a decade ago and discovered Castro Street and the promise of a new age.

There, with a middle-aged camera shop owner named Harvey Milk, Bill had learned the nuts and bolts of ward politics. He had learned how to walk precincts, study election maps, and forge coalitions. He had seen how everyone had power, how everyone could make a difference if only they believed and acted as if they could. This became the central tenet of his political catechism: "We can make a difference." Bill now repeated it in every speech, and on this Gay Freedom Day he felt it more strongly than ever. Everything in the last three years—Harvey Milk's election as supervisor and the first openly gay elected official in the nation, the political assassinations, and the consolidation of power after that—had conspired to convince Bill that it was true. Castro Street couldn't even get its gutters swept a few years back; today, gays were the most important single voting bloc in the city, comprising at least one in four registered voters. Bill Kraus had become president of the city's most powerful grass-roots organization, the Harvey Milk Gay Democratic Club.

The organizational power that he helped build had kept a gay seat on the board of supervisors after Harvey Milk's assassination in 1978 for a one-time Methodist minister and Milk crony named Harry Britt. Bill Kraus had replaced Britt as president of the Milk Club and now worked as his aide in City Hall. He had also managed Britt's reelection campaign in 1979, securing his reputation as the city's leading gay tactician.

The city's gay community was acquiring a legendary quality in political circles with influence far beyond the 70,000-odd votes it could boast in a city of 650,000. For the past three months, emissaries for presidential candidates had scoured the Castro neighborhood for votes. As other cities followed San Francisco's blueprint for political success, a national political force was coalescing. Bill Kraus and Harry Britt were leaving in two weeks for New York to be Ted Kennedy delegates to the Democratic National Convention. With seventy delegates, the convention's gay caucus was larger than the delegations of twenty states. This year, they would make a difference.

The gay parade had grown so mammoth in recent years that a good chunk of downtown San Francisco was needed just to get the scores of floats, contingents, and marching bands in proper order. While the parade assembled, Gwenn Craig smiled as she watched the young men mill near Bill Kraus, all thinking of some excuse to approach the famous young activist. Friends had teased Bill about his thirty-third birthday just days before; he was "l'age du Christ," somebody had joked. Bill was scarcely the scruffy malcontent with whom Gwenn had spent so many leisurely afternoons in Castro Street cafes. His once-shaggy hair was now neatly cut, and his thick glasses were replaced by contacts, eliminating an owlish stare and revealing startling blue eyes. His body was superbly toned. He carried himself with increasing confidence, much like the body politic whose ideals he was articulating.

Bill Kraus was even beginning to cut his own national reputation. Just two weeks earlier, he had delivered an impassioned plea for a gay rights plank to the Democratic Platform Committee, which was hammering together a party agenda to present at the Democratic National Convention in July. Bill had delivered the address as a gay rights manifesto, articulating the goals of the nascent political force. Gay papers across the country had written up the performance for the issues being distributed on the gay pride weekend.

The gay rights plank, Bill Kraus said, "does not ask you to give us special privileges. It does not ask anyone to like us. It does not even ask that the Democratic party give us many of the legal protections which are considered the right of all other Americans.

"Fellow members of the Platform Committee, what this amendment asks in a time when we hear much from prominent members of the Democratic party about human rights is that the Democratic party recognize that we, the gay people of this country, are also human."

⬭

The San Francisco Gay Freedom Day Marching Band blared the opening notes of "California Here I Come," and the parade started its two-mile trek down Market Street toward City Hall. More than 30,000 people, grouped in 240 contingents, marched in the parade past 200,000 spectators. The parade was the best show in town, revealing the amazing diversity of gay life. Clusters of gay Catholics and Episcopalians, Mormons and atheists, organized for years in the city, marched proudly beneath their banners. Career-designated contingents of gays included lawyers and labor officials, dentists and doctors, accountants and the ubiquitous gay phone-company employees. There were lesbian moms, gay dads, and homosexual teenagers with their heterosexual parents. Gay blacks, Latinos, Asian-Americans, and American Indians marched beneath banners proclaiming their dual pride. The campy Gays Against Brunch formed their own marching unit. A group of drag queens, dressed as nuns and calling themselves the Sisters of Perpetual Indulgence, had picked the day for their debut.

Gay tourists streamed to this homophile mecca from all over the world for the high holy day of homosexual life. Floats came from Phoenix and Denver; gay cowboys from the Reno Gay Rodeo pranced their horses down Market Street, waving the flags of Nevada and California, as well as the rainbow flag that had become the standard of California gays.

Although the parade route was only two miles, it would take four hours for the full parade to pass. Within an hour, the first contingents arrived at the broad Civic Center Plaza, where a stage had been erected in front of the ornate facade of City Hall.

Radical gay liberationists frowned at the carnival rides that had been introduced to the rally site. Parade organizers had decided that the event had grown "too political" in recent years, so the chest-pounding rhetoric that marked most rallies was given a backseat to the festive feeling of a state fair.

"We feel it definitely isn't a time for celebration," complained Alberta Maged to a newspaper reporter. She had marched with a coalition of radical groups including the Lavender Left, the Stonewall Brigade, and the aptly named Commie Queers. "You can't celebrate when you're still being oppressed. We have the illusion of freedom in San Francisco that makes it easy to exist, but the right-wing movement is growing quickly. It's right to be proud to be gay, but it isn't enough if you're still being attacked."

Many hard-line radicals, remembering the days when gay liberation was not nearly as fashionable, agreed. The event, after all, commemorated the riot in which Greenwich Village drag queens attacked police engaged in the routine harassment of a gay bar called the Stonewall Inn. From the Stonewall riot, on the last weekend of June 1969, the gay liberation movement was born, peopled by angry women and men who realized that their fights against war and injustice had a more personal side. This was the gay liberation movement—named after the then-voguish liberation groups sweeping the country—that had taken such delight in frightening staid America in the early 1970s.

By 1980, however, the movement had become a victim of its own success. Particularly in San Francisco, the taboos against homosexuality ebbed easily in the midst of the overall sexual revolution. The promise of freedom had fueled the greatest exodus of immigrants to San Francisco since the Gold Rush. Between 1969 and 1973, at least 9,000 gay men moved to San Francisco, followed by 20,000 between 1974 and 1978. By 1980, about 5,000 homosexual men were moving to the Golden Gate every year. The immigration now made for a city in which two in five adult males were openly gay. To be sure, these gay immigrants composed one of the most solidly liberal voting blocs in America, but this was largely because liberals were the candidates who promised to leave gays alone. It was enough to be left alone. Restructuring an entire society's concept of sex roles could come later; maybe it would happen by itself.

To the veterans of confrontational politics, the 1980 parade was a turning point because it demonstrated how respectable their dream had become. Success was spoiling gay liberation, it seemed. Governor Edmund G. Brown, Jr., had issued a proclamation honoring Gay Freedom Week throughout the state, and state legislators and city officials crowded the speaker's dais at the gay rally. For their part, gays were eager to show that they were deserving of respectability. The local blood bank, for example, had long ago learned that it was good business to send their mobile collection vans to such events with large gay crowds. These were civic-minded people. In 1980, they gave between 5 and 7 percent of the donated blood in San Francisco, bank officials estimated.

The Ferris-wheel gondola rocked gently as it stopped with Cleve Jones at the apex, staring down on the 200,000 milling in front of the majestic City Hall rotunda. This was the gay community Cleve loved. Tens of thousands, together, showing their power. Marches and loud, angry speeches, an occasional upraised fist and drama, such drama. This was what being gay in San Francisco meant to Cleve Jones.

"This is my private party." He grinned. "Just me and a few thousand of my closest friends."

From the time he was a fourteen-year-old sophomore at Scottsdale High School, Cleve Jones knew that this is where he wanted to be, at gay rights marches in San Francisco. He had suffered through adolescent years in which he was the class sissy and the locker room punching bag. But, as soon as he could, he had hitchhiked to San Francisco and marched in the 1973 gay parade. For the rest of his life, he would know that he had arrived at the right place at the right time.

San Francisco in the 1970s represented one of those occasions when the forces of social change collide with a series of dramatic events to produce moments that are later called historic. From the day Cleve walked into Harvey Milk's camera shop to volunteer for campaign work, his life was woven into that history and drama. Political strategists like Bill Kraus recalled the 1970s in terms of votes cast and elections won; Cleve Jones, the romantic, framed the era as a grand story, the movement of a dream through time.

Cleve remembered 1978, when he had walked in the front of the parade dressed all in white, holding the upraised hand of a lesbian, who was also dressed in white, in front of a banner that showed a rainbow arch fashioned from barbed wire. Death-camp motifs had been de rigueur that year because a state senator from Orange County, John Briggs, was campaigning statewide for a ballot measure that would ban gays from teaching in California public schools. The initiative brought an international spotlight both to California, where the anti-gay campaigns started by Anita Bryant in 1977 were culminating, and to the 1978 Gay Freedom Day Parade, where gays made a defiant show of strength. They had come to the parade 375,000 strong, with Harvey Milk defying death threats to ride the long route in an open convertible before mounting the stage to give his "hope speech," prodding the crowd to create the best future by coming out and announcing their homosexuality.

Such public witnessing had always been a central article of faith of the gay liberation movement, Cleve Jones knew. This, after all, would be the only way their political cause could get anywhere because homosexuality was a fundamentally invisible trait. The fact that gays could hide their sexuality presented the gay movement with its greatest weakness and its most profound potential strength. Invisible, gays would always be kicked around, the reasoning went, because they would never assert their power. On that day in 1978, never had the power been so palpable. Months later, when California voters rejected the Briggs Initiative by a ratio of two to one, it appeared to be a wonderful year.

However, three weeks after the election, Supervisor Dan White, San Francisco's only anti-gay politician, had taken his Smith and Wesson revolver to City Hall and shot down Harvey Milk and the liberal mayor, George Moscone. Cleve had helped organize a candlelight march to City Hall that night for

Harvey and George. Six months later, when a jury decided that Dan White should go to jail for only six years for killing the two men, Cleve had organized another march to City Hall—the one that turned into a riot, a vivid affirmation that this generation of gay people weren't a bunch of sissies to be kicked around without a fight. This White Night Riot left dozens of policemen injured and the front of City Hall ravaged; gay leaders across the country grimaced at the televised coverage of police cars set aflame by rampaging gay crowds.

By 1980, Cleve had helped fashion the story of Harvey and the 1970s, the Dan White trial, and the White Night Riot into one of the new legends of the fledgling gay movement, a story of assassinations and political intrigue, homophobic zealots and rioting in the streets. From it all, Cleve had emerged as the most prominent street activist in town, the most skillful media manipulator since Harvey Milk. Reporters loved the ever-so-militant pronouncements Cleve Jones was apt to make.

In recent months, Cleve had traded his blue jeans and sneakers for Armani suits to work for the Speaker of the California Assembly. It was a time when the outsiders who once marched angrily on the government were becoming insiders learning how to use the power they had gained. Cleve had spent most of the spring organizing Democratic Assembly campaigns. He split his time between Sacramento and San Francisco, where he was dating a wonderful Mexican-American lawyer named Felix Velarde-Munoz. Both knew the key players in local politics, and both loved to talk politics and liberation movements and make love and dance to the ubiquitous disco music.

That's what the summer of 1980 was to Cleve Jones. The gay community was a burst of creative energy that emanated from San Francisco and spread across America. Gays had staved off challenges that ran from bigots' ballot initiatives to political murder; now they could look forward to greater victories.

Yet like many gay activists, Cleve was troubled by the amusement park rides at Civic Center Plaza. He knew that the gay revolution was, at best, half-completed. Its tenuous gains could be wiped away by some other strongly organized force. He could understand that to a gay refugee from Des Moines, the city represented freedom beyond anything imaginable. He also knew, however, that freedom to go to a gay bar was not real freedom.

What was the right direction? Cleve asked himself. The gay movement had shifted from one of self-exploration, in which people moved through their own fears and self-alienation, to a movement of electoral politics, focused outward. Voter registration tables had replaced consciousness-raising groups as the symbol of liberation. Cleve sometimes wondered whether the new men crowding the Castro had already gone through this personal growth elsewhere or whether they had simply skipped it because being gay in San Francisco was so easy now that you didn't need to plummet to your psychic depths to make a commitment to the life-style.

Too many questions. It was nothing to dwell on today. When Cleve remembered the wonderful 1978 parade, and everything that had happened since, he felt like celebrating too. From his promontory on the Ferris wheel, he once more scanned the thousands stretched for miles around the City Hall rotunda where gay people had once marched and rioted, and where they now exerted so much power. The wheel jerked again, and slowly he began to return to the crowd, turning full circle.

◯

A new disease.

It was never a formal topic of discussion, but on that weekend, when gay doctors from across the country gathered in San Francisco, it was discussed occasionally in hallways and over dinners. What would happen if some new disease insinuated itself into the bodies of just a few men in this community? The notion terrified Dr. David Ostrow; it was an idea he tried to put out of his mind as he wandered through the crowded rally site between the whirling amusement park rides with two other doctors from the convention, Manhattan's Dan William and Robert Bolan of San Francisco.

Ostrow grimaced as a Sister of Perpetual Indulgence sashayed by. The sight rankled his midwestern sensibilities. This was all too weird, he thought. The media would play up the open display of sexuality and once again drag queens and half-naked muscle boys would be presented as the emblems of homosexual culture. People like Ostrow, who leaned toward long, steady relationships, would never get the press. The bizarre, it seemed, would always overshadow the positive things going on in the gay community, like the doctors' conference. Doctors weren't flamboyant enough to get in the headlines. They were barely mentioned in the gay newspapers, counting themselves lucky to make it a page ahead of the latest gossip about the hottest leather bar.

While strategists like Bill Kraus read the gay community's future in voter registration rolls, and street activists like Cleve Jones heard it in ringing oratory, the gay doctors had spent that weekend reading the community's prognosis from its medical chart. Like many physicians, Ostrow had been quite troubled when he left the medical conference, which had adjourned in time for the parade.

The fight against venereal diseases was proving a Sisyphean task. Ostrow was director of the Howard Brown Memorial Clinic, which provided a sensitive alternative for gay men who wanted to avoid the sneers of staffers at the Chicago Public Health clinics. The screening in Ostrow's clinic had revealed that one in ten patients had walked in the door with hepatitis B. At least one-half of the gay men tested at the clinic showed evidence of a past episode of hepatitis B. In San Francisco, two-thirds of gay men had suffered the debilitating disease. It was now proven statistically that a gay man had one chance in five of being infected with the hepatitis B virus within twelve months of stepping off the bus into a typical urban gay scene. Within five years, infection was a virtual certainty.

Another problem was enteric diseases, like amebiasis and giardiasis, caused by organisms that lodged themselves in the intestinal tracts of gay men with alarming frequency. At the New York Gay Men's Health Project, where Dan William was medical director, 30 percent of the patients suffered from gastrointestinal parasites. In San Francisco, incidence of the "Gay Bowel Syndrome," as it was called in medical journals, had increased by 8,000 percent after 1973. Infection with these parasites was a likely effect of anal intercourse, which was apt to put a man in contact with his partner's fecal matter, and was virtually a certainty through the then-popular practice of rimming, which medical journals politely called oral-anal intercourse.

What was so troubling was that nobody in the gay community seemed to care about these waves of infection. Ever since he had worked at the New York City Department of Public Health, Dan William had delivered his lecture about the dangers of undiagnosed venereal diseases and, in particular, such practices as rimming. But he had his "regulars" who came in with infection after infection, waiting for the magic bullet that could put them back in the sack again. William began to feel like a parent as he admonished the boys: "I have to tell you that you're being very unhealthy."

Promiscuity, however, was central to the raucous gay movement of the 1970s, and his advice was, as the Texans so charmingly put it, like pissing in the wind. At best, he tried to counsel the Elizabeth Taylor approach to sexuality and suggest serial monogamy, a series of affairs that may not last forever but that at least left you with a vague awareness of which bed you slept in most evenings.

The crowd cheered the parade again when the Bulldog Baths float came rolling into Civic Center. The young musclemen, in black leather harnesses, the best and the most beautiful, jumped from the cages in which they had discoed down Market Street. That night they would be at the huge Cellblock Party at the bathhouse, one of a panoply of celebrations sponsored that day by San Francisco's thriving sex industry.

This commercialization of gay sex was all part of the scene, an aspect of the homosexual life-style in which the epidemics of venereal disease, hepatitis, and enteric disorders thrived. The gay liberation movement of the 1970s had spawned a business of bathhouses and sex clubs. The hundreds of such institutions were a $100-million industry across America and Canada, and bathhouse owners were frequently gay political leaders as well, helping support the usually financially starved gay groups. The businesses serviced men who had long been repressed, gay activists told themselves, and were perhaps now going to the extreme in exploring their new freedom. It would all balance out later, so for now, sex was part and parcel of political liberation. The popular bestseller *The Joy of Gay Sex,* for example, called rimming the "prime taste treat in sex," while a leftist Toronto newspaper published a story on "rimming as a revolutionary act."

It was interesting politics, David Ostrow thought. From a purely medical standpoint, however, the bathhouses were a horrible breeding ground for disease. People who went to bathhouses simply were more likely to be infected with a disease—and infect others—than a typical homosexual on the street. A Seattle study of gay men suffering from shigellosis, for example, discovered that 69 percent culled their sexual partners from bathhouses. A Denver study found that an average bathhouse patron having his typical 2.7 sexual contacts a night risked a 33 percent chance of walking out of the tubs with syphilis or gonorrhea, because about one in eight of those wandering the hallways had asymptomatic cases of these diseases.

Doctors like David Ostrow and Dan William did not consider themselves prudish, even if they were cut from a more staid mold than the people whose pictures were in the newspaper coverage of the Gay Freedom Day Parade. But they were uneasy about the health implication of the commercialization of sex. In a 1980 interview with a New York City gay magazine, *Christopher Street,* William noted, "One effect of gay liberation is that sex has been institutionalized and franchised. Twenty years ago, there may have been a thousand men on any one night having sex in New York baths or parks. Now there are ten or twenty thousand—at the baths, the back-room bars, bookstores, porno theaters, the Rambles, and a wide range of other places as well. The plethora of opportunities poses a public health problem that's growing with every new bath in town."

Such comments were politically incorrect in the extreme, and William suffered criticism as a "monogamist." Self-criticism was not the strong point of a community that was only beginning to define itself affirmatively after centuries of repression.

Altogether, this generation of gay men was blessed by good health. Being a gay doctor was fun, William often told himself. Physical fitness was a community ritual with tens of thousands of gay men crowding Nautilus centers and weight rooms. He rarely had to go to a hospital because none of his patients ever got very sick.

David Ostrow too was haunted by forebodings as he left the parade. Between the bathhouses and the high levels of sexual activity, there would be no stopping a new disease that got into this population. The likelihood was remote, of course. Modern science had congratulated itself on the eradication of infectious disease as a threat to humankind. But the specter sometimes haunted Ostrow because he wondered where all the sexually transmitted disease would end. It couldn't continue indefinitely. He had already noticed that some Chicago gay men were having immune problems. Dan William was seeing strange inflammation of the lymph nodes among his most promiscuous patients. The swelling was curious because it did not seem to be in response to any particular infection but was generalized, all over; maybe it was the effect of overloading the immune system with a variety of venereal diseases.

Years later, Dan William would recall that it was during the days of early 1980 that he saw a man in his mid-forties recovering from a bad bout with hepatitis B. He had strange purplish lesions on his arms and chest. William referred him to Memorial Sloan-Kettering Cancer Center. The man, it turned out, was suffering from a rare skin cancer, Kaposi's sarcoma. William had to look up Kaposi's sarcoma in a medical textbook because he had never heard of the ailment. Fortunately, the book said, the man had a good prognosis. Elderly Jewish or Italian men got Kaposi's sarcoma; twenty years later they usually died of old age. The cancer itself, however, appeared benign.

$\bigcirc$

Mervyn Silverman watched the bare-breasted women in leather straps, with rings through their nipples, walk by him, and he definitely had the feeling that he was not in Kansas anymore. In his twenty years in public health, he had traveled around the world and had lived in Bangkok and South America. As he watched the passing parade of humanity at the Gay Freedom Day Parade, he knew he had never lived in a more exciting place than San Francisco, and he sensed that he would not want to live anywhere else.

With his full head of prematurely gray hair, Silverman was easily recognizable to many of the bystanders, who shook his hand and introduced their lovers. Few City Hall officials were more popular than Silverman, the director of the Department of Public Health, and few had gone out of their way to show greater sensitivity to the gay community. Within weeks of his appointment as health director by Mayor George Moscone in 1977, Mervyn Silverman had understood that being public health director in San Francisco was like nowhere else. Every community and interest group had their own advisory board to the health department—there were thirty-four of them in all—and it seemed that no decision went over his desk that was not rife with political overtones. Already, a decision over the closing of a neighborhood health center had prompted a picketing of Silverman's spacious Victorian home on Frederick Street in the Upper Ashbury neighborhood.

Something about the political tension, however, excited Silverman. He enjoyed the challenge, maintained cordial relations with the press, and carved a singularly good reputation in every corner of the city. Silverman was a popular official, and that was the way he liked it. He had avoided hard feelings by making all decisions on the basis of consensus. He had listened to all sides and forged the middle path. All public health policy was basically political, he felt; as someone who relished public approbation, he was a good politician. It was his strength as a public official.

⬭

"I am the prettiest one."

It had been the standing joke. Gaetan Dugas would walk into a gay bar, scan the crowd, and announce to his friends, "I am the prettiest one." Usually, his friends had to agree, he was right.

Gaetan was the man everyone wanted, the ideal for this community, at this time and in this place. His sandy hair fell boyishly over his forehead. His mouth easily curled into an inviting smile, and his laugh could flood color into a room of black and white. He bought his clothes in the trendiest shops of Paris and London. He vacationed in Mexico and on the Caribbean beaches. Americans tumbled for his soft Quebeçois accent and his sensual magnetism. There was no place that the twenty-eight-year-old airline steward would rather have the boys fall for him than in San Francisco.

Fog streamed over the hills into the Castro, toward the 1980 Civic Center rally. The first cool breezes of evening were thinning the throng downtown, but throughout the city thousands of gay men crowded into giant disco parties that had become a staple of the weekend-long celebration. There was the Heatwave disco party for $25 a head in the Japantown Center, the Muscle Beach party and the trendy Dreamland disco, and Alive, a funkier dance fest a few blocks away.

The hottest and hunkiest, Gaetan knew, would be among the 4,000 streaming to the chic Galleria design center, where the party was just starting when the steward and his friend arrived. Every corner of the lobby and the five-story atrium was crammed with men pulsing to the synthesized rhythms of disco music. Any redundance in the musical patterns was quickly obviated by the cocaine and Quaaludes that were a staple of such parties.

Gaetan easily made his way through the profusion of sweaty bodies with his closest friend, another airline steward from Toronto. They had met in 1977, when they were based in Halifax, Nova Scotia. Together, they had ventured to San Francisco for the 1978 gay parade, and every year they returned for the carnival. They decided that San Francisco would always be their ultimate refuge. The last weekend of every June was now set aside for nonstop partying at bars and baths.

Here, Gaetan could satisfy his voracious sexual appetite with the beautiful California men he liked so much. He returned from every stroll down Castro Street with a pocketful of matchbook covers and napkins that were crowded with addresses and phone numbers. He recorded names of his most passionate admirers in his fabric-covered address book. But lovers were like suntans to him: They would be so wonderful, so sexy for a few days, and then fade. At times, Gaetan would study his address book with genuine curiosity, trying to recall who this or that person was.

As Gaetan neared the crowded dance floor at the Galleria, various men shouted greetings, and he hugged them ebulliently like long-lost brothers. "Who was that?" his friend would ask. "I don't know," Gaetan laughed off-handedly. "Somebody."

Here, swaying and stomping to the music, Gaetan was completely in his element. San Francisco was the hometown he never had. It helped him forget the other, distant life, long ago, when he was the major sissy of his working class neighborhood in Quebec City. Being gay then meant constantly fighting taunts hurled by the other kids and being gripped by guilt, by his own conscience. But that was then and this was San Francisco. On June 29, 1980, Gaetan was the ugly duckling who had become the swan.

At the first opportunity on the dance floor, Gaetan stripped off his T-shirt and fished out a bottle of poppers, nitrate inhalants, from his jeans pocket in one swift, practiced move. Fine blond hair outlined the trim natural proportions of his chest.

He felt strong and vital.

He didn't feel like he had cancer at all.

That was what the doctor had said after cutting that bump from his face. Gaetan had wanted the small purplish spot removed to satisfy his vanity; the doctor had wanted it for a biopsy. Weeks later, the report came back from New York City, and the Toronto specialist told Gaetan that he had Kaposi's sarcoma, a bizarre skin cancer that hardly anybody got. Maybe that explained why his lymph nodes had been swollen for a year. Gaetan hadn't told friends until June, after the biopsy. He was terrified at first, but he consoled himself with the knowledge that you can beat cancer. He had created a life in which he could have everything and everyone he wanted. He'd figure a way around this cancer too.

As he felt the poppers surge through him, Gaetan realized that his high might last longer than this crowd. There were always the baths. He reviewed his choices, as he had so many times before during his regular visits to the city. The Club Baths was guaranteed to be crowded with those Anglo-Saxon men who were so well built, vaguely wholesome, and, well, so American. The fantasy rooms at the Hothouse were intriguing, as was the Bulldog Baths's promise of a Cellblock Party.

The summer was just beginning. The beaches of Fire Island and the pool parties of Los Angeles all lay ahead. Later, when the researchers started referring to Gaetan Dugas simply as Patient Zero, they would retrace the airline steward's travels during that summer, fingering through his fabric-covered address book to try to fathom the bizarre coincidences and the unique role the handsome young steward performed in the coming epidemic.

On that day in 1980, Gaetan danced to forget under the pulsing colored lights. Feeling whole again, he told himself that one day he would like to move to San Francisco.

⬭

"It looks like that guy has his arm up the other guy's ass."

Kico Govantes thought maybe the man standing between the legs of the guy in the sling was an amputee. Maybe he was just rubbing his stump next to the guy's butt.

"He does have an arm up his ass," Kico's friend said.

Kico was sickened. He had heard a lot about bathhouses since moving to San Francisco five weeks before. The local gay papers were filled with ads and catchy slogans for the businesses. The Handball Express motto was "find your limits"; the Glory Holes pledged to be "the most unusual sex place in the world"; the Jaguar sex club in the Castro hyped "your fantasy, your pleasure"; while the coeducational Sutro Baths had a "Bisexual Boogie" every weekend. The Cornholes's advertising was more pointed, featuring the unclad torso of a man lying on his stomach.

The handsome psychologist Kico had met at the gay parade had promised to take him to the largest gay bathhouse in the world, the Bulldog Baths. Decorated in San Quentin motif, the place was something of a legend in sexual circles. The leather magazine *Drummer* had gushed that the central "two-story prison is so incredibly real (real cells, real bars, real toilets . . .) that when you see a guard standing on the second tier looking down on you, you're ready to kneel down."

This is insane, thought Kico.

Kico had moved from Wisconsin to San Francisco with a clear sense of what being gay meant. He figured gay people dated and courted; you certainly never went to bed with someone you just met. Kico wouldn't mind if he had to date someone months before they consummated their relationship and settled into some hip approximation of marriage. As the scion of an aristocratic Cuban family that fled Havana when Kico was three, the young man had led a relatively sheltered life. Suddenly, he was very confused.

The Cellblock Party, just a few blocks from a rally where speakers were so loftily discussing the finer points of gay love, was like some scene from a Fellini film, intriguing and inviting to the eye, but altogether repulsive to Kico. The scene was even more alienating because these guys were so attractive, and they obviously found Kico attractive. He could sense that, physically, he fit in with these people. With his trim body and handsome swarthy features, he was what they wanted. Every floor was packed with the firm bodies of men clad in towels. Attendants cheerfully passed out free beer while disco music blared. The air felt thick and steamy, heavy with the acrid smell of nitrate inhalants.

Kico turned to his companion. Certainly, a psychologist would see that this was unhealthy, a corruption of the very gay love that this day was supposed to celebrate. The shrink eyed him curiously, as if he were a naive child. He seemed to enjoy guiding the twenty-two-year-old through the labyrinthine hallways.

"That's fist-fucking," the psychologist said.

"Oh," Kico said.

Knowing the words for the acts didn't help him fathom the meaning of what he was seeing. Where was the affection? he wondered. Where was the interaction of mind and body that creates a meaningful sexual experience? It was as if these people, who had been made so separate from society by virtue of their sexuality, were now making their sexuality utterly separate from themselves. Their bodies were tools through which they could experience physical sensation. The complete focus on the physical aspect of sex meant constantly devising new, more extreme sexual acts because the experience relied on heightened sensory rather than emotional stimulation.

Kico thought it ironic that a community so entirely based on love should create institutions so entirely devoid of intimacy. He left the bathhouse feeling horrified and disillusioned. He walked through the empty Civic Center Plaza where street sweepers were clearing the debris from the rally and muscular carny men were dismantling the amusement park rides. The fog had swept across the city on this day of interregnum. Kico was cold.

3 BEACHES OF THE DISPOSSESSED

August 1980
FIRE ISLAND, NEW YORK

Larry Kramer looked across the table toward Enno Poersch. Larry could tell from the edge on Enno's deep, broad voice that he was frantic with concern.

Enno recounted, again, the mysterious diarrhea, vague fatigue, and stubborn rashes that had devastated his lover Nick. Endless tests by countless doctors had found nothing, and the strict health-food regimen to which Nick had adhered religiously for years wasn't doing any good either. Larry was a famous author who seemed to know everybody, Enno thought; he should know something.

"Aren't there hospitals where they specialize in treating bizarre sicknesses?" Enno asked.

Larry remembered when he had met Nick on an all-gay cruise of the Caribbean.

Witty, gregarious, and handsome in a compact Italian way, Nick was a popular cruise staffer. Every day, Nick had sat away from the continuous partying to write long love letters to Enno, and at each port, packets of Enno's romantic missives waited for Nick. They were the kind of lovey-dovey letters that Larry had always wanted, and the pair's love seemed to have lost none of its luster in the eight years since they had met on a sunny Fire Island beach.

As Enno talked about taking Nick from hospital to hospital, Larry imagined Enno, a tall, broad-shouldered lumberjack of a man, cradling the small, wiry Nick in his arms while he carried him up steep, steely stairways to save his life. The image made Larry want to cry, but no, he didn't know anything about hospitals or doctors or what could be ailing Nick.

After Enno excused himself, Larry thought about how strange it was that summer. All that people seemed to talk about were the latest intestinal parasites going around. Dinner conversation often evolved into guys swapping stories about which medications stomped out the stubborn little creatures and whether Flagyl, the preferred antiparasite drug, was really carcinogenic. It was like eavesdropping on a bunch of old ladies sharing arthritis stories on shaded benches in Miami.

Later that night, Larry made his way toward the Ice Palace, where the never-ending Fire Island summer party was in full swing. He walked tentatively through the crowded doorway and saw the "Marlboro Man" saunter languorously through the disco. Larry knew that, intellectually, he could hold his own with anybody in New York, but the sight of Paul Popham, so self-assured in his model-handsome good looks, always left Larry in awe, the way you have to catch your breath after you see a movie star.

At the Y, Larry had told Paul that he had such a naturally well-defined body that he didn't need to work out, and Paul responded with a shy aw-shucks ingenuousness that reminded Larry of Gary Cooper or Jimmy Stewart. At the Ice Palace, the thumping heart of Fire Island nightlife, Larry wondered what it would be like to be Paul, to fit in so well and be accepted in a way Larry, the outsider, had never experienced. No matter where he was, Paul seemed to settle naturally among the beautiful people. On Fire Island, he lived in *the* house with Enno, Nick, and a few other handsome men who made the A-list of every major island party.

This was not Larry's summer to fit in. He hadn't even bothered to buy a house share, slipping to the island for a weekend here or there. He kept a decidedly low profile, but that didn't prevent some nasty moments. The gay man who owned the grocery store had glared at Larry when he was buying an orange juice. "You're trying to ruin the island," the grocer glowered. "I don't understand why you come here."

As the deejay turned up the volume on a Donna Summer song, Larry watched an old friend, another writer, enter the Ice Palace, glance in his direction, and purposefully walk the other way.

The antipathy, Larry Kramer knew, surrounded the book he had written about gay life in New York and on this island. Everything, from its title, *Faggots,* to its graphic descriptions of hedonism on the Greenwich Village–Cherry Grove axis had stirred frenzy among both gay reviewers and the people whose milieu Larry had set out to chronicle. Manhattan's only gay bookstore had banned the novel from its shelves while gay critics had advised readers that its purchase represented an act inimical to the interests of gay liberation.

Faggots had explored every dark corner of the subculture that gays had fashioned in the heady days after gay liberation. There were scenes of drug-induced euphoria at the discos, all-night orgies in posh Upper East Side co-ops, and fist-fucking at The Toilet Bowl, one of the many Manhattan sleaze bars where every form of exotic sexuality was explored with gritty abandon. The story climaxed with a weekend of parties and dancing on Fire Island, punctuated by cavorting in the Meat Rack, a stretch of woods that is home to some of the most animated foliage since Birnam Wood marched to Dunsinane.

Against this backdrop, lovers argued about fidelity and the plausibility of having anything resembling a meaningful commitment in the midst of such omnipresent carnality. When the book's protagonist, a Jewish screenwriter–movie producer not unlike Larry Kramer himself, sees his own hopes for love fade, he delivers a tirade that raised many troubling questions.

"Why do faggots have to fuck so fucking much?" Larry had written. "It's as if we don't have anything else to do . . . all we do is live in our Ghetto and dance and drug and fuck . . . there's a whole world out there! . . . as much ours as theirs . . . I'm tired of being a New York City–Fire Island faggot, I'm tired of using my body as a faceless thing to lure another faceless thing, I want to love a Person! I want to go out and live in a world with that Person, a Person who loves me, we shouldn't *have* to be faithful!, we should *want* to be faithful! . . . No relationship in the world could survive the shit we lay on it."

It all needs to change, Larry's protagonist told an unfaithful lover at the book's climax, "before you fuck yourself to death."

The book had proved a sensation, but ever since its publication, Larry had been something of a persona non grata on the island, returning only occasionally to visit friends and observe. It was already past 1:00 A.M. as he watched Paul Popham squire his handsome boyfriend, Jack Nau, back to the dance floor. The beautiful people, at last, were beginning to descend on the Ice Palace. Life on this long spit of sand in the Atlantic, Larry knew, was a regimen of sybaritic sameness.

Afternoons on the beaches were followed by light dinners, perhaps a nap, and then some outrageous party, before adjournment to whatever was the fashionable disco of the season. Of course, nobody got to the Ice Palace before 2:00 A.M., so you'd need some drugs to stay up. Once properly buzzed, it would be hard to get to sleep early, so you'd stop at the Meat Rack after dancing, and then you'd eventually walk home as the sun was rising over the sand. The unchanging ritual made Larry feel old. At forty-five, he didn't have the long nights in him anymore, and he wondered how the other guys could subject themselves to weekends that were more of a burnout than even the hectic pace of life in Manhattan.

At times, Larry Kramer compared the gay life of New York with San Francisco; it was another penchant that irritated the Manhattan gay intelligentsia. Larry had been in San Francisco the day Harvey Milk and Mayor George Moscone were shot, and he had wept the night that 30,000 candles glimmered outside City Hall and speakers talked idealistically of changing the world. He had been amazed to see the governor of California, the entire state supreme court, and scores of other officials at Milk's memorial service. Gays in New York had never achieved such power and respect, he thought, because they seemed more intent on building a better disco than a better social order. Being gay in New York was something you did on weekends, it seemed. During the week everybody went back to their careers and played the game, carefully concealing their sexuality and acting like everything was okay.

Of course, this was not to say that Larry was some crazy gay militant. In fact, he didn't have much use for the gay activist types in New York. The radicals seemed ensconced in rhetoric that was as passé as Chairman Mao. The more respectable gays, who talked earnestly of civil rights, seemed more intent on defending the current gay life-style than on changing it to something more meaningful. Rather than fight for the right to get married, the gay movement was fighting for the prerogative of gays to bump like bunnies.

The community seemed lost, and sometimes Larry felt lost. He had created two hits in his life and those were now behind him. First, after years in the movie business, Larry had written and produced a film based on a D. H. Lawrence novel that everybody agreed could never be made into a movie. *Women in Love* became one of the most acclaimed films of its year, winning an Oscar nomination in screenwriting for Larry and an Academy Award for one of its stars, Glenda Jackson. He had produced other films, but his next big hit as an artist, albeit controversial, was *Faggots.* And now he was fiddling with another novel and typing some screenwriting assignments, but in truth, he felt something like the gay community itself, at sixes and sevens and not really set in any particular direction.

Paul Popham had noticed Larry Kramer at the Ice Palace and thought, briefly, that he ought to give *Faggots* another try. He had managed to read only twenty or thirty pages before he got bored. He had a hard time seeing why anybody would be so deadly serious about being homosexual. Yes, Paul was gay, but it was no more an overwhelming trait than the fact he had been a Green Beret or that he had grown up in Oregon. It just was, and he didn't see any reason to talk about it much. He never felt discriminated against, never pondered suicide, nor wrestled with any guilt about being homosexual. Being gay had, at worst, been only a mild inconvenience, something he had to maneuver around.

None of Paul's private life was anybody else's damn business, he thought. None of it had much to do with politics either. Like a lot of gays on Wall Street, he voted his pocketbook as a registered Republican. This year, he wasn't crazy about the Reaganites, but Carter was a wimp. Come November, Paul had every intention of voting for independent presidential candidate John Anderson, a moderate Republican congressman from Illinois.

Paul scanned the dance floor, taking in the cream of New York gay society, the taut-bodied mustachioed men who were so beautiful you worried they might break if you stared too hard. It all made Paul regret that he hadn't taken better advantage of his share in the beat-up old house on Ocean Walk. Enno had been renting the place for years, and Paul had moved in this year to take the room of his best friend Rick Wellikoff.

Rick had mentioned last September that he had some funny bumps behind his ear. He hadn't wanted to go to the doctor, but Paul talked him into going to the famous dermatologists at New York University, where Paul was being treated for persistent psoriasis. Both Paul and Rick were stunned when the doctors said Rick had cancer, an unheard-of kind of cancer called Kaposi's sarcoma. It was even stranger when the doctor mentioned that there was another gay man with the same cancer at a nearby hospital. Rick and the second patient, it turned out, even had some mutual friends.

Rick hadn't seemed too sick until lately, and even now it wasn't that he was terribly ill. He just felt dog-tired all the time. Paul thought that maybe Rick's job as a fifth-grade teacher in a rough Brooklyn neighborhood was burning him out, but Rick insisted it was more than that. He quit his job and stayed holed up with his lover in their brownstone on West 78th Street. With a heavy load of work and the bedside visits with Rick, it was all Paul could do to get away for a rare weekend of carefree nights at the Ice Palace and days on friendly Fire Island sands.

○

Back at the house on Ocean Walk, Enno Poersch stared down at Nick's sleeping form. The idea had been for Nick to spend a relaxed summer at the beach and regain his health. Enno had stayed in the city all summer working on a major architectural drawing project. He wasn't prepared for how much Nick had changed.

Nick looked emaciated and rarely had the strength to move off the deck of the run-down, three-bedroom beach house. It was certainly peculiar that such two good friends as Rick and Nick should both be sick, Enno thought occasionally. At least Rick looked healthy enough to him. Recently, the thought had pierced the thick layers of Enno's Oregonian optimism that Nick wasn't doing as well. Enno felt as though he were breaking inside, because he loved Nick so much.

Enno thought back to their Aspen skiing trip in January, five months ago. People had said Nick's fatigue was a typical reaction to the altitude, the thin air. When they returned to Manhattan, Nick went to his Rolfing but came home a couple of hours later with the flu. He felt better the next day and went back to work, only to return again in a few hours, complaining of the same vague malaise. That was the last time he had tried to go to work. All the health foods Nick so carefully prepared and all the Rolfers and psychic healers he had consulted weren't helping.

Enno wondered again: Where could they get Nick fixed? Nick shifted restlessly and shouted something, waking himself up. He dozed back to sleep, the sheets only accenting how much weight he had lost. Tomorrow, Enno knew, Nick would mention hearing somebody shout and that it had woken him up. Maybe he'd blame Enno, and then he'd drift back into the vacant daydreams that seemed to occupy so much of his days now. Enno thought back to the warning Nick's best friend had sternly delivered a few months back.

"Nick is going to die if we don't do something."

"You're being overdramatic," Enno had said.

Saturday, August 9
NEW YORK CITY

"What do I call you?"

Senator Kennedy absently ran his hand through his graying hair while he quizzed Bill Kraus.

"Is it just gay? Or lesbians and gays? Or gay men and gay women?"

With the Democratic National Convention scheduled to convene at Madison Square Garden in just two days, the senator's fight with President Carter was coming down to the wire. The key issue was Kennedy's move for an "open convention." If Kennedy could force a rules change to permit delegates to vote their consciences and not the dictates of the party primaries, he might be able to squeak to victory. It was his last chance. The convention's Gay and Lesbian Caucus cocktail party presented a friendly audience since two-thirds of the gay delegates were already committed to the senator. As a member of the Platform Committee, Bill Kraus was the highest-ranking Kennedy delegate in the caucus, and he was going to introduce the candidate. Kennedy was trying to pick his way through the etiquette of eighties politics and get the salutation just right.

"Or is it lesbians and gay men?"

Bill rolled his eyes toward Gwenn Craig. Gwenn knew her friend was in ecstasy, squiring Kennedy around the party and not-too-subtly gloating at the New York delegates pledged to President Carter. Nobody from the Carter campaign had bothered to attend the gay event.

Kennedy settled on lesbians and gay men and started delivering his ringing endorsement of gay concerns, accompanied by a reminder that he was the first major candidate to endorse these issues. Bill couldn't believe that New York activists were arguing that it was in gays' interests to support a president who had done nothing for gay rights over Kennedy, who supported the entire gay agenda. It was typical New York gay shit, he had confided to Gwenn.

The New York gay leaders seemed to view homosexual rights as something of a driver's license—they were privileges that were doled out by the state. Bill Kraus saw the issue simply in terms of what gays deserved. They were talking about rights, not privileges, for Christ's sake. Bill would later reflect that so much of what would happen in the coming years could be understood in terms of what happened at that 1980 convention, where the split between the California and New York styles of gay politics had so clearly emerged.

It had started a month before at the Democratic Platform Committee in Washington, where Democrats drew up the statement of principles on which they would run their campaign. Bill Kraus wanted to push for the full set of gay demands. An executive order from the president could immediately end discrimination against gays by all federal agencies "with the stroke of a pen," as Bill was fond of noting. He thought it was disgusting that foreign gays could be excluded from even setting foot in this country on the ground that they were "pathological" under a law passed during the McCarthy era. He wanted a promise to change the immigration laws, as well.

The proposals horrified the Carter camp, who were worried about the increasingly contentious fundamentalists in the former Georgia governor's political base in the South. Kennedy promised enough delegates to take the issue to the convention floor in the form of a minority plank if that's what gays wanted. Bill relished the thought of a floor debate on the issue. The gay cause needed that kind of nationally televised attention if it was to be taken seriously as a legitimate social issue, he thought.

The Carter camp would have preferred not mentioning gay rights at all, but, in an attempt to avoid the floor fight, they held out the compromise of a general plank opposing discrimination on the basis of sexual orientation. New York gays supported the president, saying gays would not even get so much as this plank if they caused trouble. Bill Kraus didn't want to compromise and figured it was better to put the issue in front of 50 million television viewers than to get some nebulous statement in a document that nobody ever read anyway. With a compromise, they would get not only less than they deserved, but far less than they were politically capable of achieving. After the moderate position prevailed, Bill started talking openly of how New Yorkers were committed to "a strategy of enduring subservience." He looked forward to getting to the convention, where the greater strength of West Coast activists could take charge.

"The problem lies not in evil personalities or traitorous acts, but rather in the political orientation which believes that an oppressed group gets what it needs by being careful not to offend the powerful," Bill reported to the Milk Club after the platform compromise. "The problem lies in the desire to protect the little that we have gotten by not risking a fight for what we deserve. The problem lies in believing that what we have gotten is somehow a favor given by politicians rather than the politicians' recognition of what we have the political power to demand and to get."

The New Yorkers, Bill thought, were still unable to build the kind of power that was not dependent on the largess of the elite. It was because of all the closet cases in Manhattan, the Californians told each other. Without visibility and a concrete voting bloc, gays there would always be dispossessed and beholden to the kindness of strangers. And it would be their own fault. Begging for favors from party bosses was politics with a small "p," Bill thought. Playing Politics with a capital "p" meant using the political system to establish the long-term social change you're seeking.

For their part, New York gay leaders, led by lesbian Carter delegate Virginia Apuzzo, thought the Californians were far too militant for mainstream America. Not everybody could live like the out-of-the-closet types who were always rioting in San Francisco. You had to play the game, they thought, and that meant getting along in the real world. And Carter certainly was better than the Republican alternative who had just been nominated in Detroit, former California Governor Ronald Reagan.

Everybody applauded Senator Kennedy, who shook some hands before bustling out to another party. The gay caucus event, high above the East Side in the Olympic Tower, clearly was the "in" event for liberals that night. Gloria Steinem held court in one corner while a number of congressmen pressed Bill Kraus to be introduced. Nobody could get over how far gays had come since the 1976 Democratic Convention, where the gay caucus consisted of four delegates. Here, they had seventy-six delegates and alternates, and they had already achieved the long-elusive goal of getting their concerns written into the platform of the nation's largest political party. It was also clear that the center of the gay movement had shifted west to California, where half the gay delegates lived. Politicos from the other nineteen states represented in the gay caucus huddled around the San Francisco delegates to hear stories about Harvey Milk and how gays had engineered their political power. The gay cause now belonged to the more aggressive activists like Bill Kraus, not the moderates from the East. The next day, Bill was unanimously elected co-chair of the gay caucus.

Kennedy's defeat for both the open convention and the nomination came as a bitter disappointment to Bill and his allies. The Democrats were headed for certain defeat with a loser like Carter at the head of the ticket, Bill moaned to Gwenn Craig. Despite the large gay presence, the East Coast media also mostly ignored the new political force at the convention. Bill was still eager to get the gay cause on television and pushed the notion of nominating a gay vice-presidential candidate; that way the nominating speeches could make television. Because he wasn't the constitutionally required age of thirty-five, Bill couldn't go for it himself. But the gay delegates quickly fanned out throughout the convention and, at the eleventh hour, gathered the necessary petition signatures for the vice-presidential nomination of a black gay leader from Washington, Mel Boozer. On the morning of the final day of the convention, Bill Kraus climbed onto the podium to deliver the nominating speech.

"We are here," he said. "We are here with strength. We are here with pride. And I am happy to say we are here with friends. Many of you worked with us to pass this party's platform plank, which calls for the first time for lesbians and gay men to receive the same protection against discrimination which all other Americans enjoy."

⬭

On the flight back to San Francisco, Bill Kraus and Gwenn Craig consoled themselves with the thought that it would not be utter disaster for gays once Reagan was elected. A Democratic Congress could probably hold back the anti-gay legislation of the New Right. Although the other points on the agenda they held dear would suffer from spending cuts, the gay cause was essentially a battle for social legitimacy, not any specific spending programs. And the most basic rights of being free from police harassment and job discrimination were being won not on the federal level but in the major urban areas where gay clout was concentrated. Ronald Reagan or Jerry Falwell couldn't take away their local political power. Thank God, gays weren't after any money for social programs.

Bill nursed a vodka and tonic and fumed about the wimpy New Yorkers. If a situation ever arose in which gays needed more than reassurances of liberal tolerance, he thought, the New Yorkers would get the shaft.

Late August
VIRGINIA BEACH, VIRGINIA

The psychic sat stoically listening to Nick recount his problems. Nick's steel-gray eyes betrayed his desperation. He had been sick all year now. Would anything help?

Enno Poersch had wanted his younger lover to try the Mayo Clinic in Minnesota, but Nick instead made the trip to the psychic healer in the Shenandoah Valley. The psychic turned on the portable tape recorder and lapsed into a trance. "You are suffering from toxoplasmosis," the psychic said, finally.

Nick didn't know what the hell he was talking about.

The psychic spelled it out, but that didn't help much. Toxoplasmosis, it turned out, was some cat disease. Big help.

After his return to New York City, Nick stayed with a friend while Enno closed up the house on Ocean Walk. Though Enno remained optimistic, Nick deteriorated rapidly. Just rising from his bed required a herculean effort of thought and strength. First, Nick would consciously take some moments to make the decision to rise; there was no longer any spontaneous physical movement. Once decided, he would set about each separate act required in rising, from moving his legs, and his back, to each movement required to put on his shoes and pants. By September, such a process of rising and dressing consumed an hour. When Nick walked, every step commanded more conscious effort, placing one foot in front of the other. At times, Nick looked as though he would collapse from lack of support.

Most frightening to Enno were the bizarre changes in Nick's body. His frame seemed to be curling in upon itself. Nick became pigeon-toed while his trunk hunched over, his shoulders turning toward each other as if he were returning to some macabre and wasted fetal position.

Nick's friend was right, Enno realized. Nick was dying. He replayed the psychic's tape, trying to scour some clue that might resurrect his friend. The cassette again revealed only that strange word, spelled out slowly by the psychic: "T-O-X-O-P-L-A-S-M-O-S-I-S."

4 FORESHADOWING

September 1980
COPENHAGEN

Gasping, struggling for breath, the thirty-six-year-old fought against suffocation in his small, neat room in the *Rigshospitalet*. His palms were flushed light blue from lack of oxygen. The chart dangling from the foot of his bed had categorized the illness in a noncategory: unable to find specific diagnosis. By now, the young man's doctor, Jan Gerstoft, knew there was little he could do except watch his patient die.

Gerstoft knew why the agricultural engineer was left to so fiercely struggle for oxygen; that was not the mystery. Microscopic protozoa were filling the tiny air sacs of the man's lungs. A typical man has 300 million of these air pockets where the oxygen from inhaled breath eases into the bloodstream as part of the body's most basic fueling process. The air sacs, Gerstoft knew, also offer a warm, even tropical climate for the unseen *Pneumocystis carinii* organism.

This newly discovered protozoan had been found in guinea pigs back in 1910 by a Brazilian scientist, Dr. Carini. Three years later, doctors at the Pasteur Institute deduced that it lived quite comfortably in the lungs of ordinary Paris sewer rats. Not until 1942, however, was the tiny creature found to be living in people. A few years later, the first known outbreaks of pneumonia caused by the *Pneumocystis carinii* organism were reported in the orphanages of postwar Europe. Subsequent studies showed that the insidious protozoan, which traces its heritage directly to the most primitive one-celled animals from which all life evolved, can be found just about everywhere in the world's inhabited terrain. It is one of tens of thousands of creatures that are easily held in check by people's normally functioning immune systems.

Immune problems were what had always presaged the appearance of *Pneumocystis* pneumonia, whether among children subjected to overcrowding and poor nutrition or among people whose lymphatic systems were knocked out by cancer. When modern medicine learned how to intentionally suppress the immune system so the body would not reject transplanted kidneys and hearts, *Pneumocystis* flared sporadically, eager to take advantage of any opportunity to thrive in its preferred ecological niche, the lung. The disease, however, would disappear spontaneously once the immune system was restored. And the little creature would return to an obscure place in medical books where it was recorded as one of the thousands of malevolent microorganisms that always lurk on the fringes of human existence, lying dormant until infrequent opportunity allows it to burst forth and follow the biological dictate to grow and multiply. Humankind's evolution as a species that could survive diverse continents and climates was due in no small part to its ability to acquire immunity to such pests.

All this evolution, however, had been short-circuited for the man slowly suffocating in Copenhagen in the chilly days of autumn 1980. Something had created a deficiency in his immune system; this was the easy way to explain how the *Pneumocystis* microbe had taken such comfortable residence in his lungs.

Dr. Gerstoft had come from the State Serum Institute, Denmark's governmental research agency, to study the less easily explained part of the man's diagnosis. What had happened to this man's immune system, and, of course, what might help? Intrigued, Gerstoft performed test after test, but nothing could explain why the protozoa had reproduced so prodigiously in the man's lungs, making him sweat and strain for wisps of oxygen. A review of his recent medical history revealed nothing remarkable. He was an agricultural engineer connected with Denmark's dairy industry, and in 1979, he had visited New York City to attend training courses in the proper use of milking machines. No clue there. He also was homosexual, but in Copenhagen, one of the world's most comfortable cities for gays, this was a matter that raised neither eyebrows nor medical suspicions.

Perhaps it should have, Gerstoft thought later, because just weeks before, he had seen another gay man who, for no apparent reason, was wasting away, suffering from unexplained weight loss and a frighteningly aggressive outbreak of anal herpes. The thirty-seven-year-old man, who was well known in the theater crowd of the Danish capital, had mentioned that his lover was also mysteriously ill.

Second thoughts, of course, would come much later, because even in our advanced times it is still not uncommon for people to fall sick and even die for unexplained reasons. In any event, the agricultural engineer was the first to die, passing away that September at the *Rigshospitalet,* not far from where a surgeon named Grethe Rask had succumbed to the same pneumonia a little less than three years before.

⊂⊃

These two deaths in Copenhagen presented their own salient clue to the identity of a killer that quietly stalked three continents in 1980. In Europe, the microbe's first victims were largely linked to Africa. Just weeks after Grethe Rask was rushed from South Africa to Copenhagen, a thirty-four-year-old airline secretary from Kinshasa took advantage of her employment travel benefits to fly her sickly daughter from Zaire to Belgium. The woman's three-year-old was suffering from oral candidiasis, a yeast infection of her mouth. One of the woman's children had already died of a respiratory ailment stemming from strange problems with her immune system, problems that started with a case of this candidiasis. Within a few weeks of her arrival in Brussels, the mother was also suffering from the oral yeast infection. By mid-September, her lymph nodes were swollen, she was rapidly losing weight, and she was suffering from a severe infection of cytomegalovirus. The doctors could do nothing as waves of infection washed over the mother's body. By January 1978, as she withered away from severe diarrhea caused by an untreatable salmonella infection in her intestines, she flew back to Kinshasa, where she died a month later.

Weeks after this woman's death, baffled scientists in Cologne tried to understand why a successful young concert violinist should contract a case of Kaposi's sarcoma. The German musician was gay and had spent much of the decade traveling across Europe, but this provided no clue as to why he should fall victim to an old man's disease rarely seen in northern Europe. Nor did it explain why his lymph nodes seemed to explode three months later, as if they were fighting some unseen infection. Answers were no more forthcoming in the excruciating months ahead while doctors helplessly watched the forty-two-year-old's body be bombarded with disease after disease until finally, in January 1979, he died.

It was at about that time that Belgian doctors in Zaire began reporting an upsurge in cases of cryptococcus at Kinshasa's Memo Yemo General Hospital. By 1980, physicians could document fifteen cases of this disease. The cysts that spread cryptococcus are found in bird droppings the world over. The problem, therefore, was not the presence of new cryptococcus germs but of some weakness in the patients' immunity that let the disease take root.

In Paris, the first case of the baffling pneumonia also had an African connection, appearing in 1978 when a Portuguese cab driver suddenly experienced difficulty breathing. The short, swarthy man had returned only a year or so before from Angola, where he had served in the Portuguese navy during the Angolan Civil War and, later, as a trucker, driving Angola-Mozambique routes that cut through the narrow coastal spit of western Zaire. Dr. Willy Rozenbaum of Claude-Bernard Hospital was called in to see the man in 1979 and easily diagnosed the parasite *Pneumocystis carinii.* Unable to fathom what immune problems might have engendered the pneumonia, Rozenbaum enlisted immunologist Jacques Leibowitch to try to solve the problem. Leibowitch was accustomed to seeing bizarre diseases among people who traveled to exotic parts of the world; it seemed he was always treating some airline pilot or steward for some obscure infection. The doctor first tested the man for lymph cancer, the condition that often proves to cause such rare bouts of immune deficiency. But the tests yielded nothing, as did further blood studies. Specialists from all over Paris were trooping to the man's bedside, drawn both to struggle for a cure and to explore an intriguing medical mystery. Meanwhile, colonies of thick white fungus bloomed in the patient's mouth and throat, while warts caused by ordinarily benign papovavirus swept over his body, covering his arms and legs.

The doctors were downright awestricken when the man's brain became infected with toxoplasmosis, another rare parasite. Nothing they could do yielded any help, however, and in 1980, the man returned to his wife and five children in Portugal to die. As he was nearing death in Iberia, two women were admitted to the intensive care unit of Claude-Bernard with *Pneumocystis.* One was a Zairian woman, who, like many in the elite of that French-speaking region of central Africa, had sought treatment in the more advanced hospitals of Paris after her African doctors could find no effective treatment for her. The second woman was French, but she, too, had lived recently in Zaire.

The European fall turned to winter. By the time winter was turning to spring, all of them—the cab driver in Portugal and the two women in Paris—had drowned in the primeval protozoa that had filled their lungs.

In the United States, unexplained maladies from a mysterious new syndrome would be traced back to 1979. It was on a balmy September day in 1979 that Rick Wellikoff had been sent to Dr. Linda Laubenstein for blood studies. She duly noted the generalized rash that resisted treatment, and the enlarged lymph nodes all over his body. Laubenstein surveyed the man and assumed he had lymph cancer. Later, a dermatologist told Linda that the man's rash was a skin cancer called Kaposi's sarcoma.

"What the hell is that?" asked Laubenstein.

It didn't take her long to find out all there was to know about it because the world's medical literature on the disease didn't take much time to read. The cancer was discovered originally among Mediterranean and Jewish men in 1871. Between 500 and 800 cases of this disease had been documented in medical books in the last century. It usually struck Jewish and Italian men in the fifth or sixth decade of their lives. In 1914, Kaposi's sarcoma, or KS, was first reported in Africa, where subsequent studies discovered that it was the most common tumor found among the Bantus, the disease generally remaining within distinct geographic boundaries in the open savannah of central Africa. There, KS patients represented one in ten cancer cases.

Typically, a victim would develop some flat, painless purple lesions and die much later, often of something else. As cancers went, Kaposi's sarcoma was fairly benign. In more recent years, reports circulated of a new, more aggressive form of the sarcoma in central Africa, but that did not appear to be what had stricken Rick Wellikoff. The lesions were not rapidly covering his body and internal organs, as had been reported among the Africans. Besides, he had never been to such exotic ports. The only characteristic that made Rick mildly different from the typical New York schoolteacher his age was that he was gay.

Given the rarity of the cancer—and the novelty of a case in such a young, non-Mediterranean man—Linda decided to follow Rick closely and mentioned him to several other doctors. She would have to write it up some day.

Two weeks after she first saw the schoolteacher, she got a phone call from a colleague at the Veteran's Administration Hospital, a few blocks south of New York University Medical Center on First Avenue.

"You're not going to believe it, but there's another one down here," he said.

Laubenstein quickly went to the VA Hospital to visit the other Kaposi's patient who seemed very similar to Rick. The man was much more handsome, to be sure; after all, he was a model. But he was thirty-seven years old, homosexual, and, in the strangest twist, the pair shared mutual friends. It was uncanny.

37

Among their acquaintances, they said, was a dreamy blond flight attendant from Canada. He had an unusual name that stuck in Linda's mind.

"Gaetan. You should talk to Gaetan," the first two gay men to be diagnosed with Kaposi's sarcoma in New York City had told Linda Laubenstein in September 1979.

"You should talk to Gaetan because he's got this rash too."

October 1
DAVIES MEDICAL CENTER,
SAN FRANCISCO

Michael Maletta was curt and irritated as he was being admitted to Davies Medical Center, a major medical center on Castro Street, but he had been sick all year and he wanted to get to the bottom of it. His malaise was officially described as FUO—fever of unknown origin. His doctor, however, suspected much worse and ordered up biopsies of his liver, bone marrow, and lymph nodes. Perhaps it was a Hodgkin's disease that hadn't surfaced, his internist thought. That would explain the lingering malaise that had bedeviled the hairstylist all year. To be sure, Michael had tried to proceed with his life as normal. He still gave the best parties in town and in June had taken over all four floors of the Market Street building above his hair salon to throw the year's ultimate bash. Boys cheerfully crammed the four-story outside stairwell, swigging beers, while hundreds more squeezed into the back patios, dancing to the disco deejay. Down in the basement, scores more groped and fondled each other in a large-scale recreation of a bathhouse orgy room. And in the middle of it was Michael, the perfect host, handing out tabs of the drug MDA to all comers. These were grand times to be gay in San Francisco, Michael thought, and he relished the life-style he had built for himself since moving from Greenwich Village after the glorious Bicentennial summer. He sometimes wondered what had happened to his friends there, people like Enno Poersch and his lover Nick who had been so close. Now he wasn't hearing much from any of the old gang that had spent such hot times together in those months when the tall ships came from all over the world to New York Harbor.

UNIVERSITY OF CALIFORNIA MEDICAL CENTER,
SAN FRANCISCO

"Too much is being transmitted here."

It was getting to be the standard finale to Dr. Selma Dritz's rote presentation on the problem of gastrointestinal diseases among gay men. She felt her analysis had particular gravity at this monthly meeting of the sexually transmitted disease experts at the University of California at San Francisco Medical Center. This was one of the most prestigious medical schools in the nation, she knew. These doctors needed to know that something new was unfolding in the bodies of gay men, and they needed to be alert, to see where it might lead.

This was not how Dr. Dritz, the infectious disease specialist for the San Francisco Department of Public Health, had planned to spend the later years of her career—being one of the nation's foremost authorities on organisms that were setting up residence in the bowels of homosexual men. Her expertise had started soon after 1967, when she became assistant director of the San Francisco Department of Public Health's Bureau of Communicable Disease Control.

Normally, five or perhaps ten cases of amebic dysentery a year crossed her desk, and they were usually from a day-care center or restaurant. Now doctors were reporting that many a week. She checked the figures again. Nearly all the cases involved young single men, and an inordinate number were diagnosed at the Davies Medical Center on Castro Street. She mentioned to another health department staffer that it was odd because she hadn't heard any complaints about neighborhood restaurants. Her colleague took Dritz aside to explain that the cases were concentrated among gay men. Dritz didn't understand the relevance of the observation.

"It's oral-anal contact," he said.

"It's what?"

They didn't teach these things when Selma was in medical school in the 1940s, but she quickly learned the down-and-dirty realities about enteric diseases. Gay doctors had long recognized that parasitic diseases like amebiasis, giardiasis, and shigellosis were simply a health hazard of being gay. The problems grew with the new popularity of anal sex, in the late 1960s and early 1970s, because it was nearly impossible to avoid contact with fecal matter during that act. As sexual tastes grew more exotic and rimming became fashionable, the problem exploded. There wasn't a much more efficient way to get a dose of parasite spoor than by such direct ingestion.

Although all this was common knowledge among gay physicians, the awareness had evaded the public health profession. Earnest health officials at one point dispatched inspectors to Greenwich Village to test water after detecting unusual outbreaks of amoebas in the neighborhood.

The more expert Dritz became about the health problems of the gay community, however, the more concerned she grew. Gay men were being washed by tide after tide of increasingly serious infections. First it was syphilis and gonorrhea. Gay men made up about 80 percent of the 70,000 annual patient visits to the city's VD clinic. Easy treatment had imbued them with such a cavalier attitude toward venereal diseases that many gay men saved their waiting-line numbers, like little tokens of desirability, and the clinic was considered an easy place to pick up both a shot and a date. Then came hepatitis A and the enteric parasites, followed by the proliferation of hepatitis B, a disease that had transformed itself, via the popularity of anal intercourse, from a blood-borne scourge into a venereal disease.

Dritz was nothing if not cool and businesslike. Being emotional got in the way of getting her message across, of making a difference. Her calm admonitions to gay men about the dangers of rimming and unprotected anal sex were well rehearsed by now, although they were out of beat with that era. The sheer weight of her professionalism, however, made Dritz immensely popular among gay doctors. Her children teased her that she was the "sex queen of San Francisco" and the "den mother of the gays." Gay health had become an area in which Dritz had an unparalleled expertise because she had spent much of the late 1970s meeting with gay doctors, penning medical journal articles, and traveling around northern California to issue her no-nonsense health warnings.

But here, in 1980, among these venereal disease specialists, Dritz found her message received cooly, at best. She recognized the response. Scientists had a hard time believing that the sexual revolution had turned Montezuma's revenge and hepatitis B, the junkies' malady, into a social disease. Dritz calmly repeated the statistics: Between 1976 and 1980, shigellosis had increased 700 percent among single men in their thirties. Only seventeen cases of amebiasis were reported in 1969; now the reported cases, which were only a small portion of the city's true caseload, were well past 1,000 a year. Cases of hepatitis B among men in their thirties had quadrupled in the past four years.

These diseases were particularly difficult to fight because they all had latent periods in which they showed no symptoms even while the carrier was infectious—gay men were spreading the disease to countless others long before they knew they themselves were sick. This was a scenario for catastrophe, Dritz thought, and the commercialization of promiscuity in bathhouses was making it worse.

Dritz looked down from her slide projector to the disbelieving faces in the conference room. These med-school types didn't believe anything unless they saw it in their microscopes or test tubes, she thought. This, they argued, was "anecdotal" information and they needed data. All this talk about buggery and oral-anal contact didn't make them any more comfortable either.

Dritz tried to broaden her point, so the doctors could see that she wasn't talking so much about this or that disease, or specific sexual gymnastics.

"Too much is being transmitted," she said. "We've got all these diseases going unchecked. There are so many opportunities for transmission that, if something new gets loose here, we're going to have hell to pay."

October 31
NEW YORK CITY

Ghosts swooshed their way through the winding streets of Greenwich Village, followed by double-jointed skeletons dancing behind misshapen spirits of darkness in the Halloween parade. All Hallows' Eve had for generations stood out as the singularly gay holiday. Sociologists noted that it made sense because it was the day for concealing identities behind masks, a penchant that social conventions had long made a homosexual norm. New York, however, is one of the only cities to mark this day with a parade, which is appropriately centered in its most famous gay enclave. That last night of October was filled with all approximations of grisly death. Larry Kramer didn't take much to costumes, but he joined in the parade with Calvin Trillin and a large group of writer friends, hooting and hollering at the flamboyantly freaky costumes along the route.

○

That night, the gay hot spots came alive with masquerades and special parties. At the Flamingo, one of the choicest private clubs where A-list gays discoed to dawn, Jack Nau enjoyed the revelry and tried to pick out friends behind the costumes. His boyfriend Paul Popham was out of town, which made it all the more tantalizing when Jack saw a familiar face. A blond smiled back in a particularly winning way, and before long Jack and Gaetan Dugas slipped away from the crowd and into the night.

○

"He's had some kind of seizure."

Uptown on Columbus Avenue, Enno Poersch frantically tried to revive Nick. A friend who had been staying with the ailing youth said tearfully that he had heard a shriek from Nick's room before Nick lapsed into unconsciousness. Enno had raced over and was kneeling beside the bed, trying to raise a flicker of awareness.

"We've got to get him to a hospital," Enno cried.

Even if he's unconscious, Enno thought to himself, I should explain it to him. Nick might be aware but just unable to talk.

"We're dressing you so we can take you to the hospital," he said.

Nick threw up a clear, yellowish liquid and had a bowel movement. Enno cleaned him, dressed him, and cradled him gently as he carried his lover down four flights of stairs.

"We're taking you downstairs, out the door," Enno shouted.

Cabs raced along the Upper West Side streets. None would stop for the tall man who was holding the wasted form in his arms. Enno realized that, because it was Halloween, the cabbies probably assumed they were drunks from some costume party.

○

The next morning, Dr. Michael Lange peered into Nick's room at St. Luke's-Roosevelt Hospital. A neurologist had found three massive lesions on the young man's brain during a CAT scan. Lange had been called in as an infectious disease specialist. Nick was slumped to one side of the bed. His gray eyes were covered with a milky white film and the left side of his face seemed to sag. His fever was escalating. Nick had been dying in slow motion for a year, the doctors told Lange, and nobody could say why.

The sight lingered with Lange for years, long after such deathly visages had become familiar and Lange became an international authority about such things. Lange would always recall that first moment, staring into the hospital room at Nick, as the event that separated his Before and After. Years later, Lange could instantly remember the date, the way he could recall the anniversary of his marriage or his kids' birthdays.

It was November 1, 1980, the beginning of a month in which single frames of tragedy in this and that corner of the world would begin to flicker fast enough to reveal the movement of something new and horrible rising slowly from the earth's biological landscape.

5 FREEZE FRAMES

November 1980
UNIVERSITY OF CALIFORNIA, LOS ANGELES

Finally, something interesting.

Dr. Michael Gottlieb's four-month career as an assistant professor at UCLA had proved anything but scintillating. Fresh from his training at Stanford, the thirty-two-year-old immunologist had done what ambitious young scientists are supposed to do when they get their first job at a prestigious medical research center: He went to work with mice. Gottlieb had dutifully brought his own mice from Stanford to UCLA and planned to study the effects of radiation on their immune system, but the damned rodents kept dropping dead from viruses they had picked up in Los Angeles. Gottlieb wasn't terribly enthralled by bench work anyway, so he put out the word that his residents should beat the bushes for something interesting—some patient that might teach them a thing or two about the immune system.

It didn't take long for an eager young resident to come back with the story of a young man who was suffering from a yeast infection in his throat that was so severe he could hardly breathe. Babies born with defects in their immune systems sometimes suffered from this florid candidiasis, as would a cancer patient who had been loaded down with chemotherapy, Gottlieb knew, but he'd never seen such a thing in a thirty-one-year-old who appeared perfectly healthy in other respects.

Gottlieb and his residents examined the young man and collectively scratched their heads.

Two days later, the patient, an artist, complained of shortness of breath. He had also developed a slight cough. On a hunch, Gottlieb twisted some arms to convince pathologists to take a small scraping of the patient's lung tissue through a nonsurgical maneuver. The results presented young Doctor Gottlieb with the strangest array of symptoms he'd ever heard of—the guy had *Pneumocystis carinii* pneumonia.

Gottlieb walked a tube of blood down the hall to a lab immunologist who, like himself, was always on the lookout for something that broke the routine. This researcher was specializing in the new science of T-cells, the recently discovered white blood cells that are key components of the immune system.

Gottlieb asked for a T-cell count on the patient. There are two kinds of T-lymphocyte cells to look for: T-helper cells that activate the specific disease-fighting cells and give chemical instructions for creating the antibodies that destroy microbial invaders, and the T-suppressor cells that tell the immune system when the threat ended. The colleague ran his tests on the patient's blood, laboriously hand-counting the subgroups of T-cells. He was floored by the outcome: There weren't any T-helper cells. Figuring he had made a mistake, he tested the blood again, with the same results.

Hot damn. What kind of disease tracked down and killed such specific blood cells? Gottlieb brainstormed with residents, colleagues, and anyone with a spare hour. Nobody had a clue. Now Gottlieb was excited. He pored over his books and tracked down research on obscure immunological diseases. Nothing explained it. He also examined the minutiae of the artist's medical charts; he had suffered from a cornucopia of venereal diseases. In a conversation, the patient mentioned that he was gay, but Gottlieb didn't think any more of that than the fact the guy might drive a Ford.

After weeks of fruitless investigation, Gottlieb was still stumped. Maybe some leukemia would surface later on. In a year or two, he thought, we'll find out what's wrong.

November 4
SAN FRANCISCO

"I don't have to vote," the housewife said.

Bill Kraus, holding his neatly piled slate cards from the Harvey Milk Gay Democratic Club, tried to control his temper. As far as he was concerned, voting was like breathing: How could you *not* do it? The woman cut him short.

"Jimmy Carter was just on TV," she said. "He's already conceded the election."

"Just like that Georgian jerk to call it quits before they were even done voting on the West Coast," Bill groaned after he got back to the headquarters on Castro Street.

The national debacle shaping up was no major surprise. Ronald Reagan was sweeping the country and bringing in the first Republican Senate in nearly thirty years. There wasn't much satisfaction in the thought that, for the first time, gays indeed had been a serious campaign issue—for the other side. To be sure, the Carter camp ended up making every concession gays wanted. They had to in order to battle independent candidate John Anderson, who was even more forthcoming in his attempt to capture gay votes, which tend to concentrate in the urban centers of states rich in electoral votes. However, in the South, the Republicans had used all this to their advantage.

"The gays in San Francisco elected a mayor," announced the solemn voice in television ads aimed at southern voters. The visuals shifted from photos of deviate-looking gay rights marchers to a still of President Carter. "Now they're going to elect a president."

Religious fundamentalists, who had burst forth in 1977 specifically over the volatile gay issue, had been emboldened by their successful repeals of homosexual rights laws in a dozen cities in the late 1970s, and they organized as never before for the 1980 election. Jerry Falwell and his Moral Majority became household words, and analysts heralded the fundamentalists as the most important new political force to emerge in America in decades. Falwell and his New Right compatriots rarely let a speech go by without some dark reference to the growing clout of homosexuals, often paired with a citation from Revelation, indicating that this already had been prophesied as a precursor to the Last Days.

On television, Falwell quickly claimed credit for the Reagan landslide and announced he would push forward with his pro-family, and anti-gay, legislative agenda. Most analysts, however, pinned the conservative landslide on the sheer unpopularity of incumbent Carter and the fact that people seemed ready for a frugal government that pledged cuts in domestic spending.

Cleve Jones swept into the gay headquarters with his boss, California Assembly Speaker Leo McCarthy, while Bill Kraus, Gwenn Craig, and their cronies were assessing the impact these Baptist loonies would have on the administration. They cheerfully reminded themselves that a Democratic House could probably stall the anti-gay legislation Falwell had ambitiously proposed. Other than that, the Republican regime would largely mean massive cutbacks in domestic programs that had little effects on gays. The gay politicos turned their attention to local election results. Voters had just thrown out the city's method of electing supervisors by district. Gays had fought hard for district elections in the 1970s, largely because it seemed that no gay candidate could ever be elected citywide; there just wasn't that kind of power then. Harvey Milk had won his seat as a district supervisor, and Bill Kraus had slaved for months to engineer the election of Milk's successor, Harry Britt, in the citywide election. As aides phoned in the results from City Hall, the extent of gay entrenchment in San Francisco became obvious. Harry Britt was easily elected supervisor. Bill's strategy of building coalitions with Chinese, labor, and liberal groups had succeeded beyond his own expectations. Tim Wolfred, a former Britt aide and Milk Club officer, had also won a citywide race to the San Francisco Community College Board of Directors.

Even better, the results demonstrated that the gay neighborhoods, again, were showing the highest voter registration, feeding the highest voter turnouts in the city. Gay precincts were also proving to be the city's most liberal, churning out ten-to-one majorities for incumbent Democratic Senator Alan Cranston. Returns from big cities across the country also confirmed the wisdom of targeting gay precincts for the old-fashioned door-to-door ward politics Bill Kraus had helped fashion in San Francisco. Some of the largest Carter voting blocs in Manhattan, New Orleans, and Houston were from homosexual neighborhoods. Quick calculations showed that 62 percent of gay voters in the big cities were going for Carter, compared with 27 percent for Reagan and a surprisingly strong 11 percent for Anderson.

Cleve Jones and Bill Kraus couldn't conceal their relief at the returns. With its religious-right alliances, this would not be an administration friendly to homosexuals, but it didn't matter. Whatever happened nationally, they told each other, at least gays were dug in across the country in safe urban enclaves. Jerry Falwell wouldn't have much say in the city councils of areas where gays were concentrated. That was where the decisions that truly affected the day-to-day life of homosexuals were made.

As the crowd at the headquarters thinned, Bill shuffled through the posters, leaflets, and slate cards that littered the floor and remembered the euphoric night three years before when Harvey Milk was elected. It was a vaguely troubling thought. Back then, it had been so clear what they were fighting for. There were visible foes, like Anita Bryant and John Briggs's anti-gay school-teachers referendum. Now, in such a short time, they had already won much of what they wanted, at least in San Francisco. The votes were still there, but the fire had left the politics of Castro Street. What were they fighting for now?

November 15
ST. LUKE'S-ROOSEVELT HOSPITAL, NEW YORK CITY

Enno Poersch put Nick's hand in his own strong grip, hoping his optimism might course into the vacant man's eyes.

"This is great," said Enno. "They finally know what you have. Now they'll be able to cure you and you'll be fine."

Nick was still so exhausted from the surgery he could barely manage a smile. The white gauze still capped most of his head. The exploratory surgery had been most indelicate. The doctors had simply taken off the top of Nick's skull to try to figure out what had created the three massive lesions. The effort had at last produced a diagnosis. Nick, they said, had toxoplasmosis; yes, it could be treated.

"Everything's gonna be fine," Enno said.

November 25
SAN FRANCISCO

Ken Horne had always wanted to be a dancer, performing a dazzling array of pirouettes, entrechats, and arabesques before a rapt audience that would nod approvingly at his grace and beauty. A glowingly optimistic sort, he loved everything about the theater, with its romance and costumes and fairy-tale happy endings. Maybe he could even be a star, the guy people cheered and wrote about. That's why he had left his blue-collar family in Oregon and moved to San Francisco in 1965, when he was twenty-one, to study at the San Francisco Ballet School. A nose job had complemented an otherwise delicate face, and his body was hard and muscular from years of training. The sheer contrast between his childhood plainness and his adult beauty made Ken's introduction to San Francisco gay life rewarding. All these men liked him so much, and he so desperately wanted to be liked. Sometimes, he confided to friends, he felt like a Cinderella who had finally arrived at the ball.

Maybe that's why it was easier to let go of the dancer's dream in the late 1960s. Ken told friends a vague story about the ballet director decreeing that all the single men had to get married or engaged to stay in the company, something about hating to be embarrassed by all the dancers' arrests in gay bar raids. In any event, Ken dropped out of the ballet school, assuring friends he would get back into it once he got his finances straightened out. In 1969, he took a clerical job at the Bay Area Rapid Transit system and found he liked the regular paycheck as well as a work week that was a dream compared to the regimen of 6 A.M. to 9 P.M. he'd followed with the ballet. He had more time to go out at night now. "This isn't so bad after all," he told a friend. "I'm having fun."

Ken soon fell in love with a German sign painter and lost touch with his early San Francisco friends, who recalled a sweet young kid who loved romance. They were surprised five years later to happen into Ken at the Folsom Prison, a leather bar. His hair was cut severely and he sported a close-cropped, narrow beard that followed the line of his jaw like a chin strap on some Nazi helmet. His old friends were floored, not only because he was so thoroughly the proto-type of the black leather machismo then sweeping San Francisco, but also because he looked so wasted. His hair had gone gray and his eyes looked glazed. Ken complained about how tough it was in this "city of bottoms" to find a man who would screw him.

His friends decided that Ken had fallen into the trap that had snared so many beautiful gay men. In his twenties, he had searched for a husband instead of a career. When he did not find a husband, he took the next best thing—sex—and soon sex became something of a career. It wasn't love but at least it felt good; for all his time at the Cinderella ball, the prince had never arrived.

As the focus of sex shifted from passion to technique, Ken learned all the things one could do to wring pleasure from one's body. The sexual practices would become more esoteric; that was the only way to keep it from getting boring. The warehouse district alleys of both Manhattan and San Francisco had throughout the 1970s grown increasingly crowded with bars for the burgeoning numbers of leathermen like Ken Horne. By 1980, it was a regular industry.

Life is a disappointment, Ken was thinking as he walked into San Francisco's largest medical office building on the morning of November 25, 1980. It was an ironic thought for a man who was taking his first steps toward finally becoming someone that people would write about.

$\bigcirc$

"My life is falling apart," Ken Horne told Dr. James Groundwater.

Groundwater was a dermatologist, involved in a course of work that did not lend itself to such dramatic confessionals. But the forty-three-year-old physician had the fatherly manner of someone to whom you'd spill your guts, and as Ken anxiously took off his shirt, the doctor heard his story.

For two years, he'd been feeling tired and always a little sick to his stomach.

There was also this diarrhea, off and on, since 1978. It was horrible. And then, last month, Ken said, came these funny bumps.

Groundwater examined the bluish-purple spots. One was on Ken's left thigh, the other was near his right nipple.

"What's happening to me?" Ken pleaded.

He was angry that years of visiting doctors had not made him one bit better, or even told him what was wrong.

Groundwater was surprised at the size of Ken's lymph nodes. They certainly had something to do with those spots.

Ken continued his story as the doctor examined him: His bosses had been making unrealistic demands, so he went on disability this month. He had also started seeing a shrink; he'd do anything to get his life back together.

Groundwater pondered what could be wrong with the thirty-seven-year-old patient. It could be lymphoma, which would explain the swollen nodes but not the spots. Groundwater drew some blood and cut off a sliver of the lesion for a biopsy. They'd figure this out.

Thanksgiving Day, November 27
ORANGE COUNTY, CALIFORNIA

Canadian winters were so tedious that Gaetan Dugas was overjoyed at the invitation to spend Thanksgiving weekend in southern California. The new object of Gaetan's affections, a hairdresser, was equally thrilled at the catch. Normally, the hairdresser was content to cruise the Boom-Boom Room in Laguna Beach. His trip to the 8709 Club in West Hollywood had been only his second or third time at a bathhouse, and he'd hooked this gorgeous airline steward who was coming back for seconds, maybe even thirds. What a wonderful weekend they'd have. The baths weren't so bad after all, he thought.

Gaetan briefly examined himself in the mirror. Yes, a few more spots had had the temerity to appear on his face. The doctors said there was no treatment, but that didn't matter. He felt fine, and pushing back his sandy hair just so, he smiled at the thought: "I'm still the prettiest one."

December 5
SAN FRANCISCO

Desperation haunted Ken Horne's sunken eyes as he slowly pulled off his shirt to show Dr. Groundwater the two new purple spots on his chest. No, not another biopsy, he told the doctor fiercely. He wanted some answers.

The blood test assay that had come in from the lab was also disconcerting. Something was wrong with Ken's white blood cells. Even more startling was the lack of reaction to a series of routine skin tests Groundwater had given the BART station manager during his last exam. The tests, little pricks with needles infected with benign germs, normally swell up to hard red bumps. This means the immune system is manufacturing the antibodies to fight the germs. No bumps on Ken. The immune system had just ignored the needle pricks.

Ken repeated his complaints of nausea, fatigue, and diarrhea, leaving the dermatologist mystified. The man sounded sick, very sick, but from a lab point of view, there wasn't really *that* much wrong with him. Blood tests are off all the time, and sometimes the skin tests don't take—but such immune fluctuations don't leave you so incapacitated. All Groundwater could do was order more tests. He persuaded Ken to let him do a biopsy of a lymph node, which would show whether there was some kind of lymph cancer. The doctor also drew extra blood and sent it to the lab with special instructions to scan the serum for every exotic viral disease they could imagine.

There is an answer to this, Groundwater thought. There always is.

December 9
LOS ANGELES

"What are we doing to ourselves?"

It was the question that Dr. Joel Weisman felt compelled to ask himself as he checked out the nervous, thirty-year-old advertising manager. The guy was sick. He had a painful eczema, persistent diarrhea, and endless fevers. Even worse, he'd been sick for six weeks now and was seeing Dr. Weisman on a referral from his normal internist. After ordering up tests, Weisman wrote his tentative diagnosis on the patient's chart: "Patient has problems that appear to be secondary to immune deficiency."

Mysteriously ill people aren't all that rare in a medical practice, Weisman knew, but this was not isolated. In October, another young gay man had gone to Weisman's associate with a strikingly similar disarray in his immune system. The constellation of diseases was startling. White fungi grew around the man's fingernails, fluffy candidiasis was sprouting all over his palate, and he too was suffering from rashes, prolonged fevers, swollen lymph glands, and low white blood counts. Hospitalization brought a brief respite from the skin problems, but by early December, the patient's nightsweats were soaking through the sheets of his bed and the rashes had returned. Weisman's partner first thought the man's blood had been bombarded with both bacterial and viral infections, but by December he also diagnosed "immune deficiency."

On top of these two cases, another twenty men had appeared at Weisman's office that year with strange abnormalities of their lymph nodes. That's how the ailments of these two more seriously ill patients had started. Weisman had half-expected something more serious when he started seeing the lymphadenopathy, or abnormal enlargement of the lymph glands. New studies were showing that 93 percent of gay men were infected with cytomegalovirus, a herpes virus that had been linked to cancer. The gay sexual revolution had also made the Epstein-Barr virus, a microbe also linked to cancers, pandemic among homosexual men. There were only so many viruses a body could battle before something went horribly awry. Now Weisman worried that he was seeing what could happen in the frightened eyes of the advertising manager who had been far too young and healthy last year to be so sick today.

The dean of southern California gay doctors, Weisman had pondered how to start telling gay men to slow down, that all this sex might end up being hazardous to their health. This was not a community that took kindly to stern reprimands, especially about sex, the doctor knew. These men had often been bruised by the painful proddings of parents and priests. This was not a time or place to be judgmental, because most of these men had fled their homes for cities like Los Angeles precisely to escape judgment. Yet the strange mix of taboos and newfound freedom had created a social climate that was wonderfully tailored for aggressive little viruses. So, as Weisman reassured this young man that they'd give him back his health, he was wondering to himself, "What are we doing to ourselves?"

It was the end of 1980, a year when the top movies were *Coal Miner's Daughter* and the second Star Wars fantasy, *The Empire Strikes Back.* The top musical album was *The River* by Bruce Springsteen, filled with sad songs of economic dislocation and moral confusion about where a once-secure America was going. Meanwhile, a new virus was now well-entrenched on three continents, having moved easily from Africa to Europe and then to North America. Later surveys would show that in the United States fifty-five young men had been diagnosed with some infection linked to the new virus by the end of 1980. Ten others had been diagnosed in Europe, while many more were ailing among the uncounted sick of primitive Africa. Slowly and almost imperceptibly, the killer was awakening.

December 23
NEW YORK CITY

Rick Wellikoff's rapid deterioration stunned his doctors no less than his friends. Kaposi's sarcoma wasn't supposed to act this way, Dr. Linda Laubenstein knew, but nonetheless Rick was dying. The doctors put it to him bluntly: His lungs were filling up with something. They didn't know what. They could keep draining the fluid through the tube they had inserted in his chest, and they could, of course, keep him alive on the machines. That, however, would be all they were doing—keeping him alive.

Rick mustered his courage and said, no, he didn't need the machines. He wanted to go home to his brownstone on the Upper West Side. He checked out of the New York University Hospital two days before Christmas. Paul Popham wanted to go home with him. It was what a friend should do. But that night John and Wes, two of the men with whom they shared the house on Ocean Walk, were throwing their holiday party. Go to the party, Rick insisted.

As the night wore on, Rick's lover sat at Rick's bedside and listened to his breaths grow shorter and shorter until, deep in the night, he stopped breathing altogether. In those first hours of the day that Danes observe as the Feast of the

Hearts, the thirty-seven-year-old fifth-grade teacher passed away in a flat on West 78th Street, becoming the fourth American to die of what would later be called Acquired Immune Deficiency Syndrome.

BETH ISRAEL MEDICAL CENTER, NEW YORK CITY

With a sense of weariness, Dr. Donna Mildvan studied the autopsy report of a thirty-three-year-old German chef to whom she had devoted so much of the past five months. His death had been particularly grisly. Plagued by the cytomegalovirus that had spread its virulent herpes throughout his body, the young man had simply curled into a ball and finally died one day, as the late December cold descended on Manhattan. Mildvan grimaced as she surveyed the last CAT scan of the man's brain. It was shrunken and atrophied, like the brain of a senile old man. She wondered whether she would ever understand what she had missed, what had so cruelly torn away this man's life.

Two weeks later, a Beth Israel nurse appeared in the emergency room, suffering from *Pneumocystis.* Within ten days, he was dead. It turned out that he was also homosexual. When the pathologist told Mildvan that an autopsy had revealed widespread infection with cytomegalovirus, the physician's thinking crystallized quickly: There were too many coincidences. Two men had died of infections that should be mere nuisances, not brutal killers. Their immune systems had collapsed. This also explained why she had ten other patients, all gay men, who were suffering from a strange enlargement of their lymph nodes. Something was wrong with their immune systems too.

Mildvan quickly arranged a meeting with the city's best-known gay physician, Dan William.

"I'm very concerned too," said William. "I have lots of patients with lymphadenopathy."

Mildvan went quickly to the point. This was all connected, she was convinced, and in the early weeks of 1981 she became one of the first doctors to begin conceiving a larger picture.

"Whatever that lymphadenopathy is, I think it's the same thing that just killed those two other guys," Mildvan said. "There is a new disease going around in homosexual men."

PART III

PAVING THE ROAD 1981

As in most crises, the events surrounding Andromeda Strain were a compound of foresight and foolishness, innocence and ignorance. Nearly everyone involved had moments of great brilliance, and moments of unaccountable stupidity. It is therefore impossible to write about the events without offending some of the participants.

However, I think it is important that the story be told. This country supports the largest scientific establishment in the history of mankind. New discoveries are constantly being made and many of these discoveries have important political or social overtones. In the near future, we can expect more crises on the pattern of Andromeda. Thus I believe it is useful for the public to be made aware of the way in which scientific crises arise, and are dealt with.

—MICHAEL CRICHTON,
The Andromeda Strain

6 CRITICAL MASS

January 15, 1981
ST. LUKE'S-ROOSEVELT HOSPITAL, NEW YORK CITY

Enno Poersch watched the white foam bubble out of Nick's mouth. Foam oozed from his ears and nostrils. For a few days after his mid-November diagnosis, it had looked like the young bartender was improving. The swelling in his brain receded. Nick and Enno even joked occasionally. But Nick never regained his strength after the diagnostic surgery. He had a heart attack, was revived, and was put into the intensive care unit with a tube down his throat and into his lungs to make sure he'd breathe.

He slept most of the time, though sometimes his eyes would open and he'd look at Enno, tall and strong and utterly helpless. Enno was convinced Nick was trying to communicate, but then his eyes would close again. When they pulled out the tube and simply cut a hole in his throat to ease the labored breaths, Nick didn't have the energy to talk. He had two more heart attacks, but the nurses and the machines had kept him from death. The doctors said a herpes virus, cytomegalovirus, was running wild in his body, inundating every organ, and he had some lung infection too. Nobody could say exactly what it was.

Enno and Nick's sister were keeping vigil over his bed on the brisk Thursday morning of January 15 when one of the nurses commented, "It's like he's trying to hold on for somebody." And Nick's sister turned to Enno and said the inevitable: "Why don't we turn it off?"

As the machines were disconnected, Enno looked down at the young man he had met on a Fire Island beach so long ago. He had been so handsome and vibrant. Enno was still staring down at the bed when the machines stopped bleeping and Nick's chest heaved one last time, and he was dead.

Enno made the trip to Nick's Pennsylvania hometown for the big Italian funeral. After the long trip back, he walked listlessly into his 80th Street apartment. He had never felt so alone. The phone rang and an anonymous caller started talking dirty. Enno couldn't believe what he was hearing.

"My lover just died, you asshole, and I just now got back from the funeral," he shouted.

"Oh God," said the voice in tones of genuine contrition. "I'm sorry."

February 1
CENTERS FOR DISEASE CONTROL, ATLANTA

In her tiny office in the cluster of red brick buildings that serve as nerve center for the federal government's monitoring of the public health, technician Sandra Ford did a second take on the pentamidine request form. Pentamidine was one of the dozen drugs that were used so rarely that the federal government stockpiled the nation's supply through a special arrangement with the Food and Drug Administration. Not only were the drugs not yet officially licensed for widespread use, but not enough profit existed in their production to interest commercial firms. When doctors needed them, they called Sandy Ford.

The thirty-year-old Ford had spent the last two years in the cramped Room 161 of Building 6 at the CDC, processing pentamidine requests and sending out small bottles of the drug in reinforced cardboard boxes covered with RUSH stickers.

She wasn't going to save the world at this job, she thought, but she was where the action was and she prided herself on her thoroughness. That's why she looked twice at the pentamidine request from a New York City physician. The form said he needed the drug to treat a case of *Pneumocystis carinii* pneumonia. Nothing unusual about that, because *Pneumocystis* was the disease that pentamidine was most frequently used to cure. Unlike most other requests, however, the doctor didn't say why the patient had this rare pneumonia. You only got *Pneumocystis* when something had kicked the bottom out of your natural immunities, Ford knew. Her drug requests almost always mentioned some underlying cause of immune suppression. Most typically, childhood leukemia patients being treated with chemotherapy needed the drug. Others were people with lymphomas or patients on drugs used to stop the body from rejecting a transplanted organ. Sandy made a mental note about this unusual request, methodically filed the form away, and filled the order.

RAYBURN HOUSE OFFICE BUILDING, WASHINGTON, D.C.

"Are you for the president or against him?"

Every Republican on Capitol Hill seemed to be echoing the line in the early days of February. The country seemed downright giddy over its new president, who had been able to announce the end of the humiliating Iranian hostage crisis only moments after pledging, in his friendly way, to cut and hack the federal budget to size. Battered by the loss of the Senate and the defeat of an incumbent president, the Democrats collectively seemed as insecure as a teenager who was stood up on the night of the senior prom. In the first months of 1981, they didn't appear to have the gumption for much fight.

The long-feared Reagan budget was handed to Tim Westmoreland moments after it arrived in his office. This, everyone knew, was to be the opening volley in the new Reagan administration's war on domestic spending. The book was still warm to the touch from the printing presses as Westmoreland quickly leafed to the sections on health programs. As chief counsel to the House Subcommittee on Health and the Environment, he would be the key congressional staffer to defend the Democratic health agenda. Westmoreland was thankful that his boss, Los Angeles Congressman Henry Waxman, rarely wavered from a thoroughly liberal commitment to federal health spending.

Slapped together quickly in the days after the Reagan inauguration, the book was a hodgepodge of handwritten margin notes. The Carter administration had held a tight line on health spending. Under Reagan, Westmoreland could see, it would be worse. The National Institutes of Health did not fare too poorly under the Reagan proposals, losing only $127 million of Carter's proposed $3.85 billion. Westmoreland sighed, however, when he saw the Reagan plan for the Centers for Disease Control. The executive Office of Management and Budget, or OMB, wanted to cut the Carter budget's recommended $327 million in CDC funding to $161 million.

None of this was particularly surprising. President Reagan had gone into office promising that federal programs would be turned over to the states. About half the money cut from the CDC budget would go to the states in block grants so they could administer comparable programs locally. Westmoreland, however, worried that the slashing of the CDC budget courted disaster. The CDC was the frontline in any public health emergency that might befall the country. In the past decade, it had been called upon to tackle Legionnaire's disease and Toxic Shock Syndrome. These weren't pork-barrel special interest programs or social engineering schemes by pointy-headed liberals. The CDC usually got involved when people were dying.

NEW YORK UNIVERSITY

Dr. Linda Laubenstein immediately recognized Paul Popham as a friend of Rick Wellikoff, the schoolteacher who had died last December after contracting the rare skin cancer. Paul was at NYU being treated again for psoriasis. Now there were six cases of that cancer, Kaposi's sarcoma, she mentioned to Paul. Funny thing, she added, all of them were gay men.

UNIVERSITY OF CALIFORNIA,
LOS ANGELES

The fungus on the fingers, the diarrhea and herpes, those had been around for a long time, the young man explained carefully to Dr. Michael Gottlieb. The fevers had been running at 104 degrees for three months now, and he had dropped thirty pounds, he said. But the shortness of breath was something new.

Dr. Joel Weisman had sent the patient to UCLA in hopes that they could figure out what was so mercilessly haranguing his body. As Michael Gottlieb began studying test results, he was struck by how similar this man's symptoms were to those of another young man he had treated late last year. Coincidentally, this second patient was also gay. Gottlieb still was taken aback when the lung biopsy indicated that the thirty-year-old, like last year's patient, was suffering from *Pneumocystis*. Even more striking was the depletion in his T-cells, just like the other patient.

◯

Michael Gottlieb thought Joel Weisman looked anxious as they sat down with two other specialists to talk about the case in Gottlieb's office at UCLA. Of course, Weisman was anxious: He hadn't told Gottlieb yet that he had still another patient with precisely the same bizarre constellation of symptoms, right down to the rare pneumonia that suddenly didn't seem so rare anymore. Two cases was something to be concerned about. Three cases, he felt, were a big deal, a harbinger of more to come.

Weisman offered that the men's immune systems might have been shattered by some new cytomegalovirus or some combination of CMV and the Epstein-Barr virus, the cancer-linked microbe that most commonly causes mononucleosis. The new patient's blood certainly showed elevated levels of CMV that were rising and falling daily. Something was going on with that virus, Gottlieb agreed, and he would work it up further, but he still wasn't sold on the idea that CMV was causing it. The virus had been around for years and was reported to have infected as many as 93 percent of gay men. Something that ubiquitous just doesn't pick on a handful of people to start brutalizing. It needed careful study, they decided. Weisman soon sent Gottlieb his second *Pneumocystis* patient, the third such case at UCLA. Like Weisman, Gottlieb now knew something important was going on, even if he wasn't sure what. He started poring over books on CMV, immune problems of transplant patients, and anything else he could find on immune suppression. He began framing a scientific paper on the miniepidemic of pneumonia.

ST. LUKE'S-ROOSEVELT HOSPITAL, NEW YORK CITY

Not many Haitians can afford to whisk themselves up to a fancy Manhattan hospital for treatment, Dr. Michael Lange thought, but the house staff confided that the patient was a bodyguard to President-for-Life Jean-Claude Duvalier. The patient, Lange noted, was positively ravaged, suffering from severe candidiasis, and even worse, tuberculosis that had spread throughout his body. The fellow's immune system appeared to be shot, and there didn't appear to be any reason for it. In another room, Lange was probing a similar mystery—a drug addict suffering from *Pneumocystis*. Talk was that a hospital in Queens was treating an outbreak of the pneumonia in intravenous drug users.

March 3
UNIVERSITY OF CALIFORNIA,
SAN FRANCISCO

The doctors lifted the baby boy gently from the mother's womb. Not only was the birth complicated by the cesarean section, but this was an "Rh baby." Because of an unusual genetic complication, his body had antibodies to its own blood. Only complete transfusions would save the infant's life, and within the next week, his entire blood supply was replaced six times.

A week after the baby's birth, a forty-seven-year-old man came into the Irwin Memorial Blood Bank to donate blood. The donor seemed fine and healthy. Before the day was over, his blood was broken into components. On the next day, one of those components, special cells that help blood to clot, were transfused into the ailing baby at the UC Medical Center on Parnassus Hill.

CASTRO STREET, SAN FRANCISCO

Shortly after they met, Kico Govantes told Bill Kraus about his first night at a bathhouse on the day of last year's Gay Freedom Day Parade. Bill laughed and hugged Kico, and told him he was hopelessly naive. Kico's wholesomeness had been a source of amazement and attraction for Bill since the day they had met.

Kico knew he was in love the minute he saw Bill standing at the hip dance bar, The Stud, in his chinos, tennis shoes, and the knit polo shirt that showed off Bill's pectorals and flat stomach.

"I work at City Hall," Bill had said proudly, sliding the subject of politics into the conversation as soon as he could.

"Where's that?" Kico asked.

"I can't believe I'm talking to somebody who doesn't know where City Hall is," said Bill. "I work for Harry Britt."

"Who's that?"

"That's who took Harvey Milk's place," said Bill, as if that should explain it all.

Kico had never heard of Harvey Milk.

"We live in two different worlds," said Bill, somewhat pleased with the idea.

Bill couldn't believe that Kico had lived six months in San Francisco and had never gone to bed with anybody. He laughed at the earnest twenty-four-year-old when he saw the Hindu religious book, the Bhagavad Gita, by Kico's bed.

"You're just like a little kid," concluded Bill after they made love.

"What other way is there to be?" Kico asked.

Kico was enchanted by the earnest politico who seemed so caught up in helping people and making a difference in the world. Bill explained all kinds of things to Kico, about gay politics, the importance of coalitions, and his new plan to foster gay clout by placing key gay activists in the offices of various political leaders.

"You don't get power by just having these people come to your cocktail parties," Bill would lecture. "You need to be on the inside."

Bill seemed to take a most wicked pleasure, however, in shocking the recent émigré's sensibilities, explaining the nuances of cruising and the rituals of such hallowed gay institutions as bathhouses.

"It's dirty," Kico said flatly of the raucous bathhouse sexuality.

"It's not dirty—that's a value judgment," Bill answered. "If that's what a person feels good doing, it's not dirty."

"Why would somebody want some stranger's hand up their ass?" Kico asked. "What does that have to do with love?"

"You've got these people from Moline," Bill explained. He always had a hard time being calm when he felt an argument coming on. "They've been repressed all their lives, and now they're going to be a little extreme, a little weird, but it will swing back. It's like straight sailors when they get off a ship after a long time."

When Bill got backed into a corner, he rarely admitted to the inadequacies of his own arguments. Kico sensed that Bill was being overly sensitive and defensive about the commercialization of gay sex, as if he were trying to justify the excesses to himself. Kico wouldn't push the subject any further that day.

Indeed, the arguments came when Bill was having a more difficult time reconciling the gay community's sexual Disneyland with the political aspirations he wanted his minority to achieve. The sex had started off with such camaraderie. There was a warmth and brotherhood to it. When he went to a bathhouse for the first time in Honolulu, he had felt very liberated. Here was a place you could do anything you wanted with nobody to slap your hand and call you a pervert. But in the mid-seventies, when red hankies sprouted from everybody's pockets, something about it offended Bill's native midwestern conservatism. "Is this what these people want to communicate to the world?" he wondered. "That they want to get fist-fucked or have someone piss on them?"

The gay sexual scene became progressively depersonalized: At first you'd sleep with a person, hug all night, talk and have omelettes in the morning. Then, you skipped the breakfast because just how many omelettes can you make before it gets boring? Then you wouldn't spend the night. With the bathhouses, you wouldn't even have to talk. The Glory Hole and Cornhole clubs came into vogue next. There, you wouldn't even have to see who you had sex with. Bill's leftist inclinations blamed it on corruption of money and businessmen. These places were created because there was money in them. Bill personally appreciated the convenience of the sex, sometimes making his way down to the giant bathhouse on 8th and Howard for Tuesday's buddy night. Politically, however, the dehumanization of sex was troublesome.

Even more problematic was what happened when you got straight people into the act. In early 1981, Bill was at the center of a controversy around the Jaguar Bookstore, a sex club in the heart of the Castro district. The Jaguar was one of a dozen gay private sex clubs in San Francisco, doing far less business in books than in membership fees that allowed patrons to wander around dark back rooms. There, men could be found engaging in proverbially unnatural acts at just about any time of the day or night. The store wanted to expand to a third floor, but neighborhood heterosexuals had rallied against the zoning variance the expansion would require. As an aide to Supervisor Harry Britt, Bill Kraus had championed the sex club's arguments, and Britt had accrued substantial criticism in conservative neighborhoods. To Bill, it was a matter of territorial imperative. If gays couldn't call the shots in the Castro, their only liberated zone, where could they exert their power?

Still, the debate left him with a sour taste for the entrepreneurs of the gay sex industry. While the Jaguar owner had publicly pleaded that he was the victim of horrible anti-gay bigotry to rally gay political support, he showed no further interest in city politics once he got his variance. As far as Bill was concerned, the guy was a pig who was only interested in making money. He still didn't regret the politicking, however, if only because he was convinced that straight people had no business getting involved in gays' sex lives. It had taken a decade to build this sexual freedom in San Francisco, and they couldn't give an inch or else it all might be taken away.

Kico thought that whole line of reasoning was stupid after Bill explained it to him one afternoon as they strolled down Castro Street.

"I still think it's dirty," Kico said.

March 30
ST. FRANCIS HOSPITAL,
SAN FRANCISCO

The pain pounded on both eyes, like heavy wooden mallets. Any movement increased the pounding, as if somebody wanted him to sit there and suffer through each excruciating pulsation.

Dr. James Groundwater knew this was serious stuff and immediately ordered Ken Horne to the hospital on a foggy Monday morning. Groundwater was now one of a panoply of specialists thoroughly baffled by Ken's failing health. Groundwater had seen a lot of skin in his day, and he knew what was benign and what wasn't. Whatever was causing Ken Horne's purple spots certainly was not benign. Never was this more clear than on that cloudy Monday morning when he admitted Ken to the hospital.

Ken had been suffering from unrelenting fevers for weeks now and complained of increasingly severe headaches and, today, that pounding pain. Ken had become testier with each passing month. He didn't want any more tests; he just wanted to be told what he had. Meanwhile, he deteriorated. New lesions appeared on his face and palate in February. In early March, they began covering his lower back.

Groundwater thought it might be a blood vessel tumor and had sent specimens to a lab in Michigan, which was unable to make a diagnosis. A cancer specialist wasn't helpful either. Within hours of Ken's admission to the hospital, a neurologist was checking out his complaints of weakness. She ordered a lumbar puncture. The test revealed an even more baffling malady—cryptococcus.

Groundwater thought he would drop when he heard the diagnosis. It explained the headaches but nothing else. Cryptococcus, he knew, was a parasite most commonly found in bird feces. Cryptococcus-infected pigeon droppings had fallen on San Francisco every day for a century. Why in March of 1981 should somebody suddenly come down with cryptococcus?

◯

The first diagnosis of Kaposi's sarcoma in San Francisco arrived in Jim Groundwater's office on April 9, 1981, from a pathologist at the University of California at San Francisco. Ken Horne's lesions were "consistent" with the disease, the pathologist said. The tumor also had invaded Ken's lymph nodes. But Ken, Groundwater knew, was not suffering from classical KS. This was not the benign skin cancer that old Italians lived with for ten years. Groundwater started comparing notes with every pathologist and expert he could contact. Something else was ailing Ken, and he was going to die if Groundwater didn't find out what.

7 GOOD INTENTIONS

April 4, 1981
CENTERS FOR DISEASE CONTROL,
ATLANTA

This guy should go back to medical school if he can't find some simple neoplasm, Sandra Ford thought. Maintaining her professional air, however, Ford asked the doctor again, in a different way: How did he come to have not one but two patients with *Pneumocystis carinii* pneumonia who needed pentamidine? This was a simple question, Ford thought. What was the underlying cause of immune suppression that had brought on the pneumonia?

The Manhattan physician, again, answered he didn't know why the two young men had PCP. In fact, there didn't seem to be any reason for their immune systems to be so out of whack. Still, they needed pentamidine because they weren't reacting well to the sulfa drugs more commonly used for *Pneumocystis*.

Ford figured the doctor was either incompetent or lazy. He probably didn't have the patients' charts in front of him and didn't want to move his overpaid ass into another room to get them. But in the last eight weeks, she had filled five orders for adult male patients with unexplained *Pneumocystis*. All but one of them lived in New York.

UNIVERSITY OF CALIFORNIA,
LOS ANGELES

The fourth *Pneumocystis carinii* pneumonia patient at UCLA appeared in April, a black man suffering from what Dr. Michael Gottlieb could now identify as all the typical symptoms: swollen lymph nodes, fevers, weight loss, and a wicked case of candidiasis. Like the other three PCP sufferers, this man showed dramatically elevated levels of cytomegalovirus in his blood. The thirty-six-year-old was referred to Gottlieb by a distinguished West Los Angeles internist who had heard Gottlieb was studying gay men with just such immune problems. Gottlieb marveled at how fast news spread on the gay medical grapevine.

Dr. Joel Weisman had told him that the miniepidemic might be some strain of CMV gone wild or some new combination of CMV and another virus. No matter what it was, Gottlieb felt that with four patients, he didn't have the luxury to collect data for the next two years before writing up an august article for a medical journal. People had to find out about this, Gottlieb thought frantically. He'd only been in L.A. since July, but he had one key contact.

Dr. Wayne Shandera answered the phone in his cramped downtown office at the Los Angeles County Department of Public Health and immediately recognized Gottlieb's voice. The two doctors had been friends and residents together at Stanford and had both moved south in July. Shandera had ended up in L.A. on the first leg of a two-year stint with the Epidemiological Intelligence Service, the field investigative corps for the Centers for Disease Control. After three years in the San Francisco Bay Area, Shandera hated Los Angeles, though his spirits lifted whenever he and Gottlieb talked about collaborating on some project. Long before Gottlieb's call, Shandera had suggested studying the immune response to infectious agents.

"Wayne," Gottlieb said, "there's something going on with *Pneumocystis carinii* pneumonia and CMV in homosexual men. Can you look into it?" Gottlieb was relieved Shandera was his friend, because somebody he didn't know would probably think he was a crank caller.

Gottlieb described the cases. It sounded to Shandera as if the pneumonia victims must have had chemotherapy that had wiped out their immune systems. Once off the phone, Shandera mentioned the call to a colleague. She looked a little surprised and pointed to his desk.

"You've got a report of a CMV death sitting right there," she said.

Shandera scanned the report. A twenty-nine-year-old attorney had died of cytomegalovirus pneumonia in Santa Monica last month. Health authorities had written it up for its novelty; CMV didn't normally kill people. Wayne walked upstairs to the health department lab, where specialists were growing CMV cultures from the dead lawyer's lung to see if there was anything unique about the CMV strain that had killed him.

This was important, Shandera knew, and the very reason he had volunteered for work in the medical world's version of the Peace Corps. He would have preferred to be in some underdeveloped nation helping the truly disadvantaged, but, as he relayed his findings to Gottlieb, he sensed that what he was doing now was significant.

Armed with his county health department power to pull any patient's medical records, Shandera launched his car down the crowded Santa Monica Freeway toward the hospital where the attorney had died. An autopsy, it turned out, had found another organism in the man's lungs, something that wasn't mentioned on the death certificate. Maybe it was because a diagnosis of *Pneumocystis* would have made the death seem even stranger.

Any unusual outbreak of a disease is, in medical jargon, an epidemic. With five cases of *Pneumocystis* diagnosed in five gay men over the past few months in just one city, the phenomenon Gottlieb and Shandera were studying fit the necessary criteria for an epidemic. One man was already dead. Gottlieb had the queasy feeling that there was something bigger, something catastrophic lurking behind this. Five cases of an uncommon illness in just a few months meant that the disease was no longer uncommon among gay men, Gottlieb thought, and chances were that it was going to get a lot more common in the months to come.

He also knew it would be good to get out a medical journal report on this before anybody else did. He called the nation's most prestigious journal, the *New England Journal of Medicine,* and talked to an associate editor.

"I've got something here that's bigger than Legionnaire's," he said. "What's the shortest time between submission and publication?"

The editor explained it would take three months to send the story around to a panel of expert reviewers who would make sure that it was scientifically sound. There would be another delay between the time the review was finished and the publication date, he said. He didn't need to tell Gottlieb about the ironclad rule that the journal, like virtually all major scientific publications, maintained about the secrecy of material about to be published. If there was any leak whatsoever to the popular press about the research, the journal would pull the story from its pages.

"We'd like to see it," the editor concluded. "Sounds interesting, but there's no way we can guarantee that it will be published."

But this is an emergency, Gottlieb thought as he hung up the phone in frustration. You don't just run business as usual in an emergency.

It was an observation Gottlieb would recite almost daily in the difficult years ahead. For this young doctor, about to be credited with the discovery of the public health threat of the century, the thought became a grim mantra for the AIDS epidemic.

April 14
Centers for Disease Control,
Atlanta

Sandy Ford wanted to scream at the stupid doctor. For the second time in ten days, the same Manhattan physician was ordering pentamidine for two men with unexplained *Pneumocystis.* Not only that, these were the same two men who already had been treated with the drug. Sandy filled eighty or ninety pentamidine orders a year, and she never had filled two orders for the same person. The drug works and the *Pneumocystis* goes away. She also knew that the Food and Drug Administration reviewed the records she collected on drug orders. The antibiotic was only available on an investigational new drug license. Its uses were strictly controlled, and too many unexplained diagnoses on her annual FDA report would raise questions. She was sending in too many incomplete forms, and she didn't know what to do about it.

April 17
Los Angeles

As the naked body stirred beside him, Cleve Jones reflected on his favorite aspect of gay life, that you could meet someone and in such a short time become so intimate. Cleve never viewed his sexual adventures as conquests, like many of his friends; instead, they were little romances, brief studies into another idea of what a human being could be. At twenty-six, Cleve still had never had what he could call a long-term relationship, but his life was filled with romances, like the affair with Frank, the handsome lawyer from Long Beach. They had met at the state Democratic Convention in Sacramento last year. Frank was a successful attorney involved in gay politics, very bright, and most importantly, very progressive. Cleve had gone to work for San Francisco Assemblyman Art Agnos and was trying to line up party regulars for a state gay civil rights bill that Agnos had introduced to every legislative session since 1977. Frank recognized Cleve from a CBS documentary on gay politics in San Francisco. Cleve loved the idea of another romance, and they were off. Of course, it couldn't go anywhere because Frank had his lover back in Long Beach, but they had stolen afternoons when Cleve was in L.A., like today, and possibly, some more weekends in San Francisco or at Democratic gatherings.

Cleve was fresh from an affair with a prominent Democratic legislator from a midwestern state, and, a week after Frank returned to Long Beach, Cleve fell for an independent filmmaker who lived in Marin County. That's the way romances passed for Cleve.

Frank wasn't feeling well that day, Cleve recalled later, which is why Cleve never forgot that warm afternoon in Los Angeles when they made love, after a leisurely lunch. It was April 17, 1981. Good Friday.

April 22
UNIVERSITY OF CALIFORNIA,
SAN FRANCISCO

The sunny morning turned warm and pleasant. From the crowded huddle of concrete and glass medical buildings, one could see the Golden Gate Bridge and the Marin headlands, which were turning deep green after heavy winter rains. Dr. Marcus Conant walked the half-block to the hulking gray UCSF Ambulatory Care building from the office where he had run his thriving dermatological practice for eleven years. He couldn't get last night's phone call from his old friend, Alvin Friedman-Kien, out of his head.

Alvin said he had discovered a new outbreak of Kaposi's sarcoma in New York. He had embarked on the research after he had seen two KS patients within a matter of days in his office at New York University. He started checking with other doctors and quickly learned that a number of Manhattan hospitals were treating men suffering from this cancer. The victims were all gay, he confided, and a lot of them were into pretty heavy stuff like fist-fucking.

Conant immediately thought back to 1969 when he was studying for his dermatology boards. He remembered repeatedly reviewing the pathology pictures of KS, worrying that the tumor was so rare that it would be just the slide he wouldn't recognize on the test. Since then, he'd seen KS maybe half a dozen times in his career, usually at symposia or presentations.

The cancer was particularly interesting to both Marcus Conant and Alvin Friedman-Kien because they were herpes experts and African KS had been linked to a herpes virus, CMV. This research was intriguing in that it might establish one of the first links between a virus and cancer, something scientists had sought for years. They talked about the Kaposi's sarcoma–cytomegalovirus connection, and Conant promised to ask about KS the next day, when he was the featured speaker at the monthly UCSF conference of dermatologists.

Jim Groundwater was stunned when Conant asked if anyone had seen any unusual cases of KS. Groundwater had struggled for months before finally getting a KS diagnosis on Ken Horne just two weeks ago, and now the same thing was turning up in New York.

"I've got a case of KS in a gay man over at St. Francis Hospital right now," he told Conant.

Oh God, Conant thought. This means trouble. At that moment, the realization was born that a new epidemic had arrived in San Francisco.

The next day, Groundwater called Friedman-Kien to tell him about Ken Horne. Groundwater was surprised at how similar Ken's life-style was to the stricken New Yorkers', right down to the habit of fisting. That afternoon, a letter arrived in the mail from the eminent New York dermopathologist with whom Groundwater previously had consulted.

"It is difficult to determine whether the infectious agents play any role in inducing this lesion," wrote Dr. A. Bernard Ackerman, who added with surprising prescience, "We have recently seen numerous cases of Kaposi's sarcoma in young homosexual men and, it is our opinion, that these lesions may well be induced by an infectious agent."

April 24

After talking to Jim Groundwater, Dr. John Gullett, an infectious disease expert who had been treating Ken Horne, decided to call Atlanta to report Ken's Kaposi's sarcoma and *Pneumocystis* pneumonia to the Centers for Disease Control. None of the CDC doctors he talked to, however, seemed particularly interested in his story. Gullet got the feeling he was being treated as a crank caller. At the CDC, nobody would later recall the day that Ken Horne became the first reported victim of a frightening new pestilence.

FIRE ISLAND, NEW YORK

A brisk breeze blew off the ocean and over the sand where Paul Popham and a small cluster of friends trudged, carrying a small box. Tourist season wouldn't open for another month, so they had the island to themselves, except for a few merchants and homeowners out to check the damage from the winter storms. Paul looked toward Bob, who was holding the ashes of Rick Wellikoff. He never knew what to say at times like this so he didn't say anything at all. The group had walked past a boarded-up disco and the tightly shuttered houses, out to where there is just sand and sky and sea. That's where the fifth-grade teacher from Brooklyn had wanted his remains to be spread, off the beach of the island he had loved so much. As the sun began its westward tumble toward twilight, Bob poured out the white gritty ashes, and Rick was gone into the cold gray Atlantic. Maybe now, Paul thought, he could put this behind him.

April 28
CENTERS FOR DISEASE CONTROL, ATLANTA

"What do you think about those five cases of bone sarcoma in homosexuals they're investigating at State University of New York?" the doctor asked Sandy Ford.

Ford said she had never heard of any such study. After she hung up, the conversation gnawed at her. They were investigating something about homosexuals in Queens at the same time she was getting all these strange pentamidine orders. There had been two more orders in the past two weeks for patients with unexplained immune suppression. One of them was from the Manhattan doctor who previously had seemed so inept to Ford. He alone had now made five orders for pentamidine in three weeks. Since February, she had filled nine orders that were all tinged with similar shades of mystery.

The unknowns went against the methodical streak in her attentive nature, so on that Tuesday afternoon, Sandy wrote a memo to her boss, the deputy director of parasitic diseases, and told him about the nine drug orders and the gossip about the bone sarcoma. That was how the thorough GS-7 drug technician in Room 161 of the Centers for Disease Control's Building 6 alerted the federal government to the new epidemic.

Sunday, May 17
WEST LOS ANGELES

Michael Gottlieb and Wayne Shandera sat at Shandera's dining room table surrounded by stacks of medical charts in neat manila folders. Gottlieb had heard that Alvin Friedman-Kien was working on a Kaposi's sarcoma study in New York, and he was eager to get his paper out before Friedman-Kien's. Shandera hit on the idea of publishing the PCP reports in the Centers for Disease Control's weekly newsletter, the *Morbidity and Mortality Weekly Report,* known to doctors just as the *MMWR.* The 6 × 8½-inch booklet was mailed every Friday to thousands of hospitals and health agencies internationally. Everybody who was anybody in public health or infectious diseases read its updates on every blip in the nation's physical well-being, along with the weekly state-by-state breakdowns on every new case of just about every infectious disease, from anthrax to rabies and typhoid. Although the publication did not carry the scientific prestige of, say, the *New England Journal of Medicine,* publication required virtually no lead time. In early May, Shandera had called Dr. Mary Guinan, an old friend at the CDC venereal disease division, and she said she'd get whatever report they wrote into the right channels.

The report required a case-by-case detailing of this new phenomenon. Gottlieb talked through the charts while Shandera put the information into the dry, turgid prose that the *MMWR* preferred. The report noted the links between PCP, CMV, and the oral candidiasis that commonly preceded the pneumonia, and stated: "The fact that these patients were all homosexuals suggests an association between some aspect of homosexual life-style or disease acquired through sexual contact and *Pneumocystis* pneumonia in this population."

The next day, Shandera phoned in the report, entitled simply *"Pneumocystis pneumonia in homosexual men—Los Angeles."*

CENTERS FOR DISEASE CONTROL, ATLANTA

Dr. Mary Guinan sent the paper to Dr. James Curran, her boss at the VD division. He sent the paper back to her with a four-word note: "Hot Stuff. Hot Stuff."

Word spread around the agency about the paper CDC was going to publish on PCP. Guinan got another call from a CDC staffer in parasitic diseases. "There are a lot of people dying of PCP in New York City, but nobody will tell us about it," he said. Apparently, the doctors had some paper that was in the review process for a scientific journal, and they couldn't breathe a word about the PCP outbreak for fear of losing their shot at the prestigious publication credit. Already, a Manhattan gay newspaper, the *New York Native,* had published a story about the rumors of a new killer pneumonia striking gay men, but the CDC liaison with the local public health department had pooh-poohed the gossip, telling the paper that the rumors were "unfounded."

This isn't right, Guinan thought. We'd better investigate.

May 30
SAN DIEGO

Congratulations were in order, thought Dr. David Ostrow as he prepared his speech for the CDC's annual sexually transmitted disease conference. The gay community had played a key role in the development of a vaccine for hepatitis B, a major international health problem, and it was time the medical world took notice. For the past three years, thousands of gay men had cooperated with the CDC research that gave the world both the first definitive hepatitis B epidemiology and, finally, a vaccine against the disease, a major killer of children in Africa and Southeast Asia. Tens of thousands of blood samples from these gay men remained frozen in the refrigerators of the CDC for use in future studies. The new vaccine could save millions of lives worldwide, and it was coming into production courtesy of the gay community. Moreover, Ostrow thought, CDC plans for widespread vaccination of gay men would start the long process of eliminating the disease from the gay population.

Things were looking up, Ostrow told the conference in his presentation on gay sexually transmitted diseases. This story had a happy ending. Personally, Ostrow hoped that he'd be able to get out of the STD business altogether, now that the biggest of gay venereal diseases had been effectively beaten.

That was when Dr. Jim Curran stood up. Ostrow recognized Curran from years of work on both the hepatitis study and gay VD issues. Curran start talking about the five cases of *Pneumocystis carinii* pneumonia in Los Angeles. The CDC would be publishing an *MMWR* on *Pneumocystis* next week, he said, and they'd soon be setting up a task force.

◯

Later that night, Ostrow, Curran, CDC veteran Harold Jaffe, and a few gay doctors caucused in Dave Ostrow's hotel room at the Harbor Holiday Inn. A light spring breeze blew over sailboats rocking gently in the marina outside the window. Ostrow mused on the years he had spent getting Curran and Dr. Jaffe acculturated to the gritty details of gay sexual habits, from rimming to fisting. Curran had seemed uptight at the start, Ostrow thought, but he buckled down to his work. Both Jaffe and Curran were unusual in that federal officials rarely had any kind of contact with gays, and the few who did rarely wanted to learn the detailed gymnastics of gay sex.

Maybe the pneumonia was the effect of some bad batch of drugs, Ostrow hoped aloud. Something easily taken care of. Curran agreed that there might be some environmental factor that could explain the outbreak. Maybe some bad nitrate inhalants. That was one of the two major hypotheses. There was another hypothesis, far more frightening: "It could be an infectious disease."

◯

On Friday, June 5, 1981, the Centers for Disease Control *Morbidity and Mortality Weekly Report* published what would be the first report on the epidemic, based on the Los Angeles cases of *Pneumocystis* that Drs. Michael Gottlieb and Joel Weisman had seen in the previous months. In the week before publication, skittish CDC staffers debated how to handle the gay aspect of the report. Some of the workers in the venereal disease division had long experience working with the gay community and worried about offending the sensitivities of a group with whom they would clearly be working closely in the coming months. Just as significantly, they also knew that gays were not the most beloved minority in or out of the medical world, and they feared that tagging the outbreak too prominently as a gay epidemic might fuel prejudice. As it was, the fact that the hepatitis vaccine project had been largely a homosexual effort was downplayed for both Congress and the administration for fear that it would squash the program.

The report, therefore, appeared not on page one of the *MMWR* but in a more inconspicuous slot on page two. Any reference to homosexuality was dropped from the title, and the headline simply read: *Pneumocystis* pneumonia—Los Angeles.

Don't offend the gays and don't inflame the homophobes. These were the twin horns on which the handling of this epidemic would be torn from the first day of the epidemic. Inspired by the best intentions, such arguments paved the road toward the destination good intentions inevitably lead.

8 THE PRETTIEST ONE

June 9, 1981
MEMORIAL SLOAN-KETTERING CANCER CENTER,
NEW YORK CITY

"What's going to happen to me?"

Dr. Jim Curran stared at the patient who was such a reflection of himself. Like Curran, the man was thirty-six years old and the product of an Ivy League education. He was even raised near Detroit, Curran's hometown. And he was a successful professional, having carved out a career in New York as an entertainer. The man wasn't like Curran at all in that he was homosexual and had lived in Greenwich Village for the past fifteen years.

Married and the father of two, Curran's decade in the Centers for Disease Control had forced him to shift from city to city before landing in Atlanta, where he headed up the CDC's venereal disease prevention services. That was why it was only yesterday he had attended the first meeting of an ad hoc task force hurriedly put together to investigate the outbreaks of *Pneumocystis* and Kaposi's sarcoma. He'd taken a morning flight to New York City to talk to Alvin Friedman-Kien and see some of these patients for himself. The performer was the first victim of this unlikely new battery of diseases Curran had ever met.

Though he knew he was supposed to act like the big expert doctor from the CDC, Curran didn't know what to say when the man asked him what would happen. Like most doctors, he was loathe to admit he didn't have all the answers. Today, however, he didn't have much choice. This epidemic was only three days old.

"I have no idea what will happen," said Curran.

He felt embarrassed to be examining the man, stripped down to his underwear, as if he were a lab animal. The lesions, however, got him back to business. Whatever this was, Curran thought, it wasn't the benign African KS in all the textbooks. This disease was far more aggressive.

Curran was also struck by how identifiably gay all the patients seemed to be. After years of working with the gay community, he knew that you couldn't tell homosexuals by looking at them. These clearly must be patients who put a high personal stake in their identification as gay people, living in the thick of the urban gay subculture. They hadn't just peeked out of the closet yesterday.

It was strange because diseases tended not to strike people on the basis of social groups. Epidemics could be restricted geographically, like the Legionnaire's epidemic of 1976, hitting a group of conventioneers at a particular hotel in Philadelphia. Diseases might appear in a group bound together by physiological similarities, such as women who had physical reactions to Rely tampons and suffered from Toxic Shock Syndrome. To Curran's recollection, however, no epidemic had chosen victims on the basis of how they identified themselves in social terms, much less on the basis of sexual life-style. Yet, this identification and a propensity for venereal diseases were the only things the patients from three cities—New York, Los Angeles, and San Francisco—appeared to share. There had to be something within this milieu that was hazardous to these people's health.

Curran returned to Atlanta, where the Kaposi's Sarcoma and Opportunistic Infections (KSOI) Task Force was chasing down leads with a vigor that had earned the CDC its reputation as the world's foremost medical detective agency. With all the overlapping infections, the mysterious immune defects, and the unprecedented sociological issues, nothing about this epidemic fit into any neat category. About a dozen staffers from all the disciplines potentially involved with the diseases volunteered for the working group. They included specialists in immunology, venereology, virology, cancer epidemiology, toxicology, and sociology. Because the outbreak might be linked to the Gay Bowel Syndrome, parasitologists were called in. With Curran, Harold Jaffe, and Mary Guinan, the task force was weighted with people from venereal disease studies. Curran was designated the KSOI Task Force chair, in large part, he figured, because he was the only member important enough to have his own secretary, who could type minutes.

As the task force met daily to share notes, the two potential causes of the epidemic emerged with greater clarity. First, there could be some substance common to the environment of these patients causing their immune problems. The leading candidate was poppers, or nitrate inhalants, though almost any bad batch of drugs might be to blame. The second explanation, of course, was that this was the effect of some infectious agent, either one new virus or some combination of old microbes working together in a new way. Though the two hypotheses gave latitude for a nearly infinite range of answers, most of the CDC staffers had no doubt that a smoking gun would emerge. They had tackled epidemics before, and they would again. It would take old-fashioned, shoe-leather epidemiology, and the symbol of the CDC was an old shoe with a hole worn through the sole.

When they weren't fielding the onslaught of phone calls coming in from around the country in response to the *MMWR* report, the CDC doctors were calling contacts. Since the first *MMWR* article only discussed pneumonia, the most common comment was, "I'm seeing the *Pneumocystis,* but I'm also seeing Kaposi's sarcoma in gay men too." Whatever was happening to the PCP cases in Los Angeles was somehow related to these KS patients in New York.

Mary Guinan went down the street to the medical library at Emory University and checked out an immunology text so she could get a handle on Michael Gottlieb's finding that the pneumonia victims were strangely deficient in T-helper lymphocytes. The book didn't have anything about any kind of T-cells; their discovery was too recent. Guinan called her friend Donna Mildvan at Beth Israel Medical Center in New York. Mildvan told her about the immune problems in gay men she'd been seeing since last July. These people get horrible infections, Mildvan said, and then they wither up and die.

On a hunch, Guinan called a drug company that manufactured medicine for severe herpes infections. They told her about a New York City doctor who had been seeing still more dreadful herpes infections in gay men. This doctor told Guinan that he thought the ravaging infections were related to PCP. He hadn't told anybody about the cases, however, because he had written a paper that was under submission at a medical journal.

Guinan was shaken by her investigation. She was accustomed to dealing with venereal diseases, ailments for which you receive an injection and are cured. This was different. She couldn't get the idea out of her head: There's something out there that's killing people. That was when Mary Guinan hoped against hope that they would find something environmental to link these cases together. God help us, she thought, if there's a new contagion spreading such death.

$\bigcirc$

After the publication of the *MMWR* report on *Pneumocystis,* the news services carried a dozen or so paragraphs on the pneumonia outbreak. Most gay papers across the country carried the item well off the front pages since it seemed, at best, to be some medical oddity that was probably blown out of proportion by homophobes in both the scientific establishment and the media. It was in the gay press, however, that the complicated phraseology of *Pneumocystis carinii* pneumonia was first simplified to a term that fit better into headlines. Gay pneumonia, it was called.

June 12
CLAUDE-BERNARD HOSPITAL,
PARIS

The gay man arrived at Dr. Willy Rozenbaum's examining room, complaining of a severe weight loss and a shortness of breath. Again, Rozenbaum made the diagnosis of *Pneumocystis,* as baffled about the cause as he had been for the Portuguese cab driver, the Zairian airline employee, and the French woman who had spent time in Central Africa. That afternoon's mail brought from the United States the *MMWR* describing the pneumonia outbreak in Los Angeles. This was related to the man he had seen this morning, Rozenbaum knew, and there was only one explanation. It couldn't be anything in the environment; Los Angeles was virtually on the other side of the world. It had to be a new infectious agent.

June 16
CENTERS FOR DISEASE CONTROL
HEPATITIS LABORATORIES, PHOENIX

Although he was only thirty-eight, Dr. Don Francis was one of the most eminent experts on epidemics at the CDC, having been among the handful of epidemiologists who literally wiped smallpox off the face of the earth in the 1970s. In recent years he had worked with the gay community on the hepatitis vaccine project, which he was now wrapping up.

Don called his old Harvard mentor, Myron Essex, as soon as he heard about how PCP and Kaposi's sarcoma victims suffered from a strange depletion in T-lymphocytes. It was with Essex that Francis had studied the mechanisms of feline leukemia virus for his virology doctorate.

"This is feline leukemia in people," Francis began.

Essex knew Francis had a penchant for quick conclusions stated in the most dramatic terms; he also knew that his former student had gained an international reputation for singular brilliance. After spending eight years studying feline leukemia, the major cause of cat deaths, Essex was more than casually interested in links between this disease and human disease. He and Francis were among the small minority of scientists who believed that viruses would one day be linked to cancer and other serious human ailments. Together, they had published eight articles on feline leukemia as well as a controversial piece suggesting that some human lymphomas, leukemias, and cancers of the immune system might be linked to viral infections. Essex settled back to listen to Francis's logic.

Cancer and immune suppression, Francis said. Both feline leukemia and this new gay disease were marked by a trail of opportunistic infections that seemed to take advantage of an immune system weakened by a primary infection. In cats, the infection was a leukemia virus that knocked out the cats' immune systems and left them open to a number of cancers. Clearly, some similar virus was doing the same thing to these homosexual men, and they were getting cancer too. Secondly, feline leukemia has a long incubation period; this new disease must have long latency too, which is the only way it was killing people in three cities on both coasts before anybody even knew it existed.

His years of battling epidemics in Africa, Asia, and America had imbued Francis with the idea that viruses were crafty little creatures constantly trying to outsmart humans in their bid for survival. Long latency periods were one of the most clever ways to thwart detection and extermination. Francis didn't think the gay health problems were being caused by cytomegalovirus or the other familiar viruses under discussion. They had been around for years and hadn't killed anybody. It was something new; it could even be a retrovirus, Francis said.

Essex was intrigued, although he knew most scientists would consider Francis's suggestion farfetched. As a small subgroup of viruses, retroviruses were, at best, an obscure microbe. Last year, a National Cancer Institute researcher, Dr. Robert Gallo, had shown that a retrovirus caused a leukemia common in Japan, the first time any virus had been linked to cancer. That was something of a backward scientific affair, however. Gallo had first discovered the virus and then searched worldwide for a disease that it might cause. By chance, Japanese researchers were studying the T-cell leukemia, assuming it was a contagious cancer, but they hadn't identified a viral culprit. Identifying Human T-cell Leukemia virus, or HTLV, as the cause, had forged a major scientific breakthrough in virology; it also had frightened scientists because of its long incubation period. Such a virus could be spread all over before it caused disease and anybody would even know it existed.

Many scientists remained dubious about the future of retroviral research, however, and many still believed retroviruses to be animal bugs because virtually all of them were linked to diseases in chickens, pigs, or cats. Essex figured that this was wishful thinking. Francis's idea, Essex thought, was a hypothesis that bore watching.

Francis was already convinced. He quickly became the leading CDC proponent of the notion that a new virus that could be spread sexually was causing immune deficiencies in gay men.

June 28
SAN FRANCISCO

Bill Kraus looked embarrassed by all the attention, but he obviously enjoyed the party Kico Govantes helped organize for his thirty-fourth birthday. Cleve Jones and Gwenn Craig and all his cronies from the Harvey Milk Club were there. Everybody toasted Bill with champagne before going downtown to march in the 1981 Gay Freedom Day Parade.

The mood was more somber than in years past, veteran parade observers noted; there were no amusement park rides at Civic Center this year. The theme was "Front Line of Freedom," a reference to the popular local idea that San Francisco was the front line of the nation's gay movement and battle lines were shaping up between them and the new religious conservatism in the Reagan administration. The parade drew a throng of 250,000, a typical turnout for the annual foray; in New York City that afternoon, 50,000 marched in the gay parade, making the march one of the largest gay demonstrations ever held in Manhattan.

A special issue of the San Francisco gay paper, *The Sentinel*, carried five paragraphs on gay pneumonia that day. More prominently featured was an editorial raising questions for a San Francisco gay community awash with its own gaudy mixture of insecurity and self-confidence. "What are the goals of the gay movement?" the editorial asked. "Where are we going?"

July 1
SAN FRANCISCO GENERAL HOSPITAL

Struggling to stay awake through lonely nights as a postdoctoral intern at the University of Utah Hospital in Salt Lake City, Paul Volberding had sometimes watched the taillights of cars heading west on the freeway toward San Francisco. He had never been there, but he knew that's where he would go once he finished his internship. He knew that as certainly as he had known for years that he was going to be a retrovirologist. Growing up near the Mayo Clinic, on a dairy farm in rural Minnesota, had long ago enchanted him with medicine. By high school, he found a refuge in lab work, experimenting with plant viruses. In college, the stability of the laboratory gave him a respite from the revolution happening on the radical University of Minnesota campus; he spent his hours away from the noise, intrigued by unseen bits of genetic information that could have such a devastating impact on a human being. It was in college that he heard about retroviruses, and he knew he would devote his life to trying to understand them.

Paul Volberding would have been in bench research today if he hadn't started meeting cancer patients in his residency. He fell in love with cancer patients. He loved the honesty that cut through all the superficial crap. In other parts of life, there was so much miscommunication. People said things they didn't mean and heard things they really didn't understand. That didn't happen with cancer patients; there was nothing trivial in the talk. Paul noticed that the viruses that bring disease also seemed to bring out the best in people.

After three years at the retrovirus lab at UCSF, Volberding was starting his dream job as chief of oncology at San Francisco General Hospital. He was young for such a position—thirty-one years old. He was nervous and excited and not sure what to think when the veteran cancer specialist slapped him on the back on his first day at work, July 1, and pointed toward an examining room.

"There's the next great disease waiting for you," he said. "A patient with KS."

Volberding had never heard the term "KS" before. He didn't know what the old-timer was talking about. Volberding walked into the room and, for the first time, saw one of the people who would merge his interests in retroviruses and the terminally ill into a career that would consume much of his life.

A friendly down-home accent identified the twenty-two-year-old patient as from the South. He was an attendant in a San Francisco bathhouse and had been admitted to the hospital a few days ago with diarrhea and weight loss; the Kaposi's sarcoma diagnosis had been confirmed just the day before. Volberding had never seen anything like this in such a young patient. Emaciated and covered by lesions, the young man looked like a patient who was, perhaps, in the advanced stages of a stomach cancer. It was hard to look more advanced than this fellow, Volberding thought; he looked like someone who was going to die.

The youth didn't have many friends in San Francisco and lived in a lonely apartment in the seedy Tenderloin neighborhood. He was estranged from his family, and he didn't understand why he had lost so much weight or where the purple spots had come from. He was frightened and isolated, dependent and needy. The sight of him left a memory with Volberding that stuck with him for years.

Hearing that other cases of this strange cancer were appearing in New York,

Volberding called Michael Lange at St. Luke's-Roosevelt Hospital, and the pair compared notes about treatments. Volberding read all the papers in the medical libraries on Kaposi's sarcoma and started the patient on the recommended chemotherapies. None worked. Volberding didn't know what to do; none of the KS experts in the country knew what to do. In the months that followed, Volberding simply became a helpless witness to the young man's excruciating and lonely death, the first of the hundreds to follow at San Francisco General Hospital. It truly was to be "the next great disease."

July 2
UNIVERSITY OF CALIFORNIA,
SAN FRANCISCO

In his office above the UCSF Medical Center, Marcus Conant jotted a memo to the handful of other local specialists who had expressed an interest in the outbreak of Kaposi's sarcoma. He now knew of six KS cases in San Francisco; because it was a gay mecca, he figured the city would have more as the months developed.

"If Alvin Friedman-Kien is correct, we should see 40–50 cases of Kaposi's sarcoma in males here in the next 12–18 months," Conant wrote. "Half of these patients will have fulminant disease and may die. While planning is contrary to our national genius, I feel that it may be wise to put together a multidisciplinary task force to decide how we will investigate this disease as cases are referred here to us."

At the Faculty Club a few days later, Conant proposed a KS clinic. The doctors agreed it was a rational way to proceed. The centralization of local cases would both aid physicians who were trying to understand the baffling phenomenon and help patients secure the most expert care. Within weeks the clinic was established, if for no other reason than that it seemed the most intelligent medical solution to a medical problem. Perhaps, Conant subsequently reflected, that's why it took four years before hardly any other medical institution in the United States began working in earnest on their own clinic. The new epidemic would rarely be dealt with as simply a medical problem.

$$\bigcirc$$

The first official report on the outbreak of Kaposi's sarcoma was released in the *MMWR* of July 4, 1981, five years to the day after the tall ships from fifty-five nations had amassed in New York Harbor for the Bicentennial celebration. The title of the report was "Kaposi's Sarcoma and *Pneumocystis* Pneumonia Among Homosexual Men—New York City and California." In the driest possible prose, the report outlined the common symptoms of the KS patients, twenty of whom lived in New York City and six in California. Four of the KS patients had suffered a bout with *Pneumocystis;* others had suffered from severe herpes, candidiasis, cryptococcal meningitis, and toxoplasmosis. The report also announced ten new cases of PCP among gay men, including six in the San Francisco Bay Area.

"The occurrence of this number of KS cases during a 30-month period among young, homosexual men is considered highly unusual," the report noted. "No previous association between KS and sexual preference has been reported. The fulminant clinical course reported in many of these patients also differs from that classically described for elderly persons. . . . That 10 new cases of *Pneumocystis* pneumonia have been identified in homosexual men suggests that the 5 previously reported cases were not an isolated phenomenon. In addition, CDC has a report of 4 homosexual men in NYC who developed severe, progressive, perianal herpes simplex infections and had evidence of cellular immunodeficiencies. Three died, 1 with systemic CMV infection. . . . It is not clear if or how the clustering of KS, pneumocystis, and other serious diseases in homosexual men is related."

Days before the publication, Dr. Paul Weisner, chief of the CDC's sexually transmitted disease section, collared CDC director Dr. William Foege for the first of many conversations about getting more money for the harried KSOI Task Force. "I think this is bigger than we think," he said.

The day the *MMWR* was released, Jack Nau was admitted to St. Vincent's Hospital in Greenwich Village with strange pains and a numbness in his legs. The doctors diagnosed Jack's disease as a rare kind of lymph cancer that usually strikes children.

The day after Jack's admission to the hospital, Paul Popham read about Kaposi's sarcoma in *The New York Times.* He had broken up with Jack a month ago, but he still cared for his former lover. He immediately sensed a connection between the rare cancer that had hit Jack and the skin cancer that had killed his best friend, Rick Wellikoff, six months ago. Including Rick and Nick, Jack was the third guy from the Fire Island house on Ocean Walk diagnosed with a bizarre disease.

July 5
1040 ASHBURY STREET, SAN FRANCISCO

Fuck the doctors, Ken Horne thought, I'm not going back.

Outside his window, the purple twilight sky faded to black, and headlights snaked their way across the Golden Gate Bridge. Ken's pet cockatiel was pacing nervously around its cage. Ken's stomach rose briefly, but he forced the foul taste back. Seven days before, he had been released from his third stay at St. Francis Hospital. They said he had some kind of pneumonia that was just as strange as his skin cancer, and now there was talk that this was going on in L.A. and New York too. He was weak, and he felt like he was going to throw up again. But he couldn't call Jim Groundwater because the doctor would want to put him back in the hospital, where they would poke, prod, and test him, and tell him again that he was very sick and not tell him why. The phone was ringing, long, blasting shrieks that split his head, and he stumbled as he started walking toward the sound.

It was nearly midnight when Ken's sister let herself into the apartment. She found Ken lying on the floor of his bedroom, his lip bloodied where he had hit it on the bedside table as he'd fallen to the floor. She touched his forehead; he felt hot.

In the emergency room, Ken refused to talk to the doctors, staring vacantly away while they took his pulse and blood pressure. Once in bed, he lapsed into a demented babbling confusion, occasionally screaming out. Nurses rushed busily in and out of his room. At times, he stirred and pleaded and then fell silent.

"Please," the nurses heard him cry from his darkened room. "Please. Please. Please."

The *MMWR* announcement about KS received a one-day infusion of press attention, garnering the obligatory stories in *The New York Times* and the *Los Angeles Times*. This ensured that all the wires would carry the story into most of the nation's major newspapers. The writing was crafted so as not to offend and not to panic. The notion that there might be a new infectious agent was downplayed in favor of hypotheses involving some environmental factor, mainly poppers, or some new strain of an old virus, particularly the cytomegalovirus that the *MMWR* discussed in detail. This day in the limelight, however, was the most attention the new epidemic would receive for the next year. After the first week of July, the outbreak faded from newsprint and became an item of interest largely to gay men.

In San Francisco, Bill Kraus attributed the reports of the new diseases to anti-gay bias in the press. Reporters never talked about the constructive things the gay community did, he thought, but let a few people get sick and they're all over it.

Cleve Jones clipped out the wire story that appeared in the morning *Chronicle* and pinned it to his office bulletin board under his handwritten headline: "Just when things were looking up."

TORONTO

If Gaetan Dugas had an obstacle, he decided on the quickest way to overcome it and confidently set about the task. When he resolved to get out of the hairdressing business and be an airline steward, he studied the requirements carefully and got to work. Air Canada required that flight attendants be bilingual, so Dugas, who had never lived outside the parochial confines of the French-speaking Quebeçois, moved to Vancouver without knowing a word of English. Immersed in the new language, he quickly acquired the skill necessary for the job.

When he saw the first story about Kaposi's sarcoma, he researched the best American centers for treatment and made a beeline for New York University, where Alvin Friedman-Kien and Linda Laubenstein were seeing the most KS patients. He was going to beat this, he told friends. His Canadian doctors hadn't done anything for him. Within days, he had lined up an appointment at NYU.

Paul Popham was leaving the Trilogy Restaurant in Greenwich Village when he thought he recognized Gaetan Dugas walking down Christopher Street. God, that guy is handsome, Paul thought. He couldn't blame Jack Nau for picking him up last Halloween. The pair had also spent a few weekends together after that, Paul knew.

"Jack's at St. Vincent's Hospital," Paul said. "I'm sure he'd like to see you."

Gaetan smiled and chatted but didn't mention why he was in town.

A few days later, Gaetan cajoled an airline steward friend to go with him to St. Vincent's to visit an old trick. The friend had come from Toronto to help Gaetan through his first week of chemotherapy. Gaetan, who had already checked into the apartments used for ambulatory NYU patients, was in good spirits on the trip over to St. Vincent's. Neither of the young men were prepared for how wasted the once-handsome patient would be.

"Maybe next week, I'll get up," Jack sighed.

It was obvious to both visitors that Jack wasn't going anywhere, not next week and probably not ever again.

Gaetan sat in stony silence during the cab ride back to NYU. For the first time, his friend thought, he's seeing how serious this really is.

Gaetan moved back to Montreal when he finished his chemotherapy. He had taken a leave from Air Canada and decided to adopt a more leisurely life, using airline passes he still held to do the coastal hopping he enjoyed so much. He returned to NYU once a month for more treatments. When his hair began falling out, he simply shaved his head so nobody would notice. His Yul Brynner look was quite attractive. As he traveled between San Francisco, Los Angeles, Vancouver, Toronto, and New York, he realized that if he kept to bathhouses where the lights were turned down low, nobody would ask him about those embarrassing purple spots. He was still the prettiest one.

9 AMBUSH POPPERS

July 1981
CENTERS FOR DISEASE CONTROL, ATLANTA

Jim Curran finally got the official word that he would be detailed to the KS and PCP outbreak for three months. The assignment meant he could work the epidemic full time in what he knew was a very bad environment for a new health problem. It wasn't that his bosses weren't interested. He met weekly with the director of Centers for Disease Control; even the nation's top health official, Dr. Edward Brandt, the Assistant Secretary for Health of the U.S. Department of Health and Human Services, called periodically for updates. But Brandt, like other top administration officials, supported the CDC budget cuts, believing that states could better handle their own health problems.

The cuts in funds meant a major reduction in force, Curran knew, and just about everybody working KS and PCP was sure of being fired any day. That included some key people. Harold Jaffe, for example, was an experienced veteran of work in gay sexually transmitted diseases and was rapidly emerging as the coordinator for the KS epidemiology. But he had lost seniority when he took a University of Chicago fellowship a year ago, and Curran had to pull every string he could to save Jaffe's job.

Against this backdrop, Curran realized he couldn't expect to hire any new people. He'd have to pillage other departments for his staff. Fortunately, a new mystery brought out the Sam Spade in the generally young and enthusiastic corps at CDC, and few problems the CDC had tackled were as mysterious as the emergence of these bizarre infections in such widely separated locales.

Countless leads needed to be tracked down. Hypotheses needed to be eliminated. Was the *Pneumocystis* outbreak really new or merely a phenomenon that had been unreported? Early investigations of the Legionnaire's outbreak in 1976, for example, revealed that the pneumonia had been around for years; it just had never been detected until it so dramatically invaded the American Legion convention in Philadelphia and seized twenty-nine lives.

Drug technician Sandra Ford, with her methodical speed, went back through all her old pentamidine files to see whether there were previous PCP cases that might fit the disease's new pattern. Sure enough, she found drug orders for nine patients who fit the new PCP victims' profile perfectly—all cases reported during the last six months of 1980. Her search failed to turn up any gay pneumonia patients from much before 1979, strong support that this was something new.

Researchers also sought to determine whether the disease was indeed geographically isolated in the three gay urban centers. Did the detection of cases in the three centers make the patients appear to be only fast-lane gays because gay life tended toward the fast track in those cities? Was the disease all over gay America but in such low numbers that it had not been detected? The task force decided to check cities with high, middle, and low ranges of gay venereal disease as points of comparison. Los Angeles and New York ranked at the high end of the spectrum, Atlanta and Rochester, N.Y., were picked for the middle, and Oklahoma City and Albany, N.Y., for the low end of the scale. Officers from the CDC's Epidemiological Intelligence Service, or EIS, interviewed dermatologists, oncologists, infectious disease experts, and internists, and scoured hospital records in those cities for possible unreported cases. They returned with the expected findings. Dozens of new cases were found in Los Angeles and, particularly, New York City, but few appeared in the middle- and low-range cities.

The CDC also needed a standard definition of what they were studying. After much arguing among members of the task force, a case definition of the still-unnamed syndrome would include people with Kaposi's sarcoma, or *Pneumocystis* pneumonia among patients not undergoing chemical immune suppression. They had to be older than fifteen, to make sure no congenital immune cases were mistakenly included, and younger than sixty, so that none of the classic KS cases among elderly men were erroneously mixed in.

Like most of the task force, Curran hoped passionately that the diseases could be traced to poppers. After all, one bad batch of the inhalants could have triggered the immune problems. This would explain why the diseases appeared limited to just three cities; the contaminated vials could easily make the LA-SF-NY circuit given the bicoastal life-styles some affluent gays led. Everybody who got these diseases seemed to snort poppers. If it did turn out to be the drug, the CDC could simply turn into antipopper zealots. They would get the stuff banned, break all the bottles, and end the epidemic. That would be that.

The less hopeful side of Curran was dubious that this would be the answer. After all, some five million doses of nitrate inhalants were sold in America in 1980 alone; everybody in the gay community was using them, so it wasn't surprising that these first cases should be doing it too. And, Curran sensed, the popper theory was too easy. This did not look like it was going to be an easy epidemic.

What they needed, the members of the task force agreed in July, was a case-control study. They would match up the KS and PCP cases with controls who did not have the disease. The differences between the cases and controls would point the way toward what was causing the epidemic. Harold Jaffe called the expert epidemiologists at the National Cancer Institute to get advice on getting the case-control study in gear. It was simple, they explained: Spend a year developing the interview document and deciding whom to use as controls.

Conduct the interviews in the second year and spend the third year analyzing data and putting it together for a splendid article in a medical journal.

"In three years, we could do a good study on this," the National Cancer Institute experts told him.

Jaffe wondered whether the experts had heard that, away from the comfortable laboratories of the NCI, people were actually dying of this thing. Such a process might be all right for delving into the problems of breast cancer or melanoma, but Jaffe was worried about the possibility that this disease was infectious. The CDC was not accustomed to the luxurious pace that characterized research at all the National Institutes of Health.

"We want that study in three months, not three years," he said.

It was clear, however, that it would take weeks to get the questionnaire and protocol worked out for a case-control study. With eight of the forty-one first reported cases already dead—and many more obviously nearing death—the task force didn't feel it had that amount of time. Curran and the task force made their decision in the second week of July: Get investigators into the field and talk to every single patient in the United States they could collar. Harold Jaffe, a California native, packed his bags for San Francisco; Brooklyn-born Mary Guinan flew to New York.

July 17
NEW YORK CITY

It had been another typical day of gay cancer studies for Mary Guinan. She had awakened at 6 A.M. to breakfast with gay doctors and community leaders and asked, again and again, "What's *new* in the community?" What new element might have sparked this catastrophe?

She visited hospital rooms and sick beds throughout Manhattan for the rest of the morning and afternoon before returning to her hotel room at 7:30 P.M. Usually, she'd make phone calls that would last another four hours, but tonight she had promised to go out for an anniversary dinner with her husband, who had flown to New York for the occasion.

Over champagne, Guinan confided to her husband that this was the most emotionally draining assignment she had ever tackled in her public health career. With her leggy good looks and long blond hair, Mary Guinan looked considerably younger than forty-two. Her harsh Brooklyn accent and straightforward demeanor belied a maternal sensitivity that flavored her concern about the epidemic. Maybe that's why she was such a good field investigator, colleagues thought. She came across as both strong enough to hear the blunt truth and empathetic enough to let you know she really cared. As the summer turned Manhattan hot and sticky, Guinan could feel her heart break a little more with each interview.

It was horrible, she said. The guys were young, bright, talented people, and incredibly cooperative. They struggled to resurrect every detail that might be helpful. At the end, they'd ask, "What's the prognosis?"

Guinan would have to say she didn't know. Like many cancer patients, a lot of the men were convinced that there was some cure out there; they just hadn't been linked up with it. When they were, they'd beat this bug and it would just be some ugly nightmare that would fade slowly from their memory. Two weeks later she'd get a call telling her the patient was dead.

Guinan felt helpless and frightened. This was the meanest disease she had ever encountered. She strained to consider every possible nuance of these peoples' lives. The CDC, she knew, needed to work every hypothesis imaginable into the case-control study. Had they been to Vietnam? Maybe this was a delayed effect of Agent Orange. Did their grandmother ever have cancer? Maybe this was some genetic fluke only appearing now. Or perhaps it was some health food fad gone awry.

Several of the cases, it turned out, weren't gay men at all, but drug addicts. At the CDC, there was a reluctance to believe that intravenous drug users might be wrapped into this epidemic, and the New York physicians also seemed obsessed with the gay angle, Guinan thought. "He says he's not homosexual, but he must be," doctors would confide to her.

The problem was that the drug addicts didn't seem to get Kaposi's sarcoma; they got the far more virulent *Pneumocystis*. Most of them were dead before they even got reported to the CDC. Guinan carefully interviewed surviving addicts about their sexual habits. It was the most significant lead she developed in her weeks in New York City. Her drug addicts were not taken very seriously back in Atlanta, but years of syphilis interviews had given Guinan a sixth sense about when people were lying and when they were telling the truth. She didn't feel that these people, so close to death, were lying about their sex lives. Hepatitis B struck both gays and intravenous drug users, she knew; as she had believed for several weeks, it was reasonable to assume a new disease might do the same.

The analysis had the ring of biological plausibility. A virus like hepatitis B could spread sexually among gay men and be transmitted through blood contact among intravenous drug users. Guinan had already made a mental note to watch for cases among hemophiliacs and blood transfusion recipients. As other prime victims of hepatitis B, they could be expected to pick up this bug too through blood products.

There was another point, or perhaps just an odd coincidence, Guinan had noted. She had walked in on one of her interview subjects as he was stepping out of the shower in his room in the ambulatory care apartments at New York University. Guinan was a bit embarrassed at first, but he was so charming with his soft French accent that she got on with her questions.

He had been quite sexually active, he confided rather proudly. The patient, a French-Canadian airline steward, had a sex life much like that of the other gay men Guinan had interviewed. Including his nights at the baths, he figured he had 250 sexual contacts a year. He'd been involved in gay life for about ten years and easily had had 2,500 sexual partners. In fact, one of his old tricks was in a New York hospital with something strange now, Gaetan Dugas said.

Guinan later mentioned the conversation to the task force, but nobody made too much out of it, even though Gaetan's comment about sleeping with Jack

Nau was the first time that two victims of the new epidemic were ever linked sexually. Because Gaetan was Canadian, the first person in his country to be diagnosed with AIDS, he was lost to immediate follow-up by the CDC. The case-control study included only those in the United States.

July 29
New York University Medical Center, New York City

Larry Kramer was startled to see David Jackson in Dr. Alvin Friedman-Kien's waiting room. An antique dealer, David was a friendly, nondescript man in his late thirties who sold odds and ends from a shop on Bleecker Street. Larry had come to talk to Friedman-Kien because he was frantic about the new cancer he had read of in *The New York Times.* Friedman-Kien was the doctor who had put together the early KS epidemiology for the CDC. None of his friends seemed that concerned, but Larry had more than a philosophical interest in the subject. He had a history of sexually transmitted diseases not unlike the KS victims he had read about in the paper. So did almost everyone he knew, leading Larry to think this could be something major. Still, the author wasn't prepared to actually run into somebody he knew the moment he arrived at the office of the big expert. David started talking, almost to himself, as if he were trying to straighten everything out in his own mind.

"I was walking the beach at Fire Island and decided to turn over a new leaf," David said. "I was going to eat right and watch my nutrition."

His voice trailed off, and he looked pleadingly toward Larry and told him about seeing these funny purple spots.

"I don't have any friends," David said. "I'm ashamed to tell anybody about this. Will you come and visit me?"

⊂⊃

This was only the tip of the iceberg, Friedman-Kien told Larry Kramer. It was going to get bigger, and studies had to get started right away.

"I don't think anybody's going to do anything about it," the doctor said. "You've got to help. I need money for research. It takes two years to get grants."

Larry had heard of some other guys who had come down with the disease, friends from Fire Island. He promised Friedman-Kien he would get them together in his apartment to try to raise some money.

"What can I do to not get this?" Larry asked, trying to keep the lingering hypochondria out of his voice.

"I know what I'd do if I were a gay man," said Friedman-Kien.

Larry thought it was an odd thing for the doctor to say, but he listened intently for a prescription anyway.

"I'd stop having sex."

On the way out of Friedman-Kien's office, Larry was jolted to see Donald Krintzman, a fund-raiser for the Joffrey Ballet and the on-again, off-again lover of one of Larry's good friends. He was Friedman-Kien's next appointment.

"Don't tell me you've got it too?" Donald asked.

"No," answered Larry, not sure what to say.

"I've got it," Donald said comfortably. He was just in for blood tests.

Over the next few days, Larry called Donald Krintzman and Larry Mass, a doctor who wrote medical news for the *New York Native*—the city's most important gay publication—as well as Paul Popham, whose best friend, Larry had heard, died of KS last year, to discuss plans for a small fund-raiser at Larry's apartment.

NATIONAL CANCER INSTITUTE, BETHESDA, MARYLAND

When it was introduced a year earlier, most immunologists considered the new Fluorescent Activated Cell Sorter, or FACS, to be one of the most expensive scientific toys ever created. The sorter did by computer what people once did by hand, separating the T-helper lymphocytes from the T-suppressors and then counting them to see if they were in a proper ratio. In a normal person, there were, say, two helper cells for each suppressor, making a normal helper-suppressor ratio of 2:1. This quick counting didn't make the FACS that handy a tool. After all, the subsets of T-lymphocytes themselves had only been recently discovered, and scientists weren't that sure what the lymphocytes did or how significant the ratios were. According to lab chatter, it would be another five to ten years before those mysteries were fathomed. Only then would the expensive white elephant of a cell sorter have any practical value.

Still, Dr. James Goedert was glad the National Cancer Institute had invested the half-million to buy one of the first FACS machines available, because he had a new patient with the same kind of rare skin cancer he had first seen last December. The institute's FACS was so new it hadn't even been used until Goedert ran blood from the two KS patients he was treating. The helper-suppressor ratios were so far off that the lab technicians were suspicious of their results.

On a hunch, Goedert drew blood on fifteen apparently healthy gay men from the Washington area. Half of them, he found, had similar abnormalities in their immune system. The results gave him the kind of sinking feeling one gets watching television footage of an airplane making that gentle arc in the first moments of a crash landing. Whatever was causing these immune problems, Goedert knew, was very widespread. Jim was leaning toward a toxic agent and suspected poppers. He began outlining a study of gay men to test the idea.

Dr. Harold Jaffe looked nervously toward the barroom door. Even with a stiff summer breeze, the air was redolent with something thickly acrid, like a strange mixture of battery acid and vegetable shortening. The Ambush looked as seedy as Jaffe had heard, the kind of place where your feet stick to the floor. It was also the source of the poppers about which the gay men in San Francisco couldn't rave enough. The Ambush's own brand of poppers, sold discreetly in an upstairs leather shop, didn't give you headaches, patients told Jaffe. In fact, virtually all the city's AIDS cases reported using Ambush poppers, leading Jaffe and Carlos Rendon, a city disease-control investigator, to the seedy leather bar on Harrison Street.

"I'm not sure I want to go in that place," said Jaffe.

"I'll go in," offered Rendon matter-of-factly. "What should I ask for?"

"They call it the real thing," Jaffe said. "Ask for the real thing."

Rendon returned with an unlabeled amber bottle that Jaffe tucked away for chemical analysis back in Atlanta. Like Mary Guinan, Jaffe was out to explore every possible explanation with a focus on the two leading hypotheses: Either the syndrome came from exposure to some toxic substance, like Ambush poppers, or it was part of the spread of a new infectious agent.

Jaffe didn't believe he would find the solution in poppers. If the puzzle was that simple, somebody would have solved it by now, he thought. Instead, one of Jaffe's basic motives was to try to grasp what these new diseases were. Like the growing numbers of doctors involved in the outbreak, he was struck by how sick the sufferers were. They were so emaciated that they looked as though they had been dragged out of some sadistic concentration camp; many were so weak they needed to rest between questions. The thirty-five-year-old CDC epidemiologist had seen people with advanced cancer before, but they were never so young as these.

The severity of the illness as well as the number of cases also convinced Jaffe that this was not some discrete outbreak, like Legionnaire's, that would strike and then fall quietly back into the woodwork. This epidemic was something novel, something that was only beginning to define itself and take shape. All his interviews gave Jaffe only two substantive leads: Ambush poppers and, of course, numbers of sexual partners. The typical KS or PCP patients had had hundreds of partners, most drawing their contacts from gay bathhouses and sex clubs, the businesses whose profits depended on providing unlimited sexual opportunity. The vials of Ambush poppers might offer an environmental clue to the outbreak, but the highly sexual life-style of the early victims was beginning to persuade Jaffe, as it had Jim Curran and Don Francis, that a sexually transmitted bug might be behind the unexplained cancers and pneumonia.

◯

Mary Guinan had a terrible headache on the flight back to Atlanta. Something stank terribly on the plane and it was splitting her temples wide open. On her arrival, she pulled her purse from under her seat, heard the clatter of small glass bottles, and noticed that the stench followed her through the Eastern Airline terminal. It was those poppers, she realized. She had gone to every porno bookstore she could find to buy every conceivable brand of nitrate inhalants, picking them up herself because none of the men who worked for the New York City Health Department would walk into the places.

When one of Mary Guinan's gay contacts suggested that the disease might be caused by a mixture of poppers and Crisco, a popular lubricant among the fist-fucking aficionados, Guinan dispatched a gay friend to collect popper-tainted globs of Crisco from various bedrooms throughout Greenwich Village for chemical analysis back at the CDC. Nothing was too farfetched to check out.

Both Jaffe and Guinan returned to the CDC in time to hear the unsettling news of the proliferation of Kaposi's sarcoma and *Pneumocystis carinii* pneumonia. In the four weeks after the *Morbidity and Mortality Weekly Report* on KS, 67 more cases of either the cancer or pneumonia were reported to the CDC. Now there were 108 cases nationwide. Of these 43 were dead.

Of the 82 cases for which a date of diagnosis was known, 20 became sick in 1980, while 55 were stricken just in the first seven months of 1981. Curran was preparing a new *MMWR* update on the diseases, the last that would appear for the next nine months.

The task force pored over Jaffe and Guinan's studies. Guinan was convinced it was a new infectious disease. Some of the guys she interviewed didn't use poppers. Certainly, somebody who gets a rush from heroin isn't going to toy around with something as lightweight as disco inhalants. Jaffe ran the lab work on Ambush poppers and discovered that their popularity rested on the fact that they were not the isobutyl nitrites usually packaged for gays, but genuine amyl nitrate, the kind you can only get with a prescription, unless, of course, you know the right leather bars in San Francisco. This prescription amyl had been around for a century without killing anybody, Jaffe knew.

Bill Darrow was alarmed by the preliminary data Jaffe and Guinan had collected. A twenty-year veteran of VD work, Darrow was generally deferred to as both the most eminent sociologist at the CDC and an expert in the gay community. At forty-two, he was pretty much the old man among the CDC staffers, who tended to be in their early thirties, and he had a calm, professorial way of analyzing a crisis. That was why people were shaken with his analysis of the thirty-one patients interviewed in New York and California.

"It looks more like a sexually transmitted disease than syphilis," he concluded bluntly.

Hepatitis and amebiasis could be contracted in other ways than by sexual contact, like infection through food, or, as with hepatitis, through shared needles or by blood transfusions. The epidemiology was much more cut and dried with the new victims, Darrow said. The only thing that seemed to matter in these cases was number of sexual partners, which, not coincidentally, was about the only thing that mattered in charting the risk of someone with any sexually transmitted disease in a low-prevalence situation.

In early August 1981, Bill Darrow and perhaps six or seven people in Atlanta were worried; across the country, there were, maybe, a dozen or so other clinicians and gay physicians who also saw the implications of what was beginning to unfold. The trouble, Darrow thought, was trying to convince the other 240 million Americans that they had something to be concerned about too.

◯

The next weeks were spent acculturating the CDC field staff to the complicated gay sexual scene. Local epidemiologists like Selma Dritz of the San Francisco Department of Public Health were flown to Atlanta and given instruction on how to administer the twenty-two-page questionnaire for the case-control study. Invariably, as task force members explained that some victims would have as many as 2,000 lifetime sexual contacts, somebody's jaw would drop and he or she would ask, "How on earth do they manage that?"

August 1981
CASTRO STREET, SAN FRANCISCO

Gary Walsh ushered Joe Brewer, the gay psychologist with whom he shared an office, through the swinging doors of the Badlands saloon a few doors off Castro Street.

"I'm going to teach you to cruise," Gary explained with his characteristic decisiveness. "Anybody can do it."

Joe had spent the spring moping about the breakup of his seven-year relationship, and the ever-ebullient Gary had had enough of his friend's depression.

"See that gorgeous guy over there," Gary said, pointing toward a blond in jeans that fit so snugly one couldn't help but notice he was wearing no underwear. "First, somebody else will walk up to him and try to strike up a conversation. He won't talk much to him, though. Remember, never be the first guy to go up to someone."

Gary gave Joe a significant look to make sure he understood.

"People won't go home with the first person to talk to them—it makes them look too hard up," continued the thirty-six-year-old psychotherapist. "It's the second person who gets the shot."

Joe leaned back toward the wall as he watched Gary's prediction unfold perfectly. Gary pulled Joe away from the wall.

"No, no, no," Gary prodded, like a nun lecturing an errant altar boy. "Never stand by the wall. Always stand out a little, and keep yourself sort of turned, so people notice you."

Although he had been a psychotherapist in gay San Francisco for seven years, Joe was still amazed at the intricacies involved in gay cruising. Joe had always tended toward long relationships, while Gary was the horniest person Joe had ever met. Joe and Gary were so different in so many ways; that probably was why they had been best friends almost from the day they met in 1977.

Gary Walsh saw the Georgia-bred Joe Brewer as a southern gentleman who understood life's finer qualities; for his part, Joe liked Gary's straightforward midwestern informality, the legacy of a working-class Catholic childhood in

Iowa so vastly different from Joe's southern Methodist roots. Gary seemed to envy Joe's ability to maintain long, sizzling relationships; Joe couldn't fathom how Gary kept up his active sexual pursuits even after he was settled down with a wonderful boyfriend. Professionally, Joe and Gary made a good pair. They were among the pioneers of gay psychotherapy in San Francisco, and they had virtually invented gay couples' therapy.

Gary barely held back a wicked smile as he slipped into sample poses guaranteed to increase Joe's cruising yield. Brewer mused on the irony that he and Gary were guiding couples through the difficulties of maintaining relationships in the biggest sexual candy store God ever invented, even while they were having problems in their own love lives. Joe was single now, and he hated being single. Gary, meanwhile, was struggling with his lover Matt Krieger over all the typical issues of monogamy and individualization. Matt wanted to be married but Gary wanted to fuck around, so Matt would fuck around just to show Gary. To his psychologist's eye, Joe thought it was typical male competition. But then, so much of the gay community's sexuality, right down to the whole cruising ritual, seemed more defined by gender than sexual orientation, Joe noticed.

Joe Brewer's early memories of the Castro were of romantic bubble baths after lovemaking. He was not long from the closet when he came to the Bay Area in 1970, and not far from the times when he had pleaded with a psychiatrist to make him straight. Shedding his guilt in the frolicsome first days of the Castro boom was liberating, and the sex was so brotherly. Slowly, the relational aspects of the sexual interaction dropped away. Intimacy disappeared and, before long, people were wearing outward signs of sexual tasks, hankies and keys, to make their cruising more efficient, and the bathhouses became virtual convenience stores for quick cavorting, 7-Elevens for butt-fucking.

About 3,000 gay men a week streamed to the gargantuan bathhouse at Eighth and Howard streets, the Club Baths, which could serve up to 800 customers at any given time. Joe figured that the attraction to promiscuity and depersonalization of sex rested on issues surrounding a fear of intimacy. Joe knew these were not gay issues but male issues. The trouble was that, by definition, you had a gay male subculture in which there was nothing to moderate the utterly male values that were being adulated more religiously than any macho heterosexual could imagine, right down to the cold, hard stares of the bathhouse attendants. Promiscuity was rampant because in an all-male subculture there was nobody to say "no"—no moderating role like that a woman plays in the heterosexual milieu. Some heterosexual males privately confided that they were enthralled with the idea of the immediate, available, even anonymous, sex a bathhouse offered, if they could only find women who would agree. Gay men, of course, agreed, quite frequently.

Too frequently, Joe sometimes thought. Stripped of humanity, sex sought ever-rising levels of physical stimulation in increasingly esoteric practices. Joe preferred the bubble baths and wished he were in love again.

Gary Walsh had a far less complicated view of gay sexuality. A passionate devotee of sexual liberation, Gary believed that promiscuity was a means to exorcise the guilt and self-alienation ingrained in all gay men by a heterosexual society clinging to the obsolete values of monogamy. Privately, Gary thought people who didn't like a lot of sex were just plain boring. Life was for learning, he lectured Joe, and sex was as legitimate a learning tool as anything else.

Over lunch, the pair planned a weekend trip to the gay resort area on the Russian River, an hour's drive north of San Francisco. Joe wasn't surprised when Gary later canceled, complaining of a yeast infection in his mouth. Gary always seemed to be getting something.

August 7
SAN FRANCISCO

By early August, there were eighteen cases of gay men suffering from the baffling immune deficiency in the San Francisco Bay Area; two had died.

"No one yet knows the extent of this potential danger, but playing it on the safe side for a few weeks cannot hurt," *The Sentinel,* a local gay paper, editorialized. "Just a few short years ago, the government dropped millions of dollars into research to determine the cause of Legionnaire's disease, which affected relatively few people. No such outpouring of funds has yet been forthcoming to research the how's and why's of KS, a rapidly fatal form of cancer that has claimed far more victims in a very short time than did Legionnaire's disease."

August 11
2 FIFTH AVENUE, NEW YORK CITY

Twilight brought no respite from the humidity as eighty men streamed into Larry Kramer's apartment on the edge of Washington Square. Paul Popham was there with his Fire Island housemate Enno Poersch; KS victim Donald Krintzman came with his lover. The men milled around the apartment, sharing the latest rumors about who was sick and who didn't look well. Larry scanned the crowd and noted, with some relief, that none of the political crazies were there. Present, instead, were la crème de la crème of New York's A-list gay nightlife, the hottest guys you'd see on the island or at the trendiest discos. The conversation abruptly ended when Larry introduced a short balding man who mounted a platform in the center of the comfortable living room.

"We're seeing only the tip of the iceberg," said Dr. Alvin Friedman-Kien in what would become the all-encompassing metaphor for the AIDS epidemic for years to come.

He didn't know what was causing the epidemic, but he knew that the people who got sick had lots of sex partners and a long history of VD. (Larry noticed a lot of the men shift uncomfortably in their Topsiders.) The word needed to get out, Friedman-Kien warned; people needed to take it seriously. The doctor added that he needed money for research—now.

For most of the people in that apartment, the brief stunned silence that followed Friedman-Kien's talk represented the moment between their Before and After. The days of their lives would be counted from this time when they realized that something brutally unexpected had interrupted their plans. For Enno Poersch, this was the moment it dawned on him that the horrible death Nick had suffered seven months ago might be related to Jack Nau's and Rick Wellikoff's illnesses.

When Larry asked for volunteers to work on some larger fund-raisers, Enno stayed behind and so did Paul Popham. Paul had rather prided himself on never getting involved in gay politics, but this was different. Two friends were dead and another was dying. About thirty-five other people stayed behind to organize fund-raising tables at Fire Island for Labor Day weekend. Larry passed the hat for Friedman-Kien's NYU research and collected $6,635. That was just about all the private money that was to be raised to fight the new epidemic for the rest of the year.

Some people left Larry Kramer's apartment angry at Friedman-Kien. When one man asked him how to avoid getting this gay cancer, Friedman-Kien had repeated that he would stop having sex. The gay community didn't need some Moral Majority doctor telling them what to do with their sex lives, somebody fumed. Others suspected that the meeting was simply a furtherance of Larry's well-known distaste for promiscuity.

Still, Larry considered his new cause to be off to a grand start. He spent the next few days writing letters to alert key people to the epidemic. He dropped a note to Calvin Klein, asking for contributions to research, and he dashed off a plea to a closeted gay reporter at *The New York Times* for more coverage. Cases had more than doubled in the month since that first piece in *The Times,* and Larry hadn't seen another word since.

September 4, Labor Day
FIRE ISLAND, NEW YORK

"Are you crazy?"

Paul Popham couldn't comprehend what the guy was driving at.

"You're just making a big deal out of nothing," the acquaintance continued, giving Paul another strange look before striding purposefully toward the Donna Summer music pulsating from the Ice Palace.

How could you *not* be concerned, Paul wondered. More than 100 gay men were sick with something, many of them dead, and everybody was acting as though Paul were some major-league party-pooper out to wreck everybody's good time. Paul was downright aggravated. Lord knows, he liked to party too, but this was a time to be serious. He was asking people to put a buck or two in a can, and he was not only ignored but was often treated with unabashed hostility. Guys told him that he was hysterical, or participating in a heterosexual plot to undermine the gay community. At best, the men were apathetic.

The weekend was a disaster from the start. Larry Kramer, Enno Poersch, Paul Popham, and a handful of others had stretched a banner above a card table near the dock where everybody came into The Pines. "Give to Gay Cancer," it read.

With some of the money raised at Larry's apartment, they had printed up thousands of copies of a *New York Native* article written by Dr. Larry Mass, another volunteer that weekend, and put them at every doorstep in the island's two gay communities, The Pines and Cherry Grove. To each reprint, they attached slips explaining how people could support Friedman-Kien's research. The small band of organizers figured they'd be able to raise thousands from the 15,000 gay men who had congregated for the last blowout of the '81 season.

They were wrong.

"Leave me alone," was one typical reaction.

"This is a downer," was another.

"What are you talking about?" was about the nicest response they got.

Enno was amazed at all the smart-ass remarks. Larry was dispirited. How do you help a community that doesn't want help? he wondered. For his part, Paul felt a wholly unfamiliar sense of alienation. These are my kind of people, he thought. He knew these faces, had seen them for years dancing at The Saint, strolling around the St. Mark's Baths, sunning on the beach. They were paying $10 to get into the Ice Palace and another $50 or so for the drugs that would keep them up until dawn, not to mention the $4,000 it took to buy this summer's share in a Fire Island house rental. What was a few dollars for scientific research?

The proceeds of the weekend's fund-raising totaled $124. Paul had never thought about how frivolous people could be. He wondered what it would mean for the future, when more people were dying.

$$\bigcirc$$

Days after the Labor Day fiasco, Jack Nau died at St. Vincent's Hospital. He hadn't left the institution since he was hospitalized on Independence Day, and he had suffered the excruciating awful demise that dramatically informed doctors of how grisly a disease this gay syndrome was.

Paul Popham felt a certain hollowness when he learned Jack had died. He had loved Jack once, and now, like Rick and Nick, Jack was dead.

Later, it crossed Paul's mind that he'd have to tell Gaetan Dugas about Jack the next time he ran into him.

10 GOLF COURSES OF SCIENCE

September 15, 1981
NATIONAL INSTITUTES OF HEALTH,
BETHESDA, MARYLAND

The National Institutes of Health sprawls over 306 acres of Maryland hills, ten miles northwest of Washington, out on Rockville Turnpike. Various disease vogues and congressional initiatives had spurred proliferation of the institutes to a $4-billion-a-year enterprise that, by 1981, included the National Institute for Allergy and Infectious Diseases, the National Heart, Lung and Blood Institute, and various other institutes for eye, dental, and neurological research. The most prestigious institute is the National Cancer Institute. Unlike the other five institutes, the NCI is largely autonomous from the NIH director, with its chieftains reporting directly to the Assistant Secretary for Health. With a $1 billion annual budget, the NCI has the most lavish funding of any health research organization in the Western world.

The stone baronial mansions for the NIH director and the directors of the most eminent of the institutes stand on grassy knolls, like the stately campus homes of college presidents. That's what they like to call the NIH grounds, a campus. Here, removed from the demands of commerce, scientists are given the freedom to undertake undirected research. Pure science. That means nobody can tell them what to do. The scientists follow their own interests, and, it is hoped, they will stumble across discoveries that will benefit humankind.

The goal is thoroughly academic, but the rolling green hills of the NIH complex and the gray-haired scientists strolling at a leisurely pace also lend to the NIH the ambience of a golf course. It is a big, relaxed club where only the elite gain entrance and there isn't much need to hurry about anything.

The lack of urgency was the most striking aspect of the conference on Kaposi's sarcoma and opportunistic infections called by the National Cancer Institute for Tuesday, September 15. About fifty leading clinicians treating the problem—people like Michael Gottlieb from UCLA, Linda Laubenstein from NYU, and Marc Conant from UCSF—had flown into Washington with high expectations. Finally, the "big boys" were getting into the action. The involvement of the Centers for Disease Control was reassuring, but, everyone knew, the CDC provided only the shock troops for epidemics. As a rapid deployment force, they could be relied upon to pounce on a crisis and establish a beachhead, but it was the National Cancer Institute, with its older hands and three times the money of the CDC, that could bring in the heavy artillery.

With more than 120 cases now reported nationally and still no explanation for the patients' strange immune deficiencies, it was increasingly clear to the clinicians gathered in Bethesda that an investigation into this outbreak could become a long haul, requiring substantial NCI grants. Rumors circulated that the conference was indeed a prelude to the first extramural NIH research funding on the cancer. As the key figures among the handful working on the outbreak in America, the participants knew they would be the most likely recipients of such an accelerated granting process.

Alvin Friedman-Kien presented the epidemiological work he had recently submitted for publication, pouring out everything he had learned about the deadly new disease in the grueling five months since that first gay man with Kaposi's sarcoma walked into his office. Later, NCI's representatives took the stage. Those clinicians who were privileged to attend the briefing had already been made to understand that this was not a discussion session, so they sat dumbfounded while the NCI experts started talking about KS in Africa.

The experts explained the intricacies of the African disease and gave prescriptions on how it should be treated. There was little talk about the immune system, no interest in the relationship between KS and *Pneumocystis,* and scant discussion about possible viral causes or, for that matter, of any of the possible causes. There were just pat lectures on how doctors treated KS in Africa. Use radiation or aggressive chemotherapy on these patients, the NCI doctors said. That's what works. They didn't seem much interested in the suggestion of one New York clinician that there might be problems in treating immune-suppressed patients with therapies that are known to devastate the immune system. Thus the NCI gave its seminar and then pronounced the day a success.

Michael Gottlieb was stunned by all the talk of KS among the Bantus. It was as if nobody had told these eminent NCI researchers that benign KS in Africa seemed to bear little resemblance to the vicious skin cancer that could kill American patients. He had hoped for a plan for a multicenter study of the new disease and treatment experiments coordinated with the drug industry and physicians across the country. Instead, the only substantial development at this meeting was a vague NCI assurance that it would accept proposals for federal funding of research at some point in the future.

Knowing the delays that can encumber federal research grants, Gottlieb left the meeting crestfallen. Science was not mobilizing to fight a scourge that he felt was most certainly an infectious disease with the potential to spread across America. He had spent much of the summer methodically putting together a paper on cases of *Pneumocystis carinii* pneumonia for the *New England Journal of Medicine.* The periodical, however, did not seem overly enthusiastic about rushing the piece into print, sending it back to Gottlieb for this or that correction. The article, the first full treatment of gay pneumonia in a scientific journal, would not be published until December, more than six months after Gottlieb's first report in *MMWR.*

The NCI conference fueled Gottlieb's suspicion that no one cared because it was homosexuals who were dying. Nobody came out and said it was all right for gays to drop dead; it was just that homosexuals didn't seem to warrant the kind of urgent concern another set of victims would engender. Scientists didn't care, because there was little glory, fame, and funding to be had in this field; there wasn't likely to be money or prestige as long as the newspapers ignored the outbreak, and the press didn't like writing about homosexuals. So nobody cared, and all Michael Gottlieb could do was return to Los Angeles to preside over more deaths.

Jim Curran was not as surprised as the others. He had expected the NCI people to talk about cancer, and not the more basic problem of immune suppression that obviously was the key factor in the epidemic. Many of the federal cancer researchers, he knew, simply would not believe the CDC's assertion that the new appearances of Kaposi's sarcoma and *Pneumocystis* were even related. In the case updates Curran had forwarded to the NCI, he had created a special statistical category of the epidemic's casualties to address this, separating the cases by people with KS, others with PCP, and the growing numbers who had both KS and PCP.

Still, Curran knew that, at best, the NIH doctors had a condescending attitude toward the younger hotshots at the CDC. Curran had yet to interest anybody at the NIH in research in the gay diseases, and of course, no scientists in that land of undirected research could be ordered to work on the outbreak. All Curran could do was keep plodding up to Bethesda and hope somebody would catch on to the serious nature of what was happening. Maybe the case-control study would convince them, he thought.

University of California, San Francisco

The young parents were frantic. Their other child had been normal, what was the matter with their baby boy? They knew, of course, that his first months had been difficult, after the series of transfusions to alter his Rh factor. But now he was seven months old and he still kept getting sick. He suffered from candidiasis and an ear infection that didn't respond to antibiotics. The child's immunologists could tell the baby was suffering from some kind of immune dysfunction, but the pattern didn't fit the profile of babies born with congenital immune impairment.

Meanwhile, in another doctor's office in early October, a forty-seven-year-old man was complaining of swollen lymph nodes. He seemed tired all the time and was losing weight, probably because he just didn't feel like eating. Scarier to him was the problem with his eye—his retina had clouded over for no apparent reason. He had always been healthy before, his doctors noted. He was even a regular blood donor and had given as recently as March, when his blood was transfused into the baby now hospitalized at the UC Med Center.

October 1981
THE TENDERLOIN DISTRICT,
SAN FRANCISCO

The gay desk clerk grew more curious with each handsome young man who came to ask for Mary Guinan's room number. It didn't help when a maid mentioned that she had found a bloodstained bed sheet in the room of the pretty blond doctor from Atlanta.

The $75-a-day government limit on expenses had forced Guinan and Harold Jaffe into a seedy hotel on the fringes of San Francisco's Tenderloin, the city's highest-crime neighborhood. The desk clerk seemed reassured when Guinan said that she and Harold Jaffe were doing a study on gay cancer, and the clerk even politely told Guinan where she could go to buy new clothes when all her garments were stolen from a laundromat. For the rest of her stay, Guinan couldn't get over the idea that somebody out there was walking the streets in her underwear.

The case-control study, however, was proving to be an endurance test for everybody. During grueling sixteen-hour days, CDC doctors interviewed 75 percent of the living patients in the United States. The task force had spent the summer piecing together the form, sixty-two questions on twenty-two pages, that covered every conceivable behavior and exposure that might be involved in the epidemic, right down to what plants, pets, cleaning compounds, and photo chemicals were around the house. In an effort to cross-match for every aspect of the cases' lives, four controls were selected for each patient. One was a heterosexual of comparable age and background; another was a gay man from a venereal disease clinic who, tending toward the more sexually active side, would match sexual behaviors; another was a gay man from a private doctor's practice; and still another gay control would be a patient's friend with whom he had not had sex. This last category proved the most difficult to fill since it seemed that just about every friend of a patient was also somebody the patient had once made love to, usually as a prelude to a platonic relationship. That was simply how you tended to meet other gay men in San Francisco and New York.

The CDC staffers could tell gay from straight controls by the way they reacted to the questions about every aspect of their intimate sexual lives. Heterosexuals seemed offended at queries about the preferred sexual techniques, while gay interviewees chatted endlessly about them. One gay man flipped out a pocket calculator to estimate his lifetime sexual contacts.

The nonchalance with which doctors handled blood samples drawn from each participant would later give them nightmares. Nobody used gloves as they drew serum from patient's arms. The infectious agent talk was, after all, a hypothesis. Every day, however, the conviction settled deeper among the CDC doctors that whatever was causing this syndrome, it was not something they could see or tabulate on their neat questionnaires. The only factors that seemed to distinguish cases from controls was the number of sexual partners, the incidence of venereal disease, and attendance at gay bathhouses, which of course was the behavior that made possible large numbers of sexual partners. Maybe the computer analysis of all the detailed questions would turn up something, but the evidence for a new and deadly viral disease was becoming incontrovertible for researchers like Mary Guinan.

Guinan mentioned her fears to Marc Conant over dinner one night and was surprised to find such a sympathetic ear. She was used to being dismissed as a hysteric when she got on the subject of viral agents and pandemic spreads. This guy has a perfectly clear view of what's happening, she thought, although she was unnerved by his own projections of what a sexually transmitted killer disease might mean to San Francisco.

If we don't move fast, Conant said, thousands of people will die in this city alone. Playing in the fast lane of the freeway had merely ensured that the patients they saw would get run over first. If the virus had a long incubation period and was already widespread, it had already made it to the lesser traveled avenues of gay life, Conant warned.

$$\ominus$$

Back in Atlanta, Mary Guinan was assigned to review all those cases who claimed to be heterosexual. This was the most problematic element the case-control study had uncovered. Some patients apparently were not gay, though they did admit to being heroin users. Unfortunately, most of these addicts were dead by the time the CDC got to them, because they tended to suffer not from the slower homicide of KS but from the quick kill of *Pneumocystis*. Family members of dead patients were notoriously unreliable in confirming a victim's heterosexuality, so intravenous drug use could not be called a risk until more direct interviews established it.

Although the growing evidence for a new infectious disease startled the Kaposi's Sarcoma and Opportunistic Infections Task Force members, not everybody at the CDC was that excited over the cancer and pneumonia outbreaks. Many of the old hands were convinced that exposure to some toxic chemical had occurred, that it would not be repeated, and the disease would fade out as mysteriously as it had faded in. Maybe five years later, they'd figure out what had happened; for now, this was an interesting oddity that, ultimately, was not very important.

UNIVERSITY OF CALIFORNIA, SAN FRANCISCO

Marc Conant was always scheming to get other UC specialists interested in the "gay plague," as the gay press was ignominiously calling it, and a chance encounter at the melanoma clinic with Paul Volberding, the new cancer chief from San Francisco General Hospital, seemed particularly fortuitous. Conant saw in Volberding just the kind of doctor that would be needed in the difficult times ahead. Volberding was not trapped in some rigid specialization and was young enough not to be burdened by anti-gay biases that might cloud his scientific and medical judgments. When Volberding mentioned that he thought

KS was a particularly interesting tumor, Conant suggested they visit a patient at UCSF, one that might prefigure the shape of things to come in the epidemic.

Simon Guzman tried to smile for the handsome young doctor who walked into his room with the familiar and reassuring form of Marc Conant. A native of Mexico, Simon did not speak English well, but Volberding easily recognized him as yet another nice young gay man who appeared to be on a rapid course to a painful and early death. There were, of course, the lesions of Kaposi's sarcoma, but there was also an unrelenting diarrhea and herpes destroying the young man's body. Other infections remained undiagnosed, Conant confided to Volberding. Something was ravaging the man's gut, but they couldn't figure out what.

Volberding recalled the helpless young man he had met on his first day at San Francisco General, and promised Conant that, yes, he too would sign on to work with these strange new diseases in the clinic Conant was organizing. Conant was reassured to have the resources of the city's largest hospital behind him, as well as the nationally prominent UCSF Medical Center. Within weeks, he had appropriated several rooms used as nighttime sleeping quarters for interns, and the nation's first Kaposi's sarcoma clinic was established. Doctors from throughout northern California began referring their cases to Conant, ensuring the best treatment, study, and surveillance of the new disease. Conant would handle the dermatology and academic politicking, and Volberding would treat the patients at General.

Another young assistant professor at UCSF, Donald Abrams, also signed on at the hospital with his own agenda. Since his residency at local hospitals in the late 1970s, he had been studying the strange swelling of lymph nodes among gay patients. Already, one of these patients, a friend, had developed a lymph cancer, and another had come down with a strange meningitis. Abrams was convinced these lymph node problems were somehow related to the new diseases. In Abrams, Conant had found another doctor willing to set aside the paper writing and bench work of academic advancement in favor of trying to stop the new disease.

These early efforts, of course, were all conducted with free time pilfered from various specialists around the hilltop campus and financed in part from the earnings of Conant's private dermatological practice. But the federal money was coming, Conant told himself. It had been promised in Bethesda in September. Surely when they saw how serious this was, the government would pull out the stops.

November 1981
NATIONAL CANCER INSTITUTE,
BETHESDA

Jim Goedert mentioned his nitrate inhalant study to Dr. Bob Biggar, a staffer at the Environmental Epidemiology Branch of the National Cancer Institute, housed in an inconspicuous office building a few miles away from the major NCI offices in the rolling hills of the National Institutes of Health campus. Goedert's two KS patients piqued Biggar's interest in the new epidemic. Biggar had spent years in Africa and recognized Kaposi's sarcoma as one of the most widespread cancers on that continent. Still, he doubted the theory of poppers as the cause. There was nothing new about nitrate inhalant use in the gay community. Besides, a disease caused by a social phenomenon followed a gradual curve, increasing slowly as the behavior trend caught on. New reports of KS and PCP were coming into the CDC on an exponential curve. That was the way infectious diseases spread, increasing dramatically as the new infectious agent worked its way through the population. There had to be another way to go after this, Biggar thought, and as he plotted a course for study, his thoughts drifted toward Denmark.

Four years of studying the relationship between the Epstein-Barr virus and Burkitt's lymphoma in the jungle of Ghana for the NCI's Environmental Epidemiology Branch had convinced him that infectious agents could cause cancer. Any research on this hypothesis in an American gay urban center, however, would be tainted by the fact that some of the gay men already were infected with the disease-causing agent and one wouldn't be able to accurately tell the infected from the uninfected. Biggar figured he had to go to some place where there were gay men but where the disease had not yet struck.

Rochester, New York, at first seemed like a promising city, but it proved to be too close to New York City, the epicenter of the new disease. A more perfect research site occurred to him suddenly one day, and he quickly approached his superiors about requisitioning a plane ticket to Denmark. Aarhus, the largest city north of the fjord in Jutland, offered a fairly open gay population who would most likely cooperate, and a geographic location remote from the gay cancer centers of the United States. It also was home to an important medical center. With doctors from the medical center and uninfected gay men, Biggar could launch a study to track this new disease and fathom its seemingly unfathomable mysteries. The work would also cost next to nothing, with expenses mainly going for the plane fare and his salary.

Biggar was busily preparing the study's protocol when he received word that the National Cancer Institute chiefs would not pay for his plane ticket. Money was tight, Biggar was told privately. Studying gay cancer was not a priority.

St. Francis Hospital,
San Francisco

The last time Jim Groundwater saw Ken Horne, he couldn't help but think back to the angry young man who had stepped into his downtown office exactly one year before. The Ken Horne lying sullenly in the dark room in St. Francis Hospital no longer had the vivacity that had undoubtedly helped keep him alive through the debilitating bouts with *Pneumocystis,* cryptococcal meningitis, and widespread cytomegaloviral infections. Even though Ken had been a pest, Groundwater had come to respect his spirit and the courage with which he faced his health horrors, always somehow convincing himself that he would pull through, be cured, and get back to days at the BART station and nights at the baths.

Now, the fight was out of Ken's voice, Groundwater noted. Ken seemed reconciled to the fact that he was going to die. His once-toned dancer's body had shrunk to 122 pounds, and his fever constantly ran at 102 degrees. He was blind now too, from the CMV herpes infections that had wasted his nervous system. His mind also seemed to be going, like that of an old person suffering from dementia. But, of course, young people don't get dementia. The staff assumed that his failing mental acuity stemmed from medication or from the sheer physical stress of fighting disease after disease for the past year.

Never before had Groundwater seen anybody so consumed by any disease. He gave Ken Horne his usual pep talk that November morning about hanging in there, but as he left Ken's room he knew that death would come as a relief to that tortured body.

On November 26, after being taken off a ventilator, Ken suffered respiratory arrest. He was resuscitated and put back on the wheezing contraption that breathes for patients who are no longer able to draw their own breath. On a late November night, while a heavy bank of storm clouds shoved past the San Francisco skyline on a north wind, Ken's breath again grew heavy and pained.

At 1 A.M. on November 30, 1981, George Kenneth Horne, Jr., gasped one last tortured breath and lapsed into the perfect darkness.

⬭

Jim Groundwater wasn't surprised when he learned Ken Horne had died. The autopsy on his battered body that day, however, revealed that Ken had withstood infections far beyond what his doctors had imagined.

The primary cause of death was listed as cryptococcal pneumonia, which was a consequence of his Kaposi's sarcoma and *Pneumocystis carinii* pneumonia. Those, however, were only the obvious diseases. The KS lesions, it turned out, covered not only his skin but also his lungs, bronchi, spleen, bladder, lymph nodes, mouth, and adrenal glands. His eyes were infected not only with cytomegalovirus but also with cryptococcus and the *Pneumocystis* protozoa. It was the first time the pathologist could recall seeing the protozoa infect a person's eye.

Ken's mother claimed his body from the hospital the day after he died. By the afternoon, Ken's remains were cremated and tucked into a small urn.

His Kaposi's sarcoma had led to the discovery in San Francisco of the epidemic that would later be called Acquired Immune Deficiency Syndrome. He had been the first KS case in the country reported to a disbelieving Centers for Disease Control just eight months before. Now, he was one of eighteen such stricken people in San Francisco and the fourth man in the city to die in the epidemic, the seventy-fourth to die in the United States. There would be many, many more.

December 1
CENTERS FOR DISEASE CONTROL, ATLANTA

On the day that Ken Horne's body was cremated, Jim Curran dictated a memo to CDC Director William Foege. Curran was politically savvy enough to know that this was not a good time to be asking for more money, what with the ax falling on health budgets throughout the country, but he was also convinced that the new epidemic presented the potential of a serious health threat if it wasn't tackled.

Everybody in the Kaposi's Sarcoma and Opportunistic Infections Task Force had figured that by now reporters would be crawling all over this story. Legionnaire's disease and Toxic Shock Syndrome had, by this stage in their respective epidemics, warranted almost daily front-page treatment, which in turn engendered the interest of members of Congress, who tickled loose more money for research. Yet newspapers and television broadcasts rarely mentioned a word about the new epidemic. Instead, budgetary warfare had to be waged through discreet internal memos. In November, minutes of the task force meeting forwarded to CDC brass mentioned that the meetings repeatedly shifted, as one memo put it, to "discussions of the impact of budget cuts . . . on its own function," and attempts "to find ways to minimize disruption of the investigation if special funds were not forthcoming."

Now Jim Curran had finished his modest six-month budget proposal of $833,800 for the task force's next year of work. Foege had promised to argue for the supplemental funding, which represented only a fraction of a percent of the Public Health Service budget. Curran waited eagerly for a reply to his request.

And he waited, and he waited.

11 BAD MOON RISING

December 1981
PARIS

With a disposition tilted toward permanent agitation, Dr. Jacques Leibowitch lapsed into near-rapturous excitement long before completing Michael Gottlieb's article in the *New England Journal of Medicine* about the cases of *Pneumocystis carinii* pneumonia in gay men, and Alvin Friedman-Kien's piece in the same issue about Kaposi's sarcoma. He immediately recalled the stocky Portuguese cab driver whom Dr. Willy Rozenbaum had sent him three years ago. He too suffered from this pneumonia and he too was already dead, for a year now. Leibowitch and Rozenbaum were not close friends. A detached observer might note that they were too similar to be friendly, both with their well-toned, muscular bodies, movie-star good looks, and a professional exuberance that was altogether foreign to the staid medical profession. Both also exuded a sensual charisma, and Leibowitch preferred being the only charismatic guy in the room. Nevertheless, he couldn't restrain himself from calling Rozenbaum about the Gottlieb article.

"The epidemic—the cab driver," enthused the thirty-nine-year-old immunologist. "It's already been here. For three years."

"Yes," said Rozenbaum. "I have three other patients in the hospital now."

Rozenbaum told him of the two gay men who had come to him in the past months with the diseases, as well as two women, a Zairian and a Frenchwoman who had lived in Africa. Whatever these diseases were, they were not simply homosexual maladies, and there had to be some link with Africa, Rozenbaum said.

Given his infectious disease background, Rozenbaum wanted to start an epidemiological study of the gay men who were coming down with this to try to understand some patterns. He didn't know how kindly his hospital administration would take to studying homosexuals, but he sensed that this was big and it would only get bigger.

On a hunch, Leibowitch called his sister, a professor of dermatology at another Paris hospital. Sure enough, she was treating two more gay men with Kaposi's sarcoma. Leibowitch talked to the two men and started reading everything from the United States about the epidemic. He was taken aback at how little had been written in the popular press even though there were already so many dead and dying from this mysterious phenomenon. He was also curious to see that it was promoted as a homosexual disease.

How very American, he thought, to look at a disease as homosexual or heterosexual, as if viruses had the intelligence to choose between different inclinations of human behavior. Those Americans are simply obsessed by sex. He had no doubt it was some kind of virus. The African connection immediately suggested a viral agent; Africa was where new diseases tended to germinate. It certainly was not the poppers the Americans kept talking about. He had never heard of poppers, and certainly his cab driver had never heard of poppers nor had those two women from Zaire. If it was something that was already in the United States, France, and Africa, he realized, this was an event that could have global impact.

ALBERT EINSTEIN COLLEGE OF MEDICINE, BRONX, NEW YORK

Dr. Arye Rubinstein's soft voice was infused with a thick Israeli accent that the poor black kids from the Bronx, who made up the bulk of his patients in the immunology ward, found both exotic and reassuring. This wasn't the thick guttural English spoken among the sprawling poor tenements of a neighborhood that had for years been the very personification of American poverty. Somehow, Rubinstein sounded the way a doctor was supposed to sound. As chief of Albert Einstein's medical college Division of Allergy and Immunology, Rubinstein had seen all sorts of immune disorders among these impoverished kids, but there had been something new now for two years. He had no doubts that these kids, raised in the depths of Bronx poverty, were suffering from the same immunology problems plaguing trendy homosexual men in the chic neighborhoods of Manhattan.

It had started in 1979, he could see now, when an anxious mother brought in her three-month-old. Blood tests indicated that this child's immune deficiency clearly was different from the congenital immune problems that made up the brunt of Rubinstein's work. It had an entirely different profile, with a marked decrease of T-helper cells and other blood irregularities that one didn't see in congenital cases. For the next two years, baffled clinicians from the Bronx public hospitals started calling Rubinstein more often about kids with swollen lymph nodes and an apparent inability to fight off even the most common and benign infections. A number of them, the doctors noted, had mothers who were drug addicts.

The clincher walked into Rubinstein's office in late 1981. The mother, one of the thousands of drug addicts who used the nearby Jacobi Hospital, had swollen lymph nodes and nagging minor infections, clear indications of immune deficiency. Now, her child presented the same symptoms. There was no congenital immune deficiency in which both the mother and child had the same symptoms, Rubinstein knew. He thoroughly researched the literature. Maybe it was caused by cytomegalovirus and Epstein-Barr virus, but those infections, he learned, would behave differently. With some trepidation, he wrote on their medical charts the diagnosis he knew was correct—immune deficiency. Whatever the homosexuals had that was giving them Kaposi's sarcoma and *Pneumocystis,* it was also spreading among drug addicts and, most tragically, their children.

The doctors tending the mother and child crossed Rubinstein's diagnosis off their charts.

Although Rubinstein was an eminent pediatric immunologist, he could not get anyone else to believe his unlikely analysis. He began bringing up the cases at city immunology meetings. This is something we need to look out for, he warned. The other doctors assured him it was certainly just some new kind of congenital cytomegalovirus infection. At an immunological meeting at Cold Spring Harbor, Rubinstein presented more data, proving that what he was seeing couldn't be the work of the CMV herpes virus. This was something new, spreading not just among the elite homosexuals but in the slums of the Bronx. No, the scientists told him. Gay pneumonia and gay cancer were diseases of homosexual men.

In December, Rubinstein wrote up an abstract to present at a conference of the American Academy of Pediatrics. In his opinion, the evidence was becoming overwhelming. He had five black infants who had been thoroughly worked up. Some had *Pneumocystis* pneumonia; they all had the same T-cell patterns common to gay pneumonia victims. At least three of the kids were the children of promiscuous drug users.

The implications were clear to Rubinstein, and they needed to be shouted from the rooftops. The fact that children contracted the disease indicated that it was not from poppers or anything particular to the homosexual life-style, but that it was the effect of a new virus that mothers were transmitting to their children, probably through the placenta. Society needed to be steeled not only for a new infectious disease among gay men but also among drug addicts who could spread it to their children.

Such thinking, however, was simply too farfetched for a scientific community that, when it thought about gay cancer and gay pneumonia at all, was quite happy to keep the problems just that: gay. The academy would not accept Rubinstein's abstract for presentation at the conference, and among immunologists, word quietly circulated that the Israeli researcher had gone a little batty.

SAN FRANCISCO DEPARTMENT OF PUBLIC HEALTH

In her quiet, methodical way, Dr. Selma Dritz spent the morning rummaging through the basement of the old public health building before she came across the blackboard that would serve her purposes. It couldn't be too big or it wouldn't fit on the wall of her tiny third-floor cubbyhole at the Bureau of Communicable Disease Control. Still, it had to be big enough to hold all the names. The idea had struck her as she started noting the patterns during the long interviews she helped the CDC conduct for their case-control study. One roommate would come down with Kaposi's sarcoma and another would contract a fatal case of cytomegalovirus run wild. The latter death might not be attributed to the new epidemic, but Dritz had no doubt that it had something to do with immune defects she was seeing in gay men, so she meticulously noted the interpersonal links both in her neat black notebook and on the note cards she had started keeping in an old shoe box on her desk.

By December, there were enough links to warrant having a blackboard on her office wall, and there, with arrows between circles marked PCP, KS, and CMV, she saw the pattern emerge. There were lovers and roommates, friends and friends of friends, and all the arrows pointed toward one discomforting conclusion. Although it lacked the hard proof that elevates theory to fact, it looked to Dritz like this gay cancer was something infectious and that it was spread through sex.

The time may be coming for public health alerts and official warnings, Dritz thought. Like scientists and public health officials throughout the country, however, she waited for more evidence from the CDC's newly completed case-control study. Thousands of lives depended on it.

⬭

Other troubling conclusions were being drawn in various examining rooms in New York and San Francisco in the last weeks of 1981, though they wouldn't make much sense until later. At the UCSF Kaposi's Sarcoma Clinic, Dr. Donald Abrams had begun his own study of patients with swollen lymph nodes who were coming in with greater frequency. This lymphadenopathy was related to gay cancer, he felt, though it might be some early stage or, perhaps, some milder form of the immune deficiency. He also started studying steady sexual partners of the people with gay cancer and pneumonia, figuring they might give some clue as to whether this was an infectious disease and, if so, how long it needed to incubate before bursting forth in one of its deadly manifestations. There wasn't any money for these studies, but he managed to pilfer help here and there and add the time to his already harried schedule. The National Cancer Institute had promised grants, he knew; he could hold out until then.

CENTERS FOR DISEASE CONTROL, ATLANTA

The anecdote was precisely the story Dr. Jim Curran had feared he might hear, even though it was the kind of information that interviews with 75 percent of the living "gay plague" victims were supposed to engender: One man lives contentedly with his long-time lover in a small, remote town. He doesn't live in the fast lane of big-city gay life; he doesn't use poppers; he's dying. His lover, it turns out, is a traveling salesman who is generally faithful, except when he gets to New York, where he screws his brains out in the gay bathhouses. Shortly after his monogamous lover gets sick, the salesman gets sick too.

To prove an infectious disease, Curran knew, one had to establish Koch's postulate. According to this century-old paradigm, you must take an infectious agent from one animal, put it into another, who becomes ill, and then take the infectious agent from the second and inject it into still a third subject, who becomes ill with the same disease. That's the scientific way of proving a disease is infectious. The anecdote of the salesman and his faithful lover did not meet all the niceties of Koch's postulate, but, in an epidemiological sort of way, it added more weight to the CDC's KSOI Task Force view that gay cancer and gay pneumonia were part of a new infectious disease.

By December, the official statistics counted 152 cases in fifteen states. Including the likely cases that still needed follow-up, the toll was closer to 180, and climbing fast. Only one of the 152 cases was a woman, an intravenous drug user. Dr. Mary Guinan, who handled all the suspected heterosexual cases, was convinced that drug addicts were the next major pool of immune deficiency cases. Problems remained in saying this officially, however. The addicts tended to be dead by the time they were reported to the CDC. Health officials outside the task force often reported them as homosexual, being strangely reluctant to shed the notion that this was a gay disease; all these junkies would somehow turn out to be gay in the end, they said.

Guinan, however, wasn't convinced. If the diseases could be spread through sharing needles, there were vast public health implications not only for the United States but worldwide. Cases among addicts, Guinan thought, would certainly presage infection of hemophiliacs and transmission of the disease through blood transfusions. Moreover, such a route of contagion, so similar to that of hepatitis B, would give public health authorities a reason to issue guidelines so gay men could reduce the chance of contracting these singularly brutal diseases.

Like everyone in the task force, Guinan hoped the final tabulations of the lengthy case-control questions would provide some solid answers. But she also knew that the answers would not be forthcoming. Although the task force had been able to move quickly for the past six months by pirating other CDC budgets and diverting personnel, the lack of resources finally bogged down research at its most crucial juncture.

CDC Director Dr. Bill Foege had argued the need for new allocations for the CDC work on gay cancer directly with Assistant Secretary for Health Edward Brandt. Brandt agreed the research was important enough to warrant further funding. Sensitive to the rigid limits the administration was setting on all nonarmaments spending, however, Brandt said he'd have to try to get the money from the heftier budget of the National Institutes of Health. After all, Jim Curran's $833,800 request amounted to only one five-thousandth of the NIH annual budget. But no word came from the NIH.

Stepped-up surveillance and epidemiological studies were delayed. Any one of these studies might produce the smoking gun that could solve the epidemic, CDC officials worried, but they had to be put off.

Meanwhile, a preliminary review of the untabulated data showed one difference between the gay plague cases and the control cases—sexual activity. There was also a tendency among cases to use poppers and street drugs, but that was more a reflection of the high-paced life-style. The salience of sexual activity as a predicator of the diseases, of course, meant that it was sexually transmitted, task force members knew. And if this were the case, there was no reason to believe that it would not penetrate far deeper into the nation. Such suppositions, however, were based on cursory review. Without the case-control study, neatly analyzed, with all the scientific ratios that the general public doesn't understand, the conclusions would never stand up in a court of science. To utter them publicly would threaten the CDC's credibility.

Instead, the CDC could only issue bland assurances. Nobody need panic, they said; this would keep homophobes in check. There was no concrete evidence of contagion, they added; homosexuals could be reassured. It would always be the unwritten policy of health bureaucrats throughout the epidemic that, when in doubt, don't scare the horses.

⬭

"It's a combination of feline leukemia and hepatitis B," Don Francis told his Harvard mentor, Dr. Myron "Max" Essex, in another one of his interminable phone conversations on the gay cancer.

From the start, Francis had thought that some infectious agent caused the underlying immune suppression that made gay cancer victims susceptible to all their ailments. The talk about the case-control study had convinced Francis that this was an even neater sexually transmitted disease than hepatitis. There was no other factor confusing the epidemiology.

Years of stamping out epidemics in the Third World had also instructed Francis on how to stop a new disease. You find the source of contagion, surround it, and make sure it doesn't spread. The CDC needed to think about controlling this disease, he insisted. At the very least, blood banks should be put on the alert. If it spreads like hepatitis, he thought, it will certainly turn up in blood transfusions.

December 10
SAN FRANCISCO

"I'm Bobbi Campbell and I have 'gay cancer.' Although I say that, I also want to say I'm the luckiest man in the world."

With those words in the gay newspaper *The Sentinel*, a registered nurse became the first Kaposi's sarcoma patient to go public with his plight and start what in San Francisco would be a long and difficult effort at awakening the gay community to the threat of the immune-deficiency diseases. Before last fall, Bobbi, a Tacoma native, had led a normal enough life in the gay Valhalla, enjoying bathhouses and nightlife even after settling down with his lover in the Castro neighborhood. In late September, after a day of hiking at Big Sur, he noticed some purple spots on his feet. He figured they were blood blisters and didn't pay much attention until they got bigger. He went to see Dr. Marc Conant, who informed Bobbi Campbell that he had Kaposi's sarcoma.

The major gay newspaper in New York, the *New York Native*, was crowded with stories about the new diseases, with detailed medical writing by a physician,

Dr. Larry Mass. In San Francisco, however, the homosexual papers largely ignored the diseases, reprinting excerpts from Mass's articles if they bothered to print anything at all. So Bobbi Campbell, the sixteenth diagnosed case of the gay diseases in San Francisco, decided to launch his own personal crusade to heighten awareness, proclaiming himself to be the "KS Poster Boy."

"The purpose of the poster boy is to raise interest and money in a particular cause, and I do have aspirations of doing that regarding gay cancer," he wrote. "I'm writing because I have a determination to live. You do too—don't you?"

A longtime political crony of Cleve Jones called him off Castro Street to meet Bobbi Campbell in December. Cleve was always ready to be a bit late for work and dally over a drink, and he was curious about Bobbi's *Sentinel* columns. Bobbi showed Cleve the lesions on his feet and told him about his plans to establish a support group for gay cancer patients. He also wanted to make sure the city provided adequate services. Cleve offered to help, though he wasn't sure if there would ever be enough of these people to warrant their own program. Actually, it was the first time Cleve had ever met a gay cancer patient; it was the first time Cleve believed that this thing they were writing about in the *Chronicle* was real and not a figment of some demented headline writer's imagination.

Within a few weeks, Bobbi had jawboned the corner drugstore in the heart of the Castro to put up posters about KS in its front windows. Bill Kraus lingered long in front of the drugstore, staring at the purplish splotches. He had considered the syndrome to be a New York phenomenon restricted to sleazy fist-fuckers. It undoubtedly was being hyped by a homophobic media, yet the lesion pictures made him very uneasy; the image dogged his memory. Not long after that he stopped going to the baths. He'd been on television so much in the past year or so, he was tired of being recognized all the time, he told himself, but in his deepest thoughts he also knew that his decision to drop the baths had something to do with that picture.

⬭

Larry Kramer would maintain that from the start, gay men knew precisely what they needed to do—and not do—to avoid contracting the deadly new syndrome. The problem, he insisted, was in how gay men reacted to this knowledge, not in getting the knowledge out itself. By late December 1981, Larry was embroiled in controversy over the outspoken role he had assumed in trying to alert New York gays to Kaposi's sarcoma.

"Basically, Kramer is telling us that something we gay men are doing (drugs? kinky sex?) is causing Kaposi's sarcoma," wrote Robert Chesley, a Manhattan gay writer, in one of his several letters attacking Kramer in the *New York Native*. ". . . Being alarmist is dangerous. We've been told by such experts as there are that it's wrong and too soon to make any assumptions about the cause of Kaposi's sarcoma, but there's another issue here. It is always instructive to look closely at emotionalism, for it so often has a hidden message which is the *real* secret of its appeal. I think the concealed meaning of Kramer's emotionalism is the triumph of guilt: that gay men *deserve* to die for their promiscuity. . . . Read anything by Kramer closely. I think you'll find that the subtext is always: the wages of gay sin is death. . . . I am not downplaying the seriousness of Kaposi's sarcoma. But something else is happening here, which is also serious: gay homophobia and anti-eroticism."

After mulling the attack over with his therapist, Larry Kramer responded in kind, indelicately writing that Chesley was a spurned lover who was angry that Larry never wanted to date after their initial tryst. But most of Larry's long response was more to the point.

". . . Something we are doing is ticking off the timebomb that is causing the breakdown of immunity in certain bodies, and while it is true that we don't know what it is specifically, isn't it better to be cautious until various suspected causes have been discounted rather than reckless? An individual can choose to continue or cease smoking . . . but isn't it stupid to rail against the very presentation of these warnings?

"I am not glorying in death. I am overwhelmed by it. The death of my friends. The death of whatever community there is here in New York. The death of any visible love."

The point-counterpoint between Larry and his critics became such a regular feature in the letters column of the *Native* that one correspondent wrote to sarcastically deny rumors that "Bette Davis has been signed to play the role of Larry Kramer in the film version of 'Letters to the Editor.' "

Meanwhile, Larry was despairing over the lack of any official attention to the epidemic. Half the victims lived in New York City, but Larry's pleas to *The New York Times* for more coverage were unanswered. Even *The Village Voice,* which considered itself the arbiter of all things au courant in Manhattan, had so far failed to run a single story on the gay syndrome. When Larry called Mayor Ed Koch's liaison to the gay community about getting some public health action, the aide assured Larry "I'll get back to you tomorrow" and was never heard from again. Four months of fund-raising had netted only $11,806.

"Two new cases of KS are being diagnosed in New York each week. One new case is being diagnosed in the United States *each day.* Nothing is being done by the gay community to insist that the straight community, which controls all the purse strings and attention-getting devices, help us," Larry wrote in one of his long *Native* diatribes. "If KS were a new form of cancer attacking straight people, it would be receiving constant media attention, and pressure from every side would be so great upon the cancer-funding institutions that research would be proceeding with great intensity."

ABC Studios,
New York City

All the leg work, all the questionnaires, and all the brainstorming had yet to turn up any smoking gun as cause for this syndrome. Altogether, Jim Curran could be reasonably satisfied with the first six months of the CDC's work on the epidemic. It had taken eighteen months between the first reported cases of Toxic Shock Syndrome and the first *MMWR* report and still another month until the formation of a task force and the start of a case-control study. By comparison, it took only one month from Michael Gottlieb's notification to the

CDC about gay pneumonia until the first *MMWR* report and the establishment of the task force, and only three months to get going on the case-control study. The comparisons were less flattering when you got to the Legionnaire's epidemic. During that outbreak, resources and personnel literally gushed from Atlanta, and by a comparable phase in the epidemic, scientists had broken the mystery by finding the responsible bacteria.

The difference, Curran knew, was media attention. Once Toxic Shock Syndrome hit the front pages, the heat was on to find the answer. Within months of the first *MMWR* report, the task force had discovered the link between tampons and the malady. Back in 1976, the newspapers couldn't print enough pictures of flag-draped coffins of dead American Legionnaires. However, the stories just weren't coming on the gay syndrome. *The New York Times* had written only two stories on the epidemic, setting the tone for noncoverage nationally. *Time* and *Newsweek* were running their first major stories on the epidemic now, in late December 1981. There was only one reason for the lack of media interest, and everybody in the task force knew it: the victims were homosexuals. Editors were killing pieces, reporters told Curran, because they didn't want stories about gays and all those distasteful sexual habits littering their newspapers.

In the cab on the way to the ABC studios, Curran ran over in his mind what he would tell the interviewers on "Good Morning America." With funding stalled, Curran knew that national media coverage was essential to getting both attention and bucks to his research. Amazingly enough, this was the first time that the epidemic was making it on national network news.

The interview was supposed to last for nine minutes but it was cut to 150 seconds because of unrest in Lebanon. Curran could barely stifle a groan when interviewer Frank Gifford read aloud the startling numbers about deaths and increasing cases and began the session with a question that defied a polite answer.

"This is a terrible problem," Gifford said. "How come nobody's paying any attention to it?"

SAN FRANCISCO

As soon as Matt Krieger heard that Dr. Marc Conant was going to be distributing a brochure on Kaposi's sarcoma at the American Academy of Dermatology convention in San Francisco, he wanted to help stage a press conference. Although Matt had quit his full-time job at the UCSF News Services Bureau and divided his time between freelancing and finding a home for himself and his lover Gary Walsh, he saw gay cancer as something important, even if he couldn't explain precisely why. Marc Conant and Jim Groundwater had spent their own money putting together a full-color brochure on KS, including pictures of Ken Horne's lesions. They spent the morning before the convention's final session putting a pamphlet on every chair in the sprawling new Moscone Convention Center.

On his way home, Matt studied the pictures of Ken Horne's lesions and he thought about Gary. Matt's mind finally gave way to the wrenching terror that Gary's funny skin rashes, little health glitches, and that sore on his elbow that didn't go away for the longest time were symptoms of gay cancer.

Matt burst into the flat on Dolores Street on the verge of a full-scale anxiety attack.

"I'm afraid you're going to die," Matt told Gary.

Gary rolled his eyes.

"Don't be ridiculous."

December
AARHUS, DENMARK

Washington weather provided nothing so severe as the bitter winds blistering off the North Sea over Aarhus. At night, red hearts bobbed abruptly in the wintry blasts over doorways of crowded shops, all gaily decorated for the Feast of the Hearts. Dr. Bob Biggar preferred Scandinavia in warmer seasons, but he sensed that he could not delay his research, even if the National Cancer Institute did not consider the epidemic a priority item. Biggar had paid his own way to Denmark and had put together a group of 259 Danish gay men to study.

His research, however, had gotten off to a disquieting start. Although he had hoped Aarhus would offer an uninfected pool of research subjects, Danish authorities reported that Copenhagen already had five cases of the mysterious gay disease. Some of the particulars reconfirmed Biggar's suspicion that this was an infectious disease. One victim was the sexual partner of another. Another older man lived a closeted life in Denmark but went to New York City once a year for a month, during which he accumulated as many black male sexual partners as he could. The link to New York was the strongest argument for a probable viral cause.

As he wrapped up the first phase of the Danish study, Biggar began framing his conclusions into a scientific paper, hypothesizing a viral agent as a cause for the epidemic. "The Evidence for a Transmissible Agent" would be the most prescient work of his scientific career to that point, as well as the most widely ignored.

LOS ANGELES

The most definitive evidence for a transmissible agent appeared in an offhanded sort of way in Dr. Joel Weisman's comfortable office in Sherman Oaks. It was late 1981 or during the first weeks of 1982; the date was later lost, although it marked one of the most profound conversations of the still-unnamed epidemic.

Another friend and longtime patient had died of *Pneumocystis*. Weisman was talking with that man's lover, a chatty fellow who always knew everybody's business. He was an old friend and didn't mind sharing a number of unsettling connections he had been making in recent weeks. There were five or six guys who were sick, he said, and they had all been to these parties together. This guy had sex with that guy who had sex with this other guy, and now they were all dead or dying.

Weisman stared at the cool gray walls of his office while the man continued. Suddenly, he understood everything the man was saying. Weisman knew all the guys that he was talking about, and in his mind, Weisman began seeing the relationships, almost as if they were in little circles with arrows between them, going from one to the other.

"Oh my God," he gasped. "You're telling me something I've hypothesized. It's true."

Weisman later recalled that moment—in the office where the nation's first reported *Pneumocystis* case had walked in a year before—to be the most terrifying instant of his life. There was a new virus that was killing gay men. Jesus Christ, some of these parties happened two years ago. It could be all over the place by now. God only knew how many people were going to die.

PART IV

THE GATHERING DARKNESS 1982

. . . Small official notices had been just put up about the town, though in places where they would not attract much attention. It was hard to find in these notices any indication that the authorities were facing the situation squarely. The measures enjoined were far from Draconian and one had the feeling that many concessions had been made to a desire not to alarm the public.

—ALBERT CAMUS,
The Plague

12 ENEMY TIME

January 1982
CENTERS FOR DISEASE CONTROL, ATLANTA

Bruce Evatt enjoyed his work with hemophiliacs, and his lifetime research into the bleeding disorder had long ago made him the resident expert on hemophilia at the Centers for Disease Control. The disorder, which had plagued generations of European royalty, was determined by the hereditary information of just one molecule. Orders for this molecule's construction passed in genetic code from mother to son; the molecule determined whether or not the son's blood would clot to stop bleeding. Hemophiliac sons lacked that ability, hence the name of their disorder, hemophilia, "love of blood." Beyond the fascination with this molecule, Evatt found that hemophiliacs were simply a joy to work with. They were an intelligent, well-informed group who, in their lifetime, had experienced a scientific breakthrough that added decades to their typical life expectancy.

The invention of Factor VIII, a substance that, when injected, helped their blood to clot normally, had revolutionized thinking about longevity for America's 20,000 hemophiliacs. Before Factor VIII, a hemophiliac could expect two, maybe three, decades of a life crowded with visits to the hospital for voluminous transfusions. All the transfusions could do, however, was replace lost blood. Factor VIII, when injected into the blood with a clotting factor concentrated from thousands of blood donors, gave the necessary components that allowed the hemophiliac's blood to clot itself. The discovery gave the promise of a reasonably normal life span.

Bruce Evatt relished the optimism hemophiliacs shared. They organized, lobbied for research funding, and eagerly worked to improve their lot, not like people with cancer or chronic diseases who in despair just turned over and died.

Evatt's regard for hemophiliacs is what made the phone call from Florida so troubling in the first days of 1982. A Miami physician was convinced that Factor VIII had killed his patient, an aging hemophiliac who had died of *Pneumocystis* a few months ago. Couldn't the *Pneumocystis* protozoa have been transmitted in the clotting substance that his patient injected?

Evatt assured the doctor that the filtering process during Factor VIII preparation prevented the transmission of bacteria and protozoa. Of course, smaller microbes, like viruses, could make it through the filtering, giving hemophiliacs an inordinately high rate of, say, hepatitis B. But the *Pneumocystis* bug was big enough to be caught by the filters. Evatt's careful speech exuded an aura of kindliness; it was difficult not to believe his reassurance.

Once off the phone, however, Evatt's face folded downward toward the despairing thoughts he had been trying to hold off. Already, CDC staffers like Mary Guinan and Don Francis were predicting cases of gay pneumonia in hemophiliacs and blood transfusion recipients. This could not only be the first such case but it could provide some evidence that a virus was indeed responsible for the epidemic of immune deficiency among gay men. Evatt called the Food and Drug Administration, which has authority over blood products, to see whether they had heard of any similar problems. He also checked with the well-organized network of hemophiliac groups in case they had heard any reports of similar cases. None. Nor did Sandra Ford's records turn up any pentamidine orders for hemophiliac patients.

The Florida case itself was problematical. Although a biopsy did confirm the *Pneumocystis,* the man's death made it impossible to go for any more precise immune assay. Also, the doctors had made no autopsy, leaving the possibility that some undiagnosed tumor or lymph cancer had caused the immune suppression necessary for the pneumonia to take root.

Harold Jaffe of the Kaposi's Sarcoma and Opportunistic Infections Task Force explained the problems to CDC Director Bill Foege. An old hand at epidemiology, Foege appreciated the gravity of the case, not only for hemophiliacs and blood transfusion recipients but also for opening the way to finally nailing down *something* as the cause of the epidemic, even if it were only a generic label like *virus.* However, he knew there were too many variables.

"If it's real, there'll be another one," he told Jaffe. "And then we'll know."

Evatt told Sandy Ford to be alert for any pentamidine orders that might list hemophilia as an underlying medical condition, and the uneasy months of waiting began.

COPENHAGEN

Dr. Ib Bygbjerg had been back from Zaire for more than four years now, having returned in time to see his friend Grethe Rask die in late 1977. By early 1982, everybody in the hospital circuit was talking about the new diseases among gay men. Already, an American expert from the National Cancer Institute had been to Denmark to research the diseases. This must be something big; Danish scientists were rushing their first papers into print so they could beat out any NCI publication on the Aarhus studies.

As a tropical disease specialist, Bygbjerg had been called in late last year to treat his first case; before long, he was seeing them all, because the *Rigshospitalet* had already gained a reputation for its immunology work. As Bygbjerg, now thirty-six, studied the third Danish man to suffer from the strange gay syndrome, he was struck by a sense of déjà vu. This was so African. Here was a man whose intestines were being sucked dry by incorrigible amebic parasites, just like some

African bushman. And then there's this Kaposi's sarcoma, another disease he had seen only in Africa. There was an eerie feeling too when Bygbjerg's first KS patient died of *Pneumocystis,* and then another died of the same pneumonia. It was the protozoa Bygbjerg had wanted to study after the death of his friend Grethe, but his professors had dissuaded him with the assurance that there was no future in researching such a rare disease.

Instead, Bygbjerg had studied lymphocytes. He was glad he had, since the young men now falling ill with KS and PCP clearly had problems with their lymphocytes. The lymphocytes might even be a key to understanding what was causing their ailments, Bygbjerg thought.

But he couldn't get the notion out of his head that what was killing these men was somehow related to what had killed Grethe Rask. He still considered himself sworn to that promise he had made at the time of her death, that before he died he would understand what had taken her life. The *Pneumocystis* was a link between what was happening now and what had happened then, during the Feast of the Hearts and on the barren Jutland heath.

Bygbjerg approached his department chairman for authorization to publish a medical journal story about Grethe's death; maybe it was the piece to a larger puzzle that would help someone else see the full picture. For all they knew, it may have been in her body that some deadly new virus made its European debut.

Bygbjerg's superiors laughed off the eager young scientist's impulse to publish. You see tropical disease everywhere; you see Africa everywhere, they told him. Besides, they added, how could a disease of homosexual men with all those hundreds of sexual partners possibly be related to anything Grethe Rask might have? After all, as one friend pointed out later, the respected Dr. Rask was a lesbian who had never made any secret of her sexual orientation.

PARIS

The French study group, which Jacques Leibowitch and Willy Rozenbaum convened in early 1982, hadn't set out to discover the cause of the mysterious and still-unchristened epidemic. At first, they simply wanted to track the new diseases as they made their splashy entrances in various hospitals. Rozenbaum already had approached Parisian gay doctors but found that they simply did not believe that the new maladies were anything but some new plot to drive them underground. "Let us die," they told him. Rozenbaum decided to start his own epidemiological studies out of Claude-Bernard Hospital on the outskirts of Paris. He had set up his own hotline and would see as many patients as he could squeeze into a day. An unemployed epidemiologist looking for a gig, Jean Baptiste-Brunet, volunteered to follow the African cases in Paris. Leibowitch would keep in touch with other doctors around town.

What they had to offer, they figured, was a perspective unencumbered by America's preoccupation with divining who was homosexual and who wasn't. American scientists thought it odd to view the new epidemic as an African disease, but the French thought it unusual to view it as a homosexual disease. This was a disease that simply struck people, and it had to come from somewhere. The Parisian cases dated back three years before the first American patients, pointing toward an African genesis. Throughout northern Europe, evidence was rapidly accumulating for this theory. Belgian doctors also had been seeing *Pneumocystis* cases from such countries as Zaire and Uganda for four years.

January 6
CENTERS FOR DISEASE CONTROL
HEPATITIS LABORATORIES, PHOENIX

The horrible fever had swept seemingly from nowhere into the border region between Zaire and Sudan, on the fetid banks of the Ebola River. The disease was a blood-borne virus, wickedly spreading both through sexual intercourse, because infected lymphocytes were in victims' semen, and through the sharing of needles in local bush hospitals. The absence of modern precautions to protect doctors also spread the blood-borne disease among medical personnel through routes unimaginable in more civilized countries.

During this 1976 outbreak, local Danish doctors in the remote hospitals in Zaire, people like Ib Bygbjerg and Grethe Rask, were impressed with the vigor with which the team from the World Health Organization (WHO) had moved to stamp out this deadly disease that became known as Ebola Fever. When it became obvious that the disease was spreading through autopsies and ritual contact with corpses during the funerary process, Dr. Don Francis, on loan to the World Health Organization from the CDC, had simply banned local rituals and unceremoniously burned the corpses. Infected survivors were removed from the community and quarantined until it was clear that they could no longer spread the fever. Within weeks, the disease disappeared as mysteriously as it had come. The tribespeople were furious that their millennia-old rituals had been forbidden by these arrogant young doctors from other continents. The wounded anger twisted their faces.

On this day, as he contemplated the epidemic of immune deficiency, Don Francis could not escape the memories of the horrible Ebola Fever outbreak. The memories became particularly sharp when Francis received the Wednesday morning phone call from Dr. Guy de The in Paris, another veteran of African epidemics.

Dr. de The had reviewed the latest research from Africa. Of course, there was the stuff about the benign Kaposi's sarcoma, and Francis had already heard of the new, more virulent KS that had been reported first in Uganda in 1972. But there was more, de The said. In the western Nile district of Uganda, young men living together were getting not only the typical, easygoing Kaposi's sarcoma, but the nasty kind, like that tearing through the bodies of American homosexuals. These Africans also suffered from the lymphadenopathy that marked the early stages of the American disease, de The said. There had to be some connection.

Of course, Francis thought. A new virus from Africa. It was where Bob Gallo at the National Cancer Institute figured his new retrovirus for Human T-cell

Leukemia came from too. After all, HTLV only struck in the portions of Japan settled by Portuguese traders, who apparently had brought the microbe with them from Africa some 500 years ago. The African links reinforced Francis's hypothesis about a transmissible agent.

The talk also imbued him with a greater sense of urgency. Already, he was flying to Atlanta every few weeks to consult with the floundering Kaposi's Sarcoma and Opportunistic Infections Task Force. They had yet to be able to find any clue as to what caused this damn thing, and now their most important work, the case-control study, was hopelessly mired because they didn't have the staff and money to tabulate the questionnaires. The National Cancer Institute didn't seem terribly interested in the disease. The little bench work the cancer institute was doing focused on poppers and the sperm theory, the hypothesis that sperm deposited during sex was causing immune suppression. Although nitrate inhalants clearly did something to the body that wasn't good, the task force had all but eliminated them as a cause for the new syndrome. After all, there was nothing new about them. The sperm theory, which so enchanted the National Cancer Institute, seemed downright ludicrous to Francis. Gay men had been getting injected with sperm for centuries without getting Kaposi's sarcoma, not to mention the well-documented proclivity female heterosexuals hold for insemination.

Time is always the most formidable enemy in an epidemic, Francis thought. There wasn't time to hope that the undirected interest of the National Cancer Institute or the National Institute for Allergy and Infectious Diseases would some day fall on these new diseases. To get the serious bench work going now, Francis was plotting to set up his own laboratories to do the lab work that normally fell to the NCI. He just had to figure out how to pirate the money to pay for it.

The problems wouldn't end there, he knew, even if he nailed down what caused this disease. As he recalled the wounded faces in Sudan, he also knew that even greater difficulties lay ahead for control of the disease. Customs and rituals would have to be dramatically changed, and he knew from his hepatitis work in the gay community that customs involving sex were the most implacable behaviors to try to alter.

◯

The day after Don Francis got his phone call from Paris, Dr. Edward Brandt, who, as Assistant Secretary for Health, was the top-ranking health official in the federal government, dashed off a memo to the directors of the National Cancer Institute, the National Institute for Allergy and Infectious Diseases, and the National Institute on Drug Abuse. The Centers for Disease Control was short of funds for its research into KS and opportunistic infections. Could these better-funded agencies pick up some of the work?

The letter was in the form of a request, not an order. In the following weeks, it was simply ignored by the various chiefs of the National Institutes of Health in their comfortable offices in the rolling greens of Bethesda.

Meanwhile, across the country, researchers waited for word on the research money the National Cancer Institute had promised at the September meeting.

But it clearly was not forthcoming. The institute hadn't even issued the standard request for proposals (RFP) that call for applications for federal grants. Without an RFP, the NCI could not even begin to accept applications for the funds, much less review proposals and conduct the lengthy on-site visits required for doling out money.

Nobody at the National Cancer Institute seemed to be in much of a hurry. The new syndrome clearly was a very low priority, even as it was becoming clear to more and more people that it threatened calamity.

January 12
2 FIFTH AVENUE, NEW YORK CITY

In the meeting at Larry Kramer's apartment, everybody agreed that Paul Popham would be the ideal president of the new organization, Gay Men's Health Crisis, which was geared to raising money for gay cancer research. Some of the more salient reasons were left unspoken. Paul personified the successful Fire Island A-list gays who had never become involved in Manhattan's scruffy gay political scene. He'd help make working on this disease fashionable and something with more status than your typical gay crusade. He was also gorgeous, which would probably help attract volunteers. Unspoken too was the view that Larry Kramer's confrontational style would make him an unsuitable president of the group, even though he had taken a leading role in its organization. His very name was anathema among the crowd they needed to reach if they were to raise substantial funds. Larry had a half-crush on Paul anyway, so he joined the unanimous vote for Paul. After Paul's election, the board of directors of the new Gay Men's Health Crisis was selected, and it included Larry Kramer and Paul's longtime friend and Fire Island housemate, Enno Poersch.

The group had persuaded the Paradise Garage, one of the less popular discos, to hold an April benefit. That, they figured, would give them a chance to raise enough money for research and then they could fold up and get back to their lives. Privately, Paul had made it clear that he did not want his role in the organization to become public knowledge. Nobody at work knew he was gay, he said, and he wanted it to stay that way. Larry bit his tongue. He didn't want to be a scold about this, but Larry privately thought it boded poorly to have a president of the Gay Men's Health Crisis who did not want to say he was a gay man.

January 14
UNIVERSITY OF CALIFORNIA,
SAN FRANCISCO

Marc Conant told Cleve Jones that he needed advice from somebody political. They'd talk about it over dinner, but first there was someone Conant wanted Cleve to meet.

Simon Guzman smiled shyly at Cleve Jones when the young activist entered the room on the top floor of the UC Medical Center. As they talked, Simon pulled out a snapshot of himself from Before. Smooth brown skin was pulled taut over well-developed muscles. Clad only in a tight pair of yellow Speedos, Simon was everything that Cleve had considered hot; he knew he could have fallen for the hunky Mexican in the photo.

Simon Guzman's body now, however, was barely more than a skeleton with sallow, lesion-covered skin sagging loosely, and tubes coursing in every conceivable orifice and vein. Simon explained that he hadn't made many friends in his two years working as a printer in the suburb of Hayward. Yes, he had been popular but that kind of, uh, popularity didn't put one in line for best buddies, not in this time and place. Now he had this horrible diarrhea that wouldn't stop; the doctors couldn't even tell him what was causing it. He was embarrassed that his mother would learn he was gay because he had gay cancer, and sometimes he felt so alone he wished he would just die. It would be over then.

Cleve left the room feeling sick to his stomach. He wanted a drink.

This was real; this was the future.

⬭

Over dinner, Conant began carefully laying out what he saw ahead. He had been thinking about this since he left the National Cancer Institute meeting in September. The forty-four-year-old dermatologist leaned back in his chair. His face showed a certain weariness, but his voice never quavered. He was going through his lecture with a slow, smooth southern cadence that subtly revealed his roots in Jacksonville, Florida. Years of giving lectures as a clinical professor at UCSF had also taught him how to meter his sentences and pause to let a significant piece of information sink in.

This is an infectious disease, Conant began. The CDC case-control study may offer some definitive word on how it was spread, but that research was stalled, probably for lack of resources. We are losing time, and time is the enemy in any epidemic. *The disease is moving even if the government isn't.*

It was at this dinner that Cleve Jones first heard the technical jargon that would become the stuff of his nightmares in the years ahead—terms like geometric progression and exponential increases. Some scientist had come up with a new name for the syndrome: Gay-Related Immune Deficiency, or GRID. Conant, however, wasn't sure how gay-related this immune deficiency would stay. Viruses tended not to respect such artificial divisions among humans. Lymphocytes were lymphocytes, and clearly they were major taste treats for the new virus, whether they happened to live in gay bodies or straight.

"This is going to be a world-class disaster," Conant said. "And nobody's paying attention."

Cleve's thoughts had drifted off while he merged Conant's frightening tale of a new virus with what he knew about gay community sexual mores; hell, with what he knew about his own sexual exploits. His face turned white, and he ordered a drink.

"We're all dead," Cleve said.

Conant let the comment pass. Of course, he had harbored just such suspicions, but the gay community didn't have time to dawdle in despair. He had a plan and he needed Cleve's help.

They needed some kind of foundation, like the American Cancer Society or something, that could get warnings out to gay men and pressure the government for more research funds. In New York, gay men were trying to pay for research themselves, Conant noted. That was stupid because no private fundraising could ever begin to hold a candle to what the government could pour into research with the stroke of a pen. But the Washington money wasn't coming. It was just business as usual there even while the number of cases escalated.

This shows us that for the short term, we can't rely on Washington to save our lives, Conant said. Until the government gets going, it's going to be up to this community to save itself.

"This is the big one," he sighed. "There isn't going to be anything bigger than this."

Still, Conant told how little cooperation he had found in the gay community. He already had called the local gay churches for help in distributing brochures. They weren't interested, saying it might panic their parishioners. Gay business groups weren't interested in financing efforts that many considered alarmist. Selma Dritz, of course, was getting word out that an extremely serious health threat was coalescing, but Dritz had spent so many years warning gay men about this or that peril that it was easy to overlook her talk about GRID.

Cleve knew just where the conversation was heading, so Conant wasted no time in guiding him there. Cleve was probably the only gay leader who could claim his own personal constituency without having a title in any club or group. He was a minister without portfolio. The guys on Castro Street trusted him. Cleve also knew how to work the political system for money and favors, two things gays would be needing lots of when this GRID epidemic took off. Cleve took a last sip on his vodka tonic and sensed vaguely that he was making a commitment that would take more from him than a few nights of meetings. Then he recalled the shriveling Simon Guzman and the photograph of the man in the yellow Speedos. He stared into the melting ice and twisted lime at the bottom of his glass and said softly, "Count me in."

Marc Conant persuaded his lawyer to start writing the necessary incorporation papers for a nonprofit group called the Kaposi's Sarcoma Education and Research Foundation while Cleve Jones touched bases with political leaders. Cleve expected an enthusiastic burst of support from Pat Norman, who, as the director of the Office of Lesbian and Gay Health in the health department, was the titular leader for all things health-related among homosexuals in San Francisco. Instead, she fidgeted nervously during their meeting. We don't want to panic people, she said. She outlined the potential problems: Not only could gays be panicked but this could be manipulated to fuel an anti-gay backlash. She would see to it that appropriate information got out appropriately once she consulted various gay community leaders and arrived at a consensus agreement that what they said was . . . appropriate. For the first six months of the epidemic, Cleve knew, this meant saying almost nothing at all.

Cleve understood the dual concerns of reassuring the homosexuals while not inflaming anti-gay prejudice. Given what he knew about this epidemic, however, this twenty-six-year-old street organizer thought a little panic might be appropriate for gay men. It seemed appropriate because very few were paying even the slightest attention to the small dribble of news coverage leaking out about gay cancer and gay pneumonia.

Cleve had dinner with the KS patient he had met in December, Bobbi Campbell, the registered nurse. Bobbi and Jim Geary, a volunteer grief counselor with a Berkeley death-and-dying group called the Shanti Project, had started a rap group of KS patients, held every Wednesday night in various patients' homes. The seven-year-old Shanti Project based its approach on the works of the death guru, Elisabeth Kübler-Ross, and had been drifting without much direction in recent years. The weekly support group and Conant's KS clinic, however, were about the only services available to those stricken with the terrifyingly novel diseases. It was clear to Bobbi Campbell that as the numbers of ailing grew, many more services would be necessary, including home-health care, hospices, and massive education for the gay community.

"Nobody's doing anything," Bobbi told Cleve. "We've got to get people organized."

Cleve's time soon became split between his new work on Kaposi's sarcoma and his continuing lobbying for passage of a statewide gay rights bill sponsored by his boss, Assemblyman Art Agnos. On free weekends, he cuddled with his old boyfriend, Felix Velarde-Munoz, or with Frank, his Long Beach affair. Frank sometimes had to cancel their occasional dates, complaining of fatigue. Felix was distracted when Cleve started talking about gay cancer and seemed out of sorts lately. None of this made sense until much later; in the opening months of 1982, it was just background noise in Cleve's life, like the drone of city trolleys that you heard but never listened to.

February
LOS ANGELES

By the time Dr. Joel Weisman had called Dave Auerbach, the CDC's field man with the Los Angeles County Department of Public Health, word had also leaked from the West Hollywood Health Center that there appeared to be a number of links between the early GRID cases in Los Angeles and the heavily gay beach town of Laguna Beach in neighboring Orange County.

Auerbach then started interviewing all the GRID cases in the county. It was somewhere in these interviews that he first heard about the Air Canada steward.

There were so many airline stewards whose names came up in the investigation, Auerbach would always be grateful that this steward had an unusual appellation that stuck firmly in his mind. It was hard to forget a name like Gaetan Dugas.

St. Luke's-Roosevelt Hospital, New York City

The lab tests were so uniform that there was no denying their validity. Dr. Michael Lange had recruited the subjects from the Gay Men's Health Crisis, Columbia Student Health Service, and the gay students group at Columbia University, thinking he could get some measure of cytomegalovirus among sexually active gay men and perhaps find some link between CMV and GRID. The CMV connection was not nearly as pronounced in the first lab tests as the amazing deficiencies these men almost uniformly showed in their immune systems. Four out of five of the gay men he tested had a serious depletion in their T-helper lymphocytes. They may not be showing overt signs of gay cancer yet, Lange figured, but substantial numbers of gay men clearly have something wrong with their immune systems, and there is a disaster of great proportions lurking ahead.

Unsettling news came from every borough. Haitians were showing up at Brooklyn hospitals with toxoplasmosis, the same brain infection that had so mercilessly killed Enno Poersch's lover, Nick, just a year ago. A number of them also contracted *Pneumocystis,* implying a connection with GRID. The Haitians adamantly insisted they were heterosexual.

There were also more junkies coming down with gay pneumonia in the Bronx. At the Albert Einstein College of Medicine, Dr. Arye Rubinstein was trying in vain to get his colleagues to believe that the sick babies he was seeing were also victims of GRID. Rubinstein had sent his research paper to the *New England Journal of Medicine,* but he received no reply. He knew this was not unusual given the snail's pace of scientific publishing. But other scientists were saying that Rubinstein's hypothesis was improbable if not altogether impossible. By its very name, GRID was a homosexual disease, not a disease of babies or their mothers.

Michael Lange also found little support or encouragement for his GRID studies. He was spending tens of thousands of dollars on the expensive lymphocyte tests but had no grant money to pay for them. His already harried staff had to volunteer time for the research. Colleagues, meanwhile, counseled Lange to get off this GRID kick and return to serious lab research.

"This is nothing," he was told on several occasions. "It will disappear. You're getting off the path. Get back to research."

Lange was, they warned, threatening his scientific career with these diversions.

The young doctor wondered whether he would get such advice if an analogous epidemic was striking anyone other than homosexuals. He persevered, hoping that the National Cancer Institute or the CDC would kick in money soon. Money, he knew, had a way of bringing respectability to areas of scientific investigation.

February 22
CENTERS FOR DISEASE CONTROL
HEPATITIS LABORATORIES
PHOENIX

Don Francis had dreaded this conversation for months, although he was hardly surprised. Francis had been spending the first months of 1982 agitating for more money for lab research into GRID and wanted to start injecting primates to see whether he could track down a virus. He was convinced that some virus was behind the disease, and they'd never get to controlling it if they didn't first prove this key point. Francis wanted to use chimpanzees because their immune system was most like humans'; chimps also were the most expensive lab animals, running about $50,000 each. As chief of the Center for Infectious Diseases, Dr. Walter Dowdle was in charge of the GRID budget at the CDC, so he had to give Don Francis the depressing news on the phone.

"There is no money," he said. "This is a worst-case situation."

When Francis got off the phone, he was relieved that he was still in Phoenix and not Atlanta. He was in charge here. He called Bud the handyman and started detailing the tasks that needed to be done. Walls needed to be torn out; new labs needed to be constructed. The money will have to come from somewhere, Francis thought. Even if it cost him his job, he'd push on.

In Atlanta, staffers at the KSOI Task Force fielded calls daily from health officials eager to hear the results of the case-control study. In the highly competitive scientific world, it didn't take long for some to speculate that the CDC might be holding out their research for publication. The glory of getting their studies in, say, the *New England Journal of Medicine* might be good for a few million in research grants, everybody knew. It was almost easier for the CDC to let this gossip float than confess to the truth, that they couldn't release the results because they didn't have the nickels and dimes to hire their own statistician. Even while health officials like Selma Dritz were desperate for the study's results to see whether there was anything she could do to curtail the spread of the disease, all the task force doctors could do was assure callers that the information would be forthcoming. And week after week after week, they told everybody to call back next week.

Promising areas of investigation also were being ignored for lack of money. Sitting on somebody's desk at the CDC was the proposal from Paul O'Malley, an earnest health inspector who had headed up the San Francisco branch of the CDC's hepatitis study. In recent months, as he'd been wrapping up the hepatitis work, he stumbled across an interesting phenomenon. An inordinate number of GRID victims were among the 7,000 local gay men who took part in the hepatitis study. Of the first twenty-four GRID cases in San Francisco, in fact, eleven were in the hepatitis B cohort. O'Malley talked to Don Francis and came away agreeing that GRID could be the work of some blood-borne virus that was spread through sex. O'Malley also knew that the CDC had stored blood samples from these 7,000 men in the refrigerators of the Phoenix hepatitis lab.

This hepatitis cohort probably presents the best group in the world to study for this disease, O'Malley figured. Not only are years of their medical pasts sealed in little vials in government refrigerators, but they filled out questionnaires that detailed all their sexual habits. Most still lived in town and could be followed for the next few years to see what happens to them.

Who comes down with this disease and who doesn't? Can they go back to those blood samples from 1978 and 1979 and find where this thing started? How is it spreading? The most important clues to this epidemic could be in the CDC's own refrigerators, and they just hadn't looked.

O'Malley enthusiastically told Harold Jaffe of the CDC Task Force all about this in early 1982. Jaffe said he'd try to pry loose some funds for the study.

Two years later, he did.

⊂⊃

In late February, the Centers for Disease Control reported that 251 Americans had contracted GRID across the country; 99 had died.

February 25

The story of the first *Wall Street Journal* piece on the epidemic would later be cited in journalism reviews as emblematic of how the media handled AIDS in the first years of the epidemic. The reporter, it turned out, had long been pressuring editors to run a story on the homosexual disorder. He had even written a piece in 1981 that the editors refused to print. Finally, the reporter was able to fashion an article around the twenty-three heterosexuals, largely intravenous drug users, who were now counted among GRID patients. With confirmation of bona fide heterosexuals, the story finally merited sixteen paragraphs deep in the largest-circulation daily newspaper in the United States, under the headline: "New, Often-Fatal Illness in Homosexuals Turns Up in Women, Heterosexual Males."

The gay plague got covered only because it finally had struck people who counted, people who were not homosexuals.

UNIVERSITY OF CALIFORNIA, SAN FRANCISCO

At the Kaposi's Sarcoma Clinic, doctors raced to save lives and devise treatments for diseases that had never appeared in the textbooks. Donald Abrams, who, at thirty-one, was the youngest doctor on the GRID team, was strongly asserting that clinicians had to drop the time-tested use of chemotherapy on these KS patients. That might be what the experts tell you to do, he maintained, but the textbooks were all written before GRID. Chemotherapy worked only because it kept cells from dividing. Since cancer cells, by definition, divided most rapidly, the therapy frequently slowed the cancer. But it also slowed the normal cells that were supposed to divide, such as in the mouth, the gastrointestinal tract, and most significantly, the blood. Chemotherapy might kill the cancer, but it would also stop the lymphocytes from growing; it might kill the patient, Abrams warned. In other cities, particularly New York, the experts weren't interested in what some thirty-one-year-old whippersnapper from San Francisco had to say, so the chemotherapy continued and patients died. The experience of the San Francisco clinic was beginning to outpace that of any other hospital because it concentrated patients in one place, and soon the clinic began exploring other drugs.

Already, even in those early months, work at the clinic was taking on a nightmarish quality as stunned doctors watched patient after patient develop some new horrifying aspect of the disease before sinking toward a miserable death. For Marc Conant, Paul Volberding, and Don Abrams, few of the declines were as petrifying as that of Simon Guzman. Simon appeared to be suffering from an attack of lymph cancer in his brain, the first time the doctors had detected such a disease in a GRID patient. The Kaposi's sarcoma, meanwhile, was relentless. With his once-handsome face completely disfigured by the Kaposi's lesions and his body swollen by medications, Simon had taken on the appearance of the bloated and scarred Elephant Man. Abrams started taking monthly photos of his face to study how the disease progressed.

There was also the problem of Simon's rampant diarrhea. Repeated tests revealed nothing. Finally, an Air Force laboratory sent back test results that left the UCSF experts speechless. Simon was infected with cryptosporidium, a parasite that normally inhabits the bowels of sheep. As far as anybody knew, the diagnosis marked the first time that any human being had ever been reported to be suffering from cryptosporidiosis.

When Selma Dritz heard the report at one of the weekly discussion meetings after the KS Clinic, she felt a keen scientific thrill. This, she knew, was the cutting edge of health sciences, hearing about the first human case of a disease. She also perceived, for the first time, an even deeper dimension to the dread that lay behind the thirty-five reported GRID cases in San Francisco. The mere numbers she tabulated and the arrows and circles on the blackboard did not begin to tell the stories of the human suffering they were seeing today and the appalling misery they undoubtedly would see tomorrow.

On a hunch, one of Simon Guzman's doctors tracked down the preeminent expert of cryptosporidium at the agriculture department of the University of Iowa. Of course, he was very familiar with the cryptosporidium parasite, the Iowa professor said. The San Francisco doctor was relieved; maybe there was some easy treatment.

"What do you do with sheep that get this?" he asked eagerly.

"There is no treatment," the expert said. "We shoot them."

13 PATIENT ZERO

March 3, 1982
CENTERS FOR DISEASE CONTROL,
ATLANTA

Don Francis viewed his life as an accumulation of chance decisions that had put him in the right place at the right time. When he followed his first wife to Los Angeles, he was lucky that L.A. County–University of Southern California Medical Center Hospital was near her house and was the first place he applied for a residency, because that put him under the tutelage of Dr. Paul Wehrle, a former CDC staffer, who urged Francis to join the CDC's Epidemiological Intelligence Service as an alternative to conscientious objector work. By chance, the CDC sent Francis to Sudan, where he was able to help wipe out smallpox, giving him, at the age of thirty-three, an accomplishment he figured he would never be able to surpass. After Africa, he followed a new girlfriend to Boston and ended up studying feline leukemia virus at the Harvard School of Public Health. The CDC had hurriedly pulled Francis away from these studies to handle Ebola Fever virus. After subsequently completing his doctorate on retroviruses, Francis's next CDC assignment sent him to Phoenix, where he worked with the gay community as lab director for the CDC's hepatitis study.

By chance after chance, Don Francis felt he had been delivered to this moment in early March 1982 when it all fit together. The retrovirology, the cat leukemia, the experience with African epidemics, and long work with the gay community—it all let him see something very clearly. His object on this day at the Public Health Service's first conference on GRID was to inform concisely the representatives of the National Institutes of Health as to what was happening and, hopefully, to enlist their help.

Like many of the CDC doctors, Francis was incredulous that the National Cancer Institute was still fiddling around with half-baked theories that GRID was caused by poppers or sperm. But those were the presentations the NIH researchers made at the conference. None of them was talking about what Francis thought was the most obvious cause, a new viral agent.

During a lunch break, Francis dashed to the library and photocopied the study he had made on feline leukemia with Max Essex back at Harvard. As one of the most eminent virologists at the CDC, Francis was slated to give the last lecture of the day; he wanted to have impact.

The thirty-nine-year-old researcher presented two charts. The first traced the epidemiological work he had done in Harvard on feline leukemia. The seminal work was familiar to most in the small CDC auditorium, but Francis repeated it carefully in his soft, northern California voice to let the significance sink in.

There were 134 cats in his study, 73 of which were infected with feline leukemia virus. Of these, 63 contracted lymphomas, cancers, or various blood disorders. Only 1 was alive and healthy. Of the 61 noninfected cats, only 2 developed lymph cancer and 21 others fell ill of other causes, while most were healthy and alive. Infection with just one virus, in this case a retrovirus, could cause immune suppression that would lead to cancers and a laundry list of diseases, Francis stressed.

He pointed to his other chart, which listed the risk groups for hepatitis B, most notably the categories of gay men and intravenous drug users. Preliminary data from the case-control study showed that the risk factors were virtually identical for GRID and hepatitis, Francis said. Numbers of partners, attendance at gay bathhouses, and passive anal intercourse all seemed predictors of GRID, just as they were for hepatitis.

"Combine these two diseases—feline leukemia and hepatitis—and you have the immune deficiency," said Francis.

To Francis, the conclusions were obvious. Blood products were likely to show evidence of contamination next, and substantial lab work needed to be done to track down the viral culprit so that work on treatments and vaccines could begin. The CDC also needed to launch some educational campaigns among gays to prevent the disease.

Although most in the CDC Task Force had long been persuaded by Francis's arguments, the response from the experts at the National Institutes of Health was underwhelming. Don sensed that the various institutes felt he was making a pitch for CDC supremacy in GRID studies and that his theory was simply a way to divert research funds from the National Institutes of Health to the CDC. Clearly, the NIH doctors were going to steer their own course through the epidemic. His ideas, they told him, were, um, interesting.

He might as well be talking to a wall, thought Francis as he took down the charts. Their arrogance would cost lives, and there was nothing he could do.

CHINATOWN, LOS ANGELES

"If we don't eat, we'll be worthless."

Bill Darrow and Dave Auerbach had spent another exhausting day doing interviews on the reported connections between the first GRID cases in Los Angeles. They were supposed to be in Orange County by 8:30 that night, and it was nearly 8 P.M. already and they were still downtown. Auerbach was glad that Darrow opted for tardiness over hunger, and the pair trekked to Chinatown for some quick Mandarin food. Auerbach also was glad to have Darrow in L.A. from the CDC headquarters in Atlanta because Darrow, a sociologist, had such a keen memory. He could remember names and connections that went years back. His gentle, professorial manner also worked well in the long interviews during which gay men were asked to reveal everybody with whom they had gone to bed over the past few years.

Auerbach had returned today to that intriguing lead about the French-Canadian airline steward. His name had come up three times. But all the reports came from lovers of deceased patients, not from anybody who had actually slept with Gaetan Dugas themselves. Gaetan, of course, was just one of three airline stewards involved in this clustering. The air bridges between Los Angeles, New York, and San Francisco clearly had helped spread this virus around the country at breakneck speed.

◯

When Auerbach and Darrow finally arrived in Orange County, they were forty-five minutes late. The ailing hairdresser they were to interview led them through his well-appointed living room to a picnic table he had in the kitchen. The man was suffering from Kaposi's sarcoma. It didn't take him long to get straight to the point.

"I bet I know how I got this thing," he said directly. "I had sex with this attractive guy I had met at a bathhouse. He came over and spent the weekend. He came back to Los Angeles for a few more weekends, even stayed here for Thanksgiving, and then I never saw him again. He gave me hepatitis, and I bet he gave me this new disease too."

The man paused and then admitted, "I'm still quite fond of him."

He rustled through a book for the man's address and phone number.

"Gaetan Dugas," the man said. "He's an airline steward, and here's how you can reach him."

Bill Darrow dropped his pencil.

Auerbach shot a glance at him. The man could tell from the meaningful looks between the two epidemiologists that he had said the magic word.

He had. Finally, Auerbach and Darrow had a live person telling them he had had sex with this flight attendant. It was, Darrow said later, one of the most significant moments of the epidemic. The ball had dropped on the game show.

◯

The connections started falling into place. Of the first nineteen cases of GRID in Los Angeles, four had had sex with Gaetan Dugas. Another four cases, meanwhile, had gone to bed with people who had had sex with Dugas, establishing sexual links between nine of the nineteen Los Angeles cases. Moreover, the links bore out Don Francis's fears about the virus having a long latency period. For example, the Orange County man Darrow and Auerbach had interviewed did not show symptoms until August 1981, some ten months after Gaetan spent the weekend with him on Thanksgiving 1980. Another Los Angeles man found his first Kaposi's sarcoma lesions thirteen months after he had slept with the French-Canadian during a trip Gaetan made to southern California in February 1980.

Darrow wanted to get back to New York City so he could attempt to track this flight attendant's Manhattan escapades, but first, he made a side trip to San Francisco to see Selma Dritz's blackboard with its arrows and circles.

Like public health officers across the country, Dritz was anxiously waiting for the case-control study and couldn't fathom what was taking the CDC so long in getting this crucial information out. She was intrigued, however, when Darrow walked into her office, glanced at her blackboard and announced, "I've got nine."

Dritz immediately recognized two other Orange County names as people who lived part-time in San Francisco. At least one San Francisco KS patient had had sex with them. Again, there were the dual sentiments with which Dritz was getting so familiar during this epidemic. On one hand, there was an exhilaration when some new connection arose, some insight was gained. And there was the second, sinking feeling of despair that Selma could feel settling into her stomach now. Yes, this was intellectually exciting, but every insight only revealed more bad news, portending greater disaster ahead.

◯

On March 19, 1982, the Centers for Disease Control reported 285 cases of GRID in seventeen states. Half the cases were diagnosed in New York City and about a quarter of the cases lived in California. Five other nations, all in Europe, also reported cases of the diseases.

CENTERS FOR DISEASE CONTROL, ATLANTA

Bill Darrow called in daily to Harold Jaffe with all the latest scoops about where his cluster study was leading him. Every day added some new twist to the story, and Jaffe felt as though he were beginning to know all the victims and their lives from the complicated interrelationships Darrow mapped out. The sexual politics and, in Los Angeles, the political links with a big fund-raising dinner in 1979 seemed interwoven with these stories of party people who so casually leaped continents for their pleasures. It was like a transcontinental homosexual soap opera. The links also provided a development that, at last, *meant* something.

Darrow's work in the cluster study began coming in at the same time computer tabulations were finally being completed on the CDC's case-control study. That would be the way the CDC Task Force worked during this year of gathering darkness; no sooner was one issue laid to rest than a larger and more troubling crisis would develop, adding a new level of confusion to what had only briefly seemed resolved.

The cluster study had just that effect on the case-control study. The long-awaited comparison with GRID cases and their controls had turned up exactly what CDC Task Force members had noted in their first talks with patients last July. Patients tended to have twice the sexual contacts as the controls and to draw these contacts from among other promiscuous men, because they were far more likely to go to gay bathhouses for sexual recreation. A typical GRID case had sex with 1,100 men in his lifetime; a few counted as many as 20,000 sexual contacts. There were also correlates of having syphilis and other sexually transmitted diseases, as well as higher levels of drug use among cases, but these seemed more a part of the fast-lane life-style than predicators of immune suppression itself. The study nixed the notion that poppers or any environmental factor was behind GRID, given the fact that both cases and controls used the inhalants and were exposed to virtually the same environmental factors.

Just as this information convinced most at the CDC that GRID was a sexually transmitted disease, the Los Angeles cluster of cases added a dimension to their understanding of the epidemic. The clusters proved not only that the disease had a long incubation period between infection with the virus and the manifestation of the disease, but that carriers could spread the disease during that period. A latent carrier state of between three to six months had enabled hepatitis B to rage out of control in the major gay urban centers; the carrier state for GRID clearly was much longer, allowing even greater potential for spread by unsuspecting transmitters.

○

"Semen depositors," said Mary Guinan. "We've got to talk about semen depositors."

This became Guinan's crusade at the CDC in the spring of 1982. She talked about semen depositors the way Don Francis talked about cat leukemia. It was the logical inference from the information now bursting forth from Guinan's research.

No sooner had she convinced the CDC that intravenous drug users were indeed a category of GRID cases separate from gay men, than her field of investigations discovered the first reported GRID cases among prisoners and prostitutes. Guinan had already spent most of the spring in methadone clinics interviewing male heroin addicts and their girlfriends to establish the blood transmission of GRID among junkies sharing needles, and the subsequent heterosexual transmission from the addicts to their girlfriends. The first prison reports, however, took the attractive blond researcher to the small interview chambers of maximum security prisons.

Guards were reluctant to leave Guinan alone in the rooms with the prisoners, but she officiously insisted on one-to-one interviews, aware that she needed the most candid conversations possible if she was going to get anywhere tracking this epidemic. With prisoners that meant serious probing about their penitentiary sex lives.

"Have you ever been raped?" Guinan would ask in her frankest Brooklyn accent.

"I have lots of friends here," said one prisoner matter-of-factly. "They know I'll kill somebody if they touch me."

Guinan believed him.

The blank stares that answered Guinan's questions about poppers and fisting also indicated that those two predilections, however common among the gay patients, were unknown to these heterosexuals. Moreover, blood sampling of the intravenous drug users also revealed that, although many were infected with cytomegalovirus, the viral strains were all different. This was strong evidence that this herpes virus, which many scientists considered a strong candidate for being a causative agent, had not developed some new virulent strain. No single strain emerged, lending further weight to Don Francis's hypothesis that a new virus, not CMV, was at work.

Even as this medical hypothesis was eliminated, however, more mystery grew around the clinical manifestations of GRID in intravenous drug users. Although they suffered from the same depletion of T-4 lymphocyte cells that marked all the immune deficiency patients, they were not getting Kaposi's sarcoma. Instead, they'd get *Pneumocystis* or some other opportunistic infection. Only gay men seemed to be getting the skin cancer. This led to the suspicion that KS itself may progress from a separate cause, perhaps stimulated by some uniquely gay factor like poppers, after another virus did the initial immune busting.

Human mysteries compounded these growing medical mysteries. There was, for example, the first case of Kaposi's sarcoma in an otherwise healthy woman. The woman, a registered nurse, spurned Guinan's requests for an interview. Guinan persisted with the investigation, however. It was of national significance because it could mark the first GRID case in a health care worker. With GRID so precisely targeting the other high-risk groups for hepatitis B, federal officials held their breaths in fear of cases among health care personnel, who also were a high-risk group for hepatitis because of needle-stick injuries and blood contact. What kind of care would GRID patients get if their physicians and nurses thought they could contract the disease as easily as hepatitis B?

The nurse, it turned out, didn't want to talk because she had just gone through a nasty divorce with her husband. There were some private issues she didn't want to get into. Guinan began to understand when she traced the nurse's employment records and found that she had recently worked as a nurse in a prison. Circumstantial evidence indicated sexual transmission, and health care workers, it seemed, were safe. At least for now.

By March, ten women had contracted GRID, and Guinan's research confirmed that nearly all of them had sex with somebody in a high-risk group: a bisexual man or, most typically, a drug addict. These cases and stories like that of the prison nurse led Mary to her repeated lectures about "semen depositors." That was the key to understanding this epidemic, she said, not homosexuals. This disease was being spread through sex by people depositing their infected semen in sundry orifices of their partners. In gay men, the deposits that could get into the bloodstream seemed to be made mostly in the rectum; vaginal deposits clearly were spreading this disease among heterosexual women. Gays were just getting it more frequently because they were more active sexually and they had institutions like bathhouses that were virtual Federal Reserve Banks for massive semen deposition. The major question that remained was not whether heterosexuals would get this disease but how fast. Men could give it to women, but how efficiently could women, without semen to deposit, give it to men?

March 14
NEW YORK CITY

Jim Curran flew in from Atlanta to address the organizational meeting of the New York Physicians for Human Rights, a Manhattanized version of the four-year-old San Francisco gay doctors group. New York City Health Commissioner David Sencer, a former CDC director, had made his appearance among the 250 lesbian and gay physicians, medical students, and health professionals and was chatting casually about syphilis and gonorrhea. When it came time for the diminutive Curran to speak, he climbed on top of a chair and paused briefly as he surveyed the crowd.

Here was a cohort of physicians who were all roughly his age, in their mid-thirties, or even younger, and by now he knew what they would be spending their entire lives doing. They may not know it, Curran thought, but with the preliminary data from the case-control study and Bill Darrow's stories of the Los Angeles clusters, it was clear to Curran that all of them now had their lives inextricably bound to this phenomenon.

Curran started with his standard rap about the iceberg and how the KS and *Pneumocystis* cases were just the tip and people with swollen lymph nodes were in the middle, and how there was probably this vast reservoir of asymptomatic but infected people out there. Curran had said all this before in the matter-of-fact, midwestern way that people from Michigan talk. His voice became more tenuous as he began to escort the group from Before to After.

"It isn't going away," he said. "Even if we find a causative virus or other agent, it will be considerable time, probably years, before we can develop a vaccine or some strategy to eradicate it. We are in for a long haul."

Curran scanned the young faces that had suddenly grown so still.

"It's likely we'll be working on this for much of our careers," he said, "if not most of our lives."

Later, many of the doctors confided to each other that Curran was being a bit hysterical.

Meanwhile, at the fledgling Gay Men's Health Crisis, fights flared unpredictably between Paul Popham and Larry Kramer, such as on the night the committee received the 10,000 invitations for its upcoming April disco fund-raiser, "Showers." Paul Popham, the new president, was incensed that the invitation's return address included "Gay Men's Health Crisis."

"We can't mail this out," said Paul.

Nobody else could figure out why he was so upset.

"It says gay on it," he fumed. "You can't send something to people that has the word 'gay' on it. What if they're not out of the closet?"

Larry Kramer was not terribly sympathetic. Besides, the invitations already were late. They needed to get them out right away.

"We can strike it out with a magic marker," Paul suggested.

"Ten thousand invitations?" Larry asked.

"What about my mailman?" Paul finally burst. "He's going to know I'm gay."

Kramer was incredulous.

"What about your doorman?" he shot back. "You drag tricks up to your apartment every night. Don't you think your doorman suspects something? Why aren't you worried about him?"

The invitations were mailed out, but Kramer wondered about what would happen later, when this community really needed something and the people who were supposed to do the demanding were so ashamed of themselves that they didn't even want their mailmen to know they were gay.

CENTERS FOR DISEASE CONTROL, ATLANTA

During the final weeks of March 1982, the pace quickened in the labyrinthine corridors of the red brick Building 6 of the CDC in Atlanta. The ten people assigned to the task force barely had time to write up a new development before the epidemic took another unexpected turn that had them racing to catch up again. The latest crisis had started with sporadic reports to the CDC's parasitic disease division of toxoplasmosis in Haitians, first in Miami and then in New York City. At first, parasitologists thought this was some problem unique to the malnourished refugees who had come from the most impoverished nation in the Western Hemisphere. Others remembered reports of strange cases of toxoplasmosis among gay men in the early cases.

Dr. Harry Haverkos of the KSOI Task Force flew from Atlanta to Miami and reviewed the Haitians' medical records. The refugees were suffering not only from toxoplasmosis but also *Pneumocystis* and severe disseminated tuberculosis. There were fewer cases of Kaposi's than among gay men, but some biopsies had confirmed that diagnosis nevertheless. The patients themselves presented yet a new scene in the unfolding horror show. They tended to die quicker than the gay men Haverkos had seen, and their wasting was far more striking. He came back convinced: The Haitians had GRID.

This new risk group presented still more mysteries to the task force, which was only beginning to fathom the unknowns behind GRID cases diagnosed a year ago. There was talk of voodoo rituals that might allow blood transmissions. Investigations were made difficult by language barriers and the suspicions Haitians had of anything governmental, a not unlikely tendency after life under one of the most ruthless dictators the U.S. government had ever financed. In their crisp Creole, the patients muttered to interpreters that Haverkos, an Ohioan with a penchant for polychromatic plaid jackets, was a CIA agent. Haverkos found it nearly impossible to track down family members or friends because all the refugees had come to America illegally and few patients were willing to risk their friends' deportation.

Were these people really gay, having picked up the disease from vacationing New Yorkers? Had they given it to gay Manhattan men on holiday? Was the disease spreading through ritualistic scarring that might engender blood transmission? Haverkos was already working with Mary Guinan on prisoners and keeping track of possible cases among hemophiliacs. He had taken the Miami trip on what was supposed to be a week off between studies. He quickly mapped out a case-control study that the CDC should conduct on the Haitians. Whatever they held in common with gay men and intravenous drug users might give scientists the key to the epidemic.

As with so much in this year of lost opportunity, however, Haverkos's proposal languished among the many other projects left undone because the CDC didn't have enough money. By the time the study was begun two years later, everybody already knew what was causing the disease and the research became an academic exercise that provided interesting, but not essential, information.

◯

"Give us something else," the reporters begged Haverkos.

It was their standard line. Haverkos translated it to mean, "Give us something about the epidemic that doesn't involve gays." The science writers insisted their editors wouldn't hear of writing stories about gay diseases and gay sex. They needed an angle that was, well, legitimate. Haverkos had noted that the story didn't make the *Wall Street Journal* until it had a heterosexual angle. He wondered how reporters could honestly try to get around the fact that for all the new risk groups emerging, gay men still composed the greatest proportion of GRID cases. He also knew, of course, that lack of coverage was the most obvious single reason studies like his Haitian protocol would be left undone. Without the media to watch the federal government, the budget people would be left to finance GRID research as they saw fit. In an administration committed to cutting domestic spending, that meant virtually no funding at all.

New York University
Medical Center, New York City

Gaetan Dugas seemed quite pleased with himself as he rattled off his sexual exploits to Bill Darrow. Darrow had tracked down Gaetan through Alvin Friedman-Kien. All my beautiful lovers, the airline steward seemed to be saying, rather proudly. He paused for a moment before asking a question in what Darrow thought was too naive a tone.

"Why are you interested in all these people?"

"Some of them have been diagnosed with this immune deficiency and some haven't. We want to find out why some get the disease and others don't."

Gaetan's face dropped. He looked stunned, as if a new and horrible idea had only now taken residence in his mind.

"You mean I may have been passing this around?" he asked.

"Yeah," Darrow said, surprised that Gaetan hadn't thought of it before. "You may be passing it around or you might have gotten it from someone else."

The last part of Darrow's comment, it turned out, would probably have been best left unsaid given Gaetan's subsequent activities.

March 25
SAN FRANCISCO

After the last heart attack, Simon P. Guzman's body struggled three painful minutes before surrendering to the inevitable shortly after 11 A.M. He was the eleventh man to die in the GRID epidemic in San Francisco. His death certificate marked the first time that cryptosporidiosis, a disease of sheep, was listed as a cause of death for a human being.

March 30
ATLANTA

The NCAA basketball play-offs were starting on the tube, but Harold Jaffe had more than sports on his mind when he invited Paul Weisner over to the watch the game. As chief of the CDC's venereal disease division, Weisner was boss not only to Jaffe but to the greatest share of the Kaposi's Sarcoma and Opportunistic Infections Task Force. Jaffe figured the basketball game would give them a chance to talk, away from the constantly ringing phones at headquarters on Clifton Road. Jaffe methodically gave the growing evidence that GRID was a sexually transmitted disease. Weisner quickly saw the implications of the epidemiology.

"We're going to have to make a long-term commitment," Jaffe ventured. "We can't just keep borrowing resources. This isn't going away. It's going to get bigger and bigger."

Weisner weighed Jaffe's comments and agreed. "You've got my commitment," he answered.

Jaffe was ecstatic as he settled back to watch the game. For the first time, a person in authority was on record as favoring a permanent commitment of resources to the epidemic. In terms of the organizational chart, of course, Weisner was at best a mid-level administrator, but he was somebody who had more clout than anybody on the task force. The top CDC brass were more likely to listen to him, Jaffe figured. At this point, any sign of help was welcome.

April 1
UNIVERSITY OF CALIFORNIA,
SAN FRANCISCO

Speaking smoothly in his charming French accent, the young man seemed the personification of all things debonair. Marcus Conant was amazed that the airline steward had been diagnosed with Kaposi's sarcoma for almost two years already. He still looked healthy. He still exuded a vibrant sensuality.

Gaetan Dugas was proud that his cancer had not progressed. He was going to beat this thing, he insisted. He just wanted Conant to check him out and make sure everything was under control.

After the examination, as Gaetan was pulling on his stylish shirt, Conant mentioned that Gaetan should stop having sex.

"It's probably some virus," said Conant. "If you do have sex, make sure to avoid anything where you come inside somebody or exchange body fluids."

Gaetan looked wounded, but his voice betrayed a fierce edge of bitterness.

"Of course, I'm going to have sex," he told Conant. "Nobody's proven to me that you can spread cancer."

Gaetan cut Conant's rebuttal short. "Somebody gave this thing to me," he said. "I'm not going to give up sex."

April 2
ATLANTA

By now, a dizzying array of acronyms was being bandied about as possible monikers for an epidemic that, though ten months old, remained unnamed. Besides GRID, some doctors liked ACIDS, for Acquired Community Immune Deficiency Syndrome, and then others favored CAIDS, for Community Acquired Immune Deficiency Syndrome. The CDC hated GRID and preferred calling it "the epidemic of immune deficiency." The "community" in other versions, of course, was a polite way of saying gay; the doctors couldn't let go of the notion that one identified this disease by whom it hit rather than what it did.

Whether CAIDS, ACIDS, or GRID, the epidemic had by April 2, 1982, struck 300 Americans and killed 119. In the past two weeks, cases had been detected in two more states and two more European nations, indicating that the epidemic had now spread across nineteen states and seven countries. Of the 300 cases in the United States, 242 were gay or bisexual men, 30 were heterosexual men, 10 were heterosexual women, and 18 were men of unknown sexual orientation. Since intravenous drug transmission had yet to be proven scientifically, the cautious CDC statisticians had not yet roped off addicts as a separate risk group. By now, somebody was dying almost every day in America from an epidemic that still did not have a name.

April 8
PARADISE GARAGE,
MANHATTAN

Few nights could have been more poorly chosen for the first benefit any organization had ever undertaken to raise private funds for the epidemic. It was the second day of Passover, the night before Good Friday. Gay Men's Health Crisis had distributed tickets in stores all over town, in the bathhouses and gay card shops. But so far, they had sold only 500 tickets. Larry Kramer, Paul Popham,

Enno Poersch, and the other organizers from the Gay Men's Health Crisis nervously waited to see whether anyone would show up; so many of their friends had told them the whole subject of this gay cancer was such a downer.

Tensions had begun to surface in the committee. Larry Kramer insisted on being the public spokesman for the press. That was fine with Paul Popham since he didn't want any public role that might have repercussions for his job. Some board members, however, were worried that Kramer's rhetoric was too harsh. He was always chastising Mayor Ed Koch for refusing to meet with the group and ridiculing Health Commissioner David Sencer for not providing any educational material on the epidemic. After any fight, however, the board always got back together. There weren't that many other people who believed the epidemic was a worthwhile effort to work on.

In the past few weeks, the committee had realized that it was going to be a permanent organization, not a temporary fund-raising structure. With the city government ignoring the epidemic, somebody needed to get out educational information and coordinate volunteer efforts directed at the GRID victims, who were often left immobilized and isolated. Kramer was agitating that the committee could be a powerful pressure group to force the city into providing services, but most members were eager to avoid the kind of politics that marked the petty gay leadership scene. Besides, the medical needs seemed to be growing so fast. Dr. Michael Lange had recently appeared before the board and outlined the disaster he was convinced lay ahead. There was a lot of work to be done, he insisted, and the gay community would have to shoulder a lot of it themselves.

The lines started queuing up an hour before Paradise Garage even opened. Everybody was there, many toting checks with substantial contributions. Within a few hours, the committee raised $52,000. Enno Poersch was amazed at the turnout. These weren't political people—they were the party crowd he had danced with on Fire Island; finally, they were caring about something other than the "four D's" of drugs, dick, disco, and dish. By now, Enno had been told that Nick's toxoplasmosis was part of the GRID epidemic. Enno thought often of Nick, dead now for fifteen months. As he saw the hundreds of men swaying to disco music under the shimmering disco ball, Enno wished Nick were there to share the night and the happiness with him.

Everybody cheered enthusiastically when Paul Popham addressed the crowd in his broad, plainspoken Oregon accent.

"It may be that an equal measure of fear and hope has brought us together, but the great thing is, we *are* together," said Paul. "Most of you know someone, or someone who knows someone, who has been touched by the outbreak. I have lost two friends myself. . . . We've got to fight back. We've got to be tough. We've got to show each other and the unfriendly world that we've got more than looks, brains, talent, and money. We've got guts too, plus an awful lot of heart."

FIRE ISLAND

Paul Popham had waited all weekend in the house on Ocean Walk for the overcast skies to clear, but they kept their steely cast. Finally, on Sunday, it was nearing the time when he would have to return to Manhattan, and he couldn't wait any longer. A year ago, he had come here with the ashes of his friend Rick Wellikoff. It had been a sunny, melancholy day, warmed by the sharing of grief with Rick's surviving lover and friends. Now, Rick's lover was ailing too, the fourth person from the house on Ocean Walk to be stricken by this new plague, and Paul was alone with the ashes of Jack Nau.

Paul knew, in some corner of his awareness, that he was devoting himself so thoroughly to the Gay Men's Health Crisis in large part because he had to bury the grief he still felt so keenly both for Rick, the Brooklyn schoolteacher, and for Jack, the designer who once did the windows at the Long Island Sak's Fifth Avenue. As a harsh rain beat down, Paul again pondered the familiar imponderables. Why is this happening to me, to all my friends? Hadn't they put up with enough shit for one lifetime? Why doesn't anybody seem to care?

What a fucking nightmare.

The cold white fingers of the sea stroked the indifferent sand, littered by a winter's worth of misshapen flotsam. Paul opened the box and shook. The sea fingers reached to grab Jack's ashes and pull them into the brine. Paul gazed out to where the leaden sky met the gray Atlantic and wondered when it would all end. This can't be happening, he thought, it's simply too unbelievable.

Yet, as he shook the last of the bone dust that was once Jack Nau into the sea, Paul knew that it was happening and it was all too believable.

14 BICENTENNIAL MEMORIES

April 1982
DAVIES MEDICAL CENTER,
SAN FRANCISCO

Michael Maletta was bitter, angry, and hostile when Bill Darrow phoned him at his hospital bed. For two years he had been suffering from bizarre health problems and none of the doctors had been able to help him; for the longest time they hadn't even told him what he had. Now, some nosy doctor from the Centers for Disease Control was on the phone to ask him all kinds of personal questions about some Air Canada flight attendant he had fucked with only God knows when. And all those questions about his life in Greenwich Village. Christ, that must have been five, six years ago. He couldn't remember.

Darrow maintained his best professional demeanor. He had spent years chasing syphilis in New York City back in the 1960s after he had answered President Kennedy's call to do something for his country. Then he had been in his twenties, when he could hold on to the naive notion that just one person could make a difference. Now, Darrow was forty-two years old, with shards of gray at his temples and the sophist's cynicism that creeps into the voices of those who tend toward the academic. Once again, however, he had that old feeling that he could make a difference.

He had scented the trail distinctly after his talk with Gaetan Dugas in New York City. Gaetan had apologized about just updating his fabric-covered address book. Many names had been lost, he sighed, but one just couldn't keep them all. There'd be far too many. Nonetheless, he had seventy-three names and phone numbers of his most promising recent assignations. That led Darrow to the stories about Jack Nau and Paul Popham and the house on Ocean Walk, where so many of New York City's first GRID victims seemed to have lived. There was a second house on Fire Island with a similar concentration of dead and dying, Darrow also learned; it was the home of Paul Popham's former lover, the place where Paul had lived the summer before he moved in with Nick, Enno Poersch, and Rick Wellikoff.

The connections between Gaetan and both Michael Maletta, who was one of the first Kaposi's sarcoma patients in San Francisco, and Nick, one of the nation's first toxoplasmosis victims, were tantalizing. Nick, Enno, and Michael, it turned out, had all run with the same crowd back in the 1970s. In fact, a whole cluster of the nation's earliest cases appeared to have lived within doors of each other, south of Washington Square in the West Village. They partied together, dined together, and, friends intimated, slept together. Some people slipped in and out of this social circle over the glorious years in the late 1970s, but there was only one summer during which all the early GRID cases had been in New York at one time before they split up and went their separate ways. Unfortunately, nobody could tell Darrow which summer that was.

But Darrow felt himself getting close, being drawn to the clue that might tell him when, where, and how this sickness got into the country. It seemed beyond coincidence that a group of people, who had lived in one time and place together, should later pop up with the same disease after they had moved to such diverse parts of the nation. They must have been exposed to whatever was causing this when they were together. When was it?

Michael Maletta was grouchy at the prodding. Yes, he had moved to San Francisco in . . . well, it had to be before the end of 1977, but from there, Michael's memory and cooperation wore thin. There was a photographer whom they all ran with that summer in Manhattan too, Michael recalled. A fashion photographer.

Bill Darrow found him in a Los Angeles hospital.

LOS ANGELES

"We were together all the time," the photographer reminisced. "We did *every*-thing together."

The man searched his memory and recalled the image of soft white sails scraping a purple night sky in New York harbor.

"All I remember is that all the boats were in the harbor," he said. "All the big ships."

Darrow remembered the day immediately. Who could forget the pictures of the graceful ships and fireworks arching behind the torch of the Statue of Liberty?

"The Bicentennial," Darrow said aloud, almost to himself. "Of course. The Bicentennial."

July 4, 1976. An international festival to celebrate America's birthday with ships from fifty-five nations. People had come to New York City from all over the world.

The notion swept over him the way insights sometimes do, with each wave drawing more facts and connections into its wake. Nothing happened before 1976, but people had started getting sick in 1978 and 1979. It was clear from the other links in the cluster study that the disease could lie dormant for a long time. People were spreading it all over in 1977 and 1978, which accounted for so many cases spontaneously appearing in so many different regions of the country.

As the Bicentennial realization sank in deeper, a sense of dread overcame Darrow. People don't get this overnight; it can wait for years. It was going to be a huge problem, and it was only starting now. Decades of venereal disease work had instructed Darrow on those the disease would single out. Some of the best artists and musicians, politicians and businessmen, some of the pillars of America were gay, and they would fall down and die, and he wasn't sure whether anybody could do anything to stop it.

April 13
GAY AND LESBIAN COMMUNITY SERVICES CENTER, HOLLYWOOD

The Gay and Lesbian Community Services Center was in the heart of Congressman Henry Waxman's district. It was here that Tim Westmoreland, counsel for Waxman's Subcommittee on Health and the Environment, had engineered the first congressional probe into the growing GRID epidemic.

Westmoreland figured the hearing would draw much-needed media attention to the quiet killing caused by the gay cancer and, finally, get some of the federal bureaucrats on record as to what they were doing about the disease in the face of the Reagan budget slashing. The hearing was timely not so much because of anything happening in the epidemic, Westmoreland thought, but because of the administration's new health budget proposals. The Reagan budget men wanted to slice 1,000 grants from the National Institutes of Health and reduce positions on the Epidemiological Intelligence Service. The $5 million increase in the CDC budget barely covered inflation and gave the agency no new funds to deal with the new epidemic. Moreover, nowhere in the government budget had health officials established a line item to deal with GRID; instead, various researchers were expected to continue to pilfer and pirate money and personnel from other programs.

For the occasion, Westmoreland had written Waxman an opening statement that was meant to be a salvo in the war against federal indifference to the epidemic.

"I want to be especially blunt about the political aspects of Kaposi's sarcoma," Waxman said. "This horrible disease afflicts members of one of the nation's most stigmatized and discriminated against minorities. The victims are not typical, Main Street Americans. They are gays, mainly from New York, Los Angeles, and San Francisco.

"There is no doubt in my mind that, if the same disease had appeared among Americans of Norwegian descent, or among tennis players, rather than gay males, the responses of both the government and the medical community would have been different.

"Legionnaire's disease hit a group of predominantly white, heterosexual, middle-aged members of the American Legion. The respectability of the victims brought them a degree of attention and funding for research and treatment far greater than that made available so far to the victims of Kaposi's sarcoma.

"I want to emphasize the contrast, because the more popular Legionnaire's disease affected fewer people and proved less likely to be fatal. What society judged was not the severity of the disease but the social acceptability of the individuals affected with it. . . . I intend to fight any effort by anyone at any level to make public health policy regarding Kaposi's sarcoma or any other disease on the basis of his or her personal prejudices regarding other people's sexual preferences or life-styles."

Privately, Jim Curran of the Centers for Disease Control, who awaited his turn to testify at the hearing, cheered Waxman's statement. Like everyone at the KSOI Task Force, he had no doubt that just such prejudices regarding sexual preference were preventing everybody, from the budget people to the newspaper reporters, from taking this scourge seriously. As a federal employee, Curran had a thin line to walk between honesty and loyalty. He could not openly call for more money, but he could nudge facts toward logical conclusions, as when he talked about the familiar iceberg and, in a departure from his prepared remarks, mentioned for the first time that the epidemic would affect tens of thousands and not just the hundreds counted in the GRID stats.

"The epidemic may extend much further than currently described and may include other cancers as well as thousands or tens of thousands of persons with immune defects," Curran told the subcommittee.

With death rates soaring to 75 percent among people diagnosed with GRID for two years, the specter of 100 percent fatality from the syndrome loomed ahead, he added. Moreover, the deaths were coming at a huge cost. Curran pointed to three cases, each of which consumed at least $50,000 in medical treatment before death.

Waxman pushed Curran hard on the effect of budget cutting. Curran was evasive on specifics, noting that virtually all the KS study money had come from money redirected from other research. He pledged to "personally . . . fight to make sure the task force doesn't get compromised," while pointedly praising "my own superiors that, in spite of the threat of a reduction in force at CDC, which is quite a specter to hang over career scientists' heads, in spite of that threat, Kaposi's sarcoma was relatively spared and we surged on in spite of it."

Dr. Bruce Chabner from the Division of Cancer Treatment at the National Cancer Institute had a much tougher time eking out NCI accomplishments under questioning from the Los Angeles congressman. After pointing to the September workshop in Bethesda as a major NCI effort, he concluded that he just couldn't say what the NCI was doing for the epidemic, although he suspected that some NCI grant recipients were spending money from other projects on the new disease. "It is hard to account for the amount of money that they have invested through redirection of their grant support, but we feel it is considerable in view of the number of publications that have appeared."

At the end of his testimony, Chabner announced that the National Cancer Institute was going to release $1 million for Kaposi's sarcoma research, with one-quarter to go for treatment-directed studies and the rest for basic research. Chabner said the NCI hoped to get the money out by October.

Westmoreland grimaced when he heard the figure, thinking that Chabner should be embarrassed to mention a $1 million grant. A grant to a single research center for one project often ran beyond $10 million; it was laughable for the feds to say they were releasing $1 million to be shared by researchers across the country.

Fortunately, the president of the American Public Health Association was on hand to make just such points.

"We believe that the immunoresponse system of this country is weak, that it needs to be strengthened, and that only Congress can do it," said Stan Matek. He praised the CDC effort but added that "we are also worried about them. We don't know how close they are to the end of their rope in resolving the dangers" of the new epidemic. "We believe they cannot cope with Kaposi's sarcoma and its related syndrome. We believe their intervention abilities are so handicapped that the nation's health itself is in peril. . . . [The current work] represents, I fear, only high-level, high-caliber, 'ad-hocracy.' There is no guarantee of continuity of effort. Dr. Curran has promised us that he personally will fight to keep the effort going. Unfortunately, Dr. Curran can speak only as an individual technician and professional. The issue lies beyond him and above him; it is an issue of budget allocation. . . .

"Where is that epidemiologically essential money going to come from? It is not going to come from NIH, or at least not in any significant amounts, given the prior commitments and loss in real funding capability. If it comes from within CDC, it will come from robbing Peter to pay Paul. It will come by shifting already committed and needed resources . . . which is fine if you are Paul, but not so useful if you are Peter."

⬭

After testifying at the hearing, Drs. Marc Conant and Michael Gottlieb drove over to UCLA, where the conversation quickly drifted toward the tensions of doctoring in this epidemic. The pair were among a number of doctors in L.A., New York, and San Francisco who had created an informal support network, sharing their fears about whether they, as health workers, would join the risk groups of a disease whose transmission routes so clearly paralleled hepatitis B. Marc Conant had already devised a plan in which he could retire, build his cabin in the Sierra Nevada Mountains, and live on $30,000 a year. Gottlieb's wife, meanwhile, wanted to take Gottlieb away to Bora Bora. Conant was relieved to know that Gottlieb, a married, heterosexual, Jewish man so vastly different from himself, was going through precisely the same anxieties. Of course, both knew it was an unspeakable thing to do, to even talk about running away.

"We're not going to end up being the heroes of this epidemic," sighed Gottlieb. "We'll be the villains."

Conant saw the point immediately.

"They'll say we didn't tell them well enough, that if we had articulated what would happen better, they would have understood and done something to prevent it," said Gottlieb.

They were failing, Conant knew. People weren't listening. Nothing was more frustrating than this kind of failure, particularly for doctors, men who generally had accomplished every challenge confronting them, from the rigors of medical school to the wielding of "miracle" drugs. But this wasn't like not making an "A" in physiology, and the consequences wouldn't mean extra homework next semester.

Gottlieb's wife figured if they just got away for a couple of years, they could come back a little later, when it was all over.

Conant privately viewed the talk as extremely optimistic. There wouldn't be any getting away from this disease if you left for just a couple of years. If you wanted to get away from it, he thought, you'd better plan on leaving forever.

$$\bigcirc$$

On the flight back to Washington, D.C., that night, Tim Westmoreland was cheered that the testimony had gone so well. The dimensions of the future were clearly outlined: tens of thousands affected by a syndrome that would soon cost the society tens of millions in hospital care alone. The National Cancer Institute's embarrassing commitment of a minuscule $1 million to research for the next year should alert any science writer to the cynical lack of interest the National Institutes of Health has in the problem, Westmoreland thought, and Curran certainly dropped some hints about the vast studies that needed to be undertaken. Westmoreland waited for the media coverage. And waited.

The television networks and even the local stations, it turned out, didn't bother to cover the event. Westmoreland had hoped that at least medical journals and health newsletters would send somebody to write up the testimony since this clearly would be of interest to their targeted readerships, but the hearing was ignored. The *Los Angeles Times* wrote one of its first stories on the epidemic from the hearing testimony, but the story's lead was not on the critical public policy questions raised by the speakers, but on the only facet of the GRID story that seemed to have any interest to newspaper editors. "Epidemic Affecting Gays Now Found in Heterosexuals," the headline read.

April 18
CENTERS FOR DISEASE CONTROL
HEPATITIS LABORATORIES, PHOENIX

Don Francis was toiling to get his viral lab together on the warm Sunday afternoon when Jim Curran phoned and linked up Bill Darrow on a conference call. Darrow told Francis about Gaetan Dugas and the connections between twenty of the first GRID cases, mainly in Los Angeles. He still had some more tracking to do, but Darrow was convinced that he had the evidence the task force had been seeking to substantively prove an infectious disease. Francis was relieved, hoping that new studies might goad the slumbering National Institutes of Health into action. With proof of an infectious agent, the onus for research would shift from the National Cancer Institute to the National Institute for Allergy and Infectious Diseases. They certainly couldn't be any slower than NCI. The information also spurred his longing for a viral lab. The nation couldn't depend on the NIH to study the epidemic. Funding remained a major impediment. Francis was now flying between Atlanta and Phoenix every other week or so, and he was having a hard time finagling so much as the $150 airfare from CDC brass. With the cluster studies, Francis hoped, somebody upstairs would see how catastrophic this epidemic would become. Then they could get down to business.

⬯

By the time Bill Darrow's research was done, he had established sexual links between 40 patients in ten cities. At the center of the cluster diagram was Gaetan Dugas, marked on the chart as Patient Zero of the GRID epidemic. His role truly was remarkable. At least 40 of the first 248 gay men diagnosed with GRID in the United States, as of April 12, 1982, either had had sex with Gaetan Dugas or had had sex with someone who had. The links sometimes were extended for many generations of sexual contacts, giving frightening insight into how rapidly the epidemic had spread before anyone knew about it. Before one of Gaetan's Los Angeles boyfriends came down with *Pneumocystis,* for example, he had had sex with another Angelino who came down with Kaposi's sarcoma and with a Florida man who contracted both Kaposi's and the pneumonia. The Los Angeles contact, in turn, cavorted with two other Los Angeles men who later came down with Kaposi's, one of whom infected still another southern California man who was suffering from KS. The Floridian, meanwhile, had sex with a Texan who got Kaposi's sarcoma, a second Florida man who got *Pneumocystis,* and two Georgia men, one of whom got *Pneumocystis* and another who soon found the skin lesions of KS. Before finding these lesions, however, the Georgian had sex with a Pennsylvania man who later came down with both *Pneumocystis* and KS.

From just one tryst with Gaetan, therefore, eleven GRID cases could be connected. Altogether, Gaetan could be connected to nine of the first nineteen cases of GRID in Los Angeles, twenty-two in New York City, and nine patients in eight other North American cities. The Los Angeles Cluster Study, as it became known, offered powerful evidence that GRID not only was transmissible but was the work of a single infectious agent.

The study offered further clues into the most-feared aspect of the new disease—the long asymptomatic carrier state. By studying ten patient pairs who had contact with only one diagnosed patient, Darrow had calculated the mean incubation period of the disease for these men to be at least 10.5 months. Gaetan, for example, had infected at least one man before he had any symptoms of GRID himself. Another two had contracted it from Gaetan while he showed signs only of lymphadenopathy. Gaetan had his lesions when he spent Thanksgiving weekend with the Orange County hairdresser.

A CDC statistician calculated the odds on whether it could be coincidental that 40 of the first 248 gay men to get GRID might all have had sex either with the same man or with men sexually linked to him. The statistician figured that the chance did not approach zero—it was zero.

LUNDYS LANE, SAN FRANCISCO

He should have seen the end coming, Matt Krieger thought, as he began unpacking the crates and boxes in the cottage perched on a quiet hill overlooking the Mission District. He and Gary Walsh were supposed to be moving together into the small whitewashed home with the white picket fence. Now, Matt realized that for them, buying a home was like straight couples who have children in hopes that it will keep a failing marriage together. Gary had turned into a militant introvert in recent months, staying in his "self-expression room," writing poetry, doing sloppy fingerpainting, or just dancing around to his favorite Beatles records. He was pulling inside himself, as if he was preparing for something important, though it was never clear exactly what. Their relationship was clearly over. Matt was moving into their dream house alone.

Matt, meanwhile, had busied himself with his usual socially conscious activities. He was on the board of directors of a group that was trying to urge gay men to get the hepatitis vaccine. The campaign was a challenge. Without government support for the vaccine, companies had jacked the price up to $150 a vaccination in an attempt to pull some profit from a multimillion-dollar research program that clearly would produce nothing but losses. It was during this involvement that some doctor started talking casually to Matt about gay cancer. "It's going to get much worse," he said matter-of-factly. "This is only the beginning."

Gary, meanwhile, had turned to his old friend and colleague Joe Brewer, who was also single. The pair decided that they would try to be everything that lovers are to each other except bed partners. The worst part of being single, they agreed, was having to take vacations alone. They started planning a lavish trip to Mexico together for Christmas and organized a retreat for themselves at the Russian River resort area north of San Francisco.

At the last minute, however, Gary had to cancel. He was tired but couldn't say exactly why.

April 28
Centers for Disease Control,
Atlanta

Exactly one year after Sandra Ford wrote her memo alerting the Centers for Disease Control to unconfirmed reports of "bone sarcoma" and the mysterious orders for pentamidine, somebody made a cake for the KSOI Task Force and took it down to the narrow corridors of Building 6 where the GRID offices were clustered. People chatted briefly, drank a little champagne, and tried to avoid discussing the central reality that was emerging in their harried, overworked, and understaffed research group. The epidemic was moving faster than they were. They had no concept of where it would pop up next and no idea of how to stop it. And nobody outside this building and a handful of hospitals in a few big cities seemed to care. Finally, somebody took a butter knife smuggled from the cafeteria and cut into the icing, dissecting its legend: "Unhappy Anniversary."

15 NIGHTSWEATS

May 4, 1982
SAN FRANCISCO

Even over the phone, Cleve Jones could tell that Michael's red hair was perfectly in place, severely *Gentleman's Quarterly.* His long legs undoubtedly were stretched in one of those delicious poses that so often got him on the pages of *Blueboy* and *Torso,* Cleve thought. Cleve preferred the earnest young idealists of Castro Street to the sophisticated Manhattan scene, but there was something undeniably alluring about the aristocracy of beauty that gay men had fashioned in New York. Cleve was glad he had been accepted into their ranks, even if only as a spunky interloper, during his frequent trips to New York City. That also helped him recognize so many of the names Michael listed as among the walking wounded of this gay cancer.

"A lot of people are sick," said Michael, his voice worried. "Everybody's getting it."

Michael told Cleve about the New Year's Eve party he had attended to welcome in 1980. All the beautiful people had been there, and now a lot of those beautiful people were dead.

"Everybody at that party has gotten it except me," he said.

Cleve didn't say anything.

A note of confidence crept back into Michael's voice. "I think the government did it."

Cleve was more comfortable with this; the conversation was turning familiar.

"I don't know anybody who doesn't think the government might not have done it," Cleve confided.

By now, there were lots of theories and Cleve had heard them all. In New York, the epidemic seemed to snipe vengefully at the top of Manhattan's ziggurat of beauty. People called it the "Saint's disease" because everybody who got it seemed to be among the guys who danced all night at that popular disco. Maybe they put something in the drinks, the water, the air. In San Francisco, the epidemic spread first through the leather scene. Gay men began suspiciously eyeing barroom ionizers that helped eliminate cigarette smoke. Maybe those gadgets were emitting something else, something deadly. Theories abounded, in part because it was strangely reassuring to think that something out there had brought this misfortune on homosexuals, not something in which gay men themselves could have had any part.

Nothing seemed out of the question, Cleve thought. And everybody was worried. The visions of Simon Guzman, lying sick and disfigured, kept haunting Cleve, and sometimes, in the cool darkness of the San Francisco spring, he lay in bed sweating, terrified at what might lie ahead.

MANHATTAN

"The house staff is terrified," said the hospital chief of staff with a certain self-conscious tick. "We're getting too many of these patients. The administrator won't let me admit any more of them."

Rodger McFarlane knew what the doctor was saying, even though he wasn't saying it: No hospital in New York City wanted to become known as specializing in this homosexual disease. Given the predictions coming out of Atlanta of exponential increases, hospitals figured they'd be swamped a few years down the road if they became too well known for GRID treatment. Besides, the nurses and doctors were edgy about word that this was spread like hepatitis. Hospital staff long had been a key risk group for hepatitis, and they didn't want to become a risk group for a deadly, incurable disease.

Rodger was left arguing on what was another, typical night of his volunteer work for the Gay Men's Health Crisis. Sitting in the emergency room was a terrified patient, barely able to breathe because the *Pneumocystis* protozoa were filling up his lungs. Meanwhile, Rodger's beeper was telling him that the GMHC hotline was ringing again, and he wondered how he got involved in this mess.

Rodger McFarlane had opened the GMHC hotline on his personal answering service shortly after the Garage dance benefit. He received 100 calls the first day. The gay men of Manhattan were panic-stricken and there was nowhere else to turn. Rodger had never felt discriminated against as a homosexual in all his twenty-seven years, and he never understood the radical politics the activist types always spouted. Now, however, he could see something was wrong. People were suffering and the city wouldn't do anything about it. Half the GRID cases in the country were in New York City, and you barely heard a whisper about it from the mayor or the health officials. Gays were going to have to establish their own services or be left to die in shame, fear, and isolation. As he cabbed home, Rodger started mapping the service plans in his mind. He had always viewed management organization charts as the best cure for nebulous anxiety.

As he neared home, the beeper summoned Rodger again, this time to Beekman Downtown. Rodger phoned the medical center and talked to a mother who was terrified because the doctors said her son was crazy and hallucinating. Nobody would do anything to help him. Rodger called the doctor, hoping he'd be able to handle it on the phone. The physician didn't want to talk to some guy from the Gay Men's Whatever. When Rodger arrived at the hospital, the patient seemed utterly serene, lying in his room.

The young *Pneumocystis* sufferer, it turned out, had staged the insanity in hope of getting released from this hospital and into some psychiatric care. Then he could slip away and commit suicide. Rodger calmed everybody down and finally made it back to his apartment, where he collapsed.

A few days later, he heard that the young man had died, not by suicide but of his *Pneumocystis,* at Beekman Downtown.

May 6
CENTERS FOR DISEASE CONTROL
HEPATITIS LABORATORIES, PHOENIX

Don Francis was relieved when he got the call from Dr. Robert Gallo's lab at the National Cancer Institute. An associate of Gallo said that he had started culturing lymphocytes from a GRID patient in a special cell line Gallo had developed called interleukin-II. The IL-II, Francis recognized, was a perfect growth medium for the lymphocytes. By easily being able to grow the lymphocytes, Gallo had already overcome a formidable research barrier. Some viruses eluded decent study simply because scientists couldn't figure out how to propagate their host cells.

Don Francis, Max Essex from Harvard, and Gallo's lab were now in almost constant contact on GRID. At a scientific conference at the National Cancer Institute's Cold Spring Harbor facility in March, Essex had hypothesized that GRID was caused by a new infectious agent and suggested it might be a retrovirus similar to feline leukemia. The other doctors had given the theory only a polite reception, but Gallo had urged Essex on and started dabbling in the disease at his own lab.

Francis was glad to have the lab at work, but he worried that other major retrovirology labs needed to get to work on GRID fast and get on it full time. Francis had spent much of the spring trying to interest the virologists at the Center for Infectious Diseases of the CDC, but they just wouldn't get excited over his unlikely notion that a retrovirus was behind the syndrome. They also had other work to do. Nobody was eager to take on new projects at a time when they barely had the staff to accomplish their primary interests. At Harvard, Max Essex was working GRID part time, convinced that the CDC would come up with the answer to the GRID problem any day, as they did with Legionnaire's. Bob Gallo's lab was spending a fraction of its time on the problem. Even though Francis was grateful for any effort he could engender from the lethargic National Cancer Institute, one or two labs weren't enough, he felt. They might get off on a bum lead and retard research at a time when people were dying.

Francis decided it was time to get down to some serious groveling. Other researchers needed to get involved. People were dying. Couldn't they see how important this was?

May 12
CENTERS FOR DISEASE CONTROL, ATLANTA

Drawing largely on the work that Donna Mildvan and Dan William started in New York City in early 1981, the *Morbidity and Mortality Weekly Report* on "Generalized Lymphadenopathy Among Homosexual Males" was released from Atlanta, the first *MMWR* publication on any aspect of the epidemic in nine months. Of course, nobody knew what was going to happen to these lymphadenopathy patients, but the report noted that these symptoms already had appeared among 44 percent of the KS patients and 23 percent of the *Pneumocystis* patients diagnosed between June 1981 and January 1982. It was a bad sign.

"Causes for the persistent lymphadenopathy among patients discussed above were sought but could not be identified," the report said. Doctors should be alert for the symptoms, the article concluded, most notably fatigue, fever, unexplained weight loss, and, of course, nightsweats.

$\bigcirc$

Every week or so, a new Kaposi's sarcoma or pneumonia case would appear in some new region of the country, and the CDC would send someone to investigate the first GRID case in southwest Texas or some other remote place to see if, perhaps, that person might offer the clue. By May 18, 355 biopsy-confirmed GRID cases had been counted in twenty states. Of these, 136 were dead. New York City accounted for 158 of the cases, or about half, while California was home to 71 cases, including 40 in San Francisco. About 79 percent of all cases were among gay or bisexual men. Nearly 12 percent were among heterosexual men who were intravenous drug users, although the CDC still wasn't saying this for public consumption. Another 13 cases were among heterosexual women.

Trying to track not only the gay cases but the newly discovered Haitian cases and the growing numbers of intravenous drug users and prisoners, the CDC Task Force sometimes wondered how many cases really existed in the United States, aware that their numbers were months behind anything resembling the reality of the epidemic. Staffing shortages had forced them to rely on "passive reporting," which meant they sat in Atlanta and hoped that health officials actually were calling in their cases. They had neither the money nor the personnel to conduct the active surveillance they would have preferred. At times, their sleep too was dogged by fears of what might be out there, what they might not be seeing.

WEST 57TH STREET, NEW YORK CITY

Dr. Dan William was struck by the utter disparity among gay men facing the specter of death for the first time. Some blithely ignored the diseases, no mean task given the *New York Native*'s singularly thorough coverage of the epidemic. Others lived in unrelenting terror, racing to William's Upper West

Side office at the first fever, sniffle, or zit, and many had good cause to worry, William soon noted. The numbers of gay men with lymphadenopathy were increasing geometrically. Others just seemed dragged out and listless, while the sleep of so many more was drenched with terrifying nightsweats that left their sheets soaked with perspiration, their hair saturated with the salty fetor, and their bodies limp with exhaustion. The nightsweats themselves seemed a particularly hellish ordeal that was virtually a rite of passage into this most devilish disease.

New manifestations of the immune disorders, however, were appearing faster than William could chronicle them. The oral candidiasis, or thrush, was the most common precursor of the more serious GRID disease, William noted, often defying any form of treatment. For the past six months, people also were coming in with excruciatingly painful outbreaks of herpes zoster, known most commonly as shingles. The shinglelike growths typically appeared on the face or shoulders, spreading fulminately over the body, with each tiny scab capable of shooting a hot, piercing pain at the slightest touch. The shingles seemed most often to strike people with the lymphadenopathy, and by the end of 1981, William had begun keeping a list of his shingles patients on the personal computer in his office. He wondered what would happen to them, what this meant. In December 1981, there were eleven cases, and by June 1982, there were seventeen shingles patients. Sometime around June one of the early shingles patients came in to see William about an unusual purple spot. It was Kaposi's sarcoma.

The fear began around this time—something entirely new to worry about after eighteen months that rarely let William slip by without some new insight into the horrors that lay ahead. Maybe all these people with swollen lymph nodes were going to die. Perhaps the new virus was like some lurking jungle predator, striking the stragglers first. That would explain the extreme life-styles of the early cases; they were out dancing in the freeway, ensuring they would be the first to get run over. Their already overtaxed immune systems wouldn't put up much of a fight either. The virus would circle the rest too, William worried, bringing some fatigue and nightsweats, and then causing this or that yeast infection in the mouth, and later, say, a serious case of herpes or shingles that might go away. Then, at some unpredictable point in the future, everybody with this may just up and die.

As they would throughout the early stages of the epidemic, most doctors preferred to shove aside fears that such worst-case scenarios might materialize. Dr. Fred Siegal, the Mt. Sinai Hospital researcher who did much of the early immunology work on GRID, offered such optimism in the *New York Native*'s article on the *MMWR* lymphadenopathy report. "My hunch is that most of these patients will not go on to develop the full immunodeficiency syndrome," Siegal said. "If we're wrong, on the other hand, it would be a catastrophe."

$\bigcirc$

Seeing catastrophe ahead, William asked the owner of the St. Mark's Baths, a four-story facility that advertised itself as the world's largest bathhouse, to his apartment for dinner. William laid out his plan. He was convinced that GRID was caused by a new virus, being spread sexually. The overwhelming preponderance of his patients were people who went to the bathhouses. Obviously, bathhouses existed solely to provide the opportunity for the maximum number of sexual contacts. Nobody was saying the places should be closed down, William explained to the proprietor, but the bathhouses had a great opportunity to take the leadership role in promoting a new type of gay club.

William was quite taken with his idea. "The New Safe St. Mark's," he said. The bathhouse could take the doors off the private rooms, turn up the lights to discourage orgies, and orient the sex more toward video eroticism in which gay men could masturbate with each other but avoid the exchange of semen that probably spread this thing.

William was actually surprised when the businessman looked at him as if he were crazy.

"People can do what they want to do," he said. "I have no right to direct their behavior."

But people were going to die and die horribly, William countered.

The bathhouses weren't going to be changing, he was told.

$$\bigcirc$$

It was only later that the economic implications of his eager suggestions occurred to William. Of course the bathhouses could do nothing to suggest that a sexually transmitted disease was loose, killing their patrons. It would destroy their business. William realized that he might have been around doctors too long. He couldn't imagine anyone not wanting to act to save lives if they possibly could. The notion that some people might place personal profit above human life was utterly foreign to him.

Fortunately, William had recently signed on as a member of the medical advisory board of the Gay Men's Health Crisis. He hoped the new group would be able to start pressuring these businesses to see that their long-term survival depended on adaptation to new biological realities. The changes he had suggested were so obvious that he couldn't imagine they would not be adopted before long.

BUREAU OF COMMUNICABLE DISEASE CONTROL, SAN FRANCISCO

Amid the arrows and circles on her beat-up blackboard, Dr. Selma Dritz could now trace connections between forty-four cases of GRID in New York, San Francisco, southern California, and Canada. She had done the detective work that showed six couples in San Francisco alone were ailing from the disease. Her thoughts frequently drifted toward the bathhouses when she looked at the blackboard. She had never been overly fond of the institutions. It wasn't that she had any moral qualms; she didn't really care what people did with their lives, and she harbored a genuine curiosity about people who were preoccupied with regulating other humans' destinies. But bathhouses were biological cesspools for infection.

"Of course, from an old-fashioned textbook public health standpoint, you might go in and close the places down," Dritz mentioned to a *Chronicle* reporter one day.

"Of course, some people might argue that there were civil liberties issues involved," Dritz said, her voice trailing off in a way that suggested she did not think for one minute that civil liberties were the central issue involved here.

Such comments just fell, unharvested by the reporters and gay community leaders with whom Dritz talked. The notion that businesses might be closed was so unthinkable that it was put aside. A few dozen cases of some mystery illness did not justify such an extreme measure.

Dritz didn't push; that wouldn't be professional. Instead, she tried to engage the health and medical communities with the seriousness of what was unfolding. The future revealed itself so clearly, Dritz thought, as she looked at the charts and graphs that were the crystal balls of her career.

There was a terrible beauty in how obvious the flow of this disease was. For example, Dritz had charted a graph of the first two years of GRID cases in New York City, from 1980 through 1982, and then compared it with the San Francisco Bay Area cases. With a nearly perfect synchronicity, the curve and numbers in San Francisco followed those of Manhattan by exactly one year. The 150-plus cases New York City showed now were the 150-plus cases San Francisco would have in one year, she figured, and there undoubtedly would be hundreds, if not thousands, to follow those.

At night, in her comfortable home near the dunes of San Francisco's Pacific beaches, Selma Dritz lay awake wondering where this all would lead. She kept a small tape recorder on her neatly arranged nightstand in case she had that one insight on some sleepless night, the thought that might stop these young men from dying so horribly.

Castro District, San Francisco

Marc Conant woke up with a start, his forehead dripping in a hot sweat. Again, the incredible feeling of loss and the fear, the gnawing fear, overwhelmed him. Conant's restless Doberman paced nervously on the back porch while the dermatologist walked around his comfortable home, its lights still off, trying to clear his mind of the dream. It was recurring often now. He would be somewhere, very alone, and he would look at his skin and see the massive purple lesions of Kaposi's sarcoma spreading over his body. He was beginning to look like them, the patients he was seeing every day now in his practice, the young men so horribly disfigured by the splotches of bluish purple.

Then he would wake up in his hot sweat, seized by the impulse to run. Only a fool would stay here when you know that everybody is going to die, he thought.

Like most of the doctors working with GRID around the country, Conant had his blood tested regularly to ensure it held the proper ratios of T-helper and T-suppressor lymphocytes. It was the closest thing to a GRID test around. His lymphocytes were just fine, he knew. He didn't have gay cancer, but there were so many other things to worry about.

All day, people had been calling him about the cluster study, and every terror Conant had conceived on that April morning a year before when he first heard about Ken Horne now seemed realized. He immediately recognized Patient Zero as the suave Quebeçois airline steward who had come into his office the month before. He was the type of man everyone wanted. What everyone had wanted was bringing them death. Quite literally, Conant thought. Conant had heard that the young airline attendant was one of the more popular catches you could make at the Club Baths on Eighth and Howard these days. He might even be there now, Conant thought. People could be out there catching this now.

There were other worries. The sum total of all Conant's funding pleas was a $50,000 grant from the American Cancer Society. That was just enough to afford one harried secretary to coordinate the increasing numbers of patients using the KS clinic. The secretary ended up doing social service referrals, grief counseling, and lots of hand-holding, as well. There was nobody else.

Nine months had passed since the National Cancer Institute conference in Bethesda, and still there had not been a single gesture to intimate that the NCI was prepared to release funds. Refusing to wait for the official request for proposals, Conant had outlined his own research project on KS treatments and submitted it to the NCI. He then dashed off a letter to Assistant Secretary for Health Dr. Ed Brandt, begging him to intercede for accelerated NCI money. He received a polite reply that the United States government was deeply concerned with the problem and that both the CDC and the National Institutes of Health were doing everything possible to stop the epidemic, and thank you for writing.

The United States, Conant thought, had the know-how and resources to conquer this disease. The greatest scientific technology waited in the world's best-funded laboratories. People could be warned through a mass media network that could reach into virtually every citizen's home within a matter of minutes. This wasn't some Third World country, for Christ's sake. We could win this fight, but nobody is willing to make the effort or even acknowledge that there is a battle out there to be won.

Conant settled back into his bed, hoping the nightmare would not return, at least that night. When he was young, Conant had sometimes wondered what it might have been like to be a bright, resourceful Jewish man on the day after *Krystalnacht,* to see clearly the wholesale death that lay so soon ahead, even if the rest of the world didn't seem to care. Why didn't they run away?

Now, for the first time, Conant understood.

⬭

At the end of May, Marc Conant and Paul Volberding went to Tokyo to present their data on Kaposi's sarcoma to the World Dermatological Conference. Their Japanese hosts were polite and intrigued by the new phenomenon.

"Isn't it a shame you have the problem in San Francisco," said one prominent Japanese scientist. "It's because you have homosexuals." He paused a moment and confided, "Of course, we don't have homosexuals here."

NATIONAL CANCER INSTITUTE, BETHESDA

Robert Biggar's paper, hypothesizing an infectious agent as the cause of GRID, had now been rejected by every major scientific journal in the country. It simply went too much against the grain of prevailing theories. Other doctors were shooting up mice with semen to show that sperm actually was causing the immune suppression. Lab assistants scurried to pornographic bookstores to buy bottles of "Rush" and "Bolt" so rats could be overdosed on butyl inhalants in other experiments. Herpes experts seemed positively elated at the renewed attention to cytomegalovirus, or CMV. Other doctors posited that the collapse of GRID patients' immune systems occurred because they were overloaded with other infections. Many reviews of scientific theories on GRID etiology completely dismissed the single-agent theory as too unlikely.

Biggar's colleague, Jim Goedert, leaned toward the popper theory when the pair started putting together a large cohort of gay men in New York City and Washington, D.C., for a long-range study. Biggar was frustrated that his hypothesis was being ignored, but he also knew work must proceed. He had seen plagues in Africa, and he knew that the American infatuation for quick and easy theories, like semen or poppers, came only from naivete. No matter how affluent and civilized, humans were humans and susceptible to viruses that could come from nowhere. In fact, it was easier for a virus to come from nowhere these days.

Once, epidemics needed great movements of people to inspire their spread. The Spanish flu pandemic of 1918, which struck 20 million people, killing 200,000 Americans, directly followed the massive movements of people during World War I. Mixing Americans from diverse regions during the mobilization for World War II created a big viral mixing bowl that blended the poliomyelitis virus into people from every corner of America. The widespread outbreak of polio in the late 1940s and early 1950s was the direct result.

The popularity of air travel had eliminated the need for such dramatic world events to cast the seeds of apocalypse. It took just one person here or there to carry the right virus to the right population, and disease would strike again. Others might not see it now, but it would become obvious in time. Bob Biggar only hoped that it would not be too late.

CENTERS FOR DISEASE CONTROL, ATLANTA

Dr. Harry Haverkos of the KSOI Task Force had come up with the idea of bringing Gaetan Dugas to Atlanta. If nothing else, the flight attendant was certain to be harboring lots of virus in his blood, the CDC figured, and Haverkos had him hooked on to a plasma faresis machine so the agency could collect a half liter of his plasma for lab research.

Everybody in Building 6 was talking about Patient Zero and the cluster study, due for publication next month. Bill Darrow and Harold Jaffe wanted to get pictures of as many GRID victims as they could and start showing them to new patients. They were convinced even more connections could be established. Higher CDC officials, sensitive to gay concerns about confidentiality, vetoed the idea.

Jim Curran passed up the opportunity to meet Gaetan, the Quebeçois version of Typhoid Mary. Curran had heard about the flamboyant attendant and frankly found every story about his sexual braggadocio to be offensive. Stereotypical gays irritated Curran in much the same way that he was uncomfortable watching Amos n' Andy movies.

$$\bigcirc$$

Gaetan Dugas later complained to friends that the CDC had treated him like a laboratory rat during his stay in Atlanta, with little groups of doctors going in and out of his hospital room. He'd had this skin cancer for two years now, he said, and he was sick of being a guinea pig for doctors who didn't have the slightest idea of what they were doing.

MEMORIAL SLOAN-KETTERING
CANCER CENTER, NEW YORK CITY

Brandy Alexander kept a Rubik's Cube by his bed in Room 428A at the sprawling cancer center. Sometimes he would take the cube, with all its colors, and turn and twist it every which way with his bony, aching fingers to find the solution. But it never worked; there were no solutions.

Before the first spot had appeared, Brandy had been a brassy female impersonator who could knock 'em dead with "Over the Rainbow," "Maybe This Time," and "New York, New York." As the lesions spread, though, his brown curls turned gray and he lost twenty pounds, leaving his bones to jut out of his loose, purple-spotted flesh. Brandy's once-handsome face was covered with thick scabs wrought by an uncontrolled herpes virus. None of the standard medications stopped the herpes, so his face oozed all over with pussy discharges. Besides the KS and herpes, the thirty-eight-year-old had an array of the usual opportunistic infections, including severe hepatitis and tuberculosis of the bone marrow.

Brandy Alexander was typical of these patients, his doctors told Don Francis before he entered the room. Although Don Francis had come to Sloan-Kettering with Jim Curran on other business, he felt embarrassed that he'd been working on this disease for nearly a year and still had not met a patient. The physicians led him to Brandy Alexander, who exuded a gracious charm. He lifted his hand to Francis, as though he wanted the young blond scientist to kiss it. Francis immediately saw the large splotches of purple on the man's arm.

It wasn't even his favorite color, Brandy confided. He didn't have any bags to match.

Alone, in the room, Brandy talked honestly with Francis about his life. Brandy could tell Francis wasn't particularly shocked at anything he heard.

"The sex got to be unstoppable," he said, his eyes wandering around their hollow, gaunt sockets, trying to see the answer. "I don't know whether it was to be close to another person because I didn't want to be alone. I don't know if I just got bored with normal sex, so I'd try something new. Something more exciting. Fisting. Another rung."

The monologue was taking Brandy to a conclusion that irked the scientific side of Don Francis's mind. Brandy was trying to find a reason he was lying in pain in that bed in Room 428A about to die. The old moral teachings, Francis thought, die hard.

"I think this is a communicable disease and you got it," said Francis, matter-of-factly. "You're not being punished. A virus has made you sick."

Back with the Sloan-Kettering doctors, Don Francis got down to the purpose of his mission. Sloan-Kettering had one of the handful of retrovirus laboratories in the country. Even the CDC didn't have a retrovirus lab, and it would be months before they could get one together. They weren't set up to investigate long-latent viral diseases in Atlanta, Francis said, just the quick hits that burst forth and need a fast solution. They were floundering on GRID and needed help.

Sloan-Kettering needed to get to work on GRID, Francis prodded. There wasn't time to delay.

The doctors listened patiently and agreed this was an important problem. They'd think about it and get back to him. Of course, Francis knew then that they would never call back.

The dream came to Don Francis often during those long, frustrating nights in the gathering darkness of 1982. Just beyond his reach, a faint orange light was suspended, shimmering with promise. It was The Answer, the solution to the puzzle. He reached for it, stretching so he could draw the light toward him. But it drifted farther and farther out of reach. The answer was always there before him, tantalizingly close, and still beyond his grasp.

Don's wife usually awoke him at that point. His mournful groaning would disturb the kids.

16 TOO MUCH BLOOD

June 11, 1982
CENTERS FOR DISEASE CONTROL,
ATLANTA

Sandy Ford called Dr. Bruce Evatt, the CDC hemophilia expert, as soon as the order came in. Sandy, who had first alerted the CDC to the GRID epidemic last year, had even worse news to break to Evatt.

It had happened, Ford told him. An order for pentamidine had come in from Denver. The *Pneumocystis* victim, the doctors had said, was a hemophiliac.

That night, Evatt's associate in the Division of Host Factors, Dr. Dale Lawrence, took a flight to Stapleton International Airport in Denver.

June 14
DENVER

With his white shirts, plaid ties, black oxfords, and thinning dark hair that fell over earnest dark eyes, Dr. Dale Lawrence looked like everybody's favorite biology teacher in high school. He sounded like a serious instructor too, soft-spoken even as he strained to put his words together just right so everything he said would be easy to understand. He had to ask all these questions, he told the stunned wife of the hemophiliac patient, because so much was at stake.

Although Lawrence had worked for a year with the CDC's Division of Host Factors on issues of genetics and susceptibility to GRID, he had been to enough Task Force meetings to know what needed to be asked. He had to positively eliminate the chance that the man might have been involved in gay experiences or, perhaps, some kind of drug use or medication that could have engendered his immune deficiency. Lawrence's intense investigation the earlier few days had eliminated everything else. Just that morning, he had gone to the local blood center. Blood bank officials were very skittish about his arrival; Lawrence knew why. Just one or two documented hemophiliac GRID cases would severely shake the foundations of the blood banking industry.

Lawrence carefully drew out grids of all the different batches of the Factor VIII clotting factor that had been injected into dozens of other hemophiliacs served by the same Hemophilia Treatment Center in the Denver area. Maybe there was just one bad lot that was making people sick, and the *Pneumocystis* diagnosis was a wicked coincidence. Looking back at three previous years, however, he could find no single such lot.

Instead, Lawrence went back to the wife of the man wheezing on the ventilator at the University of Colorado Medical Center. The couple's troubled life story was laid out. The man, a janitor, had struggled against his disease for a lifetime, already living decades beyond what doctors had predicted when he was born. The uncontrolled bleeding in his joints had left him partially crippled, but he toiled to eke out a living for his wife and children just the same. Factor VIII, of course, had been a godsend, but now he was in there dying. Wasn't there anything anybody could do?

At the end of the conversation, Lawrence felt he had eliminated other possible routes of infection. Lawrence's boss, Bruce Evatt, was convinced that GRID was being spread through Factor VIII even before Lawrence returned with the final results of his investigation. Evatt had suspected it for months, after the first Florida man had died of *Pneumocystis*. The Colorado case was the clincher. Because bacteria, protozoa, and one-celled microbes were easily weeded out of the Factor VIII during its preparation process, this meant that GRID was caused by a virus, the only organism small enough to pass through the filters.

Both Lawrence and Evatt knew there would be more GRID cases among the hemophiliacs soon and blood transfusion cases would follow. Because of their exposure to vast numbers of donors, the hemophiliacs simply had the misfortune to get it first, like the gay men playing on the freeway in the late 1970s.

That Afternoon
CASTRO STREET, SAN FRANCISCO

While Dale Lawrence was wrapping up his Denver interviews on the nation's first documented hemophilia GRID case, Cleve Jones eagerly made his way to the doorway of the Castro Street building that he had leased as the headquarters for the Kaposi's Sarcoma Education and Research Foundation. Marc Conant and a couple of doctor friends had put up the money for the rent. This was the first office of any agency established specifically for the epidemic of immune suppression, and it started with one beat-up typewriter donated by a local gay bartender, office supplies pilfered from volunteers' various employers, and one telephone that started ringing within an hour of its installation. And it never stopped ringing.

Years of leading demonstrations and hanging out on Castro Street gave Cleve a vast reservoir of fellow rabble-rousers, old tricks, and prospective boyfriends from whom to cull volunteers. There was a deadly enemy out there. The fucking thing didn't even have a name.

"I don't know what to say," said friends Cleve recruited to answer the new gay cancer hotline.

Cleve sighed, "Nobody does."

FEDERAL BUILDING,
SAN FRANCISCO

Bill Kraus had respected San Francisco's Congressman Phillip Burton ever since Harvey Milk pointed out the bulky legislator at a political rally and called him "Il Patrón" of the city's liberal Democratic establishment. The congressman had created the awesome liberal clique that had dominated local politics for two decades through the weight of his wily, hardball tactics and his pioneering coalition of black, labor, and gay votes. Burton had engineered the ascension of the late George Moscone to mayor and had been a key ally to the flamboyant Assembly Speaker Willie Brown, generally regarded as California's second most powerful state politician after the governor. Burton's younger brother John represented another San Francisco congressional district. Phil Burton himself was one of the most powerful members of the House of Representatives, having missed being elected House Majority Leader in 1976 by one vote.

However, Phil Burton's obsession with playing Washington politics had weakened his San Francisco base, and never was he more vulnerable than when he sought his tenth term in 1982. The Republicans had nominated State Senator Milton Marks, the only GOP politician ever to make much of a name for himself in recent local political history. His successive wins in difficult elections, everyone knew, were because he had courted and charmed the gay community for years. Although the liberal Marks was a thorn in the side of the state's increasingly conservative Republican party, his election gave the GOP a chance to oust that troublesome Burton, so major donations from Republican political action committees flowed to Marks's coffers.

When Burton called Bill Kraus for a meeting, he was worried. Burton needed a liaison to the gay community. He wanted to win the election and get back to Washington.

"And what's the most important issue today?" Burton asked Bill.

"Gay cancer," Bill said.

The fact that the response came almost as a reflex stunned Bill. He hadn't really taken GRID that seriously in recent months. Like everybody else, he was eying his pimples more suspiciously, but fundamentally, he saw gay cancer as something that happened to other people, sleazy people with 1,100 sexual contacts. That's what he had read in the paper.

Self-conscious that he had pounced on the issue so hard, Bill laid out the political terms for the Godfather of San Francisco politics in a conversation that would have far-reaching implications for the epidemic.

He couldn't believe that the government wasn't ringing alarms and pledging tons of money to this disease, Bill explained. It didn't make sense. Look at all the hoopla they made about Legionnaire's and Toxic Shock. Bill didn't have the proof yet, but he suspected they weren't talking about it because they didn't want to spend money. They wanted to save their bucks so they could finance death squads in Central America.

When placed so sharply in the partisan terms with which Burton was most comfortable, Burton began to see Bill's point. Bill could work on this gay cancer stuff, he promised, reminding him not very gently that there was an election to win first.

○

Bill Kraus was ecstatic about his new congressional staff job. His relationship with Kico Govantes wasn't going well. He had shown Kico everything about the gay scene and defended the liberating sexuality so much that Kico was now intrigued with exploring it himself. In hopes of rekindling their fading passion, Bill had taken to escorting Kico to local baths.

Kico was always uncomfortable in those places, feeling they were dirty, even evil. And he had begun a romance with a handsome older architect, so he didn't need the release. Bill was fiercely jealous, although he and Kico remained part-time lovers, ensnared in a partnership that would never dissolve. In a corner of his mind, Bill welcomed the staff job because it would give him an escape. He never was much into alcohol or pot. Although he occasionally sniffed a line of coke, he preferred to use work to pull himself away from personal problems. The job also positioned him to work in Congress, the only elected job he felt mattered.

At night, when Kico was with his architect, Bill drove his Datsun to a desolate windswept hilltop set above the Castro District. From a craggy outcropping of Corona Heights, he could see the small, busy, gay enclave below and the tall skyscrapers of downtown set against a porcelain-blue sky. As the fog crept from the ocean and wound lazily through the high rises, a fear sometimes tugged at him. He couldn't define it, so his thoughts would drift away again to the speeches that would need to be written.

HARVARD SCHOOL OF PUBLIC HEALTH, CAMBRIDGE, MASSACHUSETTS

Dr. Max Essex eagerly took the blood samples that arrived from a Japanese infectious disease ward to his lab. The experiments to detect antibodies to the Human T-cell Leukemia virus, or HTLV, were performed easily with reagents sent from Dr. Bob Gallo's lab at the Division of Tumor Cell Biology of the National Cancer Institute. They yielded the expected results. Patients with infectious diseases in the ward, such as pneumonias and bacterial maladies, were three times more likely to be infected with HTLV than noninfected people. Essex was far less interested in what this meant for the Japanese than its implications for GRID. It proved that an infectious agent, particularly a retrovirus, was capable of engendering diseases by crippling the human immune system. The retrovirus itself could be transmitted, providing for an infectious disease of the immune system. HTLV, for example, could be transmitted in sex, through semen, or through contaminated blood products. Essex also hypothesized that some strains of this virus were more likely to induce immune suppression than others. Perhaps it was HTLV itself that was causing GRID.

Essex called Don Francis with the news. Bob Gallo's lab, Francis knew, was already poking around the lymphocytes of GRID patients in search of retroviruses. Essex decided to spend the summer testing GRID patients' blood for evidence of HTLV infection.

June 18
CENTERS FOR DISEASE CONTROL,
ATLANTA

Although just about every scientist at the CDC was convinced that the cluster study gave them precisely the evidence they needed to show that GRID was an infectious disease, its release came with a deluge of qualifiers and maybes from CDC officials.

Ironically, it was Jim Curran and the CDC Task Force who were most terrified at the implications of the cluster study. For public consumption, however, Curran and Harold Jaffe reassured reporters that no evidence existed that GRID was an infectious disease. "The existence of a cluster provides evidence for a hypothesis that people are not randomly associated with each other, and the cluster is a sexual cluster," Curran said. "It doesn't say we have evidence of one person giving to another person, certainly. The alternative hypothesis on the cluster would be that it isn't transmissible from one person to another. It's just that these people are really members of a very small subgroup among whom it might not be unusual to have sex. This is the less likely of the two hypotheses. Yet I don't think either should be discarded. We need to focus research into this. We're not prematurely releasing information that's not validated. On the other hand, we're not holding back information that might have some important health benefits."

Scientists accepted the information in the spirit that it was given. Most wanted to see more convincing evidence. Clinicians worried that such small clusterings among sexual contacts could lend credence to the toxic exposure theory because it was possible that one batch of bad drugs could have gotten into one crowd. Paraquat on one shipment of marijuana, for example, might have caused all these mens' immune disorders if the pot made it across the gay air bridges between New York, Los Angeles, and San Francisco. Of course, this argument belied the random way gay men, particularly the bathhouse-oriented men who made up most of those in the clusters, chose their sexual partners. It wasn't as though they were going to bed with each other because they were all friends. But the clinicians tended not to be sociologists, and the intricacies of the sexual 7-Elevens were lost on some of them.

Other research-oriented scientists told CDC Task Force members that they found the cluster stories intriguing, although somewhat anecdotal, and that a case-control cluster study would be necessary to prove the hypothesis of sexual transmissibility. Of course, such a study would take a few years to construct, but nobody said science worked fast.

In any event, the cluster study failed to resolve the transmissibility question as Bill Darrow and the CDC researchers originally had hoped it would. A handful of scientists and public health officials clearly saw the implications, but nobody rushed into action because the science wasn't then set in concrete.

Although the study attracted a brief flurry of national media attention, it faded fast.

VANCOUVER, BRITISH COLUMBIA

Gaetan Dugas confided to only a few friends that he was the "Orange County connection," as the study became known because of Gaetan's role in linking the New York, Los Angeles, and Orange County cases. Though on leave from Air Canada, the thirty-year-old flight attendant still had the passes that allowed him to fly all over the world for virtually nothing. He loved the travel, but he had decided to settle in San Francisco. They had an interferon program at their GRID clinic, and besides, he'd always wanted to live there.

It was around this time that rumors began on Castro Street about a strange guy at the Eighth and Howard bathhouse, a blond with a French accent. He would have sex with you, turn up the lights in the cubicle, and point out his Kaposi's sarcoma lesions.

"I've got gay cancer," he'd say. "I'm going to die and so are you."

July 2
ATLANTA

Bruce Evatt heard of still another case of immune suppression in a hemophiliac in Canton, Ohio, and now he saw clearly what was ahead. GRID was an infectious disease caused by a virus that could be spread through the blood. The nation's blood supply was already contaminated with the virus. A meeting of blood-industry officials would be needed soon; emergency measures would be needed to save lives.

July 6
CASTRO STREET, SAN FRANCISCO

Cleve Jones had spent all afternoon passing out leaflets on Castro Street for the Kaposi's Sarcoma Foundation's first public forum the next night. When he arrived at the home of his old boyfriend, attorney Felix Velarde-Munoz, he was still buzzing with talk of GRID and the new organization he was forming. Cleve couldn't believe how apathetic other gay leaders were about it. He had begged Pat Norman for a list of doctors to whom he could refer the scores of worried callers; she said she'd have to check about the right process for releasing such information.

People were dying and gay bureaucrats were worried about process. There wasn't time for process, Cleve said. Gay doctors still hadn't decided whether they'd bother to put together risk-reduction guidelines, and Cleve had spent half the day on the phone pleading with gay lawyers to sit on the board and give the organization some credibility. None of them seemed particularly interested either. They had their own political agenda, and there didn't seem anything to be gained by associating their names with some downer that was probably a lot of media hype.

Cleve took a long sip on his second vodka tonic, puffed heavily on a Marlboro, and noticed that Felix wasn't talking much. Cleve kicked himself for running off at the mouth and asked what the civil rights lawyer had been up to lately. Usually, there was some injustice that Felix was fighting in his new job at the State Bar of California. But the handsome Chicano lawyer offered little comment, complaining that he'd been tired a lot lately, just coming home after work and going straight to bed. Cleve thought it odd. They had spent the romantic summer of 1980 together, dancing hours away in the hot afternoon Tea Dances. Energy had never seemed to be Felix's problem.

The memories ended there. Cleve's peripatetic mind went back to the next day's KS forum, the new words he was learning, expressions like intubate and interferon, and the intricacies of probate with which he was becoming familiar. Suddenly, Felix excused himself from the table, dashed to the backyard, and threw up. With this, Cleve politely excused himself and headed for a bar.

⬭

Felix admitted it to no one, certainly not to old flames like Cleve Jones and not even to his best friends. Like hundreds of others in San Francisco, however, his doctor had sat him down for a serious talk. The yeast infections in his mouth, the fatigue, and those nightsweats, the doctor warned, might all be part of this new GRID syndrome. They needed to monitor his health carefully because he might come down with something worse. Somewhere, in some compartment separated from the rest of his being, Felix secreted this knowledge. There it stayed, never emerging in words to another person, haunting his sweaty sleep like a nightmare waiting to happen.

NEW YORK CITY

Rodger McFarlane and other Gay Men's Health Crisis members were training scores of hotline counselors, random volunteers collected from the board of directors' little black books. There was so much for the volunteers to learn, from the intricacies of the immune system to holding hands of healthy men who lay awake at night because a lymph node seemed just a little bigger than normal. One corps of volunteers was needed to finagle their way through the legendary red tape of getting disability and Social Security benefits. Each agency would have one or another social worker who would lend a sympathetic ear to the gay man or drug addict ailing with *Pneumocystis,* and these people needed to be discerned from among the many more who wouldn't.

Just when McFarlane would think he was going to work on long-term care plans, somebody would call and he'd have to change some man's sheets so he wouldn't be lying in shit all night. Then he'd have to talk to the guy for a couple of hours because it turned out that the family was coming the next day and they didn't even know the guy was gay, much less sick with gay cancer.

The tensions between Larry Kramer and Paul Popham were growing over the nature of what GMHC was supposed to be. Paul realized that a whole network of social services needed to be created for gay men during this epidemic. By now, it was clear that the city wasn't going to do much for a minority that wielded so little real political power in such a vast metropolis. Larry Kramer, meanwhile, wanted the group to veer into political activism and simply demand these services from the city as its just due.

Another point of conflict was over what to tell gay men. Larry was adamant that GMHC should tell homosexuals exactly what the doctors were telling board members in private meetings—to stop having sex. Or, if not to stop having sex altogether, at least to stop having the kind of sex that involves putting semen in another person's body. Most of the board members were themselves fresh from the hot summers in Fire Island bushes and long nights at spacious Manhattan bathhouses, and they had a hard time putting down the activities they had spent most of the past decade pursuing. It seemed prudish to make judgments. In the GMHC newsletter issued in July, the first nonscientific publication issued by any organization in the world on the year-old epidemic, various views of risk reduction were presented.

"A number of physicians, many of them gay as well, have advised their gay patients to moderate their sexual activity, to have fewer partners, and to have partners who are in good health," went the toughest advice. "It is the *number* of sexual partners, not sex itself, that increases risk."

Another story, by sociologist Marty Levine, however, sneered at such suggestions as "fallacious reasoning" and such advice as "panic . . . still washing over us." Levine wrote that "278 cases out of a possible 11 million (gay men in America) hardly constitutes an epidemic."

For its part, GMHC as a group decided that its job would be to give gay men the most up-to-date information about the epidemic and let them make their own decisions. This policy engendered another fierce debate between Larry Kramer and the other board members. "We don't want to get into the business of telling people what to do in bed," came the chorus against Larry. During an epidemic of a sexually transmitted disease, Larry thought, this was *exactly* what you did to save lives. He lost the arguments but remained convinced that the board ultimately would shift its position. The only question in his mind was how many people would die first.

July 13
MT. SINAI HOSPITAL,
NEW YORK CITY

Even before Dr. Jim Curran from the Centers for Disease Control started to speak, the symposium was buzzing about the *MMWR* that had just been issued a few days before from Atlanta. The report finally confirmed what doctors in New York City and Miami had known since last year—that this so-called gay cancer was all over the Haitian refugee communities in their cities. The *MMWR* documented thirty-four Haitian cases of opportunistic infections, like those striking gay men and intravenous drug users. Most Haitians suffered from either *Pneumocystis* or toxoplasmosis, although some contracted the deadly cryptococcus brain infection or disseminated tuberculosis. Unlike the stricken gay men, few of the Haitians seemed to be getting Kaposi's sarcoma. However, their blood showed the same deficiencies in T-helper lymphocytes that marked all the various risk groups.

"The occurrence of opportunistic infections among adult Haitians with no history of underlying immunosuppressive therapy or disease has not been reported, previously," the report stated dryly. In plain talk, the CDC was saying that this had never happened before and they'd be damned if they could figure out why it was happening now. The Haitians presented a new enigma in which to wrap the mystery of the growing epidemic. The worst news of the day, however, was yet to come.

When Curran started talking, a discernible chill crept through the room. There was still another new risk group, Curran said. That week, the CDC would release the case histories of three hemophiliacs who apparently contracted the immune suppression from their Factor VIII. The three cases, Curran knew, were the hemophiliacs in Canton and Denver whom Dale Lawrence had just researched, as well as the elderly Florida man who had been reported to the CDC back in January. A stunned silence greeted Curran's report.

After the lecture, somebody whispered something in the corridor to Curran about a rumored transfusion-related GRID case in Montreal. Curran's normally cool face looked plainly disturbed at the news.

Meanwhile, the doctors fell into little groups, seizing on the implications of GRID in hemophiliacs. First gays, then intravenous drug users, and now hemophiliacs. Those were the major risk groups for hepatitis B. They also knew that there was another risk group for hepatitis B: doctors, nurses, and health care workers. Hospitals were now vaccinating their entire staffs with the new hepatitis B vaccine in the first move toward eliminating that dreaded disease from the profession. Would GRID be the encore? Many doctors wondered aloud that afternoon whether the next risk group to be described in the *MMWR* would include themselves.

○

As of July 15, 471 cases of GRID had been reported to the Centers for Disease Control, of whom 184 had died. The victims now spanned twenty-four states; the pace of their diagnoses was quickening. One-third of the cases had been reported in the past twelve weeks alone. New diagnoses, which had been coming in at a rate of 1.5 a day in February, were being reported at a rate of 2.5 a day in July. Finally, the CDC was publicly calling the outbreak of immune suppression an epidemic.

"The pressure is on" to find the cause, said Jim Curran in a *Washington Post* interview published on July 18. "There may be additional groups that get it, and, in the other groups, people are going to keep on dying. . . . Somebody's got to find this thing."

17 ENTROPY

July 1982
PARIS

By the summer of 1982, officials at Claude-Bernard Hospital, a hulking collection of old brick buildings near the outskirts of Paris, had their fill of the incorrigible Dr. Willy Rozenbaum. For a year, gay patients had cluttered their hospital hallways as he engaged in an epidemiological study that had neither official sanction nor approval. The hospital was getting a reputation as the center for this disease, and its administrators were getting uncomfortable. This was not a problem decent people became involved with, and they let Rozenbaum know it. The thirty-six-year-old infectious disease specialist was given an ultimatum: Either quit studying this disease and return to a legitimate area of medical inquiry or leave.

The hospital counted itself lucky when Rozenbaum finally left that summer for a new post at Pitie-Salpetriere Hospital, where his studies would be tolerated if not enthusiastically supported. Rozenbaum knew he was risking his career by pressing ahead with his GRID studies, but he forged on anyway, establishing a position as Europe's leading authority on the epidemic. Later, the administrators who had harassed Rozenbaum would cry for experts in the disease and belatedly try to establish themselves as the city's most important facility for treatment of immune deficiency.

By the time Willy Rozenbaum left his job at Claude-Bernard Hospital, the epidemic of immune suppression had spread into eleven European nations, including Belgium, Czechoslovakia, Denmark, West Germany, Holland, Italy, Norway, Spain, Switzerland, Great Britain, and of course, France.

July 27
WASHINGTON, D.C.

If you don't abide by scientific principles, chaos will ensue.

It was a fundamental tenet of Dale Lawrence's world. It was an idea that also recurred to him after he had flown up from Atlanta to join his boss, Dr. Bruce

Evatt, and Don Francis and a gathering of leaders of the blood industry, hemophiliac groups, gay community organizations, and assorted luminaries from the National Institutes of Health and the Food and Drug Administration. The Centers for Disease Control had hoped the new evidence of blood transmission would incite the blood industry's two major components, the voluntary blood banks and the for-profit manufacturers of blood products, to move quickly to stem the tide of blood contamination.

The CDC privately preferred launching the only available preventive measure: donor deferral guidelines, asking people who fit into the high-risk groups, such as gay men, Haitians, and drug users, not to donate blood. The logical science of GRID demanded that logical steps be taken, the CDC thought, or people would die needlessly. However, as would be the case with just about every policy aspect of the epidemic, logic would not be the prevailing modus operandi.

The hemophiliac groups immediately attacked the data that linked the immune suppression to the contamination of Factor VIII. They had read that some scientists believed gay men contracted the immune suppression simply because they were overloaded with infections. With all their exposure to blood-borne viruses, hemophiliacs also might be suffering from such immune overload, they argued. Isn't it too early to say with scientific certainty that this thing is hitting hemophiliacs? The National Hemophilia Foundation was also nervous about the accusations directed at Factor VIII, the product that had done so much to improve the hemophiliacs' quality of life in recent years. Did the CDC want these 20,000 stricken Americans to go back to the less sophisticated techniques of stopping bleeding with attendant hemorrhagic fatalities?

For their part, the CDC hands wondered whether the hemophiliacs were reluctant to have their blood disorder linked in any way to a disease that homosexuals got; it created a terrible public relations problem.

Gay community leaders were even more public relations–oriented than hemophiliacs. A New York City gay physician, Dr. Roger Enlow, argued persuasively that it was too soon to push for guidelines. Any such moves would have implications for the civil rights of millions of Americans, gay leaders noted. Only Dr. Dan William argued that such deferral of gay blood donors might be an entirely appropriate step toward saving lives, and that observation marked the beginning of his loss of popularity in the gay community.

The agency with the authority to actually enforce any donor guidelines on the blood industry was the Food and Drug Administration. Already, the FDA was keenly aware of maneuvers for control of turf in this meeting. Some FDA regulators resented the CDC's brash invasion of what was plainly their territory, the blood industry. Moreover, many at the FDA did not believe that this so-called epidemic of immune suppression even existed. Privately, in conversations with CDC officials, FDA officials confided that they thought the CDC had taken a bunch of unrelated illnesses and lumped them into some made-up phenomenon as a brazen ruse to get publicity and funding for their threatened agency. Bureaucrats have been known to undertake more questionable methods to protect their budgets. Given the Reagan administration's wholesale budget slashing, this would not be all that drastic a reaction.

In the end, everybody agreed that they should do one thing: Wait and see what happens. The situation would clarify itself and then they would move. How could the government be expected to forge national policy for more than 220 million Americans just because three hemophiliacs got sick?

The meeting, however, did accomplish one memorable achievement. It was more than one year since Michael Gottlieb and Alvin Friedman-Kien had reported their cases of pneumonia and skin cancer, and the epidemic still did not have one commonly agreed-upon name. Different scientists were using different acronyms in an alphabet soup that further confused the already befuddled story of a strange new disease of unknown origin. The staffers at the CDC despised the GRID acronym and refused to use it. With the advent of hemophiliac cases, Jim Curran argued that any references to "gay" or "community" should be dropped and something more neutral be adopted. Besides, Curran thought ACIDS was a little grotesque.

Somebody finally suggested the name that stuck: Acquired Immune Deficiency Syndrome. That gave the epidemic a snappy acronym, AIDS, and was sexually neutral. The word "acquired" separated the immune deficiency syndrome from congenital defects or chemically induced immune problems, indicating the syndrome was acquired from somewhere even though nobody knew from where.

This bit of resolution, however, did not keep Dale Lawrence from fretting about the vacuum in policy on AIDS blood transmission. Immune overload didn't fit with the facts, Lawrence thought. Hemophiliacs had been getting transfusions for decades, and only now did three of them pop up with *Pneumocystis* pneumonia in a matter of months, showing identical immunological profiles to those of the gay AIDS patients.

Gays were worried about public relations and hemophiliacs were skittish about being involved with anything having to do with homosexuals. The FDA was worried about turf and was largely unconvinced there was a disease at all, much less something that merited the kind of serious scrambling those CDC hotshots wanted.

There was something else from the meeting that also troubled Dale Lawrence. Jim Curran and others discussed that AIDS cases were turning up in prisons, and a commercial plasma manufacturer had admitted that a lot of blood had been drawn in state prisons. They were a good source of plasma, he said. Lawrence could think only, "Oh God."

○

By mid-1982, there was much to be ignored; the epidemic was spreading faster than the official pronouncements indicated. Science was not working at its best, accepting new information with an unbiased eye and beginning appropriate investigations. The handful of scientists who ignored their elders' advice and worked on the newly christened AIDS epidemic found themselves not only struggling against a baffling disease but against the indifference of science, government, mass media, most gay leaders, and public health officials.

In the Bronx, Dr. Arye Rubinstein was now treating eleven babies stricken with AIDS, but few scientists would believe his diagnosis. After holding his article on the infants for six months, the *New England Journal of Medicine* had returned it to Rubinstein with the firm conclusion that these kids most certainly did not have AIDS, the homosexuals' disease. By now, at least, the CDC doctors were interested in his findings, but they were moving cautiously. Jealously watched by other federal health agencies that were worried that the CDC might use the epidemic to cut into the already restricted flow of federal money, every CDC-announced development had to be entirely sound, or enemies in the government would use it to discredit them.

In his lab at the Albert Einstein College of Medicine, Rubinstein was frantic with worry. He had to make people believe him; the science establishments' obsession with the sex lives of most of the AIDS victims was blinding it to the horror that could unfold in other pockets of America. Given the projections of new AIDS cases, it was clear that many more such babies would be born to infected mothers. Many of these mothers would die. Who would take care of their babies? How would society cope with supporting a population that seemed born to die of such a horrible disease? Yet, pondering such solutions would happen only after he had convinced somebody important that there was a problem, that these babies even existed.

August 2
NEW YORK CITY

Dan Rather put on his somber face as he stared into the cameras of the "CBS Nightly News."

"Federal health officials consider it an epidemic. Yet you rarely hear a thing about it. At first, it seemed to strike only one segment of the population. Now, Barry Peterson tells us, this is no longer the case."

The story, one of the first network news pieces to appear on AIDS, had all the right elements: Bobbi Campbell talked about how he wanted to survive; Larry Kramer said the lack of government research was because it was perceived as a gay disease; Jim Curran provided the hopeful note that solving AIDS could lead to the elimination of all cancer.

"But there is almost no money being spent so far," concluded reporter Peterson. "For Bobbi Campbell, it is a race against time. How long before he and others who have this disease, finally have answers, finally have the hope of a cure?"

Of all the sentences in this story, probably none was so pointedly directed at the fundamental problem than Rather's own lead-in, "you rarely hear a thing about it." As managing editor of the "CBS Nightly News," Rather passed the news judgment that made AIDS a disease that one rarely heard anything about. Three years later, television commentators would still be talking about AIDS as that disease you rarely heard anything about, as if they were helpless bystanders and not the very people who themselves had decreed the silence in the public media.

Because nobody heard much about this disease, nobody in 1982 really did very much about it, save for a few heroic souls. And they were too few to make much of a difference, ensuring that Bobbi Campbell, like thousands of other Americans, would lose his race against time.

August
NATIONAL INSTITUTES OF HEALTH,
BETHESDA

Now, more than a year into the epidemic, the National Institutes of Health had no coordinated AIDS plan. Everything was done on the basis of temporary assignments by the handful of doctors who happened to be intrigued by the world's first epidemic of immune disorders. At the sprawling NIH hospitals, a few doctors struggled valiantly with every conceivable medical technology to save the AIDS patients, and they failed. At Bob Gallo's lab at the National Cancer Institute's Division of Tumor Cell Biology, about 10 percent of the staff effort went into poking around the devastated lymphocytes of AIDS patients. In his lab at the NCI, Jim Goedert desperately wanted to launch full-scale bench investigations into finding the AIDS virus but ran straight into the brick wall of limited resources. The dilemma would be hard to explain to outsiders, he thought. The money was in the budget. Indeed, Congress had been generally successful at holding the budget line for health against the Reagan budget cutters. The administration, however, was retaliating by not permitting managers like Goedert to hire anybody. Goedert had enough money to pay for lab tests, to finance computer activities, and to purchase supplies, but he couldn't put any new people on board. So he didn't have the scientists he needed to steer studies, analyze data, and then write it up into papers.

In other labs, this or that contractor may have diverted NIH funds for the research, but no substantial effort was under way. It was nearly eleven months after the NCI symposium on Kaposi's sarcoma in Bethesda, and still the institute had not released its request for funding proposals or made any move to free money for AIDS investigators outside Bethesda. Researchers outside the government would have to fend for themselves.

CENTER FOR HUMAN TUMOR VIRUS RESEARCH,
UNIVERSITY OF CALIFORNIA,
SAN FRANCISCO

The hemophiliac cases convinced Dr. Jay Levy that he needed to shift from studying Kaposi's sarcoma to the blood of AIDS patients to find whatever microbe was knocking out their T-4 cells. While East Coast scientists still squabbled over the syndrome's etiology, West Coast researchers were by now almost unanimously convinced that one infectious agent was at work. The tilt toward a single agent raised an entirely new quandary for Levy. Though his tiny eighty-foot-square lab building on the twelfth floor of the Medical Sciences' had been fine for studying the skin cancer tumors of KS, the university maintained that the lab did not have the appropriate safety gear for studying an infectious disease. In order to comply with university safety standards, Levy needed to adapt a flow hood with a new $1,500 filter.

Again, Levy was at a loss as to how to comply. Like human tumor virus labs across the country, he had been bled dry by the administration's grant cuts and scientific trends that had put cancer virus research out of vogue. Many of Levy's colleagues were leaving academic medicine to get more secure jobs at private pharmaceutical corporations; some dropped out of science altogether. Levy knew that, within a few years, America would face a severe shortage of retrovirologists because of the funding cutbacks. In 1982, nobody seemed to care; that would be the nightmare of 1985. As it was, Jay Levy went to a wealthy friend in April just to meet the payroll of the only two staffers in his center, a part-time technician and a part-time secretary. He was under orders from the university to come up with grant money or leave. Now, as he was about to start what he felt would be promising research into the cause of AIDS, his efforts were arrested because he did not have $1,500 for a filter. He asked the chancellor's office for a few extra bucks but was turned down; there was no mechanism within the university that would channel him the sum.

Crestfallen, Levy talked to Marcus Conant, who continued to coordinate the efforts of the UCSF doctors. Never one for bureaucratic niceties, Conant decided on the spot, "We'll just go to the legislature." Using his growing network of gay political contacts, Conant approached the assembly speaker's office for the $1,500 for Levy's lab.

Back at the university, the hierarchy was furious with the retrovirologist. In the best of times, university officials resented any involvement at all with the political process, disdaining the shortsighted concerns of grubby politicians in the legislature. The only thing they hated more was the tendency of legislators to want to give money for this or that research, taking away the discretionary power of the university chieftains themselves. Such direct legislative funding was deemed, in the lofty towers of academia, tainted money.

Levy got his money nonetheless. One call from the assembly speaker to the chancellor took care of that. But the money came six months after he had requested it, in January 1983.

Levy could have spent those six months looking for the AIDS virus. Indeed, when his lab became one of three institutions in the world to isolate the cause of the syndrome, it was obvious that the $1,500 was well spent. It was also obvious, Levy subsequently noted, that it could have happened much faster.

The story of the $1,500 filter was just one of many that popped up in every corner of the nation in 1982.

$\bigcirc$

The lack of university enthusiasm over this homosexual disease was not restricted to retrovirology or San Francisco or Paris. In Los Angeles, Dr. Michael Gottlieb's requests for a clinic to study the burgeoning numbers of AIDS patients were still being shuffled around by administrators who remained uncomfortable with the notion of becoming a center for study of a homosexual disease. Some even seemed jealous of the attention Gottlieb had garnered in the past year.

At the CDC, Dr. James Curran, head of the rechristened AIDS Task Force, continued to cajole eminent virologists and researchers into looking into AIDS, but few were interested.

The noted lack of enthusiasm among UCSF administrators for housing the nation's only AIDS clinic prodded Marc Conant and Paul Volberding to shift the clinic's site out of UCSF and into San Francisco General Hospital, the teaching hospital associated with the university. In July, the city government approved the necessary funds to revamp a cancer clinic at the county hospital into an AIDS outpatient clinic, to open at the start of 1983. Volberding justified this first outlay of any municipal funds anywhere in the world for the AIDS epidemic by noting that between July 1, 1981, and July 1, 1982, he had seen ten cases of Kaposi's sarcoma. The city's $40,000 appropriation was based on Volberding's projection of seeing twenty more cases in the next year. The prognostication, of course, was hopelessly naive, but these summer months of 1982 were the innocent times when the names of all San Francisco's AIDS patients fit on one blackboard.

RAYBURN HOUSE OFFICE BUILDING, WASHINGTON, D.C.

In Washington, Tim Westmoreland also had spent all summer trying to get straight answers about AIDS spending from the honchos at the U.S. Department of Health and Human Services. In a July memo, the National Cancer Institute proposed to dole out $1.25 million in the next fiscal year to support three years of research for scientists outside the government. Westmoreland was flabbergasted. It would be three months before the government would even accept proposals for the funding, he realized, and probably another nine months before the money would be released. For the fiscal year coming to a close, the NCI had spent a total of $450,000 to support extramural research. Next year, they planned to spend $520,000. Out of its $1 billion budget, the NCI had spent all of $291,000 for its own studies on Kaposi's sarcoma, or about one-fortieth of one percent of its money. The total Centers for Disease Control spending for AIDS, meanwhile, amounted to about $2 million out of the agency's total $202 million budget.

Meanwhile, in an August 5 memo to Bill Kraus, the National Institutes of Health outlined their efforts. The entire undertaking from this $4-billion-a-year behemoth of health consisted of twelve different experiments being conducted at a leisurely pace by the National Cancer Institute and the National Institute for Allergy and Infectious Diseases. The complete AIDS program fit neatly on three typewritten pages, with plenty of room to spare. There was no mention of any future release of funding to outside investigators nor any plan for a coordinated response beyond their experimentation.

"This is appalling," Kraus groaned, reverting to his standard complaint: "Doesn't anyone care?"

FIFE'S RESORT,
RUSSIAN RIVER, CALIFORNIA

Gary Walsh had finally broken out of his militant introvert stage and was his old charming self, Joe Brewer thought. Lounging by the pool under the redwoods at Fife's, a popular gay resort, it seemed to Joe that their decision to be everything-but-sexual lovers was working out well. Gary had just moved into a wonderful apartment above the Castro District with a panoramic view of the downtown skyline. Matt Krieger was ensconced in the quaint home he and Gary had purchased a mile away. Joe was single too, so he and Gary commiserated on boy troubles, enjoyed the sun, and planned their Christmas trip to Mexico.

Inside the rustic log cabin, taking a private respite from the sun, Gary Walsh applied lotion to the red flaky streaks over his bushy brown eyebrows. He hated the creams and despised the constant attention he had to devote to these blemishes. But the thirty-eight-year-old was terrified at what they really were—outward manifestations of the collapse of his immune system. No doctor had come out and said it, and Gary sometimes kept the conscious knowledge even from himself. For months, however, the thought had formed, rising from his mind like a poisonous vapor, as he tossed alone in sweat-soaked sheets.

By this hot August weekend, he had stopped editing the idea from his inner monologue, even though he never spoke of it with Matt or Joe. If he did not have AIDS now, Gary knew, he was certainly about to get it and there was nothing he could do except wait.

Gary finished dabbing the hydrocortisone cream above his eyebrows and checked his smile in the mirror before leaving the cabin to join Joe again by the pool.

BELLEVUE HOSPITAL,
NEW YORK CITY

The patient, a Hispanic family man, was delirious when Dale Lawrence arrived at his bedside. His fever, fueled by severe *Pneumocystis carinii* pneumonia, was spiking and much of what he said didn't make sense. English was not his first language, creating even more problems for the interview. His doctors already had asked whether the man was gay or had used intravenous drugs; he may have said yes, but nobody was sure. His wife, however, insisted that he was neither gay nor an intravenous drug user. His physicians agreed and pointed to a more likely cause.

In January 1981, the man had received massive blood transfusions for a coronary bypass operation at Bellevue. Twelve American blood donations and eight European units of blood were pumped into the man during the surgery. None of the American donors were on the list CDC kept of AIDS patients. Lawrence realized he needed to interview the dozen New York donors to see whether any were showing early symptoms of the syndrome or whether they fit into any high-risk group. Transfusion AIDS was a disaster waiting to happen, he felt, and the nation needed to be alerted at the earliest possible moment.

Lawrence was disappointed when the officials at the New York Blood Center, the nation's largest blood bank, refused to supply him with the addresses of the donors so he could launch his planned interviews. No, the blood-banking officials maintained, there's no evidence that AIDS can be spread through blood transfusions. The legal protection of donor confidentiality could not be breached unless transfusion-associated AIDS already was an established fact. Beyond allowing the CDC to compare donor names to its AIDS roster, the blood bank would not allow the CDC to have direct contact with the donors. The center did agree to call donors and ask if they belonged to a risk group. Not surprisingly, they later reported all donors were well and not at high risk for AIDS.

Dale Lawrence's boss, Bruce Evatt, had made several trips to Washington over the summer to try to goad the blood industry into taking measures to limit donors from high-risk groups. Blood banks and the commercial manufacturers of blood products such as Factor VIII, however, could not comprehend the seriousness of the CDC's warnings about possible AIDS contamination of the blood. When moral persuasion failed to move the blood industry, Evatt mentioned the fiscal implications for blood banks. They could be open for a wave of negligence lawsuits for failing to heed the CDC advice and continuing to spread AIDS. Nothing worked.

Lawrence continued the probe as best he could. He checked on who else was in the operating room the day of the surgery, in case a health staffer might have infected the man. He checked into who shared the same ventilator, which bed the man had lain in, and even the heating duct in the room where the man slept. None of it panned out. Because the proof of AIDS transmission likely lay in the ability to interview the donors, he could not provide the necessary evidence.

There was something else that was curious about this case, although it wouldn't make sense for some time. While reviewing the patient's medical records, Lawrence discovered that the first signs of the patient's illness were not the typical symptoms of nightsweats, swollen lymph nodes, or fatigue. Instead, three months after the transfusions, the man had complained of nerve problems in his leg. He used a cane until he got better, but then he became strangely forgetful and disoriented, almost as if he were senile. One of the patient's children sighed sadly to Lawrence, "It seemed that Daddy had started to lose his mind."

18 RUNNING ON EMPTY

August 6, 1982
ST. FRANCIS HOSPITAL,
SAN FRANCISCO

The obituary the family sent to the newspapers that afternoon said the international trade consultant had died "after a long illness." Indeed, the demise of the forty-eight-year-old trade expert was recorded more to interest the socially prominent than the medical community, even though the man was one of the first local AIDS patients to die of encephalitis, another new complication of a disease that seemed chock full of grisly surprises.

Concealing an AIDS diagnosis in a death notice was nothing unusual in these times. In the first years of AIDS, obituaries disguised the reality that an epidemic was stealing the lives of the renowned, not just the better-publicized profligates. One had to read the obituaries closely to understand this, to look for the vague long illness or the odd reference to a pneumonia or skin cancer striking down someone in, say, their mid-thirties. People, especially the plutocracy, didn't die of some homosexual disease, according to the death notices; they just wasted away after a "long illness," like Camille. Wives and children were never among the survivors listed in such obituaries. Instead there were brothers and aunts, nieces and nephews, and all too often, at least one parent assigned the unnatural task of presiding at his or her own child's funeral.

Nevertheless, at 1:30 P.M. on an unseasonably sultry Friday afternoon, this graduate of Middlesex and Harvard had given a last painful groan, his head splitting from the horrible encephalitis brought on by his lack of T-4 lymphocytes, and his lungs constricted by the primordial protozoa that multiplied so prodigiously in his air sacs. And then he had died.

It made all the papers. The family pedigree was rolled out, right down to the fact that his great-grandmother had founded a famous local hospital. He was fourth generation of San Francisco high society, a member of the prestigious Pacific Union Club and all the right tennis clubs, and his services were held in the most fashionable Episcopal Church. The family preferred contributions to be sent to Harvard University, among other charities, none of which had anything to do with homosexual diseases.

The death would be little noted nor long remembered except that there was an ailing baby whose immune deficiencies were baffling an eminent pediatric immunologist at the University of California in San Francisco. Dr. Mort Cowan had ushered the seventeen-month-old infant through infection after infection, candidiasis and severe hepatitis, a swollen spleen and later the horrible *Mycobacterium avium-intracellular,* a bizarre opportunistic infection rarely seen in the United States.

It was about this time that Cowan showed the infant and all the immune mysteries his body presented to one of the nation's foremost pediatric immunologists, Dr. Art Ammann. Ammann surveyed the infant's charts and blood work and came to a quick, albeit startling conclusion. "It looks to me like this baby has AIDS," he told Cowan.

Ammann was keenly aware of the controversy his conclusion would engender. As far as he knew, he was the only doctor to arrive at such a diagnosis in an infant. Because all the prestigious journals of pediatrics and immunology had rebuffed the attempts by physicians like Dr. Arye Rubinstein in the Bronx to advance precisely this hypothesis, Ammann, 3,000 miles away, had no idea that others were cautiously coming to the same conclusion.

August 13
DALLAS, TEXAS

At the first National Lesbian and Gay Leadership Conference, the hallways were crackling with talk of who's in and who's out. Most of the major gay leaders ignored the fifty earnest organizers meeting in a small conference room off to the side in the first national AIDS Forum.

Cleve Jones had felt so isolated in San Francisco that he was ecstatic to finally meet all the people who, like himself, could see how much of the future of the gay cause lay inside the mysteries of AIDS. The forum, Cleve thought, wasn't like the dozens of other gay conferences he had attended, or even the gay leadership conference at the same hotel. He couldn't get over how cute Paul Popham from Gay Men's Health Crisis was. He also thought Larry Kramer, with his grating confrontational personality, would probably do much better in San Francisco than with all those closet queens in New York.

For his part, Larry felt like a fresh-faced, smart-assed new kid on the block. GMHC was growing by leaps and bounds, boasting over 300 volunteers now. The group would open their headquarters next month, and the organization was training scores of volunteers for a "Buddy Program" that would give the ailing people practical services. Support groups for people with AIDS and their friends and lovers would move out of the hospitals and into the new headquarters, as well. GMHC was creating an entirely new social service network, its leaders proudly told each other, and doing it completely without the self-important, politically correct bimbos who made such fools out of themselves in gay leadership conferences.

The mere fact that few of the big-time leaders bothered to take part in the AIDS Forum was itself proof of their lack of vision, Larry Kramer thought. As far as he was concerned, there was no other gay issue to be involved in. With a new epidemic beginning to erode the very core of gay political power in the big cities, the community couldn't afford the old agendas. As it was, the gay political community was running on empty in its attempts to steamroll a national gay movement; AIDS threatened to bring the whole effort to a screeching halt.

Jack Campbell looked a little worried as he handed Cleve a check for the San Francisco Kaposi's Sarcoma Education and Research Foundation. Cleve Jones understood why. From a single bathhouse Campbell had opened in Cleveland years back, he had built the legendary Club Baths chain, a franchise that ran bathhouses in every region of the United States and Canada. By virtue of their substantial largess to the always-starved gay political community, bathhouse owners long had been influential gay leaders in New York, Los Angeles, Miami, Chicago, and to a lesser extent, San Francisco. Campbell, a former chairman of the board of the National Gay Task Force, carried the most clout both nationally and in Florida, where he was the undisputed gay leader. Florida, it turned out, was one of the states hardest hit by the epidemic.

As he talked with Cleve, Campbell gently turned the conversation toward what AIDS might mean for his business.

"I think it's a sexually transmitted disease that's caused by a virus," Cleve tried to say delicately, folding the check neatly into his wallet. "Nobody has advocated closing the baths, but I think there need to be changes."

Privately, Cleve favored setting up informational pickets outside bathhouses to let patrons know they might be risking their lives in the sex palaces. But even hints toward such action were met with fierce resistance by others who still viewed bathhouses as symbols of the sexual liberation gays had fought so long to gain. Many still were not convinced that AIDS was a venereal disease. Wouldn't they just be playing into the oppressors' hands if they went and closed down businesses—gay businesses at that—and it turned out the disease was caused by poppers?

As a political issue, the bathhouses were put to rest quickly. The idea of closing them was too shocking even for those involved in the fight against AIDS, most of whom had cut their political horns in civil rights causes. Meanwhile, bathhouse owners like Jack Campbell and Bruce Mailman, the proprietor of the sprawling St. Mark's Baths in New York, showed their keen interest in the epidemic by lavishing donations on AIDS groups, the people from whom warnings about bathhouses would be expected to come. We're all in this together, everybody said.

The night after the AIDS Forum, the leading AIDS activists gathered in the hotel room of Dr. David Ostrow from Chicago to brainstorm with Dr. James

Curran, the main speaker at the forum. Like the rest, Curran was surprised that so many of the gay leaders at the conference seemed so little concerned with the epidemic that could render all other gay issues irrelevant—but he wasn't there to scold. He was there to listen. He kept asking, What's new in the gay community that might have started it?

As the group reviewed old territory, Curran was taken aback when Larry Kramer said he already knew twenty-one people stricken with AIDS. How does one person know twenty-one victims? Curran wondered. What would that be like?

Cleve watched Curran draw out the various gay leaders, tapping their ideas, not saying much himself. Being a political animal, Cleve wondered what the politics of AIDS looked like from within the government. Were they getting enough money? What was really going on at the CDC? Curran didn't talk much about that. The doctors in the group didn't ask.

$$\bigcirc$$

The week that gay leaders met in Dallas, the numbers of AIDS cases in the United States surpassed 500. The task force in Atlanta was aghast at the speed with which casualties were mounting. At least 20 percent of the cases had been diagnosed in the previous five weeks alone. At this rate, 1,000 people would be diagnosed by the end of the year, they figured. It was at this time that Bill Foege, director of the Centers for Disease Control, was heard to wonder aloud, with genuine curiosity: Why was nobody excited about this disease?

MANHATTAN

The opening of the Gay Men's Health Crisis offices only underscored how badly the growing numbers of New York City AIDS sufferers needed city services. Once immobilized by the progressive disease, many were left stranded in their New York City apartments. They needed more than support workers in the Buddy Program; they needed home nursing care. Education was also needed. Hospital workers were getting more antsy with word that AIDS was spreading like hepatitis B. They needed to have their fears quelled. Meanwhile, gays needed their fears heightened so they wouldn't be out fucking themselves to death, as Larry Kramer put it.

Attempts to meet with Mayor Ed Koch were rebuffed. It wasn't hard to see why. Koch had just lost a bitter primary fight for the New York governorship against Queens Democrat Mario Cuomo. The issue of Koch's perennial bachelorhood, of course, was badly manipulated in conservative parts of the state for Cuomo's campaign. Posters appeared in the Archie Bunker land of Queens, saying: "Vote for Cuomo, Not the Homo." Most gay leaders with any clout also had lined up for Cuomo in the state primary. Koch obviously was not about to start championing funds for a homosexual disease.

Larry Kramer urged starting an angry protest against Koch. Only a show of power would prod him into action, he said. Cooler heads on the GMHC board prevailed, arguing that would only alienate the mayor further.

In general, more gays were furious at the city's most prominent gay doctor, Dan William, than at anybody in the Koch administration. In a long essay and a subsequent interview in the *New York Native*'s voluminous AIDS coverage, William dared suggest that bathhouses should be required to post signs warning about the epidemic and promiscuous sex, the way restaurants post signs explaining the Heimlich maneuver. Bathhouses should work to change sexual behavior and reduce the risk of contracting AIDS, he said, or end up, in effect, being the "Russian roulette" parlors of the gay community.

The very suggestion of turning back a decade of sexual liberation stirred a maelstrom William could hardly have predicted. The *Body Politic,* the leading leftist gay magazine, denounced William as a "monogamist" who was "stirring panic" and an "epidemic of fear." William was surprised at the vehemence of the denunciations but understood, in a personal way, the discomfort that the entire community felt at the prospect of squarely facing a deadly new disease. In early 1981, he had been told he was suffering from a degenerative blood disease and that he could expect to live five, maybe ten years. The ailment was unrelated to the AIDS epidemic, but it let William know the desperation of denial: how, when something is so horrible you don't want to believe it, you want to put it out of your mind and insist it isn't true, and how you hate the person who says it is.

William saw that denial among some patients now, when he told them that something was wrong with their white blood cell counts and they needed to closely monitor their health. He also heard it in the angry voices raised against him. That was denial too, on a social and even political level. It was a phase the gay community would work through, just as he had found a way to work through it. The problem for the community, however, was more burning, because its denial would rob gays of time, the time when they could have begun taking AIDS seriously and time when they could have been protecting themselves. Time would always mean lives in this scourge.

$\bigcirc$

A vague awareness of something horrible had seized the collective gay consciousness by this summer, however. Businessmen were able to deal with the trend, even if politicians were not. The advertisements amounted to a blitz in the gay newspapers for astronomically priced vitamin packets called HIM— Health and Immunity for Men. The packets contained "natural vitamins, minerals and herbs for the sexually active male." The unique HIM formula, the advertising promised, helped in "maximizing the immune system to fight infection" and "maintaining sexual vitality and potency." The advertisements didn't come out and say, "Eat these vitamins and you won't die a miserable death," but that clearly was the exploitive intention as the vitamin packs became hotsellers in gay neighborhoods across the country. The sewers of Manhattan and San Francisco flowed with the most vitamin-rich urine in the nation, even as gay men trooped off to the baths, convinced that if there was really something dangerous in the business, their leaders would warn them. They were all in this together.

August 19
WASHINGTON, D.C.

The Dallas conference had drawn a dribble of coverage from the wire services, most of which grabbed the AIDS angle because of the dramatic rise in cases. Days later, Washington bureaucrats responded to the publicity the way they know best, with a press release.

"Dr. Edward N. Brandt, Jr., Assistant Secretary for Health, today directed agencies of the Public Health Service to step up activities to combat Acquired Immune Deficiency Syndrome, a little-understood syndrome afflicting increasing numbers of people in the United States."

The instructions Brandt announced that day included continuing studies of hemophiliacs, review techniques to eliminate diseases from Factor VIII, involvement of all groups affected by the epidemic in future AIDS meetings, and a call for the National Cancer Institute to "act as expeditiously as possible" in getting out $2.2 million in government and nongovernment AIDS research projects financed for the next fiscal year. Toeing the FDA line that no peril existed to the nation's blood supply, Brandt also stated, "The lung infection in three patients with hemophilia is disturbing. At this time, however, we can't be sure there is a connection between blood products used by these patients and AIDS."

Brandt's instruction for the National Cancer Institute to act "expeditiously" was chuckled over in many key AIDS research centers across the country. After all, it had been nearly a year since the money was pledged, and the grant application process was not slated to begin for another month, meaning it would be mid-1983 before any National Institutes of Health funds were released, "expeditiously."

The brief moment of official interest in the syndrome sparked a spate of further news coverage that fell into what was becoming a familiar pattern. Always eager to use an angle that did not involve perverts or addicts, *Newsweek* ran a brief story keyed to the two-month-old hemophiliac announcement: "Homosexual Plague Strikes New Victims." It was important to let people know that AIDS was hitting people who mattered, so the story's second sentence reported that "the 'homosexual plague' has started spilling over into the general population." The dozen harried CDC staffers who could barely keep up with breaking developments were transformed by *Newsweek* into a "75-member CDC task force," a number that presumably included every CDC staffer who ever sat in on an AIDS Task Force meeting. Two weeks later, a *Time* magazine story expanded the CDC Task Force to 120 members.

The inflated staffing figures, while altogether fictitious, reflected two salient problems that haunted the journalism of AIDS for years. First, reporters were willing to believe any story handed to them in a press release without the slightest inclination to discover whether the reported facts were true. Press-release journalism, out of vogue since the advent of Watergate-style investigative reporting, made a dashing comeback with the AIDS epidemic. The second tendency evident in AIDS journalism was the compulsion to lend a reassuring last note to otherwise bleak stories. Big task forces meant the problem might be solved, and every month or so, tucked away in the second section of most newspapers, a few wire-service paragraphs appeared about this or that breakthrough in AIDS research. There were headlines like, "KS Discovery Brings Glimmer of Hope," but, in truth, there were no glimmers of hope as summer faded to fall in 1982. There were just bureaucrats who thought they could both hold back domestic spending and thwart a virulent new epidemic, as well as newspaper editors who didn't care to run much about a homosexual plague and didn't care whether what they did run was true.

Meanwhile, in the last weeks of August, two more states reported their first AIDS cases. The epidemic now had swept into twenty-six states and a dozen nations.

19 FORCED FEEDING

September 1982
BUREAU OF COMMUNICABLE DISEASE CONTROL,
SAN FRANCISCO

In her cramped office, piled high with medical journals and manila folders of disease records, Dr. Selma Dritz was on the phone to Atlanta, wondering whether they understood how serious this all was. Still another disease was starting to appear among gay men, and she was convinced it was related to AIDS. As an epidemiologist, Dritz played a numbers game and she wanted the new disease included in the AIDS numbers. As usual, she was fighting with the Centers for Disease Control about it.

The first patients had gone to their doctors with lymph nodes the size of golf balls. This wasn't your garden variety lymphadenopathy. The diagnosis was Burkitt's lymphoma, a lymph cancer that was among the first human cancers linked to a virus. A number of San Francisco researchers, in fact, had once worked in Africa on studies that connected Burkitt's lymphoma to the Epstein-Barr virus, the microbe that in the United States most commonly caused mononucleosis, or the "kissing disease." Dritz was intrigued because, once again, she was seeing a tumor caused by a virus arising in the immune-deficient gay men, just as Kaposi's sarcoma had been linked to the cytomegalovirus in Africa. The immune deficiency seemed to let these viruses run wild and foster the tumors. The detection of this phenomenon had implications far beyond AIDS; the trend might offer new insight into the relationship between cancer and viruses.

When the first reports came in, casually from doctors she would be chatting with, Dritz did her homework. She checked with the California Tumor Registry in Sacramento, where all California cancer cases are recorded, and found that statisticians expected only two or three cases of the rare cancer for the entire state in two years. Dritz had eight cases, all among San Francisco gay men, in just nine months.

"Burkitt's lymphoma is a form of AIDS," Dritz told the CDC, in her most matter-of-fact Chicago voice. "We should start counting it and let people know."

The CDC demurred that they weren't hearing of it anywhere else. Of course, Dritz thought, no place else is as organized as we are in San Francisco. Health officials in other cities weren't on the phone to doctors every day to tail this horrible marauder of gay men's health. It was one of the things that made Dritz grateful for her complicated network of gay community contacts.

Dritz never nagged, but even as she hung up, the doctors at the CDC were betting that she would keep her own set of statistics now. She'd have one set of statistics that counted AIDS cases by the narrow CDC definition, and she'd have another that counted cases by the definition that gave her the most accurate profile of what was killing people in her city. They were right. The two lists were kept, making it that much easier when the CDC ultimately relented to the no-nonsense health officer and added Burkitt's lymphoma to the ever-lengthening list of AIDS ailments. By now these included fungal infections of birds, sheep, cats, and deer, as well as cancers that appeared all over the body, on the tongue, in the rectum, or most horrifically, in the brain.

September 15
FEDERAL BUILDING,
SAN FRANCISCO

"How much do you need?" asked the burly congressman flatly.

Bill Kraus had prepared long explanations with intricate details on why complicated lymphocyte research needed so much money at, say, the National Institute for Allergy and Infectious Diseases and why deeper studies of intravenous drug users needed so much more money at the Centers for Disease Control.

Congressman Phil Burton just wanted a dollar figure so he could get on with business. Kraus hesitated.

"We really have no idea, to be honest," said Kraus, sheepishly. "There's no way to find out how much you need for any health problem. There's no mechanism."

Kraus's only measure of spending had come with a Congressional Research Service report. The report found that in 1982, the National Institutes of Health's research on Toxic Shock Syndrome, a mystery that had by then been solved, amounted to $36,100 per death. NIH Legionnaire's spending in the most recent fiscal year amounted to $34,841 per death. By contrast, the health institute had spent about $3,225 per AIDS death in fiscal 1981 and $8,991 in fiscal 1982. By NIH budget calculations, the life of a gay man was worth about one-quarter that of a member of the American Legion.

The torpid pace of NIH involvement was most galling to Kraus. The National Cancer Institute still had not released an application for the more than $2 million in grants they had grandly announced last month. The promise of NCI money had, in fact, been lying dormant for more than a year now. The National Heart, Lung, and Blood Institute, which does research on blood issues, had spent all of $5,000 on AIDS in fiscal year 1982. Even after the discovery of AIDS in contaminated Factor VIII, the institute was budgeted to spend only $250,000 on AIDS in the next year. Moreover, there was no inclination within proposed budgets for either the NIH or CDC to raise AIDS funding, even though caseloads were skyrocketing with each passing month. The joke among gay congressional staffers was that NIH stood for *Not Interested in Homosexuals.*

Senator Harrison Schmidt had managed to sneak an extra $500,000 into a recent supplemental appropriations bill, earmarked especially for AIDS research at the CDC, but the administration had vetoed the bill as too costly.

While Phil Burton waited impatiently for a suggestion, Bill Kraus cast about in his mind for some nice round numbers.

"We should ask for $5 million for the CDC and $5 million for the NIH," suggested Kraus.

"Hell," countered Burton. "Let's ask for $5 million and $10 million."

Kraus realized that such numbers were nothing to Burton, who daily kept tabs on a federal budget that was counted in the hundreds of billions of dollars. But the proposal represented a 3,000 percent markup on AIDS funding, and it was soon introduced into the House.

In Washington, Tim Westmoreland, as chief staffer for the House Health Subcommittee, volunteered to put the legislation into legalese, and it was introduced on September 28. Journalist Larry Bush called it "the first gay pork barrel," and, for a movement that could barely raise the tens of thousands to finance a national organization, the appropriation seemed gargantuan. Phil Burton's bills, Kraus knew, were only symbolic, because the funding ultimately would be written into some larger spending bill, but the bills added Burton's formidable political clout to that of the House health point man, Representative Henry Waxman.

Most of the research that would come from the federal government in the next two years was financed by these bills and prodded through Congress by these two men, who in turn were sparked into action by two of the only openly gay congressional aides on Capitol Hill, Yale Law School graduate Tim Westmoreland and one-time street radical Bill Kraus. No matter what would be said about how the gay community reacted to the epidemic, it is clear that virtually all the money that funded the early scientific advances on AIDS can be credited almost solely to these two gay men.

The supplemental appropriations bill set the pattern for how Congress and the Reagan administration would deal with AIDS for the next three years. The administration, of course, opposed the extra money, dispatching its agency chiefs to argue that they had all the funding they could use. Once the money was passed by Congress, however, the administration would not put itself in the politically indelicate position of actually vetoing it. Ultimately, the money was made available, usually much later than the scientists needed it. The Reagan administration would never ask for it and insist it didn't want it, but the money would be thrust upon the government anyway. It was a ritual of forced feeding.

As he savored his ability to finally make a difference on this issue, Bill Kraus thought briefly that Henry Kissinger was right about one thing. Power did have certain aphrodisiac qualities. The boost from ensuring the first major funding for fighting the AIDS epidemic came as his spirits badly needed to be lifted. Kico Govantes had gone off with his architect, and Bill again was single. Of course, he never lacked dates, but he was feeling uncomfortable about sex and uncomfortable about the way he had lived his life during the raucous late 1970s. It was around this time that friends and colleagues started noticing his late office hours and how his conversations didn't travel much away from the new epidemic and all the things that needed to be done. Friends nodded to each other knowingly, understanding that Bill was throwing himself into his work after the end of what would always be his most romantic love affair.

September 27
SAN FRANCISCO BOARD OF SUPERVISORS CHAMBERS, CITY HALL

The supplemental appropriation sailed through the board of supervisors without a dissenting vote. Bill Kraus and Dana Van Gorder had timed the vote perfectly. Half the board was up for reelection in five weeks. Nobody would dare vote against public health money, given the fact that one in four city voters was gay. Mayor Feinstein personally felt the money should come from some other part of the health budget, but Bill Kraus knew her hands were tied as well. She was up for reelection next year and wouldn't dare veto an AIDS funding bill.

It was brute political power moving the San Francisco government to spend $450,000 to finance the world's first AIDS clinic, grief counseling and personal support for AIDS patients through the Shanti Project, and the first locally funded education efforts through the Kaposi's Sarcoma Foundation. Nearly 20 percent of the money committed to fighting the AIDS epidemic for the entire United States, including all the science and epidemiology expenditures by the U.S. government, now was pledged by the city and county of San Francisco.

October
ALBERT EINSTEIN COLLEGE OF MEDICINE, BRONX, NEW YORK

As chief epidemiologist for the AIDS Task Force, Harold Jaffe had already heard the pediatricians deriding the notion that AIDS could appear in babies. He knew that some scientists, like Arye Rubinstein, were being mocked for arguing so passionately that the epidemic had spread to infants. All the pediatric immunologists had assured Jaffe that these were congenital deficiencies misclassified as AIDS. The immune syndrome, they insisted, was a disease of homosexual men.

Jaffe could see with the first babies Rubinstein showed him, however, that they were not the victims of a congenital defect; they had AIDS. His findings were also consistent with those of Dr. James Oleske, an immunologist who had treated dozens of babies in the slums of New Jersey, where AIDS was running rampant among drug addicts. Jaffe came away convinced and started framing an *MMWR* article on AIDS in babies.

The development, he knew, strengthened the case of people who, like himself, argued that a single agent, transmitted through the placenta in this case, caused AIDS. It also directed attention toward the probability that the agent could be spread through blood transfusions, something that the CDC was desperate to prove so the blood industry would start taking precautions. Jaffe's findings also pointed to still another depressing dimension of the AIDS problem. No sooner had researchers settled on the existence of AIDS in drug addicts than they discovered it in their babies.

If Harold Jaffe was sure of nothing else in October 1982, he was sure that the numbers of people with AIDS, in all risk groups, would continue to increase. The pace of new reports was quickening every day in Atlanta. The operative term in Building 6 was "exponential."

It was during Jaffe's New York visit that somebody mentioned that there were three children, born of the same prostitute, all being treated for immune deficiency at the University of California in San Francisco. Jaffe was going to be in San Francisco later that month for an AIDS conference anyway. He wrote a reminder in his notebook: "They all have separate fathers. It doesn't fit the pattern of any known inherited immune deficiency."

⬭

The different epidemiological trails AIDS was blazing led the small group of people involved in its research to one conclusion: This thing was getting much bigger. Moreover, the spread among such diverse elements of the population meant it was going to get much, much worse before it got even slightly better.

CENTERS FOR DISEASE CONTROL, ATLANTA

The start of the federal government's new fiscal year on October 1 found the AIDS Task Force still scrambling for money. CDC budget managers had to prepare three budgets for its AIDS work before it submitted one that scaled down AIDS spending enough to be acceptable to the administration. When Wilmon Rushing, acting administrative officer for AIDS, sent the final budget to CDC management, he warned, "As you know, the attached budget is insufficient to adequately fund AIDS surveillance and epidemiologic studies. However, we will continue with the highest priority activities until additional funds become available."

At the CDC's hepatitis labs in Phoenix, Dr. Don Francis filed another memo asking for money to fund basic laboratory research. He talked up the $198,301 request as much as he could, prodding the CDC chieftains to make a quick decision. The virus was there, lurking about AIDS victims' blood, he was sure. All he needed was the basic equipment. No answer was forthcoming from Atlanta.

The only glimmer of good news for government funding broke in October when the National Cancer Institute announced it was taking applications for a $1.5 million clinical research grant. Though it came over a year after NCI officials first intimated they would put some bucks behind their often-stated fascination with the syndrome, the news brought the first traces of hope for beleaguered clinicians like Paul Volberding at the UCSF Kaposi's Sarcoma Clinic.

Then Volberding read the fine print in the cooperative agreement announcement. The $1.5 million grant was to be distributed over a period of three years at $500,000 a year. Moreover, it wasn't going to just one hospital but was intended to be shared among a number of urban AIDS centers. Volberding's heart felt leaden as he tried to create a budget request that would fit the application's demands. He had ten scientists, many of whom were eminent retrovirologists and immunologists who had put other plans on hold in hopes for this chance to work on an important disease. Now he had to figure out a way to divvy up $500,000 among them. That, of course, assumed he would get the whole grant, an unlikely scenario.

The cuts Volberding would have to make were obvious, once he realized his priorities lay with the clinic's pioneering treatments and immunology research. There would be no funding for epidemiology, even though San Francisco's centralized and cooperative gay community gave investigators the best place in the world to study the spread of this disease. Without money for epidemiology, there certainly would be no way to figure which sexual practices spread AIDS most efficiently, or how to intervene and slow the transmission of the disease through public health education.

Just writing the grant meant begging word processors at the hospital and a constant scaling-down of what Volberding knew was needed to help stop the disease.

In Los Angeles, Michael Gottlieb, who had seen the first cases of *Pneumocystis* nearly two years before, was frantically trying to pare down his grant proposal, borrowing UCLA computer time and ignoring the frowns of colleagues who continued to urge him to get out of AIDS and back into a more "legitimate" area of scientific research. As the deadline for the grants approached, he drove to Santa Monica, where he found a gay man who volunteered to do the word processing of the complex request for nothing. Of course, the grant money would not come until well into 1983, Gottlieb knew, and it would not be enough to even start decent research. He was losing time, and time meant losing lives. He wondered how many people would die before the government took the epidemic seriously. What was the threshold of death and suffering society could tolerate?

He asked himself the same question later, after the gay man who had done the word processing for UCLA's first request for an AIDS grant withered away and died of the disease.

The discovery of cyanide in Tylenol capsules occurred in those same weeks of October 1982. The existence of the poisoned capsules, all found in the Chicago area, was first reported on October 1. *The New York Times* wrote a story on the Tylenol scare every day for the entire month of October and produced twenty-three more pieces in the two months after that. Four of the stories appeared on the front page. The poisoning received comparable coverage in media across the country, inspiring an immense government effort. Within days of the discovery of what proved to be the only cyanide-laced capsules, the Food and Drug Administration issued orders removing the drug from store shelves across the country. Federal, state, and local authorities were immediately on hand to coordinate efforts in states thousands of miles from where the tampered boxes appeared. No action was too extreme and no expense too great, they insisted, to save lives.

Investigators poured into Chicago to crack the mystery. More than 100 state, federal, and local agents worked the Illinois end of the case alone, filling twenty-six volumes with 11,500 pages of probe reports. The Food and Drug Administration had more than 1,100 employees testing 1.5 million similar capsules for evidence of poisoning, and chasing down every faint possibility of a victim of the new terror, according to the breathless news reports of the time. Tylenol's parent company, Johnson & Johnson, estimated spending $100 million in the effort. Within five weeks, the U.S. Department of Health and Human Services issued new regulations on tamper-resistant packaging to avert repetition of such a tragedy.

In the end, the millions of dollars for CDC Tylenol investigations yielded little beyond the probability that some lone crackpot had tampered with a few boxes of the pain reliever. No more cases of poisoning occurred beyond the first handful reported in early October. Yet the crisis showed how the government could spring into action, issue warnings, change regulations, and spend money, lots of money, when they thought the lives of Americans were at stake.

Altogether, seven people died from the cyanide-laced capsules; one other man in Yuba City, California, got sick, but it turned out he was faking it so he could collect damages from Johnson & Johnson.

By comparison, 634 Americans had been stricken with AIDS by October 5, 1982. Of these, 260 were dead. There was no rush to spend money, mobilize public health officials, or issue regulations that might save lives.

The institution that is supposed to be the public's watchdog, the news media, had gasped a collective yawn over the story of dead and dying homosexuals. In New York City, where half the nation's AIDS cases resided, *The New York Times* had written only three stories about the epidemic in 1981 and three more stories in all of 1982. None made the front page. Indeed, one could have lived in New York, or in most of the United States for that matter, and not even have been aware from the daily newspapers that an epidemic was happening, even while government doctors themselves were predicting that the scourge would wipe out the lives of tens of thousands.

October 28
CITY HALL,
NEW YORK CITY

A policeman led Larry Kramer, Paul Popham, and the rest of the delegation from Gay Men's Health Crisis to a dark and chilly basement room in the bowels of City Hall. As the group surveyed the small chamber, furnished with a beat-up table and some straight-back chairs, the policeman mentioned that he couldn't remember the last time he had seen the room used. That was a few minutes before 11 A.M., the time of their appointment with Herb Rickman, the gay staff man for Mayor Ed Koch and liaison to the gay community.

Kramer had looked forward to the long-delayed meeting with Rickman and had neatly typed an agenda of the points the group needed to cover. Although he was dubious that GMHC would get much from Koch—they had spent well over a year just to get this audience with a low-level aide—the meeting at least would give the group a chance to set out an agenda of items the city needed to be working on.

Kramer hoped that the sheer justice of the GMHC arguments would carry the day. The week before, the group had announced that it was now offering social services to people suffering from AIDS. Since virtually all the social services were those that public health agencies normally provide, Kramer hoped the city would at least help the group finance the growing GMHC staff. Even more significantly, gay men needed some aggressive health education. That certainly was the duty of the health department, Kramer thought.

By the time Herb Rickman arrived at 12:30 P.M., bustling with his own importance, even mild-mannered Paul Popham was irritated. Yet the mayor's aide was all smiles and benevolence, apologizing for the ninety-minute tardiness and quickly acceding to all the group's proposals. If San Francisco was putting money into community groups to fight AIDS, then the city of New York would equal what San Francisco was spending, dollar for dollar, the mayor's aide said. Yes, he'd get Health Commissioner David Sencer on top of this epidemic right away, and of course, the mayor would issue a proclamation for an AIDS awareness week in the spring. The city's commission on real property would find a building for the group, Rickman promised, and the mayor's liaison to Washington would call the White House.

Even the ever-implacable Larry Kramer seemed in a good mood as he left the meeting that marked the first official attention the municipal government of New York City had lent to the epidemic. "We've finally got our foot in the door," the men told each other.

"Considering how slowly the wheels of government move, we are making some progress," Paul Popham told the *New York Native*. After the year of delay and the months of unanswered phone calls and bureaucratic runarounds, it all seemed too good to be true. And it was.

PARIS

Drs. Francoise Brun-Vezinet and David Klatzmann had gone to the New York University symposium on AIDS in September to present their data on "AIDS in France: The African Hypothesis." Their theory was that AIDS had come out of Africa, since so many of the early cases were among Africans and Europeans who had been to Central Africa shortly before falling ill. The African connection was all the talk of European AIDS researchers. Not too many months before that, Copenhagen's Dr. Ib Bygbjerg, recalling the horrible death of his friend Grethe Rask, was derided for linking AIDS to infectious tropical diseases. Now, scientists in Brussels and Paris raced to be the first doctors to publish on the cases of *Pneumocystis* and virulent Kaposi's sarcoma from the late 1970s.

Two distinct waves of the AIDS epidemic were sweeping Europe—the first dating back at least five years to Africa, and the second, more recent, among gay men who had contacts with American homosexuals, usually in New York City.

What had excited Brun and Klatzmann, however, was the scientific gossip about Human T-cell Leukemia virus, or HTLV, as the cause of AIDS. Dr. Robert Gallo at the National Cancer Institute had long hypothesized that HTLV had an African origin, being carried to Japan by Portuguese who had stopped in Africa on their way around the Horn in the late fifteenth century. HTLV was also endemic to the Caribbean, where the disease was festering among Haitians. Brun found the theory intriguing, given her studies into HTLV under Dr. Luc Montagnier at the Pasteur Institute. Klatzmann, meanwhile, had spent much of the past year working up immunological profiles on Willy Rozenbaum's AIDS patients.

Brun and Klatzmann were also part of the working group on AIDS that Dr. Willy Rozenbaum and Jacques Leibowitch had organized early in the year. After returning from New York, the researchers eagerly shared the talk about HTLV at the next European group meeting. They decided to try to enlist retrovirologists to study the hypothesis, hopefully at the Pasteur Institute, France's most respected scientific institution.

In the long brainstorming in the weeks that followed, Brun and Klatzmann also arrived at the idea that any search for such a virus would best be started not in the blood of AIDS patients but in the lymph nodes of men with lymphadenopathy. If anything marked the blood work of AIDS patients, Klatzmann said, it was the virtual absence of T-4 lymphocytes. The virus appeared so deadly that it killed its host cells, which might render fruitless a search for the virus in the blood. Given the fact that lymphadenopathy appeared to be some kind of early symptom of AIDS, it made more sense to try to find the culprit while it was still proliferating and not after it had delivered the coup de grace to so many T-4 cells.

This line of inquiry turned out to be one of the most momentous in the scientific history of the AIDS epidemic. Nothing seemed certain then, however, except that the French doctors finally had a tangible plan and, most importantly, that they needed a big retrovirus lab to see whether it would pan out.

On October 28, the Centers for Disease Control reported that 691 Americans were documented as contracting AIDS in the United States, of whom 278 were dead. Nearly one in five of the cases had been reported in September or October. The epidemic had swept into four more states in those past two months with the reports of the first cases in Alabama, Kentucky, Vermont, and Washington. Twenty states, largely in the South and Rocky Mountain regions, still reported no cases. Three more nations reported their first AIDS cases in those two months. Altogether, 52 cases had been reported in fifteen foreign nations, largely in western Europe.

October 30
UNIVERSITY OF CALIFORNIA, SAN FRANCISCO

Dr. Marc Conant had organized one of the first national conferences on the AIDS epidemic, and Catherine Cusic, a respiratory nurse, eagerly took her place in the crowded auditorium for the session on epidemiology. For a year, she had been treating AIDS patients, putting tubes down their throats when they went on ventilators, holding them as they wheezed and coughed through the night. An active member of the Harvey Milk Gay Democratic Club, Cusic also had been bending Bill Kraus's ear about the lack of local educational programs for AIDS prevention. She hoped the new epidemiology might nudge Kraus's attention away from strictly federal issues and into local public health concerns.

Pediatric immunologist Art Ammann's presentation at the conference on his AIDS babies gave final proof to Cusic's conviction that AIDS was an infectious disease. The three children of the intravenous drug–using prostitute, all suffering from immune problems, established blood transmission that, together with the drug addicts themselves and the cluster study, was all the evidence Cusic needed to bolster her fears about the epidemic spreading among gay men. Epidemiologist Michael Gorman was droning on about census tracks and diagnosed cases when Cusic heard a statistic that made her sit bolt upright in her seat.

"In a central part of the city, one percent of gay men have been diagnosed with AIDS," Gorman said cautiously.

Cusic interrupted him: "What central part of the city?"

Gorman looked flustered.

"A central part of the city," he repeated.

Cusic knew immediately what he didn't want to say. The central neighborhood of the city was, of course, the Castro Street District. One percent of the men there were diagnosed and nobody had told them? For Christ's sake, she thought, half the guys she talked to remained convinced that AIDS was some media hype. This study could go a long way toward letting gay men know it was serious business.

"What are you going to do with this study?" Cusic demanded. "This is a phenomenal rate."

The information had been submitted to a medical publication in England, Gorman explained. It couldn't be released until it was published there, he said. Of course, the statistics were now available to every participant at the conference, and they quickly became the talk of the gay leadership.

Catherine Cusic started goading Bill Kraus to get the study into the newspapers so people would know how serious AIDS already was. Things had to get moving, she said. Kraus started checking around and was surprised that the consensus of gay leaders was to withhold the information. "It could destroy the Castro," he was told.

After his presentation at the UCSF conference, Harold Jaffe from the CDC huddled with Dr. Art Ammann to check on reports of more pediatric AIDS cases. The CDC was preparing an article about the AIDS babies in New York and New Jersey. Jaffe knew that Ammann's substantial reputation among pediatric immunologists would help give the report more credibility. It was during the conversation about the three children of the prostitute that Ammann mentioned another infant. Neither parent was an intravenous drug user or in any AIDS risk group, Ammann said, but the baby had undergone extensive transfusions at birth.

Jaffe knew immediately what Ammann potentially had—the first documented case of AIDS contracted through a blood transfusion. As soon as he returned to Atlanta, Jaffe called Dave Auerbach in Los Angeles for the most important AIDS investigation since Auerbach's work on the cluster study.

Back in San Francisco, Ammann called Selma Dritz and told her the particulars of the baby's health. Dritz contacted the Irwin Memorial Blood Bank, which had supplied all the baby's blood.

In the early days of November, the bank completed its records search and came up with thirteen donors whose blood had been transfused into the baby in March 1981. Dritz's eyes froze on the name of one donor. She recognized it as the socially prominent international trade consultant who had died of encephalitis in August, the one who so vehemently had denied being gay.

"Oh, God," she sighed. The familiar feelings returned to her: the excitement of being on the cutting edge of one of the most intriguing phenomena anyone in her profession could ever hope to experience, and the sadness because of what her insights meant for the society whose health she had spent a lifetime trying to protect.

She called Jaffe in Atlanta.

"You won't believe this, but one of the donors is a man who was diagnosed with AIDS," she said.

"It's finally happened," Jaffe thought.

20 DIRTY SECRETS

November 1982
CLUB BATHS,
SAN FRANCISCO

Gaetan Dugas examined himself closely in the steamy mirror of San Francisco's most popular bathhouse. He had always been looking for someone, he thought. As a child he had searched for his mother, not the woman who had brought him up in Quebec City, but his real mother. As soon as he was old enough to understand that he had been adopted into that rough-hewn life of the French-Canadian working class, he had dreamed of the day he would meet his true mother. He knew he was meant to be born into a better life, far from the brawny bullies who called him a faggot and rubbed snow in his face during those bitter Canadian winters.

He could see the difference in his face; he was meant for something better. He loved his family and adored his older sister, but they were dark and plain looking while he had always had delicate features and light, winsome hair. He was like the prince taken up by the farmers, he thought. When he did finally meet his natural mother, he told friends they fought. She wouldn't say who his father was and she didn't seem like a princess, and suddenly Gaetan had stopped talking about searching for his parents. Anyway, he had found his own niche in the royalty of gay beauty, as a star of the homosexual jet set.

Now, as he searched the mirror, oblivious to the smiles aimed at his still-handsome body, he was thinking about another search. Who had done this to him? Certainly somebody had. They had passed him the virus that meant he was going to die, and he couldn't get over wondering who it was, the way he once could not stop wondering what his real mother looked like.

Gaetan stood back to give his smooth body another appraisal. He was thirty years old, the age he had never thought he would make. But he was triumphing. He was living in San Francisco, where he had always wanted to live. He had outlived all the doctors' predictions and felt quite nice, thank you, two and a half years after he was told that the small purplish spot near his ear was Kaposi's sarcoma. True, he was a bit more tired these days and sometimes breathing came hard. He would win, nevertheless, and enjoy his evening here at the baths.

Of course, those assholes at the CDC might scream at him for being here, but he had told them to fuck off. They were bothering his old boyfriends with phone calls and nosy questions. The other doctors could fuck themselves, too, with all their warnings that he might be spreading this thing. Everybody knew you couldn't catch cancer. He wanted to see proof. Besides, Gaetan had told the doctors defiantly, somebody gave this to him.

Gaetan peered down the long hallway of cubicles, some with their doors open. Inside, men lay on their stomachs, usually with a can of Crisco and a small bottle of poppers at their side. Gaetan surveyed the material and made his choice. He edged into the small cubicle and waited for the ritual nod that indicated he would be welcome. Without a word, the assignation was set. Gaetan pushed the door shut.

UPPER ASHBURY, SAN FRANCISCO

Paul Volberding looked down at his long fingers. They were bony now. His full frame, made strong through a childhood of chores at his parents' Minnesota dairy farm, was gaunt and emaciated. He was like all the rest, now. The breaths were coming harder as he lay in his home in Upper Ashbury, above the Castro District where so many of the others had lived and died. And now Paul Volberding was dying too. Had he given it to his child? What would happen to his wife? This was the time that Volberding usually woke up.

The dream was recurrent in the last months of 1982, settling a layer of dread on each night, because Paul never knew when the nightmare would return. On his first day at San Francisco General Hospital back in July 1981, when the veteran oncologist had told him that the "next great disease" awaited him, Volberding had seen AIDS as a curiosity. By early to mid-1982, it was an intriguing phenomenon. Now, Volberding saw, it was turning into a catastrophe.

Just a few months before, he had known all the names of the local AIDS cases when he sat down with Marc Conant, Selma Dritz, Don Abrams, and the handful of other involved doctors who regularly went to Conant's biweekly meetings for updates on the epidemic. Now cases were mounting rapidly, far outstripping Conant's own depressing projections. Volberding's AIDS outpatient clinic would open in January, but he had not foreseen the rapid increase in the rate of new cases and wondered whether his budget could handle it.

His concerns were not only professional. The Orange County cluster, the hemophiliacs, and now talk of a transfusion case at UCSF had convinced Volberding that this certainly was a viral disease that could be spread like hepatitis B. Already, some nurses had reconciled themselves to gallows humor about their vulnerability to the disease. There would soon be a fifth "H" to add to the "Four H's" of the disease risk groups—homosexuals, heroin addicts, hemophiliacs, and Haitians. The fifth "H," they said, would be house staff. In New York, there were reports that some nurses were simply refusing to work with AIDS patients, leaving food trays at their door and allowing them to lie for entire shifts in sheets stained with defecation.

Volberding's own nightsweats had started in the waning weeks of autumn, coming on like any viral infection with high fevers and the wrenching, sheet-soaking perspiration all night. Volberding knew AIDS had a long incubation period. Was it incubating in his body? Had he given it already to his baby boy? A spot had appeared on his body. Marc Conant had assured him it wasn't a KS lesion, but was there another splotch of purple now growing silently on his back, where he might not see it?

Paul knew his fears were not unique. His assistant director, Don Abrams, had spilled some liquid nitrogen on his hand, causing a big purple spot, and had also become convinced he was going to die, even though the discoloration was easily shown to be the legacy of the nitrogen. A prominent Harvard clinician had called Volberding, complaining of fevers and shortness of breath. "Do I have *Pneumocystis?*" he asked.

CLUB BATHS, SAN FRANCISCO

Back in the bathhouse, when the moaning stopped, the young man rolled over on his back for a cigarette. Gaetan Dugas reached up for the lights, turning up the rheostat slowly so his partner's eyes would have time to adjust. He then made a point of eyeing the purple lesions on his chest. "Gay cancer," he said, almost as if he were talking to himself. "Maybe you'll get it too."

NEW YORK CITY

For Enno Poersch, the terror settled in as department stores began erecting their cheerful Christmas displays. In the first year after Nick's death, Enno hadn't worried much about catching whatever killed his younger lover. Toxoplasmosis, he heard, wasn't a contagious disease. But now, nearly two years after Nick had died, Enno was scared. At the Gay Men's Health Crisis board meetings, he had heard about a man who had sex with all these guys who died in Los Angeles and about how it was spreading through hemophiliacs. When the Christmas decorations went up, the idea overtook him. He'd never live to see Christmas. AIDS would kill him too, the way it already had killed so many friends—Rick Wellikoff, the schoolteacher, Jack Nau, the window dresser, and of course, Nick, the man with whom he had spent eight blissful years in love.

CASTRO DISTRICT, SAN FRANCISCO

The large gray Victorian stood proudly over the sidewalk, as if it graced the street by its presence. Gary Walsh had always loved the gingerbread trim on these grand remnants of 1880s tract housing, and he was thrilled that he and Lu Chaikin, a lesbian psychotherapist, had bought their own offices in the Castro.

"It's like we're married professionally," teased Gary, his green eyes sparkling at the fifty-seven-year-old Lu Chaikin.

Lu gave him an affectionate shove and considered that they were indeed an odd couple, the laid-back lesbian nearing sixty and the handsome, hot psycho-therapist in his prime. Privately, Lu worried that their relationship was unequal. Gary seemed so often to be the nurturer and teacher, almost in the traditional female role, while Lu, former tomboy from Flatbush, had the rougher male role.

In November, Lu and Gary decorated the new offices and waiting room they would share. Gary groused a bit during all the shopping, complaining of fatigue, but he was excited about the move and about his planned Christmas trip to the Yucatán with Joe Brewer. However, Gary remained run down, and when he went to the drugstore to pick up some medication, he admitted to Lu that he was "very worried."

Lu didn't understand why. She knew Gary had recently suffered a case of salmonella so severe that he was hospitalized for a few days, but most of her clients were gay men and it seemed they all had parasites at one time or another. Gary looked impatient at Lu's naiveté.

"AIDS," he said, confiding his deepest fears for the first time. "These are all symptoms of AIDS."

Lu dismissed the thought. AIDS was some exotic disorder, something far from her life.

"If you get AIDS," she joked, "I'll kill you."

Irwin Memorial Blood Bank, San Francisco

Dr. Herbert Perkins looked like a man whose cocker spaniel puppy had been run over by a truck. Selma Dritz understood Perkins's despondence. He was the medical director of northern California's major blood bank—the source of the blood products transfused into the ailing baby at UCSF. Dritz knew, of course, that the announcement of the nation's first AIDS-by-transfusion case would batter the blood industry. Both could predict what would follow. There would be calls to ban gays from giving blood. The suggestion ran counter to both doctors' sensibilities, but Perkins added in another factor. A drop in gay donors would have a terrible effect on the region's always-tenuous supply of blood. Between 5 and 9 percent of Irwin's donors were gay, he told Dritz. "They are very good donors," he sighed.

Dritz was sympathetic, but she had the public health to worry about and there was still a troubling aspect to this case. The donor, the blue-blood who had died in August, insisted to the end that he was heterosexual. The case for blood transmission of AIDS had to be made as clearly as possible if health authorities were going to get about the business of saving lives, Dritz thought. The man's disputed sexual orientation only muddied the scenario. He certainly was not a prime suspect for sharing needles in some shooting gallery. He was probably gay, like 98 percent of the city's other AIDS cases. Dritz needed to talk to the family and try to find the truth. Perkins provided what information he could.

Dr. Dave Auerbach, one of the CDC's Epidemiological Intelligence Service officers, went to see the donor's brother. Like Dritz, Auerbach also had previously interviewed the recalcitrant AIDS sufferer who had so vehemently denied being gay during their various epidemiological investigations. The brother was more cooperative, telling Auerbach about sifting through the dead man's personal effects after his death in August. That was when he found this, he said, showing Auerbach a small black address book.

Back at Public Health, Dritz leafed through the pages eagerly, thankful once again that she was born so nosy. Under "B," Dritz saw a name she recognized.

Practicing out of Davies Medical Center on Castro Street, Dr. Bud Boucher was one of the first local physicians to direct a practice specifically at gay men. Like all the gay doctors, Boucher had known Dritz for years because of her parasite preaching. He pulled the patient's files without hesitation. The donor only came to Boucher for those messy little troubles that he didn't want to tell the socially prominent physician handling his routine medical care. Among those problems was a case of rectal gonorrhea back in 1980. The mystery was solved.

⬭

Gaetan Dugas's eyes flashed, but without their usual charm, when Selma Dritz bluntly told him he must stop going to the bathhouses. The hotline at the Kaposi's Sarcoma Foundation was receiving repeated calls from people complaining of a man with a French accent who was having sex with people at various sex parlors and then calmly telling them he had gay cancer. It was one of the most repulsive things Dritz had heard in her nearly forty years in public health.

"It's none of your goddamn business," said Gaetan. "It's my right to do what I want to do with my own body."

"It's not your right to go out and give other people disease," Dritz replied, keeping her professional calm. "Then you're making decisions for their bodies, not yours."

"It's their duty to protect themselves," said the airline steward. "They know what's going on there. They've heard about this disease."

Dritz tried to reason further but got nowhere.

"I've got it," Gaetan said angrily. "They can get it too."

Gaetan Dugas was not alone among AIDS patients at the bathhouses. Bobbi Campbell, who had made his self-avowed role as a KS Poster Boy into something of a crusade, was also going to bathhouses, although he denied having sex with people. Gay doctors had told Dritz that several other patients still went as well. The situation was intolerable, Dritz thought, and she had no doubt as to what she would like to do. There was only the question of whether it would stand up in court. These people should be locked up, particularly Gaetan. Dritz started talking to city attorneys to see what laws existed to empower such action.

⬭

Two more states reported their first cases of Acquired Immune Deficiency Syndrome in the month of November. Altogether, 788 AIDS cases in thirty-three states had been reported to CDC since the epidemic was first detected in June 1981. About 400 of these cases were in the New York City area, accounting for half the AIDS diagnoses in the country, while 10 percent more were in San Francisco, the second hardest-hit city. The AIDS casualties had quadrupled in the first eleven months of 1982. It was exactly one year since Ken Horne, the first AIDS case reported to the CDC, had died in a dark hospital room on November 30, 1981; by November 30, 1982, nearly 300 were dead nationwide.

December 1
NATIONAL CANCER INSTITUTE,
BETHESDA

Robert Gallo was supposed to be the star of the day, but there was growing interest in AIDS, so the National Cancer Advisory Board put Jim Curran on the agenda of their regular Wednesday meeting as a prelude to Gallo's talk. It was just as well because the peripatetic Gallo was late. He came in while Jim was in the midst of his thirty-minute dissertation on the iceberg and the vast numbers of asymptomatic carriers who were probably spreading AIDS now without even knowing about it. Toward the end of the meeting, Gallo finally walked to the front of the room, clearly relishing the applause of his colleagues. It was a sweet vindication for his work. After Gallo's problems in the late 1970s, when his career took a nosedive because of a mistake in his cancer studies, he had become the fading star of the NCI. But he had hung in there and made his Human T-cell Leukemia virus discovery and was fresh from winning the prestigious Lasker Award. Now he was, inarguably, one of the nation's foremost retrovirologists.

Curran had spent much of the year trying to jawbone such prominent scientists into working on AIDS, with little success. Curran also was filled with talk from Don Francis, who kept insisting that AIDS could well be caused by a retrovirus, like feline leukemia. As the applause faded and Gallo approached the lectern, Curran made his move. "You've won one award," he told Gallo, loud enough to be heard in the microphone. "You should come back when you win another award for working on AIDS."

Gallo smiled graciously as he shook Curran's hand. Curran wondered if he had overstepped his bounds. In the hierarchy of government science, he knew, the CDC was considered the minor league to the NCI's New York Yankees. There was the hint of the brash upstart in his comment.

For his part, Gallo had had it up to here with this goddamn disease. At the prodding of Max Essex, who had found HTLV antibodies in the serums of two AIDS patients, Gallo's lab had searched through AIDS blood in hopes of finding some retrovirus. He later estimated that perhaps 10 percent of his lab time in 1982 had been spent on the baffling disease. He considered that quite enough. If the truth be known, AIDS had always created some discomfort for Gallo, who hailed from traditional Italian-Catholic stock in New Jersey. There was all this dirty talk of 1,100 partners, fist-fucking, and other exotic sexuality; frankly, Gallo found it embarrassing to talk about. Besides, the lab research had been so damned frustrating.

The work had turned up one intriguing clue. Because retroviruses are constructed of RNA, and not the DNA ladders that make up the typical virus, they create a special enzyme to reproduce. This reverse transcriptase enzyme pulls the DNA molecules to the retrovirus' RNA structure to let it replicate. By November, Gallo's lab had found evidence of reverse transcriptase in the infected lymphocytes of AIDS patients. This enzyme, in effect, had left the footprints of a retrovirus all over the lymphocytes. But it was impossible to find the damned retrovirus itself.

That was the rub. Gallo's staff couldn't keep the lymphocytes alive long enough to find any retrovirus. Any leukemia virus, Gallo knew, caused the proliferation of cells, not their death. People with leukemia died because they had too many white blood cells. When Gallo's staff added the blood from AIDS patients to their lymphocytes, however, the cells would die without any proliferation. The frustration was galling and, by November, Gallo had made what would prove to be among the most important decisions of his career. He gave up. Sure, he would let his name go on some research papers that were to be published in the spring, linking HTLV to AIDS. But his research wasn't getting anywhere. In November, his lab staff took the AIDS cultures they'd been studying and slipped them into the round metal freezers of Gallo's Tumor Cell Biology Laboratory. For the time being, at least, he was done with AIDS research.

PASTEUR INSTITUTE, PARIS

"Is there a retrovirologist in the house?"

The audience gave a collective groan. By now, many of the doctors in attendance had heard about how the unorthodox Dr. Willy Rozenbaum had to change hospitals because he refused to give up his studies on this strange new disease. He was respected as the continent's foremost clinical authority on the epidemic, but he was also known to be thoroughly wrapped up in his own almost childlike enthusiasm. He couldn't resist the play on the old Groucho Marx line, "Is there a doctor in the house?," when he gave his lecture on SIDA, as the French called AIDS, at the august Pasteur Institute.

Toward the end of the talk, he got around to explaining his opening joke. Some researchers at the NCI and the CDC were hypothesizing that a retrovirus caused AIDS. His working group on AIDS was trying to recruit laboratory assistance to help find the virus. "Is there a retrovirologist in the house?" he asked again.

After the talk, Francoise Brun-Vezinet approached Rozenbaum with an idea. She had studied under Dr. Jean-Claude Chermann, one of France's most famous retrovirologists. She'd ask him for help.

Brun-Vezinet quickly called Chermann. Meanwhile, by coincidence, officials were approaching the Pasteur Institute's leading virologist, Dr. Luc Montagnier, about AIDS. The Pasteur Institute's pharmaceutical company, which generated a good portion of the revenue that financed the privately run institute, was frantic over rumors about the hepatitis vaccine. Pasteur Production had the license to manufacture the vaccine in France. The vaccine was derived from the plasma of gay men, and with the hemophiliac cases, people were worried that the inoculations might transmit AIDS. Although Montagnier learned that an American researcher, Dr. Don Francis, already had done research on the vaccine and found no link between AIDS and the inoculations, Montagnier agreed he would look into it further. The inquiry from Brun-Vezinet was fortunate; both Montagnier and Chermann agreed to make the Pasteur's retrovirus labs available to the research.

21 DANCING IN THE DARK

December 9, 1982
SAN FRANCISCO CITY HALL

The reporters walked swiftly down the long, oak-paneled hallway leading into Mayor Diane Feinstein's office. She had called the press conference today because once again the San Francisco Board of Supervisors had enacted a law that no other municipal governing body in the nation had even considered, and the mayor did not like it one bit. At issue was Supervisor Harry Britt's "domestic partners' ordinance," more indelicately called the "live-in lovers' law," which recognized the legitimacy of unmarried relationships, most notably homosexual relationships. The law extended to domestic partners of city employees the same benefits as those granted to spouses of married employees. The ordinance also established a legal procedure through which unmarried couples could record their relationship with the city clerk's office and gain some form of legal recognition for their partnership. Given the times, Britt had also drafted a clause that gave unmarried partners the same visitation rights as spouses in city hospitals and bereavement leave to attend a lover's funeral. Mayor Feinstein had decided to veto the law.

"On a personal level, this legislation causes me deep personal anguish," the mayor told the reporters. "I would like to be able to sign legislation that recognizes the needs of single persons, but such legislation must not divide our community."

By "divide our community," Feinstein was talking about the maelstrom that had enveloped the proposal in recent days. Just one day before, Roman Catholic Archbishop John Quinn made a rare foray into city politics by publicly prodding Feinstein to veto the law, saying that "to reduce the sacred covenant of marriage and family by inference or analogy to a 'domestic partnership' is offensive to reasonable persons and injurious to our legal, cultural, moral, and societal heritage." The proposal, Quinn said, was a "radical repudiation of fundamental values and institutions."

Virtually every other religious leader had also lined up against the measure. The Episcopal bishop noted that "marriage as an institution has been under such heavy pressure," while the Board of Rabbis of northern California also urged a veto, with the group's president saying he would "look askance upon any legislation that would attempt to equate nonmarried adults, heterosexual or gay, to what our society deems as a marriage between a man and a woman." Speaking for the city's black churches, the city's most politically powerful black minister, the Reverend Amos Brown, cast the issue in racial terms when he insisted that, "We, as blacks, particularly, come out of the extended family. It's the only way we've been able to make it."

In her veto message, Feinstein talked about the bill being poorly drafted and not specific enough, but the real issue, everyone knew, was whether homosexual relationships would be granted the same legitimacy as heterosexual relationships. To Bill Kraus, who had begun engineering the ordinance's passage before leaving Britt's office to work for Congressman Phillip Burton, there was no other point to the measure. Its intent was to frame into law a basic tenet of the gay liberation movement—that homosexuality as a life-style is equal to and on a par with heterosexuality. The veto, of course, was simply a reaffirmation of the fact that, as far as church and state were concerned, gay people had not yet achieved that equality; moreover, the veto underscored that the notion that homosexuals and their relationships should be granted such recognition was still repugnant to this society. Gay relationships were meant to be dirty secrets, and nothing more.

A spontaneous demonstration of 500 people coalesced on Castro Street that evening and thundered down to City Hall, chanting "Dump Dianne." Feinstein's appointees on various city commissions toyed briefly with the idea of a mass resignation. The talk was short-lived. Feinstein's appointees, by definition, came from the more moderate wing of gay Democrats and were not given to the dramatics popular among members of the Harvey Milk Club.

Condemnations of the veto continued to pour in from gay activists around the country. Much of the criticism descended into vicious ad hominem attacks on Feinstein, characterizing her as a nasty bigot. Some politicos whispered that she had vetoed the ordinance because she was trying to lure the 1984 Democratic National Convention to San Francisco, where she hoped to be installed as a vice-presidential candidate. All this, of course, missed the point that, of all the big-league Democrats in the United States, Feinstein was undoubtedly the most consistently pro-gay voice. Two lesbian friends had held a sort of marriage ceremony in Feinstein's backyard, outraging conservative voters. As a supervisor, she had authored the nation's first gay rights ordinance in 1972, long before any other prominent politician had learned to even utter the G-word. Feinstein also talked convincingly of tolerance and civil rights. Indeed, the very political power she had helped nurture in more uncertain days a decade ago was the very reason she was stuck dealing with a "live-in lovers' law" in the first place; no other mayor had even to come close to touching such an issue.

"We have been through a lot over the last twelve years," said Feinstein in an interview she granted once it was clear that the veto was probably the singly most controversial act in her career. "But San Francisco remains an open, tolerant city, and on the subject of gay rights, it is probably the most enlightened city anywhere."

Few could deny she was telling the truth, but the statement said less about how good things were for gays than how bad. For all the acceptance gays had gained, homosexuality still was not accepted as equal in the city they called Mecca. A prevailing morality that viewed homosexuals as promiscuous hedonists incapable of deep, sustaining relationships ensured that it would be impossible for homosexuals to legitimize whatever relationships they could forge. Prejudice has a way of fostering the very object of its hate.

In December 1982, at a time when gay people more than ever needed to be encouraged into relationships, they were told their partnerships were valueless by institutions that later scratched their heads and wondered why gays didn't settle into couples when it was so clear their lives were at stake.

December 10

Dr. Dale Lawrence was in Washington when he got the conference call from his boss, Bruce Evatt at the CDC's Division of Host Factors, and Drs. Harold Jaffe and Walt Dowdle. Lawrence knew that the call must be important to warrant the involvement of Dowdle, chief of the Center for Infectious Diseases. Evatt told Lawrence to get back to New York and interview the donors from that Bellevue Hospital transfusion case in the summer.

Lawrence recalled the case, immediately. He also remembered the fierce resistance the New York Blood Center, the nation's largest blood bank, had put up at the notion of letting Lawrence contact their blood donors.

"Why the sudden turnaround?" Lawrence asked.

The first transfusion case was being announced that afternoon, the callers explained. The San Francisco people planned a press conference to issue warnings. The CDC was rushing a report of the case into its *MMWR* for release that day. They needed a strong case to present to the blood bankers. Evatt had met with the Food and Drug Administration's blood advisory committee, made up largely of blood industry people, the Saturday before in Bethesda to tell them about the UCSF baby. As they had done all summer, the FDA officials and blood bankers insisted they needed more proof to believe the threat of AIDS from transfusions. Lawrence knew that Bruce Evatt had a reputation for planning his chess moves far in advance. Evatt had been concerned since the first word about hemophiliac cases nearly a year before; now he was going to prove that it was all real.

That Afternoon
UNIVERSITY OF CALIFORNIA,
SAN FRANCISCO

The press conference, with Selma Dritz and Art Ammann flanking Dr. Herbert Perkins from Irwin Memorial Blood Bank, sent a collective shudder through the conference room on Parnassus Hill.

"The etiology of AIDS remains unknown, but its reported occurrence among homosexual men, intravenous drug abusers, and persons with hemophilia suggest it may be caused by an infectious agent transmitted sexually or through exposure to blood or blood products," the *MMWR* had reported carefully that morning. "If the infant's illness described in this report is AIDS, its occurrence following receipt of blood products from a known AIDS case adds support to the infectious-agent hypothesis."

This first public announcement that AIDS might be in the blood supply brought an angry reaction from blood bankers in the East. The CDC had, of course, meant the day's *MMWR* to be a one-two punch to the blood industry, releasing not only the report on the first transfusion case but an update on five new cases of AIDS in hemophiliacs. In spite of that, Dr. Joseph Bove, who headed the FDA's blood advisory committee and served as an officer of the American Association of Blood Banks, went on network television to say flatly that there still was no evidence that transfusions spread AIDS. Privately, some blood bankers thought the CDC was overstating the possibility of transfusion AIDS to get publicity and, therefore, more funding. The scientific community was aware of the severe problems health agencies were having in securing adequate funding under the Reagan administration. Some blood bankers, including some officials of the FDA, remained unconvinced that AIDS even existed.

$$\bigcirc$$

The barrage of publicity given to the first transfusion AIDS case resulted in less notice of a report in that day's *Journal of the American Medical Association* on evidence that strange brain disorders were appearing among AIDS patients. Often, neurological problems were the only early symptoms of AIDS, scientists had reported at a meeting of the American Neurological Association. Upon closer examination, three in four AIDS sufferers showed evidence of some brain damage. Doctors frequently missed the damage to the central nervous system, writing off the often-vague symptoms of dementia as related to stress or depression. Nevertheless, some patients were dying of brain disorders, their cerebral matter sometimes reduced to "a boggy mass."

There was a doctor from New York University who had written an extensive study on the apparent infection of the central nervous system, but he refused to tell the reporter from the American Medical Association journal about his work because he had submitted his paper to a neurological journal, where it had been accepted for publication. The neurological journal might throw out the story if he publicly discussed his findings with the press, and that would hurt the doctor's career in the publish-or-perish world of academic medicine. It was science as usual, and the *Journal of the American Medical Association* would just have to wait until the research was published in six months.

The Next Day
CASTRO STREET, SAN FRANCISCO

The petitioners appeared on the corner of 18th and Castro streets with the rush of morning shoppers. Their scruffy long hair and unkempt demeanor were antithetical to the gay men whose own casual appearance was so entirely studied, but the people with their petitions stood under a sign that brought smiles to the gay faces. "Dump Dianne," it said, and gay men did not hesitate to sign petitions to recall Dianne Feinstein as mayor.

For six months, members of the local White Panther Party had tried to scrounge enough signatures to put the recall on the San Francisco ballot. Their principal agenda was fervent opposition to Feinstein's support for a local ordinance to outlaw handguns in the city. Although enacted, the law had been thrown out by a federal appeals court. That didn't stop the remnants of this sixties radical group, known for taking occasional potshots at police officers who tarried too long near their Haight-Ashbury commune. They wanted to recall Mayor Feinstein simply for suggesting that guns should be outlawed. Their efforts, of course, were dismissed by the professional politicians, so nobody really noticed their appearance on Castro Street two days after the veto of the domestic partners' ordinance. However, they filled petition after petition with the responsibly registered voters of the neighborhood.

○

The stranger stopped Gaetan Dugas as he walked casually past the window of All-American Boy, the quartermaster depot of the "Castro clone" look, where even the manikins had washboard stomachs. He grabbed the flight attendant's arm and wouldn't let go when Gaetan tried to jerk away.

"I know who you are and what you're doing," the man said. "You'd better leave town if you know what's good for you."

Volunteers at the Kaposi's Sarcoma Foundation help line, who had long been apprised of Gaetan's bathhouse escapades, were now hearing that a group of gay men had decided to drive the "Orange County connection" out of town for so purposefully spreading his disease.

Gaetan tore away from the menacing face and said something defiant before ambling back down Castro Street. These people are hysterical about AIDS, he told himself.

It was around then that he confided to Canadian friends that he was thinking of moving back to Vancouver.

December 12

Dana Van Gorder, Supervisor Harry Britt's aide, called Bill Kraus in his congressional office with the news. Mark Feldman, whom Bill Kraus had dated some time ago, had been diagnosed with both Kaposi's sarcoma and *Pneumocystis carinii* pneumonia. Bill was stunned. It wasn't that they were great friends as much as the fact that Mark was so much like Bill. He was successful, handsome, and politically involved to the point that he publicly announced his dual diagnosis with KS and PCP only days after he got the word from doctors. He wanted to raise peoples' consciousness about the disease, he said. Like Bill Kraus, Mark Feldman was young, healthy, and strong. They even worked out at the same gym together, and now, Mark had suddenly started dropping weight and looking as though he were aging rapidly. Intellectually, Bill had always tried to banish the idea that the illness was some kind of metaphor, something that only the sleaze-balls who fist-fucked on Folsom Street contract. That idea, he knew, wasn't politically correct. Still, the shock at Mark Feldman's diagnosis educated him as to how much he had seen AIDS as the problem of other people. Sure, he had worked on it as an issue and had repeatedly instructed Phil Burton that it was the top-priority gay issue, but Bill had never seen it as an issue for himself, except in some dark corner of his imagination.

In the days that followed, Bill Kraus contemplated his own future and his own fear that some day a doctor might tell him he had this sentence to die. He did double-takes on this or that spot, found while he was scrubbing his shoulder in the shower; the fear was pervasive. Bill always remembered that day of early fear, December 12, 1982, because it was the last time he ever had a sexual encounter that involved the proverbial exchange of bodily fluids.

⬭

A number of San Francisco physicians would remember the end of 1982 as an invisible demarcation line for their patients. There weren't any formal studies, but, in their evaluations of patients, doctors noted that gay men who had stopped getting inseminated by the end of 1982 tended to avoid infection with the AIDS virus; those who were infected tended to be those who carried on into 1983 and beyond. It was just a rule of thumb, of course, because later studies indicated that at least 20 percent of San Francisco's gay men were probably infected with the AIDS virus before the end of 1982. The most recently infected would constitute the swelling caseloads and mortality statistics of 1986 and 1987. Such numbers meant that, by 1983, it would be very difficult to be at the receptive end of semen deposition and not get this virus.

In New York City, where the virus apparently arrived first and was probably more widespread, a fierce debate had already consumed the gay community in the final weeks of 1982, precisely on the issue of promiscuity and AIDS. Two people with AIDS, a rock singer named Michael Callen and one-time hustler Richard Berkowitz, had fired the first volley with an essay in the *New York Native* called "We Know Who We Are."

The piece blasted all the fashionable talk about how the gay community was getting a bad public relations rap with the discussion about sexual activity and gay cancer. When Callen made media appearances to talk about his AIDS diagnosis, he was counseled by the Gay Men's Health Crisis to say, "I don't know," if he were asked how he got the disease. Callen had no doubt how he got the disease. He had frequented every sex club and bathhouse between the East River and the Pacific Ocean and had gathered enough venereal and parasitic diseases to make his medical chart look like that of some sixty-five-year-old Equatorial African living in squalor. He had spent much of 1982 going to support groups for other AIDS patients, many of whom were still attending their old pleasure parlors in the bowels of Greenwich Village.

The politically correct line, emerging from a handful of "AIDS activists," maintained that talking about the gay community's prodigious promiscuity was part of a "blame-the-victim mentality." Michael Callen saw a fine line between blaming the victim and taking responsibility, and he thought it was time for some straight talk about the disease if gay men were to survive. Merely moderating sexual behavior, as most gay doctors and health officials counseled, was not enough, he and Berkowitz wrote in the *Native*. Strong measures needed to be taken; it was time to think about closing the bathhouses, they wrote. "If going to the baths is really a game of Russian roulette, then the advice must be to throw the gun away, not merely to play less often."

Callen and Berkowitz were quickly denounced as "sexual Carrie Nations," and the letters column of the *Native* was filled with angry rebuttals. Writer Charles Jurrist responded with his own *Native* piece, "In Defense of Promiscuity," which highlighted the popular party line that a gay man was more likely to be killed in a car accident than by AIDS. An infectious agent might be hypothesized, Jurrist wrote, ". . . but that's all it is—a theory. It is far from scientifically demonstrated. It therefore seems a little premature to be calling for an end to sexual freedom in the name of physical health."

The disputes over sexuality also gnawed at the board of directors of the Gay Men's Health Crisis. Many board members were outraged at what they perceived as prudery on the part of Callen and Berkowitz. Although they were on the forefront of educating people about AIDS and had largely cut back on unsafe sex themselves, the GMHC board thought that issues like bathhouse closure presented profound civil rights questions. You might start by closing baths, but what would happen next? they asked.

Meanwhile, Larry Kramer was growing more militant in his stance that GMHC needed to get down-and-dirty with the facts about AIDS and tell people that, if they wanted to survive, they should just stop having sex. He also was edging toward the position that bathhouses should be closed.

GMHC board meetings often degenerated into heated battles with Larry Kramer on one side and everybody else on the other. Kramer was just continuing his vendetta against the gay fast lane that he had started with *Faggots* years ago, other board members thought. Some privately worried that the arguments might end up as the subject of some new literary effort by Kramer. Everybody knew that a number of his friends had formed the basis for characters in *Faggots;* some had never spoken to Kramer again. Worry that board members might end up in *Faggots II* did nothing to ease the growing tensions.

December 13

The New York Blood Center's records on a suburban matron who contracted AIDS in August turned up a donor who was an intravenous drug user. Dr. Dale Lawrence interviewed him on the Monday morning after Friday's announcement in San Francisco. Maybe he shouldn't have donated blood, the man confided, but there was a blood drive at work and he didn't want his boss to know that he once had been in a methadone program. No, he didn't have any AIDS symptoms, but one of the guys with whom he had shared needles had come down with a strange blood disease, he said.

Lawrence checked the other man's name with the master list in Atlanta—he was a diagnosed AIDS case. They now had substantiated a second transfusion case. Other investigators were checking out more reports, and at the CDC's prompting, the U.S. Public Health Service had called for a meeting with blood bankers and representatives of AIDS risk groups for the first Tuesday in January. CDC virologists were racing to do studies to determine whether there were any existing blood tests that might help screen out AIDS-infected donors. The agency hadn't been able to do much to actually control the spread of AIDS among gays, officials knew; at least with the blood industry, which was firmly under federal regulations through the FDA, they had a chance to save lives if they moved fast.

December 15
CASTRO DISTRICT, SAN FRANCISCO

Joe Brewer knew something was wrong as soon as Gary Walsh called and said they had to have lunch. For Christ's sake, Joe thought, their respective offices were next door to each other. Why did they need lunch? Joe was busy enough, pulling together their trip to Yucatán for the weekend, having to tend to extra details because Gary just hadn't had the energy to pull his end.

"The doctor tells me I can't go to Mexico," said Gary sullenly, not looking at his friend.

"Why?"

"He's sort of worried that I might get intestinal parasites," said Gary, staring at the floor during a pause that seemed far too long. "He's worried I might be pre-AIDS."

Joe Brewer knew Gary's stolid, conservative doctor and knew that if he was "sort of" worried about something he actually was extremely worried. He would never do something as drastic as tell Gary to cancel a trip unless something was very wrong.

"He's afraid if something happens down there, away from good hospitals . . ." Gary let the sentence drift off.

Gary was going to die.

Even in his numb state, Joe knew that, and all the hints he had never fleshed out suddenly sprang into a life of their own. Of course, he should have seen it; now it was real. Gary had AIDS and he was going to die.

That evening, at Gary's comfortable apartment on Alpine Terrace, Gary finally told Joe about the skin problems he had suffered, the different salves he had to use. Gary opened his mouth to show his friend the white spots. Candidiasis, the doctor had said, more commonly known as thrush. Joe began to realize how sick Gary was, how sick he had been.

Time was important now, Joe thought. They couldn't waste it. Joe quickly began putting together an alternative plan. They could go to Key West. That was tropical and still near all the conveniences of modern medicine. Within an hour, Joe had booked the last open flight reservations to Key West and lucked into the last two available rooms at a popular gay guest house. They'd make a trip after all; life would not end.

As Joe drove from Gary's house, perched on the hills over the Castro District with the dark silhouettes of downtown skyscrapers in the distance, he realized their lives would never be the same. December 15, 1982, was his point of demarcation. From then on, he cast his life in terms of Before this event had happened and, now, After.

December 17
CENTERS FOR DISEASE CONTROL,
ATLANTA

For the second consecutive week, the small, innocuous-looking *Morbidity and Mortality Weekly Report* contained a bombshell in its gray pages with the report: "Unexplained Immunodeficiency and Opportunistic Infections in Infants—New York, New Jersey, California." Even in the dry prose of the *MMWR,* each case read like a horror story.

There was, for example, the black-Hispanic baby, born in December 1980, who had grown slowly in his first nine months and then stopped growing altogether. At seventeen months, he suffered thrush, various staph infections, and severe calcification of his brain. His bone marrow was swimming with *Mycobacterium avium-intracellular,* a horrible fungal infection normally seen in birds. The baby's mother was a junkie who seemed healthy at the child's birth but developed candidiasis and decreased T-cells in October 1981, only to die of *Pneumocystis* a month later. The infant, now orphaned, was itself hovering near death. There was another, Haitian baby, who in just thirty weeks of life had contracted *Pneumocystis,* cryptococcus, severe cytomegalovirus and a panoply of other infections before lapsing into respiratory failure. Altogether, the CDC had reports of twenty-two babies who seemed to fit no existing category of inherited immune defect; all were children of people in high-risk groups for AIDS, either intravenous drug users or Haitians.

The report was not cheerful reading, but the CDC staffers hoped it would pound another nail in the case they were still trying to prove to a reluctant scientific establishment—that a new infectious agent was making substantial inroads into diverse corners of American life and threatening unimaginable tragedy.

$\bigcirc$

As the Friday evening newscasts carried the first sketchy details of the startling new reports from Atlanta that day, Joe Brewer and Gary Walsh were on their way to San Francisco International Airport for the flight to Miami. Joe was incredulous that everything had worked out perfectly but, on the plane, Gary was moody, staring out the window as he watched the city twinkle below, like a chest of diamonds that had been tossed haphazardly on a black velvet blanket. San Francisco became very small and receded in the darkness, leaving Gary with the question he would ask again and again.

"Why me? Why me?"

◯

With nonhomosexual victims of AIDS to report, a spate of media attention dutifully noted the new twists in the epidemic. AIDS made rare appearances in *Time* and *Newsweek,* as well as on television networks and wire services. In the entire last quarter of 1982, only thirty articles on AIDS had appeared in the nation's leading news magazines and newspapers, and most of those were in the year's final days, reporting on the babies and transfusion threat. In the third quarter of 1982, only fifteen stories had appeared in these eminent news organs.

All this was about to change suddenly, of course, but the reporting that did exist had already set a pattern for how the disease would be reported: The focus was on the men in the white coats, who were sure to speak innocuously. The stories were carefully written not to inspire panic, which might inflame homophobes, or dwell too much on the seamier sex histories of the gay victims, which might hurt the sensitivities of homosexuals. The pieces always ended on a note of optimism—a breakthrough or vaccine was just around the corner. Most importantly, the epidemic was only news when it was not killing homosexuals. In this sense, AIDS remained a fundamentally gay disease, newsworthy only by virtue of the fact that it sometimes hit people who weren't gay, exceptions that tended to prove the rule.

This is what all the talk of "GRID" and "gay cancer" had helped accomplish in the early months of 1982; AIDS was a gay disease in the popular imagination, no matter who else got it. It would be viewed as much as a gay phenomenon as a medical phenomenon, even by gays themselves, although they were the last to admit it. And the fact that it was so thoroughly identified as a gay disease by the end of 1982 would have everything to do with how the government, the scientific establishment, health officials, and the gay community itself would deal—and not deal—with this plague.

December 29
RAYBURN HOUSE OFFICE BUILDING,
WASHINGTON, D. C.

The new reports of babies and blood transfusions only heightened Tim Westmoreland's apprehension about the epidemic ahead. Congress was in its Christmas recess, but Westmoreland was still riding the National Institutes of Health for more data on exactly what they were doing about AIDS. Two days before the end of the year, the Congressional Research Service sent over the report he had been seeking for months. The basic mortality statistics were startling enough, the service found, far worse than the 40-percent-dead figure that always made the papers. Of the handful of cases diagnosed in 1979, 85 percent were dead, about the same level of mortality as for cases reported in 1980. For cases reported in 1981, 60 percent already were dead, while one in four patients diagnosed between January and June of 1982 had died. Moreover, the rate of new cases reported had tripled in the past twelve months and was expected to increase further.

Westmoreland looked carefully at the dollars spent. In the first twelve months of the epidemic, June 1981 through May 1982, the CDC had spent $1 million on the outbreak, compared with $9 million on Legionnaire's disease. In the past week, Congress had allocated $2.6 million earmarked for AIDS research at the CDC. Although the Reagan administration had said it didn't need the money and opposed the supplemental appropriation, once passed, it became law. This would be the scenario for the next three years: Congress would have to discern for itself how much money government doctors needed to fight AIDS. The administration would resist but not put itself in the position of an on-the-record funding veto. The epidemic's research would survive from continuing resolution to continuing resolution, a game that would ultimately achieve some funding for the doctors while disabling any attempt to plan ahead for studies that might be needed as the scourge continued to grow.

It was the end of 1982, a year in which a movie about a lovable space alien, *E.T.,* had topped all box office records, and two movies about people dressing in drag, *Tootsie* and *Victor/Victoria,* had been surprise smashes. The class movie of the year was a film about Mahatma Gandhi, exploring issues of prejudice and brotherhood, the power of love and the allure of hatred. Paul McCartney had topped the record charts with a perky duet with Stevie Wonder, "Ebony and Ivory," a song about racial bias. Despite the cultural obsession with androgyny, homosexuality, and prejudice, 1982 marked the beginning of the time, commentators would later note, when America started feeling good about itself again. Old-fashioned red-white-and-blue patriotism was coming back into vogue. Certainly, nobody was paying much attention to an epidemic among people like homosexuals and Haitians, even though by the end of the year, the Centers for Disease Control reported that the number of documented AIDS cases in the United States had risen to nearly 900.

The truth was that, at the end of 1982, there were 1,000 or 2,000 people, at most, in the United States who truly understood the dimensions of the crisis that was unfolding. For these people, it would be a restless New Year's.

December 31
THE EVERGLADES, FLORIDA

Gary Walsh and Joe Brewer had decided to leave Key West and check out the Everglades because neither had ever been there and it seemed like an adventure. Gary, however, begged out of the evening early, saying he was too tired to stay up until midnight. For the first time, Joe could see Gary's weakness. The energy with which Gary was constantly able to hype himself was draining away.

Gary climbed into his bed in their sticky room while Joe, feeling dismal, mixed himself a martini and stared out the window. Darkness had enveloped the end of the year and darkness would soon envelop his friend, and there was nothing to be done. In the distance, the clamor of celebrants greeting the New

Year echoed. Joe lifted his glass in the direction of where Gary now slept, growing more distant with each hour. "Happy New Year," Joe whispered to himself.

"Happy New Year, Joseph."

CASTRO DISTRICT, SAN FRANCISCO

Cleve Jones clapped his hands enthusiastically when "KS Poster Boy" Bobbi Campbell made his entrance at Cleve's New Year's Eve party clad in a rhinestone tiara and a silver lamé, floor-length gown. The nurse was now a member of the Sisters of Perpetual Indulgence and had rechristened himself Sister Florence Nightmare. He looked ravishing, Cleve thought, even if his ever-present "I Will Survive" button clashed with the lamé. Sister Boom-Boom, Sister Vicious Power Hungry Bitch, and Sister Missionary Position had already arrived and were dancing habit to holster with the gay police officers who were grinding away in the cleared-out living room.

Everybody was there, Cleve beamed. Dozens of volunteers from the KS Foundation had come, along with an anybody-who's-anybody list of gay politicos and a good sprinkling of the city's heterosexually powerful. A San Francisco supervisor was snorting cocaine in Cleve's bedroom. Supervisor Harry Britt had come with Bill Kraus, who was collecting accolades for his role in passing the first supplemental money for AIDS research.

Bill Kraus was thoroughly single again, Cleve could tell, and, oh, how he could work the crowd. Yet, like Cleve, Bill seemed a little quiet. He told Cleve they'd have to talk, something about AIDS, in the next few days. Then, Bill disappeared into the throng.

The specially made tapes reached a disco frenzy, and the house shook with the synthesized beat of the year's top dance hit, Laura Branigan's "Gloria." When the party neared midnight, Cleve allowed himself some champagne. He hadn't been drinking all night, aware that once he started drinking he was not likely to stop and he'd end up embarrassing himself in front of all these politicians. The smooth flow of champagne, however, made Cleve feel withdrawn. He wasn't unhappy, just detached.

He had carved himself a wonderful niche in nine years, he realized as he surveyed the crowd. His job as an aide to Assemblyman Art Agnos gave him a headstart on whatever political career he chose to pursue. Agnos was being a virtual saint by letting him spend all his time at the KS Foundation. All this gave Cleve a warm feeling, but it still did not make him feel like partying. There was something else that, for once, Cleve could see as bigger than himself and his own ambitions. The horror. He couldn't escape the sense of impending doom.

The clock struck midnight and it became 1983, but the friends, the midnight dancing, the wonderful music, and even the champagne couldn't melt the stone in Cleve's stomach on that New Year. He knew a dark secret. Something they didn't know. When he looked at Bobbi Campbell, he saw more than the tiara flashing; Bobbi would die and so would thousands more. It had all been one big party and, now, it was about to end.

PART V

BATTLE LINES JANUARY – JUNE 1983

In this respect our townsfolk were like everybody else, wrapped up in themselves; in other words they were humanists: they disbelieved in pestilences. A pestilence isn't a thing made to man's measure; therefore we tell ourselves that pestilence is a mere bogey of the mind, a bad dream that will pass away. But it doesn't always pass away, and from one bad dream to another, it is men who pass away. . . .

—ALBERT CAMUS,
The Plague

22 LET IT BLEED

January 3, 1983
PITIE-SALPETRIERE HOSPITAL, PARIS

They would not need much of a lymph node, Dr. Willy Rozenbaum told the gay fashion designer who was suffering from mild lymphadenopathy, just a scrap the size of the top of your little finger, enough to try to culture, to find out what was causing SIDA, the French term for AIDS. Rozenbaum wasn't performing the excision, but he wanted to be on hand to make sure nothing went wrong. Dr. Francoise Barre from the Pasteur Institute also sensed this was something important. She roused herself on the brisk morning the biopsy had been ordered, toting the supplies she needed to preserve the specimen for the trip across town to the institute in the Latin quarter.

Barre peered over her oversized tortoiseshell glasses at the brief procedure and smiled at Rozenbaum's agitation. He was always so excitable. Minutes later, she packed the small piece of lymph node on ice and rushed from the hospital. Back at the Pasteur Institute, Dr. Luc Montagnier put the tissue into a cell culture of T-lymphocytes and gave instructions to Barre to monitor its growth over the next weeks.

Dr. Barre hardly needed the guidance. Quiet and methodical, the thirty-four-year-old researcher had spent most of her career in viral labs, from the Pasteur Institute to the National Cancer Institute, and had earned a reputation for her thoroughness. Both Barre and Montagnier suspected that they would find a retrovirus like the Human T-cell Leukemia virus, or HTLV. Barre had once studied under the NCI retrovirology whiz, Robert Gallo, who had proposed HTLV as a possible cause of AIDS. If the virus in the lymph node behaved like HTLV, they should soon see a proliferation of lymphocytes in the growth culture. Though such viral stimulation typically took weeks to accomplish, Barre decided to start checking the culture every three days, just to keep things under proper scrutiny. This was a new disease, she thought, you never knew what you might find.

January 4
CENTERS FOR DISEASE CONTROL, ATLANTA

Don Francis pounded the table with his fist. The other officials from the Centers for Disease Control exchanged vaguely embarrassed glances. The blood bankers were becoming visibly angry.

"How many people have to die?" shouted Francis, his fist hitting the table again. "How many deaths do you need? Give us the threshold of death that you need in order to believe that this is happening, and we'll meet at that time and we can start doing something."

As far as Francis was concerned, the assembled leaders of the blood banking industry were about to take a course of action that could, at best, be termed negligent homicide, although Francis was known to drop the word "negligent" in private discussions on the issue. The blood banks refused to believe that transfusion-associated AIDS existed, and now they were going to kill people because of it, Francis thought. It was that simple.

Privately, almost all the officials from the Centers for Disease Control agreed with Don Francis, although they were groaning to themselves that he had shown so little politesse as to say it aloud.

The meeting of this ad hoc advisory committee for the U.S. Public Health Service had been fashioned to embrace every group with an interest in the burgeoning epidemic, including the American Red Cross, the American Association of Blood Banks, the National Hemophilia Foundation, the National Gay Task Force, and the Pharmaceutical Manufacturers Association, which represented the commercial blood-products makers, as well as the representatives from the National Institutes of Health and the Food and Drug Administration, the one federal agency that has regulatory power over the blood banks. Congressional aide Tim Westmoreland was there too, as well as reporters from most of the major medical journals and the *Philadelphia Inquirer,* the only major newspaper to provide thorough coverage of the meeting.

The CDC had hoped the assembly would produce some action to arrest the threat the new syndrome posed to the nation's blood supply. Even before the meeting opened, however, it was clear that each group had come with its own agenda, and on most lists, stopping the potential spread of AIDS was secondary. Blood bankers were openly skeptical of the CDC claim that AIDS could be transmitted through blood. Some FDA officials remained unconvinced that AIDS even existed. Gay groups already had condemned any call for screening of blood donors as "scapegoating" homosexuals. The San Francisco Coordinating Committee of Gay and Lesbian Services, chaired by Pat Norman, issued a policy paper asserting that donor screening was "reminiscent of miscegenation blood laws that divided black blood from white" and "similar in concept to the World War II rounding up of Japanese-Americans in the western half of the country to minimize the possibility of espionage."

As Tim Westmoreland saw the players assemble in the CDC's Auditorium A, all facing off at tables positioned in a large square, he sensed that this would not be a polite meeting of scientists engaged in the usual academic one-upmanship. There were interests to guard and turfs to protect. In most reminiscences, the participants would simply refer to the conference as "that horrible meeting."

Jim Curran described the two options the blood industry could take. They could either adopt guidelines to keep people at high risk from donating blood or they could start testing blood to try to weed out likely AIDS carriers. Curran gave the blood bankers a sobering conclusion to his talk: There was at least a one-year incubation period for AIDS. No matter what course the blood industry took that day, it would have no effect for another year, during which still more cases of blood-borne AIDS would incubate and emerge.

It was left to immunologist Thomas Spira, one of the CDC's top virologists, to make the case for the testing of all blood products, the route that the AIDS Task Force desperately hoped blood bankers would follow. Although no test for AIDS itself yet existed, Spira had spent his past weeks testing the blood of AIDS patients for other markers. The trait that distinguished the blood of AIDS sufferers was not difficult to find, considering that virtually everybody in AIDS risk groups—gay men, intravenous drug users, and hemophiliacs—had also suffered from hepatitis B at some point in their lives. Although the hepatitis virus usually disappeared after recovery, the blood still harbored antibodies to the core of the virus. Thus, Spira had found that 88 percent of the blood from gay AIDS patients contained hepatitis core antibodies, while all the blood from AIDS patients who were intravenous drug users had the antibodies, and 80 percent of people with lymphadenopathy carried the antibodies. The test might not screen out all AIDS carriers, Spira suggested, but it would eliminate enough to sharply reduce the threat of transmitting AIDS through transfusions.

CDC officials hoped the data on the testing for a surrogate marker would point the discussions toward what blood banks and commercial blood-products manufacturers could do about AIDS. Instead, the discussion turned into a heated debate about the reality of transfusion AIDS.

"Don't overstate the facts," said Dr. Aaron Kellner, president of the New York Blood Center. "There are at most three cases of AIDS from blood dona-tion and the evidence in two of these cases is very soft. And there are only a handful of cases among hemophiliacs."

Besides, Kellner said, the proposed testing would cost his center $5 million to implement. False-positive test results would result in the unnecessary disposal of blood that wasn't infected with AIDS. "We must be careful not to overreact," he said. "The evidence is tenuous."

Dr. Joseph Bove, director of the blood bank at Yale University Hospitals and chair of the FDA advisory committee on blood safety, joined in the objections. "We are contemplating all these wide-ranging measures because one baby got AIDS after transfusion from a person who later came down with AIDS and there may be a few other cases."

Assistant CDC director Jeffrey Koplan was taken aback. "To bury our heads in the sand and say, 'Let's wait for more cases' is not an adequate public health measure," he argued.

Dr. Bruce Evatt of the CDC tried to reassert the data about hemophiliacs. AIDS simply did not happen among these people before 1982. In only the past year, however, 6 of just 100 hemophiliacs in Ohio were dead of AIDS and 3 more were suffering from severe blood problems associated with the syndrome. Nearly 10 percent already were sick with something having to do with AIDS, Evatt said. What kind of proof did the blood banks need?

Dr. Selma Dritz from the San Francisco Department of Public Health sympathized with the blood bankers. She knew that vast sums of money were involved with any surrogate testing of blood. She also knew that a more moderate proposal to screen out groups at high risk for AIDS from blood donors would severely hurt urban blood banks that relied on civic-minded homosexuals as an essential part of their donor pool. Still, Dritz had the health of her city to tend to and a board of supervisors to answer to. Like so many health officials, her data was hardly reassuring to the blood bankers. "Of 140 (AIDS patients), 10 or 11 had donated whole blood in the previous few years," she said. "We don't know how many others sold their blood or plasma at commercial centers."

At the very least, all people at high risk for AIDS should be ordered to stop giving blood, Dritz thought. Given the fact that carriers could be perfectly healthy while donating a fatal dose of blood, as was the case with the San Francisco baby, Dritz felt that all gays should stop donating.

As the blood bankers got back to arguing the specific case histories of CDC's transfusion AIDS victims, Don Francis started shouting about the "threshold of action." The evidence that the latency period might be long, much longer than anyone suggested, fueled Francis's conviction that the job of the CDC was not merely to monitor the spread of AIDS and count its victims, but to control the disease. "We can't constantly be reacting," he pleaded, "and be constantly behind the eight ball."

Everybody could tell now the meeting was going badly, very badly. The blood bankers were worried about money and the costs of drawing new donors; they were also suspicious of all the reporters covering the conference. Was the CDC trying to pressure them into action? FDA representatives were also wary of the CDC and were slightly irritated that the FDA's turf had been so brazenly invaded by the hotshot epidemiologists from Atlanta. Blood policy was FDA terrain and would stay that way.

Representatives from gay organizations sided with the CDC on surrogate tests of blood but firmly opposed taking any action to screen blood donors, saying the screening would pose serious civil rights questions.

"So-called 'fast-lane' gays are causing the problem and they are just a minority of male homosexuals," offered Dr. Bruce Voeller, representing the National Gay Task Force. "You'll stigmatize at the time of a major civil rights movement a whole group, only a tiny fraction of whom qualify as the problem we are here to address. . . . Also, many gays don't self-identify as such and won't respond to the questionnaire."

Representatives from hemophiliac organizations were stunned by the gay perspective. What about a hemophiliac's right to life? they asked.

After a lunch break, the blood bankers returned even more resolutely opposed to blood testing, arguing almost solely on fiscal grounds. Although largely run by non-profit organizations like the Red Cross, the blood industry represented big money, with annual receipts of a billion dollars. Their business of providing the blood for 3.5 million transfusions a year was threatened. Already the high cost of blood had created new markets for self-donation. Prices had to be competitive, blood bankers knew. The cost of testing for hepatitis antibodies, Kellner from the New York Blood Center suggested, would be $100 million annually for the entire nation. That was simply too much. Instead, he proposed, perhaps, some pilot studies in New York, Los Angeles, and San Francisco.

The for-profit blood-products manufacturers, however, did not enjoy the cartel on their merchandise that the non-profit blood centers held. With the fear of direct competition for their market, the spokesman for Alpha Therapeutic Corporation announced that his firm, which manufactured Factor VIII, would immediately begin screening donors and exclude all people in high-risk groups, including all gays, whether or not they appeared to be "fast-lane." The position infuriated the gay representatives.

⬭

The goal of the meeting was to forward some consensus recommendations to Dr. Edward Brandt, who, as Assistant Secretary for Health of the U.S. Department of Health and Human Services, headed the Public Health Service. At the end of the meeting, CDC's Jeffrey Koplan, who was chairing it, began proposing consensus recommendations. Bruce Voeller suggested a resolution opposed to deferral of high-risk donors; the proposal was defeated soundly on a voice vote. Other proposals met similar fates or were modified so extensively that they were rendered meaningless. The meeting adjourned with no recommendation or agreed-upon course of action. Things would simply go on as they were, as if nothing was happening.

⬭

Don Francis was enraged. The blood banks were going to kill people, he fumed, and the FDA wasn't going to do a damn thing about it.

Harold Jaffe was not given to such dramatic pronouncements, but he was equally disappointed. He couldn't believe what he had heard from the blood bankers. They did not want to believe their industry could be involved in something as horrible as AIDS, so they had simply denied the problem existed. To a large extent, the same thing was happening in the gay community, Jaffe knew, but the blood bankers were doctors and scientists of a sort. They were supposed to be rational and most had sworn to uphold the Hippocratic oath.

It had been a year since Bruce Evatt had heard of the first suspected AIDS case in a hemophiliac. He had expected more cases at that time, but the problem was growing much faster than anyone had expected. He had not anticipated that the CDC would be so definitively thwarted in its influence on public policy. The CDC had stood alone and lost. In history, he knew, it would all go down as a stupid mistake, a terribly stupid mistake.

The year 1983 was going to be that kind of time for the AIDS epidemic. There would be denial on all fronts, leading to stupid mistakes that would cost thousands of lives in the short term and tens of thousands in the long term. The lost opportunities of 1982 would be explained later with the chorus: "How were we to know?" This had no meaning in 1983. By then, vast numbers of people knew better, but confronted with knowledge and the chance to do something, they usually did the wrong thing, if they did anything at all. At the time, their postures seemed like the right thing to do in order to preserve civil rights or, say, the economic viability of the blood industry. The problem, of course, was that such considerations constantly overshadowed concerns of medicine and public health.

Two days later, after the fateful meeting in Auditorium A, the American Association of Blood Banks convened a Washington meeting with all the major blood banking organizations, as well as the American Red Cross, the National Gay Task Force, and the National Hemophilia Foundation. Under prodding from gay representatives, the groups issued a joint statement reiterating the blood banking industry's opposition to donor screening. "Direct or indirect questions about a donor's sexual preference are inappropriate," the statement said. Dr. Roger Enlow, a New York City gay physician and a leader of the American Association of Physicians for Human Rights, heralded the policy. "We've preserved not just gay rights," he said, "but the human right to privacy and individual choice."

January 6
RAYBURN HOUSE OFFICE BUILDING,
WASHINGTON, D. C.

Tim Westmoreland returned from Atlanta more convinced than ever that AIDS was the very public health crisis he had feared when he first read of the Reagan administration's proposed health budget cuts two years ago. He pressed his investigations of CDC and NIH funding harder. The revelations about transfusion AIDS had created an unprecedented level of media attention to the epidemic, finally. How would the NIH respond to questions about its dismal handling of the epidemic, Westmoreland wondered.

The answer was between the lines of a memo from the National Institute for Allergy and Infectious Diseases, or NIAID, that arrived in the health subcommittee's office that Thursday morning. The memo claimed that NIAID had financed a "large effort" in the past fiscal year, doling out $22 million for the study of immunoregulation, another $2.4 million for immune deficiency conditions, and $1.3 million for research into cytomegalovirus. Altogether, the NIAID position paper concluded, "The level of support of NIAID's portfolio for studies relevant to patients with AIDS is approximately $26 million."

The phrase "studies relevant to patients with AIDS," Westmoreland knew, was the operative lie of the document. Buried in another paragraph was the agency's admission that it was devoting only $750,000 of funds directly to intramural AIDS research. Since a bout with the common cold technically involved the immune system, NIAID simply was claiming that such studies were "relevant to patients with AIDS," even if the research was only tangentially related to the syndrome.

That week, Bill Kraus talked to Dr. Robert Gordon, one of a long succession of NIH coordinators for AIDS, to ask whether there were any problems with AIDS funding. Congress would be no barrier to getting more money, Kraus said.

No, answered Dr. Gordon, the NIH funding for AIDS was "more than adequate."

January 7

The *Morbidity and Mortality Weekly Report* on AIDS among female sexual partners of male AIDS sufferers established what would be the last major risk group for Acquired Immune Deficiency Syndrome. Mary Guinan had been railing about "semen depositors" for more than a year, but the publication of the two case histories of New York women with AIDS finally put a "heterosexual contact" category on the CDC's official list of AIDS risk groups. One thirty-seven-year-old woman, suffering from *Pneumocystis,* lived for five years with an intravenous drug user who had died in November, the *MMWR* reported. A twenty-three-year-old Hispanic female with lymphadenopathy had no risk for AIDS other than living for the past eighteen months with a bisexual who had developed both Kaposi's sarcoma and *Pneumocystis* in June 1982. The account also noted that the CDC had received reports of forty-three other previously healthy women who had developed either *Pneumocystis* or other AIDS-related opportunistic infections, mainly after having sexual relations with intravenous drug users. Although none of the men had contracted AIDS, the CDC concluded, "Conceivably these male drug abusers are carriers of an infectious agent that has not made them ill but caused AIDS in their infected female sexual partners."

Another summary in that issue of the *MMWR* also hinted at the shape of things to come, with the first official report on the growing problem of AIDS in prisons. Most of the ten New York state prisoners discussed in the narrative were intravenous drug users, as were all of the New Jersey AIDS prisoners. In fact, prisoners accounted for six of the forty-eight AIDS cases in New Jersey.

Both *MMWR* reports gave greater weight to the idea that gay cancer wasn't so gay anymore. Now AIDS became more newsworthy, particularly as the implications of transfusion AIDS sunk in. Because any chance accident might put one in need of a transfusion, just about everybody was now at risk for AIDS, it seemed.

Pressure mounted on the blood industry in the weeks after the Atlanta meeting to protect "innocent victims." The National Hemophilia Foundation enraged gay activists by calling for "serious efforts" to bar all gay men from donating blood. The for-profit blood-products manufacturer soon fell in line with the foundation, unable to take the commercial risk of offending hemophiliacs, a major market for blood products. The non-profit blood bankers, however, continued to oppose such deferrals as "premature." Meanwhile, gay groups across the country were organizing to oppose what they called the "quarantine" of gay blood.

Blood bankers were quick to pick up the gay rhetoric. At an AIDS study group at the University of California in San Francisco, where Dr. Marcus Conant was trying to engineer a strong university position for hepatitis antibody testing, the staid medical director of San Francisco's Irwin Memorial Blood Bank took his arguments against surrogate testing straight from the lexicon of militant Gay Freedom Day speeches. The hepatitis testing would end up marking gay men with a "biological pink triangle," said Dr. Herb Perkins, alluding to the emblems gays wore in Hitler's death camps. "If 95 percent of gay men are antibody core positive, do we want them marked to exclude all blood with this marker?" he asked.

Conant was unimpressed by Dr. Perkins's oratorical flourishes. He knew more than civil rights was involved with the blood banks' refusal to test blood or defer donors. It was dollars and cents, both in increased testing expenses and for the larger recruiting drives needed to replace gay donors. Conant had no doubt that self-deferral of donors could prove to be a disaster. Too many gays were in the closet, and those who weren't tended to view AIDS as a problem for sleaze-bag gays, the bad homosexuals, not themselves.

Within two weeks, Conant had enlisted the major AIDS experts from UCSF, as well as the highly respected dean of the medical school, to issue a public plea to blood bankers in New York, Los Angeles, and San Francisco to start hepatitis core antibody testing.

The blood banks ignored the statement. Perkins insisted that the call for surrogate testing was "not based on any rational evidence that it would screen out everyone with AIDS, or anyone who was incubating AIDS."

23 MIDNIGHT CONFESSIONS

January 13
SAN FRANCISCO CITY HALL

The ragtag cluster of White Panthers smirked at the voter registrar's clerks when they presented their grocery boxes of petitions for certification. Word swept through the broad marble corridors of City Hall, stunning political veterans who had long ago written the Panthers off as scraggly gun-toting malcontents. The voter registrar confirmed, however, that they had collected some 35,000 signatures, largely from the heavily registered precincts around Castro Street. This was far more than the 19,000 signers needed to put the recall of Mayor Feinstein on the ballot, and the special recall election was set for April.

Upstairs, in her large paneled office, the mayor broke down and wept when she learned that she would be the first San Francisco mayor in thirty-six years to face a recall. Although she referred to it publicly as a "guerrilla attack on our system" by a "small eccentric fringe group," she had no doubts about where the recall organizers had drawn their support in those angry days after the veto of the domestic partners' ordinance. As gay leaders gathered for their weekly meeting with Feinstein that afternoon, she chided, "Well, you've had your revenge."

Even some of Feinstein's longtime supporters chortled, enjoying the fact that they truly had exacted some retribution for the domestic partners' veto. Few could have imagined the impact the recall election would have on the lives, and deaths, of thousands of San Franciscans for years to come.

January 18
PASTEUR INSTITUTE,
PARIS

Francoise Barre peered at the cultures where the tissue from the biopsied lymph node had been set fifteen days before. She was at a loss to understand why, but her lymphocytes seemed to be dying off. This was the opposite of what the scientist expected. When HTLV infected lymphocytes, the virus caused the white blood cells to replicate madly, creating the overabundance of lymphocytes that is called leukemia. Barre added new lymphocytes to ensure that the culture stayed alive. She worried that she might be doing something wrong, but persevered in her calm, methodical way.

That Afternoon
UNIVERSITY OF CALIFORNIA,
SAN FRANCISCO

Marcus Conant knew the minute he saw the first lesions that Gary Walsh had Kaposi's sarcoma. Conant had worked up Gary completely just a few weeks ago, right before Gary left for Key West. Conant had examined every inch of his skin. The three small spots, two on his right calf and one on his left, were new.

"I'm not going to play games with you," said Conant. "I think it is KS. We're going to have a biopsy. It may take ten days to confirm it. I understand that this will be ten days you spend in limbo, but we have to make sure."

Gary was anxious as he dressed to leave. In the hallway, Conant quietly told his nurse to write on Gary's chart that he had Kaposi's sarcoma.

January 23
ATLANTA

As president of the nation's largest gay community AIDS organization, Paul Popham was making the circuit of appearances at the new AIDS groups sprouting up around the country to provide information and support services for victims of the new disease. Paul enjoyed the opportunity to travel. The fledgling AIDS activists in the hinterlands always came away from his talks all gushy about the hunky guy from New York who was out there in the trenches, still keeping his cool.

The debate over the civil rights aspects of blood donations raged everywhere; it was the first topic of conversation between Paul Popham and CDC's Jim Curran as the pair waited their turn to speak at the Aid Atlanta organizing event. Paul echoed the fears Curran was hearing so much lately, about how AIDS might be used as a medical pretext to round up homosexuals and put them in concentration camps.

"I know I'm not going to get AIDS, and I'll be damned if I'm going to spend the rest of my life in some camp," said Paul, in his friendly Oregonian way.

Curran thought the train of thought was curious. After all, nobody had suggested or even hinted that gays should be in any way quarantined for AIDS. The right-wing loonies who might propose such a "final solution" were not paying enough attention to the disease to construct this Dachau scenario. Still, it was virtually an article of faith among homosexuals that they would somehow end up in concentration camps.

In fact, such talk had been around even before AIDS, back when Anita Bryant and California State Senator John Briggs had mounted their campaigns to protect children from homosexual teachers.

PASTEUR INSTITUTE, PARIS

Every three days, Francoise Barre returned to her lymphocytes to see what might be growing from the lymph node tissue. It was late on this Sunday afternoon when she got around to running the radioactive test to detect the presence of reverse transcriptase, the chemical that retroviruses secrete to enable their reproduction. She found the radioactivity to be 7,000 counts per minute. The level was significant but still was not proof that a retrovirus was indeed growing in the culture. She may have been measuring some extreme background radiation. Three days later, the harder proof came. The radioactive assay now measured reverse transcriptase at a rate of 23,000 counts per minute.

This was not background radiation; this was a retrovirus. Moreover, it did not seem to be the Human T-cell Leukemia retrovirus. Although the reproduction of the retrovirus seemed to be peaking, it was killing off her cell line. Had she not added the new lymphocytes earlier, Barre would have missed seeing the virus altogether because all the cell line would have been killed by the extraordinarily lethal retrovirus. That, she would learn later, was what had happened in the laboratories of both the Centers for Disease Control and the National Cancer Institute. The viruses had killed off the cell lines again and again while the scientists waited for the infected lymphocytes to proliferate, the way white blood cells proliferate when infected with the Human T-cell Leukemia virus.

Barre explained her discovery to Luc Montagnier and Jean-Claude Chermann. She had a human retrovirus, she said, but it was not behaving like HTLV. It was a new retrovirus.

New human viruses aren't discovered very often; the scientists knew that they would have to present exhaustive evidence to have their claim believed. Moreover, it would take more evidence to establish that they had found the virus that could be the cause of the "mystery disease," as SIDA was most commonly called in those early months of 1983. A number of tests needed to be run to validate their results. They needed to get antibodies to Robert Gallo's HTLV to ensure that theirs was not the previously discovered virus. Ultimately, the researchers would need to take a picture of the virus through electron microscopes and characterize its genetic properties.

Montagnier decided to hold off telling the excitable Dr. Rozenbaum about the discovery until they were more certain; he didn't know whether he could stand the young doctor's unrestrainable enthusiasm just yet.

January 24
CASTRO DISTRICT, SAN FRANCISCO

The weeds grew wild and rangy in the summer here, on this desolate outcropping of granite that jutted above Castro Street; in the winter, they turned brown, jerking stiffly in the cold January wind. Among them, Gary Walsh could see new buds as well, the harbinger of spring growth. Gary came to the promontory when he was troubled. He'd stare at the little village of Castro and the larger city that lay far beyond, shimmering by San Francisco Bay. Tomorrow morning, he would leave his Alpine Terrace apartment and see Dr. Marcus Conant again, and although he hoped Conant would grin broadly and tell him it was a false alarm, he knew that wouldn't happen. The spots on his legs were not a false alarm. He had AIDS and, tomorrow morning, Marc Conant was going to tell him that the biopsy confirmed Kaposi's sarcoma.

As Gary surveyed the village below him and watched the weeds in the wind, he was surprised at how much more he was seeing, how every sight had extra color and more palpable texture. Intellectually, he understood why. He might never see another winter. As if for the first time, he was actually taking in the feeling, the entire sense of the moment as he had never before. It was what he had long been seeking in his years of self-exploration and his career in psychology—to be so totally in touch with the moment, with now. In a strange way, he began to feel as blessed as he was cursed.

◯

Matt Krieger was ebullient when Gary Walsh called. He had made Gary a photo album of a trip they had taken together to Mexico. He had wanted to give the album to Gary for Christmas, but Gary had been in Key West. Gary dallied in pleasantries only briefly.

"I'm calling because I want to tell you something," he said. "I have AIDS and I want to tell you myself. I don't want you to hear about it on the grapevine."

They talked briefly. Matt wanted to tell Gary how much he loved him, how he wanted them always to be friends even if they weren't lovers. But he didn't want to push too hard on his independent former lover. Not now.

For the rest of the night, Matt was devastated. This was what he had warned Gary about over a year ago, after organizing that press conference with Marc Conant, and now his most fearful nightmare had become reality.

◯

Late that night, Gary poured himself a snifter of cognac, put Beethoven's Fifth Symphony on the stereo, and pulled out his small cassette tape recorder.

"There have been some incredibly special times during the past few months that leave me very, very rich: spots I could not have gotten to without the spots that are on my leg," said Gary. "It seems amazing to me how rich this time can be, how much I've enjoyed touching that inner self. It's like it's never been touched before. . . . And all the hell you bear along the way, including this fucking disease, it all seems to be helping to get me to a spot where I can rest peacefully, whether it's living or whether it's dead. I want this spot, this connection with the beauty around me more than I've ever wanted a lover—because it is my lover. It's what you can always carry with you, where you can understand everything. . . ."

The strings of the Beethoven symphony played dramatic crescendos as Gary planned his approach to his disease, the way he'd explain it in a therapy session.

"It's important for me to keep a very close watch on this time. It would be so easy to think I'm not even going through this. It's an interesting time. I would not miss it for the world—what it's like to go through this unfolding."

The Next Morning
UNIVERSITY OF CALIFORNIA, SAN FRANCISCO

Gary Walsh was visibly agitated when he stepped into Marc Conant's examining room. Conant hated giving out these diagnoses. It wasn't the kind of talk dermatologists usually have with their patients. Conant confirmed the diagnosis and the pair talked about possible therapies. Gary said he'd talk to his own internist about the further course and get back to Conant.

Gary slipped out of the office. Conant glanced down at the chart. There would be a lot of Gary Walshes in the years to come, he knew, and they were all going to die. Conant had to remain fixed to this reality, even as friends and colleagues sometimes told him that he was overly pessimistic. It would be even worse if he really believed he could save these people, Conant felt, because it would make it that much worse when they died. He put the chart aside. In the next waiting room was another bright young man, not unlike Gary Walsh, who had come in worried about some purplish spots he had found the day before on his thigh.

The confirmation of Kaposi's sarcoma on January 25, 1983, made Gary Walsh the 132nd San Franciscan diagnosed with Acquired Immune Deficiency Syndrome.

That same morning, Dr. Don Francis again submitted a budget request for a modest $198,301 to establish a laboratory for AIDS at the Centers for Disease Control. It was the same request Francis had made months ago, with no reply, and he had doubts as to whether the resubmission would meet a kinder fate. "It still stands as our request," Francis wrote the assistant director for management of the Center for Infectious Diseases. "The purpose of this input would be to search for an etiologic agent by electronmicroscopy, cell culture, and serologic testing. They are badly needed if we are to be successful in this pursuit."

January 31
SAN FRANCISCO

All day, clients left Gary Walsh's office crying. In the waiting room that Lu Chaikin shared with Gary, her clients were very impressed.

"He must be wonderful, to get people so moved," one client told Lu.

Upstairs, Joe Brewer was in tears most of the day, even as he shepherded his clients through their increasing anxieties about the epidemic that suddenly was making the newspapers and nightly newscasts. Was it real, they wondered, or just homophobic media hype?

That night, Lu and Gary went out for a drink at Fanny's, a popular restaurant with a small cabaret on the street level, just a few doors down from the Victorian offices the gay psychotherapists shared. While the cheerful music wafted around them, Gary talked about returning to his practice in a few months, once he was rested. Both of them knew this would probably never happen, but neither said it aloud. The fifty-seven-year-old Lu Chaikin would not deprive her friend, or even herself, of the brief comfort of denial, that first stage in accepting any terminal diagnosis.

February 1
CENTERS FOR DISEASE CONTROL
HEPATITIS LABORATORIES, PHOENIX

Frustration swept over Don Francis in waves. The Centers for Disease Control was behaving in an entirely reactive mode, he thought. There was no planning, no efforts at actual control of the disease, and precious little long-range vision. In his windowless office in Phoenix, he began laying out his own long-range plans for getting ahead of the epidemic.

A broader laboratory approach was necessary, even beyond the establishment of the lab he had proposed months ago. The CDC needed to hire personnel in San Francisco and New York to start collecting specimens for lab analysis. Francis also wanted an advisory group of immunologists and retrovirologists from outside the CDC. In a terse memo to Dr. Walter Dowdle, director for the Center for Infectious Diseases, Francis thrust as nimbly as he could at the dilemmas that current underfunding of AIDS research might pose.

". . . Given the seriousness of the disease, I think it deserves a large commitment of resources," Francis wrote. "Nevertheless, many important CDC studies of other diseases have already been curtailed or stopped to do AIDS work. To avoid cutting more into important existing programs, it seems wise to add now to our efforts with additional staff and funds. . . . The total cost of this would be between $250,000 and $300,000 a year. This may seem expensive now, in times of tight budget, but with increasing cases, increasing public and congressional pressure, I predict we will have less trouble finding funds in the future than explaining our inadequacies."

Francis's second memo outlined the most crucial component of his long-range plan for AIDS. Even given the mysteries of the disease, the CDC knew enough about the syndrome to start large-scale campaigns to halt its spread now, particularly among gay men, who were well-educated and far more likely to heed government warnings than other risk groups such as intravenous drug users or Haitians.

"I feel that to control AIDS we are obligated to try to do something to modify sexual activity. No doubt neither the fear of gonorrhea nor syphilis nor hepatitis B has decreased the numbers of sexual partners among homosexual men. But the fear of AIDS might. It seems mandatory for CDC to spread word of AIDS to all areas of the country. We have the network of VD clinics by which this word can be spread. Why not try?"

Why not try?

Years later, many people would ask that question.

Don Francis never received any written replies to his memoranda of February 1, 1983.

○

Dr. Selma Dritz at the San Francisco Public Health Department's Bureau of Communicable Disease Control promptly reported the Kaposi's sarcoma diagnosis of Gary Walsh to the Centers for Disease Control, where it was included among the new reported diagnoses released on Wednesday morning, February 2. It was the week that the number of AIDS cases in the United States exceeded 1,000. By this time, the nineteen-month-old epidemic had stricken 1,025 nationally, including 501 in New York State and 221 in California. At least 394 Americans were now dead from the syndrome. Nearly one in four cases had been reported to federal officials over the past two months alone; more than 100 had died in the past eight weeks. Since December, two more foreign countries had reported their first AIDS cases, putting the epidemic officially in sixteen nations worldwide.

24 DENIAL

February 7, 1983
CAPITOL,
WASHINGTON, D.C.

Mary Kraus Whitesell smiled as she stepped carefully into the office of Congressman Phil Burton on that blustering February morning. She was so proud of her son Billy she could burst. Of course, Bill had always shown an interest in politics. That could be laid to his father, Mike Kraus; Bill was so much like Mike in every way, right down to his infernal stubbornness.

Even though Bill had earned top grades and was named a National Merit Scholar in his senior year at Cincinnati's St. Xavier High School, Mary knew he had been an unhappy child. When both sons separately moved to San Francisco and announced that they were gay, Mary wondered whether they could truly be happy in this life-style that she didn't know much about. Mary hadn't told many of her friends in Cincinnati that her sons were gay; they wouldn't understand.

More recently, Mary, who had remarried, had been reading about AIDS. It made her vaguely worried, so she paid sharp attention to anything that appeared in the papers or the Cincinnati television newscasts. Bill said he was in Washington now to get more money for AIDS research. Mary noticed, however, that Bill avoided telling her much about the disease itself and what it might be doing in San Francisco.

Bill Kraus beamed when Congressman Burton hunkered through the waiting room and insisted that Mary come into his own spacious office. Burton was considered a political tiger on Capitol Hill; Bill couldn't believe he could turn into such a teddy bear for his mom.

"I want you to know how helpful Bill has been to me—I don't know what I'd do without him," Burton said, smiling.

Mary could tell from the way Bill talked about the congressman that Burton had become something of a father figure to her younger son.

Bill took Mary and her husband Ernie to the Capitol dining room for lunch. Mary still couldn't get over how proud and excited she was for Bill, who had grown so handsome and self-assured over the past few years. After so much unhappiness, he finally had made it.

◯

Bill Kraus hadn't realized what a mess AIDS lobbying was in until he assembled the Capitol's half-dozen or so openly gay congressional aides with the leaders of the two national gay groups for a meeting on this snowy Monday morning. Most of the work on behalf of AIDS funding came from three people: Bill Kraus in Burton's office; Michael Housh, another Milk Club activist who worked in the office of San Francisco's second congressional representative, Barbara Boxer; and Tim Westmoreland in his pivotal role as the Health Subcommittee's counsel. The seven-year-old Gay Rights National Lobby, or GRNL, had not grasped the severity of the epidemic as a congressional issue, so the gay community's one full-time lobbyist on the Hill, Steve Endean, had spent 1982 and early 1983 pursuing the agenda he had for years, signing up sponsors for a federal gay rights bill. GRNL had achieved success in enlisting seventy-one co-sponsors for the legislation, but both Bill Kraus and Tim Westmoreland knew the measure would not pass Congress for years, perhaps decades, and that more short-term efforts were needed for AIDS funding. GRNL, however, wasn't interested.

The nation's second national gay group, the National Gay Task Force, or NGTF, had divided up Capitol responsibilities with GRNL by announcing it would handle the gay community's relations with the executive branch of the government. Bill Kraus was at a loss as to what that meant at a time when the executive branch was aligned with raving anti-gay fundamentalists, but agendas were slow to change in a community that had long viewed civil rights as its priority issue. Bill assembled congressional aides from Los Angeles, San Francisco, and New York for the first such meeting of gay aides ever held in the Capitol. This fact alone worried Bill, who was convinced that East Coast closet cases would be the death of the gay movement.

Bill had amassed the depressing statistics on AIDS funding and presented them to the group. The president's new budget called for a 7 percent real decrease in money for the CDC, once inflation was factored in. Under the current budget for the fiscal year ending in September 1984, the entire National Institutes of Health had proposed spending only $9.4 million on AIDS, or about two-tenths of one percent of the agency's budget.

Even more aggravating to Bill Kraus was the delay in National Cancer Institute grants, the money that researchers had been waiting for since September 1981. Privately, NIH officials had told Bill that the proposals were not up to normal standards. They were not "focused," Bill kept hearing. So far, the National Cancer Institute had released only $340,000 in funds to applicants for the extramural grants. Scientists, meanwhile, told Bill that the low approval scores on unapproved grants was merely another example of National Institutes of Health dillydallying on the AIDS epidemic. How can you "focus" a grant application concerning a disease that has been known to exist for only twenty months? Any attempt to get such a focus would be highly artificial, given the fact that nobody knew even what caused the disease, much less how to focus research against it. The NIH was applying its ordinary standards to an extraordinary situation, they said. A lot of research would have to be shooting in the dark. To all this, NIH officials would wink that AIDS research involved a bunch of amateurs—hardly any of them were over thirty-five years old—and you couldn't expect the federal government to throw money at a problem. Not in these days.

To make matters worse, Bill Kraus had heard rumors circulating among AIDS researchers nationally about internecine warfare at the NIH. The always-simmering rivalry between the National Cancer Institute and the National Institute for Allergy and Infectious Diseases had apparently exploded over AIDS. Now that AIDS was established as an infectious disease, NIAID wanted more of the action; the NCI argued that it had been working on the disease first, back when NIAID was ignoring it. Neither agency was talking much to the other, hampering anything like a concerted NIH assault on AIDS.

"We've got to get to work on this," moaned Bill. "Doesn't anybody up here care?"

Bill Kraus wanted to start making noise, hold angry press briefings, and begin militating for more funds. Tim Westmoreland was impressed with Bill's street-politician smarts but considered his approach to Congress "blunt-instrument politics," as he later confided. You just don't walk into the U.S. House of Representatives, start screaming, and hope to prevail because you are right. Moral indignation did not win House appropriations. These things took ma-neuvering, said Tim Westmoreland, the consummate congressional insider. And they took time. Bill was relieved when the meeting was over. God, how he hated to be diplomatic, he told Michael Housh, especially with those fools who didn't see AIDS as the top item of the gay agenda. What good were gay rights if they were all dead?

The next day, officials of the National Institute for Allergy and Infectious Diseases took Bill Kraus and other gay leaders on a three-hour tour and briefing on NIAID's efforts against AIDS. With elaborate pie charts and complex scien-tific language, an eight-page memo showed that NIAID already had "pro-pelled" a "large effort" against the epidemic. The memorandum used many of the bloated numbers about tens of millions of dollars in immune system research floated to Tim Westmoreland the month before. Now, however, the NIAID portfolio of "studies relevant to patients with AIDS," the memo stated, "is approximately $27 million." Somehow millions more had been added to the month-old numbers given to Tim Westmoreland.

Washington was all white and virtually paralyzed by the blizzards that swept across its broad avenues and majestic monuments on the last day of Bill Kraus's visit. Bill stayed with Michael Housh and his lover Rick Pacurar. The three played together like children in the snow, making snowmen and snow angels. That night, however, Bill turned serious, recalling the snow that had drifted around his father's freshly dug grave exactly twenty-five years ago that month.

Michael Housh had always noticed a dark side to Bill Kraus. It came out not only in his cynical humor but also in a certain downcast view he extended to his life in general, whether it was his inability to keep a relationship going or his frustrations with AIDS funding. Only now, however, could Michael trace the darkness back to something in Bill's life.

His father's death was very painful, Bill said. He was only ten years old and had felt so alone; it was even worse when the family moved away from bucolic Fort Mitchell, Kentucky, to nearby Cincinnati. And there was that memory, that awful visual image that returned to his nightmares, of the Kraus family plot in the Milwaukee graveyard buried deep in drifting snow the day they buried his dad. Ice. The frozen-hard ground into which they lowered the casket. Once Bill had seen an Ingmar Bergman movie in which a casket was being lowered into the ground of a cold Swedish winter, and Bill had bitten his knuckles so hard that they bled. It was so much like that awful February day twenty-five years ago, the day that was the end of his childhood.

He had never communicated well with his mother, Bill went on, and never really knew happiness until he went away to Ohio State University. He paused, his eyes following the ornate woodwork in Rick and Michael's living room.

"I think I'm going to get it," Bill said.

Michael didn't know what he was talking about.

"I think I'm going to get AIDS," Bill continued. "I've known it for a while."

"A lot of people are worried about AIDS," Michael said. "You're being melodramatic. You're perfectly healthy."

Bill shook his head. "I just know it. Before this is over, I'm going to have it."

PASTEUR INSTITUTE,
PARIS

Willy Rozenbaum could not contain his excitement. Days before, Professor Luc Montagnier had called, saying: "We've found something. Can you come over and tell us about this SIDA?"

Rozenbaum, Montagnier, Francoise Barre, Francoise Brun-Vezinet, and Jean-Claude Chermann had gathered in Montagnier's office on the Pasteur campus. A new human retrovirus had been discovered, Montagnier announced. He said they would test the new virus to see whether it was HTLV, but it didn't appear to be like the leukemia at all. It was cytopathic, dramatically killing the T-lymphocytes.

Rozenbaum laid out all that he knew about SIDA, describing some of the horrible deaths that had unfolded. All he could do was watch helplessly, he said. Treating one disease did no good because another disease would erupt a day later and kill the patient. Until they knew what caused the actual immune deficiency, there could be no effective treatment for SIDA.

Although he knew the idea lacked scientific proof, Rozenbaum had no doubt that the Pasteur team had discovered the cause of SIDA. A retrovirus—it made perfect sense.

Much work needed to be done, Montagnier cautioned. The group needed to start meeting weekly, every Saturday, in Montagnier's office. They would start preparing a paper on this new human retrovirus for medical journals.

○

At the next meeting of the working group of doctors that Willy Rozenbaum and Jacques Leibowitch had assembled a year earlier, Rozenbaum enthusiastically explained the Pasteur's findings. Leibowitch was immediately doubtful that the Pasteur people had found anything but HTLV. By then, of course, the flamboyant doctor's antipathy for the Pasteur Institute was well known. In the fall, Leibowitch had applied for an immunologist's job at Pasteur Production, the commercial arm of the institute. He was turned down for the post and was still furious.

At the study group meeting, the scientists argued bitterly over the significance of the discovery. Rozenbaum felt the Pasteur Institute had found the cause of AIDS. Leibowitch was certain that nothing of any significance could come from Pasteur. The National Cancer Institute—now there was a major-league institution, Leibowitch said. As for Willy Rozenbaum, Leibowitch thought privately, he was like a child.

○

Across the country, the blood issue also was drawing battle lines among gay community leaders. A split had engulfed the Bay Area Physicians for Human Rights and its national parent group, the American Association of Physicians for Human Rights (AAPHR), after the Bay Area leaders revealed they would urge gay men to cooperate with the local blood bank in screening themselves out as blood donors. As a compromise, however, the Irwin Memorial Blood Bank did not directly ask whether donors were gay, instead inquiring only whether people giving blood were suffering from swollen lymph nodes, nightsweats, and other overt signs of immune deficiency.

At its national convention, AAPHR issued its national policy, calling for hepatitis B core antibody testing and opposing the elimination of gay men from the donor pool, except for those "who think they may be at increased risk for AIDS." Said the AAPHR statement, "We object strongly to the attempts by some members of the blood products and banking community to identify gay men by questionnaire and exclude them from blood donation. These attempts are an unnecessary invasion of individual privacy and grossly misrepresent the issues to the American people." In Washington, gay leaders were successful in persuading Red Cross officials to back off from their plans for sexual-orientation questions and, instead, to work with gay activists to develop a donor policy the gay politicians could support. One longtime veteran of gay politics, Frank Kameny, said he would "advise fellow gays to lie" if the local blood bank officials proceeded with screening.

In New York, the National Gay Task Force rounded up virtually every gay leader in Manhattan to stand on the steps of the New York Blood Center for a press conference denouncing efforts to screen donors. As he scanned the group, Michael Callen, a leader in the newly formed New York chapter of

People With AIDS, relished the irony of the press conference. He knew that virtually every gay man there had had hepatitis B and that most had engaged in the kind of sexual activities that put them at high risk for AIDS. Not one of them could in good conscience donate blood, Callen thought, and here they were, exuding self-righteous indignation at the thought that someone would suggest they did not have the right to make such donations.

⊂⊃

The question of risk-reduction guidelines was even more problematical for gay groups. At its national convention, AAPHR released its tepid proposals for "healthful gay male sexuality." Sensitive to concerns that the group not be "sex-negative," the guidelines assured gay men that there was nothing wrong with having sex, but that they should check their partners for KS lesions, swollen lymph nodes, and overt symptoms of AIDS. It might be a good idea to have fewer partners, the guidelines also suggested tentatively. The Gay Men's Health Crisis in New York had put the accumulated wisdom of homosexual physicians in one phrase: "Have as much sex as you want, but with fewer people and HEALTHY people." Complicated considerations of asymptomatic carriers— the people who looked perfectly healthy while they deposited a dose of AIDS virus—were not weighed for the guidelines, even though they were well documented in the medical literature.

In San Francisco, the more cautious Bay Area Physicians for Human Rights was still holding committee meetings to wrangle over every phrase of risk-reduction guidelines. Some doctors were squeamish about the very idea of telling people what to do in bed. The remainder felt it best to take their time and be prudent so they didn't say anything wrong. Meanwhile, calls still deluged the KS Foundation from people wondering what they could do to protect themselves. Foundation leaders could only suggest they call back, once the gay doctors finished their committee meetings.

In Washington, friends told Tim Westmoreland he was turning gloomy because of his propensity for warning them about their sex lives and AIDS. The disease was a problem of New Yorkers and San Franciscans, friends told him. Westmoreland started to feel like a guy talking airline safety in a crowded airport. In a guest editorial for the local gay paper, the *Washington Blade,* he wrote a long warning about the ramifications the epidemic could have for years to come. There may come a time when insurance companies refuse to insure gay men or try to eliminate AIDS diseases from insurance protection, Westmoreland warned. "To some extent the insurance industry exists to discriminate among risks and to pool or avoid them," he wrote. For this, other gays denounced Westmoreland as an alarmist.

ORLY INTERNATIONAL AIRPORT, PARIS

The airline steward eyed the thermos warily while the handsome young scientist took his seat. Passengers craned to see from where the smoke was coming.

Jacques Leibowitch explained to the supervising attendant that he was a scientist taking specimens to the National Cancer Institute in Bethesda. This was top-priority science. The smoke was only liquid nitrogen. No, he couldn't open it. The young scientist's charm prevailed and he settled into his seat, with the smoking thermos beside him.

Pasteur Production had paid his way to Bethesda, not to deliver these specimens, he laughed to himself, but to pick up the antibodies to HTLV for Drs. Luc Montagnier and Jean-Claude Chermann. Leibowitch also carried a letter from Montagnier explaining the French discovery.

Jacques Leibowitch desperately wanted to prove the Pasteur Institute wrong. He'd do anything he could to help Dr. Robert Gallo prove that his virus, HTLV, was the cause of this epidemic. Leaving nothing to chance, he had even taken biopsies of lymph nodes from one of his sister's Zairian AIDS patients that he planned to hand-deliver to Gallo. Oh, how he loved getting one over on those assholes at the Pasteur Institute.

TIJUANA, MEXICO

The holistic healers had promised that the amino acid and DMSO treatments would cure Gary Walsh. They had cured AIDS patients before, they assured him. Moreover, the medical establishment *knew* the treatments were effective; that was the very reason they were illegal in the United States, they said. Doctors would go out of business if they let people get about the business of really curing disease.

The reasoning appealed to Gary's iconoclasm. In the days before leaving for San Diego, his hope burned fiercely.

He didn't have a deadly disease, he told himself. That was a lot of bunk, he thought as he walked into the clinic for the first of his ten days of treatment.

Almost immediately, Gary felt better. The holistic practitioners told him that with the help of the amino acid injections, his healthy cells would consume his Kaposi's sarcoma lesions. Sure enough, by the end of the regimen, it looked to Gary as though the lesions were getting smaller. Thank God, he thought. I'm going to live.

February 25
SAN FRANCISCO

Marc Conant was not surprised at the letter he received from Gary Walsh in the morning mail; he'd seen this all before.

"My KS lesions are going away," Gary wrote. "I'm feeling much better. The healthy cells are dissolving the cancer cells."

Gary wrote that he might not need to see Conant again if the trend continued. He expected to recover.

Gary Walsh was not Conant's first patient to go traipsing off to Mexico for a miracle cure. The amino acid clinics were making a killing from desperate

AIDS victims seeking a reprieve from their death sentences. The fact that you had to leave the country for treatments rejected by the medical establishment only made them seem all the more tantalizing. Patients recently diagnosed with a fatal illness tended not to be wild about anything that smacked of official medicine.

Conant's own psychologist, Paul Dague, had tried the amino acid route, going to the same clinic that was made famous by its promotion of laetrile for cancer patients. It was Paul who suggested the amino acid treatments to Gary. Other patients returned from healers, usually in Mexico, and chatted excitedly about how their lesions were disappearing even while Conant could measure a substantial growth in the tumors. It was all part of the process of accepting a terminal illness, Conant knew. First, denial.

For Paul Dague, one of the early well-known community organizers to contract AIDS, the search for a cure took one final bitter turn when, in the last days of his life, he flew to the Philippines for "psychic surgery." Marc Conant visited Paul days before his departure. Although near death, Paul was sitting in a chair when he greeted Conant. He was forced to sit, Conant knew, because a Kaposi's sarcoma lesion the size of a ping-pong ball was dangling on the inside of his throat. If Paul lay down, the lesion would fall into his windpipe, choking him. Conant thought it was particularly cruel that God would not even let the man lie down to die, that he would spend his final months always sitting.

Paul hesitated briefly after he told Conant about his travel plans for the Philippines, as though he were waiting for Conant's blanket condemnation of such alternative therapies. Conant instead wished Paul the best of luck.

"I'm not going there for a cure," Paul said. "I'm going for a miracle."

$\boxed{25 \text{ ANGER}}$

March 3, 1983
DEPARTMENT OF HEALTH AND HUMAN SERVICES, WASHINGTON, D.C.

Throughout February, pressure had continued to mount on the federal government to move to protect the blood supply. The nine-month stall on a national blood policy, dating back to the discovery of the hemophiliac cases, could not be sustained. Sensitive to the demands of hemophiliacs, virtually all the private pharmaceutical companies had fallen in line with the National Hemophilia Foundation's guidelines restricting donations from gay men and other high-risk groups. The federal government, meanwhile, had to steer its policy through turf wars between the Centers for Disease Control and the Food and Drug Administration, as well as the pressures exerted by blood bankers, easily agitated gay groups, and congressional representatives promoting their various interests.

The Centers for Disease Control took the hard line in their proposed guidelines, calling for both blood testing and mandatory exclusion of all people in high-risk groups, not merely the voluntary self-deferral the blood banks wanted. Taking its cues from the blood industry, the Food and Drug Administration favored more moderate restrictions. The blood bankers were worried that they would not have enough blood and would suffer economically if all gays were restricted; they also fretted about accusations that they would look like anti-gay bigots if all homosexuals were summarily rejected.

The government's final recommendation was as broad a compromise as could be worked out. It was issued as the policy of the U.S. Public Health Service, the umbrella agency for the CDC, NIH, and FDA. "As a temporary measure, members of increased risk for AIDS should refrain from donating plasma and/or blood," the guidelines said. High-risk people, however, did not include all gays, according to these guidelines, but merely those who were sexually active, had overt symptoms of immune deficiency, or had engaged in sexual relations with people who did. There would not be the hepatitis antibody blood screening that the CDC wanted. Instead, the guidelines called for studies to evaluate screening procedures. With the weight of the Public Health Service behind them, the American Red Cross, the American Association of Blood Banks, and the Council of Community Blood Centers had no choice but to announce that they would comply.

The Public Health Service guidelines came seven months after the CDC first had proposed policy for the AIDS blood problem in July 1982, and two months after "that horrible meeting" in Atlanta. Between that January 4 meeting and the March 4 publication of the guidelines in the *MMWR,* nearly one million transfusions were administered in the United States.

$\bigcirc$

The Public Health Service pronouncements on AIDS also included the first risk-reduction guidelines ever issued by the federal government. The PHS saw fit to offer only two sentences of guidance to gay men eager to avoid the strange new disease, despite reams of data collected in the still-unpublished case-control study. "Sexual contact should be avoided with persons known or suspected to have AIDS," the PHS wrote. "Members of high-risk groups should be aware that multiple sexual partners increase the probability of developing AIDS."

That statement represented the sum total of the U.S. government's attempt to prevent the spread of acquired immune deficiency syndrome among gay men in March 1983, more than twenty months into the epidemic.

CASTRO STREET, SAN FRANCISCO

Gary Walsh picked through his pasta salad at the Village Deli on Castro Street, looking out the broad plate-glass windows at a passing parade of men, all buttoned up in thick wool jackets. Joe Brewer could see that the disease had skimmed the extra fat from Gary's body. Where he was once cheeky, his face now displayed prominent cheekbones. Although Gary's eyes occasionally flashed their old merriment, they were deeper set now, in gaunt sockets, making them look larger and more open.

Gary speared a spinach pasta curl on his fork and watched it slip around as he finally said what he wanted to say:

"What do you think of suicide with extreme illness?"

"I think it's wrong," said Joe, surprising himself at how automatic his answer was. "It's a disrespect of the life force to end it. That's playing God, to end it before it ends itself."

"I don't know," Gary said, unconvinced.

After the meal, the pair made their way to Gary's apartment on Alpine Terrace. Joe studied the cityscape that spread below the bay windows while Gary made coffee in the kitchen. Joe, of course, knew how bitterly disappointed Gary had been with the amino acid therapy. Gary had felt better for a week but, within days, the fatigue and aches had returned, and he had angrily canceled a check for $1,000 that was to be his final payment for the treatment. He hadn't wanted to see any of his friends for days after that. He had moved from denial into depression, Joe thought. Gary would be better off once he got to anger.

Gary sat down on the couch and continued his thought. He had spent most of his life in pain, from the time he was hit by a car when he was seven years old. Finally, just a few years ago, he had found relief with corrective back surgery, but recovery from the surgery had required him to be bedridden for three months, again in chronic pain.

"I know all too much about pain," Gary said, "and I might not want to follow this all the way to the end."

Joe recalled those agonizing days after Gary's back surgery and understood his point. Besides, it was Gary's decision to make.

"All right," Joe answered, reluctantly. "I'll do whatever it takes to help you."

March 7
NEW YORK CITY

"If this article doesn't scare the shit out of you we're in real trouble. If this article doesn't rouse you to anger, fury, rage and action, gay men may have no future on this earth. Our continued existence depends on just how angry you can get. ... Unless we fight for our lives we shall die. In all the history of homosexuality we have never been so close to death and extinction before. Many of us are dying or dead already."

With those words, Larry Kramer threw a hand grenade into the foxhole of denial where most gay men in the United States had been sitting out the epidemic. The cover story of the *New York Native*, headlined "1,112 and Counting," was Kramer's end run around all the gay leaders and GMHC organizers worried about not panicking the homosexuals and not inciting homophobia. As far as Kramer was concerned, gay men needed a little panic and a lot of anger.

Kramer built his story around the burgeoning statistics, the fears of doctors who were at a loss as to how to handle the new caseloads, and the first rumors of suicides among gay men who preferred to die rather than face the brutal, disfiguring disease. He lashed out at the delays in grant funding by the National Institutes of Health and chided the CDC for falling behind on gathering epidemiological data. "There have been so many AIDS victims that the CDC is no longer able to get to them fast enough. It has given up," Kramer wrote. "This is a woeful waste with as terrifying implications for us as the alarming rise in case numbers and doctors finally admitting they don't know what's going on. As each man dies, as one or both sets of men who had interacted with each other come down with AIDS, yet more information that might reveal patterns of transmissibility is not being monitored and collected and studied. . . . How is AIDS being transmitted? Through which bodily fluids, by which sexual behaviors, in what social environments? For months the CDC has been asked to begin such preparations for continued surveillance. The CDC is stretched to its limits and is dreadfully underfunded for what it's being asked, in all areas, to do."

On the local level, Larry Kramer attacked *The New York Times* for its scant AIDS coverage and the "appalling" job of health education conducted by city Health Commissioner David Sencer. Kramer's sharpest barbs were directed at Mayor Ed Koch, "who appears to have chosen, for whatever reason, not to allow himself to be perceived by the non-gay world as visibly helping us in this emergency. Repeated requests to meet with him have been denied us. Repeated attempts to have him make a very necessary public announcement about this crisis and public health emergency have been refused by his staff. . . . With his silence on AIDS, the mayor of New York is helping to kill us."

The gay community received no better marks. Kramer said that the New York gay doctors, as a group, have "done *nothing.* You can count on one hand the number of our doctors who have really worked for us." And he noted that the only national gay newsmagazine, the *Advocate,* "has yet to quite acknowledge that there's anything going on."

"I am sick of guys who moan that giving up careless sex until this thing blows over is worse than death," Kramer wrote. "How can they value life so little and cocks and asses so much?"

At the end of the story, Larry Kramer listed friends who had died, people like Nick, Rick Wellikoff, Jack Nau, Michael Maletta, and the two men he had seen that first day in Alvin Friedman-Kien's office, David Jackson and Donald Krintzman. Kramer knew twenty-one people who had died—"and one more, who will be dead by the time these words appear in print. If we don't act immediately, then we face our approaching doom."

<hr />

Larry Kramer's piece irrevocably altered the context in which AIDS was discussed in the gay community and, hence, in the nation. Inarguably one of the most influential works of advocacy journalism of the decade, "1,112 and Counting . . ." swiftly crystallized the epidemic into a political movement for the gay community at the same time it set off a maelstrom of controversy that polarized gay leaders. Endless letters poured into the *Native,* denouncing Kramer as an "alarmist" who was rabidly "sex-negative" and was using AIDS to deliver his post-*Faggots* "I told you so." Even as the issue sold out on Manhattan newsstands, Kramer laid plans for wider publication of the piece around the country, where it would prove to have a far greater impact on AIDS policy, particularly in San Francisco.

The New York AIDS Network timed the release of its own demands for city services to Mayor Koch to coincide with Kramer's piece. "It must be stated at the outset that the gay community is growing increasingly aroused and concerned and angry," its statement said. "Should our avenues to the Mayor of our City, and the Members of the Board of Estimate not be available, it is our feeling that the level of frustration is such that it will manifest itself in a manner heretofore not associated with this community and the gay population at large."

To drive home the point, the *Native* printed a request for 3,000 volunteers to be instructed in civil disobedience such as sit-ins and traffic tie-ups to force city officials to confront AIDS concerns.

<hr />

Two days later, on March 9, Mayor Ed Koch and Health Commissioner David Sencer hurriedly announced the formation of an Office of Gay and Lesbian Health Concerns under Director Dr. Roger Enlow, an architect of the low-profile handling of AIDS in the gay community. Dr. Enlow, gay leaders knew, would not rock any boats.

○

On the same day, in a simple but tasteful ceremony in Washington, a new secretary for the U.S. Department of Health and Human Services was sworn in. Like her predecessor, Richard Schweiker, Secretary Margaret Heckler came to her job with moderate-to-liberal political credentials after serving for eight terms as one of the only Republican congressional representatives from Massachusetts. Just four months before, she had lost her bid for reelection to Boston State Representative Barney Frank in a campaign that, in the desperate end, featured a whispering campaign by Heckler supporters that Frank was gay. Pundits, however, said Heckler's appointment was an attempt by the Reagan administration to polish its image in the social policy area after two years of brutal budget cuts in spending for the poor.

Over at the Rayburn House Office Building, Congressman Henry Waxman noted, with some concern, that the president had managed to appoint a person who, in all her years in Congress, never seemed to have much interest in issues related either to health or human services. Moreover, Heckler was not known as an intellectual giant or as a person of sufficient will to stand up to an administration dedicated to dissecting the very programs she was sworn to administer.

○

On the day that Secretary Heckler was administered her oath of office, the Centers for Disease Control released new figures showing that AIDS had stricken 1,145 Americans, killing 428. One in five of the diagnosed cases in the United States had been reported since January.

March 12
VANCOUVER, BRITISH COLUMBIA

Everybody who came to the AIDS forum had vague concerns about this new disease that people in the United States were talking so much about; that's why they had come. Nobody expected much of this gorgeous hunk in a plaid shirt, faded jeans, work boots, and a beautiful mustache—a definite "10," they agreed. Yet he was billed as leader of the Gay Men's Health Crisis in New York City. And few were unmoved when he talked about his friends who had died, and about how death was spreading in New York and San Francisco, Toronto and Los Angeles, and that it would come here too.

Paul Popham had accepted the invitation for the organizational forum of AIDS Vancouver because of the chance it would give him to visit the Northwest and see his family in Oregon. After his talk, he was startled when a familiar figure walked up to the audience microphone for the question-and-answer session.

"People say you can spread this through sex," said Gaetan Dugas. "Are there any studies that actually prove this can be passed? How can people say this can be passed along when they don't even know what causes it?"

Paul Popham had never seen the normally affable Gaetan Dugas so angry. He let the doctors field most of the questions. It wasn't clear from the bickering, however, who knew more about AIDS, the doctors or Gaetan. Gaetan had spent the past two years reading positively everything he could grasp on the strange disease with which he had been diagnosed for three years. He hadn't read anything that gave him hard, solid facts to support the idea he couldn't have sex, Gaetan said.

Of course, other comments from the floor were also challenging Paul Popham and the doctors on the podium. Leftist gay radicals insisted that all this attention to the U.S. disease would foster homophobia. Gay bathhouse owners were angry at the local gay newspaper for running a health page; this obsession with a handful of sick people in the United States was bad for business. Yet it was the contentious Quebeçois, standing there in his black leather outfit, who captured the attention of forum organizer Bob Tivey. There was something else about him, something familiar. Toward the end of the evening Tivey realized that he knew Gaetan from at least ten years before, in the hot discos of Toronto. Gaetan was older now, but he was the same man. It must have been 1971 or 1972, and Gaetan was always the hottest party guy in Ontario, Tivey remembered, very fashionable and always charming. He was the man, it had seemed then, that everyone was looking for in those long nights at the gay bars.

Bob Tivey reintroduced himself to Gaetan at the end of the forum while taking the names of people who might provide or need social support services. Gaetan confided that he had been one of the first people in North America to be diagnosed with Kaposi's sarcoma. Yes, he'd like support services, Gaetan said, but no, he did not have AIDS. He had skin cancer. Gaetan started getting angry again, talking about the doctors who said he shouldn't be having sex. Who ever heard of cancer being infectious? Tivey detected that Gaetan was almost a textbook case of denial and anger, and he figured it would be easy to provide counseling for him.

Meanwhile, a gay newspaper in Edmonton had already written a story about an airline steward with AIDS who was popping into Alberta and screwing people in the bathhouses—but Bob Tivey hadn't heard those stories. Not yet.

◯

Paul Popham couldn't believe how well Gaetan looked, considering how long it was since he had been diagnosed. Gaetan confided that he had suffered a bout of *Pneumocystis* that winter and had gone back to Quebec City for care. All his West Coast friends had thought they'd never see him again, but now he felt great. His hair was growing back now that he was off chemotherapy. Paul told Gaetan about the wonderful circus GMHC planned as a fund-raiser at Madison Square Garden the next month. He also mentioned that Jack Nau had died about a year and a half before.

Not far below the surface of the conversation, Gaetan's anger continued to simmer. Suddenly, he blurted, "Why did this happen to me?"

In March 1983, the first case of AIDS was diagnosed in Australia—an American visitor. Australian public health officials now waited for their first homegrown cases, aware that tens of thousands of men from Down Under had taken advantage of the cheap "Skytrain" flights to San Francisco in the early 1980s. In France, AIDS researcher Jacques Leibowitch began calling AIDS "the charter disease," because so many of the early European gay cases were among the men who had boarded the inexpensive charter flights to New York and San Francisco.

March 17
NEW YORK UNIVERSITY,
MANHATTAN

Marc Conant picked up a copy of the *Native* with "1,112 and Counting . . ." from a newsstand and showed it to Paul Volberding while the two San Francisco doctors shared a private moment at a New York University AIDS conference. They were standing on a campus patio; Conant could see the scores of other doctors milling about inside, sharing their latest insights on whether this or that form of chemotherapy worked best on Kaposi's sarcoma.

"Kramer's right," said Conant. "Here we are working on people who are already sick, people for whom it's already too late. We need to be out there screaming to gay people that, if they don't stop, we're all going to die." The pair decided to call a meeting of gay community leaders when they returned to San Francisco. It was time to sound major alarms.

Paul Volberding was grateful he didn't have to contend with the politicalization of AIDS medicine in San Francisco. In New York the gay doctors seemed to make everything into a political issue. At one session of the conference, Volberding had noted that San Francisco General Hospital planned to open a ward for AIDS patients in the summer. The rationale for the AIDS ward was the same as for the city's AIDS clinic. Presenting such a complicated array of disorders, the syndrome demanded that new specialists be created, people who understood the nuances of treatment for a *Pneumocystis* patient who might simultaneously be suffering from ulcerating herpes in the rectum and KS lesions coating the stomach. Dealing just with the medicines and symptoms generated some of the most intricate clinical problems in the history of medicine, drawing on virtually every medical specialty. At San Francisco General, they were literally writing the textbooks on AIDS care because of their clinic. It made medical sense to have such a ward, Volberding said, both for the patients and for the doctors who wanted to find a way out of the AIDS nightmare.

Paul Volberding was astonished at the vehemence with which Dr. Roger Enlow, the new coordinator of New York City's Office of Gay and Lesbian Health Concerns, denounced the plans for the AIDS ward. It would be nothing more than a leper colony, he said. Dr. Enlow vociferously argued that AIDS patients should not be treated separately; it was everything they were trying to avoid in New York.

○

That afternoon, Congressman Phillip Burton introduced a resolution in Congress asking for an additional $10 million in funding for the Centers for Disease Control for AIDS research. Congresswoman Barbara Boxer, the other representative from San Francisco, introduced a parallel bill to allocate $20 million to the National Institutes of Health for AIDS studies. The money bills were calculated and written by the Capitol's three most prominent, openly gay aides, Bill Kraus, Tim Westmoreland, and Michael Housh from Boxer's office. The Reagan administration, of course, was still solemnly insisting it did not need more money for AIDS research. Scientists had all the funds they needed, they claimed. For the three gay aides, however, the bills were just the opening salvo in the funding wars. Westmoreland already was planning a Health Subcommittee hearing on AIDS for May, while Manhattan's Representative Ted Weiss, who chaired an oversight committee on government operations, was considering a full-scale hearing to delve into the government's entire response to the epidemic.

We've finally got things moving, thought Bill Kraus as he typed Phil Burton's press release on the AIDS bills.

○

The three-day NYU conference on AIDS offered the embattled blood industry a chance to draw its battle lines against further government demands for blood testing. Dr. Joseph Bove had by now become the leading spokesman for the blood industry, given his roles as chair of the FDA blood advisory panel, chief of the blood bank at Yale–New Haven Hospital, and chair of the American Association of Blood Banks Committee on Transfusion-Transmitted Disease. With the Public Health Service blood guidelines less than two weeks old, Bove worried aloud that the "CDC—now more aggressive and independent"— would want even more action from blood banks in its compulsion to "do something." Bove mocked the CDC's evidence of blood transmission, insisting the action could not be warranted until the CDC showed definitively that an infectious agent caused AIDS. "The evidence for nearly all this is inferential," said Bove, a professor of laboratory medicine at Yale. "I wish it were better."

Moreover, in only one transfusion AIDS case could the CDC pair a transfusion recipient with a donor who actually had AIDS. In the other six cases under investigation, the donors were in high-risk groups showing early AIDS symptoms, but none had one of the diseases the CDC required to substantiate a case of full-blown AIDS. The report of the San Francisco baby appeared in the *MMWR*, Dr. Bove added, not a standard peer-reviewed medical journal. Bove chose not to dwell much on the fact that such peer-reviewed publication takes six to nine months. "Nothing exists in the peer-reviewed medical literature— not one case!" said Bove. ". . . Evidence for such [blood] transmission is lacking."

Years later, when it was clear that hundreds were dying because the blood industry and federal regulators at the FDA heeded the calls of people like Joseph Bove, the doctor would pull a copy of his speech from his shelf at Yale to show that his 1983 presentation at NYU was, technically, accurate. "I wrote 'evidence is minimal,'" said Bove. "I was extremely cautious about my choice of words. I didn't want to go on the record either way. I was smart enough not to say it wasn't there. Technically, I was not inaccurate."

On the day the NYU conference opened, the San Francisco gay newspaper, *Bay Area Reporter,* published Larry Kramer's broadside of anger and outrage. The issue also included an editorial that contained some startling confessions from editor Paul Lorch. "This space—for that matter, the entire paper by editorial fiat—has been sparse in its coverage of what has come to be known as AIDS," Lorch wrote. "The position we have taken is to portray that each man owns his own body and the future he plots for it. And he retains ownership of the way he wants to die. . . . [Now] we have made a very deliberate decision to up the noise level on AIDS and the fatal furies that follow in its wake."

CASTRO STREET, SAN FRANCISCO

Gary Walsh and Joe Brewer were enthralled by the Larry Kramer story. Gary couldn't stop reciting the litany of complaints Larry raised. There wasn't enough government funding. The newspapers weren't paying attention. Nobody cared; there was no outrage.

Joe was pleased to see Gary get worked up about AIDS; he hadn't seen Gary's famous temper since his diagnosis.

"We've got to do something—something dramatic," Gary said.

Candles, Gary thought suddenly. The candlelight march.

It was the perfect idea. The candlelight march from Castro Street to City Hall in 1978 on the night of the assassinations of Supervisor Harvey Milk and Mayor George Moscone had been one of the most dramatic moments of their lives. Gary had even left the march to call his parents and dramatically announce he was gay, prompting his mother to worry openly that Gary would not go to heaven.

A stream of candles glimmering down Market Street, Gary thought. It would be such a gentle, nonthreatening battle line. The demands could be made, not in an ugly confrontational way, but in a way that invited the best in people. Besides, the media could not avoid taking long, lingering shots of homosexuals holding candles. It would be a smash.

Gary got on the horn to other people with AIDS. It was going to be *their* march, they decided, articulating their needs as the people most intimately struggling with the horrors of the new disease. There was no more talk of suicide as Gary busied himself with his new project and started boning up on AIDS facts for the media appearances and political lobbying he planned.

Joe Brewer began putting together notes for a series of articles he wanted to put in the local gay newspapers to give gay men the psychological tools to start changing their sex lives. His denial about AIDS had been shattered too late, only when Gary was diagnosed. He could date his practice of strictly no-risk sexuality only to his Christmas trip to Key West. All the AIDS groups, like the Shanti Project, the KS Foundation, and especially the San Francisco Department of Public Health, were obsessed with keeping gay men from panicking. From his own experience, and from conversations with clients, Joe figured gay men could use a little panic now if they were going to change their sex lives and survive.

VANCOUVER, BRITISH COLUMBIA

When Gaetan Dugas's best friend moved from Toronto back to Vancouver, he felt like he had landed in the middle of Peyton Place. Everybody was talking about Gaetan as "the Orange County connection," going out to the bars and having sex with people. It hadn't helped when Gaetan made a scene at the AIDS Vancouver forum, arguing about whether AIDS actually could be spread through sex. Gaetan's sexual prowling had reached near-legendary proportions since then. He made little effort to conceal his medical problems, casually rolling up his sleeves as he quaffed beers at pubs, despite the lesions on his forearms.

According to one story, one tryst of Gaetan's was so furious when he heard that Gaetan had AIDS that he tracked the former airline steward down to confront him. By the time they were done talking, Gaetan had charmed the man back into bed.

The friend from Toronto sat Gaetan down for a talk. They had known each other for years, since they were Air Canada stewards together in Halifax and had escaped to San Francisco for the Gay Freedom Day parades and parties. He genuinely loved Gaetan, knowing him as a kind and caring friend, not just somebody to party with. If a friend were sick, Gaetan could be relentless in his attentions, and there never seemed to be an end to the little considerate gestures Gaetan doled out to the people close to his heart. Still, the friend suspected that the rumors might be true. Asking Gaetan to give up sex, he knew, would be like asking Bruce Springsteen to give up the guitar. Sex wasn't just sex to Gaetan; sex was who Gaetan was—it was the basis of his identity.

Gaetan at first denied he was having sex with anyone. His friend didn't let it end at that. He suggested to Gaetan that anyone with AIDS should stop having sex. Period.

"They can't tell me that having sex is going to transmit it," said Gaetan. "They haven't proved it yet."

"Yes," his friend countered, "but if there's even the slightest possibility, then you shouldn't do it."

"Yes, I suppose you're right," Gaetan shrugged.

The friend wasn't sure that Gaetan agreed at all. He recalled the conversations they had had years before in Halifax, deciding whether they could hit the bars on the nights after they had shots for gonorrhea. The doctors always said to wait a few days, but Gaetan figured that since somebody gave it to him, he could give it right back.

"This is incurable," Gaetan's friend pushed. "You don't just get a shot. It would be so incredibly unfair to give it to someone."

Yes, Gaetan said, so unfair.

26 THE BIG ENCHILADA

March 20, 1983
79 URANUS STREET,
SAN FRANCISCO

Rain beat against the redwood deck outside the sliding glass doors; winter was leaving northern California reluctantly that year. The core of gay political activists who had been closest to Harvey Milk sat around the kitchen table, a copy of "1,112 and Counting" lying nearby in case anybody hadn't read its call to action. Among others were Bill Kraus, Cleve Jones, and Dick Pabich, the aide who had rushed into Harvey Milk's tiny office on the dark November day five years before to discover the group's political mentor lying facedown in a pool of blood.

Dana Van Gorder, aide to Supervisor Harry Britt, laid out the problem on the city level. The Department of Public Health still had not produced one piece of informational literature on AIDS. Endless committee meetings were being held to determine the politically correct way to say what had to be said. The simplest suggestions, like Dana Van Gorder's old proposal for bus signs on the city-owned transit system, also were bogged down in process. There was no sense of emergency at the health department.

There was also the question of the study. As early as October, epidemiologists from the University of California in San Francisco, working in conjunction with San Francisco General Hospital, had been talking about data that compared the incidence of diagnosed AIDS cases with census tracts counting unmarried males. By the end of December, 1 in 333 single men over age fifteen in the Castro neighborhood already was diagnosed with AIDS. Factoring out heterosexual single men and the delay in reporting diagnoses, this meant that perhaps 1 in 100 gay men in this area already had AIDS. A person having twenty sexual contacts a year had 1 chance in 10 of making it with an AIDS sufferer. The odds shot up astronomically when larger numbers of infected but asymptomatic gay men were included.

The researchers, Drs. Andrew Moss and Michael Gorman, had given their incidence study to the Bay Area Physicians for Human Rights and other gay political leaders in January, figuring they would release the statistics and sound alarms to gay men. However, these gay doctors and activists, assuming they knew what was best for the city's homosexuals, had done nothing. Instead, they were pondering how to deliver the information. . . . appropriately. They feared that the study results would have a devastating impact on the Castro neighborhood and prove a major public relations nightmare, and they managed to intimidate the researchers with that argument. The epidemiologists, fearing they would lose the community cooperation that was the key to their studies, agreed to hold off releasing their results until the study was published in April in the form of a letter to the British medical journal *Lancet.*

Public Health Director Dr. Mervyn Silverman had done nothing to disseminate the study's findings in the weeks since his meeting with Supervisor Harry Britt, who informed him of the study. Rather, Silverman seemed content to simply lay the responsibility for education on gays themselves. It was the liberal thing to do. It was politically savvy as well, because no gay leaders would be offended this way. Bill Kraus noted that this also was the cheapest course for the health department, requiring no commitment of departmental staff time or educational resources.

"Okay, we have to do an end run around these people," Bill said to the group gathered at 79 Uranus Street. "We'll just do it like a political campaign. We'll get the message out about safe sex, and repeat it and repeat it until it sinks in. Targeted mailings. Brochures that speak to the audience. We've done it all before."

Also, the study needed to be emancipated from the gay-leader types, Bill decided. Fuck process. When people see how serious this is, they'll change. Who did these leaders think they were, deciding the life and death of the community?

Over the next two hours, the group mapped out an educational plan. Since the health department wouldn't send out brochures, Bill Kraus would get Phil Burton and Barbara Boxer, who also was aligned with the Milk Club, to send out their own brochures using their congressional franking privileges. The mailings could be directed to the computerized mailing lists of single, male voters in heavily gay precincts. The Harvey Milk Club, meanwhile, could do another brochure that was much more explicit than anything congressional representatives could issue. Gay men needed simple direct messages about what to do, and not do, for the community to survive.

After these tasks were assigned, Bill pulled Cleve aside into a guest bedroom. He had this spot on his leg, he said, pulling up the cuff on his pants. Cleve examined the discoloration and pronounced it a garden-variety liver spot.

"That's what happens to you older men," he joked.

Bill looked only mildly relieved. Cleve wondered to himself if they all were going to spend the rest of their days like this. His lymph nodes had been slightly swollen for months, and he had taken to examining every visible square inch of his body during his morning showers. Half his friends were doing the same thing; the other half were going to the baths as they always had.

March 22
901 MISSION STREET,
SAN FRANCISCO

The *San Francisco Chronicle* is housed in a building with a tower and a big clock at Fifth and Mission streets. Not far from the financial district, the neighborhood had become a refuge of winos and derelicts who petitioned passing reporters to spare change. Having run that gauntlet, on this morning, a young reporter approached an assistant city editor with the copy of a study leaked to him by a "congressional source." The bold "CONFIDENTIAL" stamp piqued the editor's curiosity, as did the reporter's confirmation from an official "high in the health department" that the study was accurate. It wasn't Merv Silverman, of course, and a feminine pronoun strategically slipped out along the way, leading the editor to accurately assume that the high official was the no-nonsense Selma Dritz who, in news circles, was considered only slightly less credible than God. Reporters don't have to tell editors their sources, but it doesn't hurt to hint during lobbying for a story. The *Chronicle* was running more AIDS stories than any newspaper in the United States. This, however, wasn't saying very much. AIDS stories still needed a careful marshaling of editorial support to clear the various hurdles toward publication.

"It's definitely a story," the editor agreed, casting a calculative eye toward the news editors to whom he needed to sell the piece. "Let's go."

⬭

"We don't want the data released," said Dr. Michael Gorman, the study's co-author, when contacted about the study. "You have no right to release it. It's marked confidential."

At the SF Department of Public Health, Pat Norman was upset when she was told the *Chronicle* was going to publish the study. "I've only known about it for two weeks," she said abruptly. She was on the verge of announcing her candidacy for the board of supervisors, and it wouldn't pay to look like part of a coverup. She obviously was unaware that the reporter had seen the letter, dated two weeks before, in which Dr. Andrew Moss alluded that Pat Norman was already opposed to the data's release.

It wasn't her job to release medical studies, Norman reasoned. It was the job of the director of the Bureau of Communicable Disease Control, and he hadn't let the information out either. "There was never a question of whether we were going to release this information," she said. "We wanted to release it in a reasonable way. Appropriately, so as not to cause panic."

Back in the newsroom, the reporter had written two paragraphs of his story when the phone rang. It was Randy Stallings, who was president of the Alice B. Toklas Memorial Democratic Club and co-chair, with Pat Norman, of the Coalition for Human Rights, the umbrella group of all the city's gay organizations.

"I'd never ask a reporter not to do a story," he said, adding that there were many reasons not to publish the information. Instead, he said, it should come out in an . . . appropriate way.

"They'll put barbed wire up around the Castro," said Stallings. "It will create panic. People won't go to gay businesses in the Castro. It will be used to defeat the gay rights bill in Sacramento."

After the reporter had written three more paragraphs, Dr. Moss called from London, pleading that the study not be printed. He clearly was worried that gays would not cooperate with future studies if their leaders denounced his research.

"This already has gone out to the appropriate channels," said Moss, referring to gay leaders and the Bay Area Physicians for Human Rights. The reporter needed to give "very serious thought" to whether to write the story.

Two paragraphs later, Selma Dritz called the reporter, chuckling over an appearance that Pat Norman had made in her office. Stop the *Chronicle* from running the story, Norman had requested. "I don't know what she's worried about," said Dritz. "It's true." Dritz then went on the record confirming the study's accuracy.

NEWARK, CALIFORNIA

Rick Walsh always remembered his Uncle Gary as a wonderful storyteller. In the basement of the Walsh home in Sioux City, Gary would talk on and on, making up his stories as he went along. Ever since then, Gary had been Rick's favorite uncle. He was never condescending to Rick and had always treated him as an equal. During the four years that Gary didn't talk to his parents because of Grandma Walsh's unfortunate comment about going to heaven, Rick was the conduit for family news. Rick and Gary had remained close, even after Rick married and settled into a quiet cul de sac in suburban Newark, California.

On that March evening, Rick was happy to hear Gary's voice, although he could tell his uncle wasn't going to share jokes.

"Have you heard about AIDS?" Gary asked.

"I think so," said Rick, not liking the drift of the conversation.

"I've got it," said Gary. "I could die in two years or less. Nobody has ever been cured."

"Awesome," said Rick.

Rick couldn't believe Uncle Gary would have something so serious. He didn't know what to say. After a long pause, he blurted out the first thing that came to his mind.

"I don't know what to say except that I love you."

Gary's parents in Sioux City were another matter.

"That's what you get from all that," his mom said, not bringing herself to utter the words she meant. "Why don't you leave that city?"

Gary hung up shortly after she suggested he go to confession.

March 25
FEDERAL BUILDING,
SAN FRANCISCO

Making a difference was the raison d'être of Bill Kraus's politics and his life. His arm-twisting with the Social Security Administration was yielding results, and Bill looked forward to the call he was about to make to the sister of an AIDS patient. She had called months before, telling Bill about the Social Security case workers who had denied her brother disability payments. Yes, he had *Pneumocystis carinii* pneumonia, but he looked well enough to work. He did not fit the Social Security requirements for disability, they said. He had appealed his case but lost.

Bill Kraus had been calling bureaucrats for months on the case. Again, he felt fortunate to be working for Phil Burton, who signed any letter Bill put in front of him when it concerned AIDS. In Congress, Bill knew, Burton was the only representative who didn't blanch at the gay jokes that inevitably came up during any cajoling on the epidemic. He had become the leader on the issue, and at Bill's request, fired off letters to top Social Security administrators to make an AIDS diagnosis presumptive evidence of disability. The bureaucrats were not so recalcitrant as they were slow.

Concentrating on the specific case of the ailing San Francisco man, Bill first secured cooperation from a local official who then referred the matter for approval in Sacramento. Now, months later, the man finally was qualified for disability.

The sister's voice was hollow when Bill called with the good news.

"Thanks," she said, "but my brother died last night."

Eventually, Bill's lobbying secured a national directive declaring AIDS a presumptive disability. Even years later, however, Bill could not manage to tell the story about the man and his sister without crying. It seemed to sum up so much of 1983.

March 31
PACIFIC HEIGHTS, SAN FRANCISCO

"All of you represent different constituencies in the gay community," said Marcus Conant, scanning the huge room where an anybody-who's-anybody inventory of the city's gay politicians were seated. "Things have to change and change fast, or you won't have any constituents left."

The politicos shifted uncomfortably in their chairs. By and large, they were unaccustomed to this kind of talk. They were much more familiar with discussions about discrimination and liberation, co-sexuality and heterosexist oppression. Now there were new, disconcerting terms like cytomegalovirus, clusters, incubation periods, the hepatitis B model, and of course, geometric progression. When dealing with AIDS at all, most gay political leaders preferred framing the epidemic in familiar concepts. This is why condemning the federal government had become so popular. One could use the conventional rhetoric, including discrimination and prejudice. Now, however, doctors were tossing the ball squarely into the gay leaders' court, and most of the activists weren't sure what they should do, or more accurately, what was the politically correct thing to do.

This was the mobilizing meeting Marc Conant and Paul Volberding had decided to orchestrate when they were at the AIDS conference at New York University, when Conant read "1,112 and Counting." These were the leaders who could ring the alarms, Conant thought.

Lia Belli, a longtime proponent of gay causes and wife of the city's most prominent and bellicose lawyer Mel Belli, had offered the playroom of her Pacific Heights mansion for the event. The playroom, it turned out, was the entire top floor of the palatial home; a lot of the activists privately conceded they had come just to see what the house, at one of the most fashionable addresses in the city, looked like. When she introduced Marc Conant, Lia Belli pleaded that the epidemic demanded the gay community's "immediate action" and that it was "an issue that's above politics." Conant had assembled every major AIDS researcher in town to recite a litany of horror about the years that lay ahead.

By current estimates, the incubation period was as long as eighteen months, Conant said, meaning the AIDS cases of tomorrow were out there spreading the virus around today. "The 1984 AIDS victims have already contracted the disease," said Conant. "Even if we had a vaccine today, there is nothing we could do to prevent these cases."

Selma Dritz gave the latest update on numbers, reporting 207 Bay Area cases, "as of today," and the probability of hundreds more by the end of the year. Andrew Moss showed his census tract charts that identified Castro Street as ground zero of the local epidemic. Moss's line graphs showed a near-vertical curve of cases that wouldn't begin to level off, he noted, until well after gay men started changing their sexual activity.

Paul Volberding talked about the Los Angeles cluster study and Patient Zero. The study indicated that you didn't need 1,100 sexual contacts to get AIDS anymore, he said. It was just a matter of luck. Sex as a lottery. "When the disease first started, it probably took more contacts in order to get it, because there was less incidence of the disease," he said. "That's not the case anymore."

Questions focused largely on one issue: Did the doctors *really* know how AIDS was transmitted? Anal intercourse could be a major problem, the scientists said, given the hepatitis B model of transmission. The virus, obviously present in semen, could be injected directly into the bloodstream through fissures in the rectal lining. Nobody, however, seemed particularly enthralled with Conant's suggestion that gay men start wearing condoms. The CDC case-control study had indicted promiscuity, a word quickly denounced by gay leaders as "judgmental," but the doctors could offer little direct advice on which practices spread the disease. Because of federal funding shortages, no subsequent epidemiological studies had been undertaken to investigate this issue, even though they were precisely the inquiries that could most directly have saved lives. Now doctors, who were trying to urge a reluctant gay community to change, were bearing the burden of the shortfall.

"Bodily fluids," suggested Dr. Robert Bolan of the Bay Area Physicians for Human Rights.

It was the first time the gay community had heard the expression; and it wouldn't be the last.

"You have to avoid contact with bodily fluids," said Bolan, who had emerged as the most militant AIDS fighter in the gay doctors' group. "That would include semen, urine, saliva, and blood. And I mean avoid them. This is the big enchilada, guys. You don't get a second chance once you get this."

Hearing this, San Francisco Supervisor Carol Ruth Silver, a close, longtime ally of the gay community, made what she considered a logical suggestion: "If you're saying that this can be spread through sexual contact, it makes sense to me to have the public health department get a court order to shut down the gay bathhouses. That would probably save lives."

A chorus of boos and hisses greeted Silver's recommendation. The gay leaders were prepared to, perhaps, think of AIDS as a big enchilada, but they were not ready to swallow a combination plate. Such action would have profound political ramifications, they warned. The sheer volume of the heckling cowed Silver into silence, as it would every other civic leader. Not only was closing the bathhouses something that could not be done, it was something that could not even be discussed.

As the leaders slowly filed out, they invariably told Marc Conant or Paul Volberding what fine work they were doing. Keep it up, they said. Conant had a sinking feeling as he walked down the mansion's twisting, baronial staircase to leave. He had hoped the leaders would agree on a call to arms to fight the epidemic within the gay community. Instead, they seemed preoccupied with the politically correct thing to do. Conant feared that people were going to die because of it.

⬭

Bill Kraus preferred long yellow legal pads for writing, jotting down his ideas carefully in longhand with no punctuation other than dashes. He had hoped some kind of consensus might emerge from the Belli meeting on what to do, but instead the conflicts had become clearer. AIDS could not be fought effectively if gay people continued to think in terms of the old gay community, Bill thought. The rhetoric of the old gay movement—the sexual liberation movement—also needed to be revised. It was not anti-gay to be pro-life, he thought. Bill Kraus began writing his manifesto, one that drew the battle lines on which he would wage his fiercest political fight.

"We believe it is time to speak the simple truth—and to care enough about one another to act on it. Unsafe sex is—quite literally—killing us. . . . Unsafe sex with a number of partners in San Francisco today carries a high risk of contracting AIDS and of death. So does having unsafe sex with others who have unsafe sex with a large number of partners. For this reason, unsafe sex at bathhouses and sex clubs is particularly dangerous. . . .

"If the gay movement means anything, it means learning self-respect and respect for one another. When a terrible disease means that we purchase our sexual freedom at the price of thousands of our lives, self-respect dictates it is time to stop until it once again is safe. . . ."

Cleve Jones and Ron Huberman—Bill Kraus's best friend and the vice-president of the Milk Club—both signed the letter with Bill. When Huberman took the letter to the *Bay Area Reporter,* publisher Bob Ross joked that a lot of his advertisers wouldn't like its tone. And it was six weeks before it was published.

◯

Meanwhile, three Castro-based psychologists—Leon McKusick, Thomas Coates, and William Horstman—were tabulating results from a sample of 600 gay men surveyed in mid-March as to their sexual behavior. Although it did not draw on a randomly selected population, the study was the most extensive ever attempted. The results were culled from questionnaires handed out in the early evening at gay bars and to men leaving gay bathhouses and sex clubs late at night. Another 200 respondents were gay couples, filling in the surveys mailed to them. The sampling revealed how vast the task would be for public health educators.

Only 15 percent of the respondents said they had stopped passive anal intercourse, one-third said their level of that activity had remained the same, and 28 percent said they were doing less. About 20 percent of respondents said they were rimming less often, while one in nine were rimming new partners at the same level as the previous year. Twenty-eight percent had stopped rimming altogether. The most difficult behavior to change, it turned out, was oral sex. Although one in three men said they were sucking less, only 5 percent had stopped altogether, while 55 percent were partaking at the same rate as before the epidemic.

Even worse, bathhouses and sex clubs clearly remained a major center of gay sexual activity. One in four gay men went to bathhouses at least once a week, while one in five others went once a month. The popularity of the sex palaces was ironic given how health conscious gay men had become. Two-thirds of the respondents had visited their physician in the ten weeks before the sampling. Only one in twelve had not seen their doctor in the past year.

Also disconcerting was the survey's finding that one in six men agreed with the following statement: "Since I found out about AIDS, sometimes I get so frustrated that I have sex that I know I shouldn't be having."

Altogether, the study was alarming on a number of points. First, it showed that gay men knew what put them at risk for AIDS. That message had gotten out. However, 62 percent still engaged in high-risk sex at the same frequency— or more often—than before they found out about AIDS. Only 30 percent had reduced their risk behaviors, although not even all of these men had eliminated all activities likely to put them in the path of the AIDS virus. Secondly, the study showed the dangerous role bathhouses played in the spreading epidemic. Men who went to bathhouses were far less likely to have changed their sexual behavior than the other groups sampled in the survey and were far more likely to be infected with a sexually transmitted disease. Sterner messages needed to be delivered to prevent more deaths, the doctors concluded.

"As the rate of infection is climbing exponentially while this report is being submitted, it is evident that measures gay men are currently taking to avoid infection have begun but are still inadequate," the authors wrote. "As the survey indicates, the gay men surveyed are still poorly informed about disease transmission or are unwilling or unable to change sexual patterns in a manner that will place them at lower risk."

March 31

The analysis of the first quarter's AIDS incidence figures in San Francisco indicated how widespread the risk had become. The report on the AIDS case-load as of the end of March found that 1 in 250 single men between the ages of thirty-five and forty-four living in the Castro Street neighborhood had been diagnosed with AIDS, while 1 in 150 of the same age group living in the adjacent Duboce Triangle area was now stricken. Assuming that some of the men living in the neighborhood were heterosexual, Dr. Andrew Moss concluded that "in some cohorts of gay men in San Francisco, AIDS incidence rates in the thirty and forty-year-old groups are now of the order of 1 to 2 percent."

Only later would studies show that by this time in 1983, the 62 percent of gay men who still engaged in risky sexual behavior had at least a 25 percent chance of being intimate with someone infected with the new virus. Hellish odds in this lottery of death.

◯

By the end of March 1983, it was also clear that the epidemic was taking on different faces as it spread through different parts of the country. In New Jersey, for example, epidemiologists found that gay or bisexual men represented a minority of AIDS cases reported to state authorities as of March 28. Instead, intravenous drug users accounted for 44.2 percent of the state's AIDS casualties, with Haitians making up another 4 percent. AIDS was rapidly becoming a disease of the poor and the non-whites in the sprawling ghettos bordering New York; 68 percent of New Jersey AIDS cases were black or Hispanic. In fact, researchers later marked the spread of AIDS in concentric circles, pulsing out of the center of Manhattan to include larger and larger rings of land and population in the impoverished outlands of metropolitan New York City. This proliferation of AIDS through the East Coast corridors of poverty heralded the start of the second AIDS epidemic in the United States, distinct from the epidemic in gay men.

In Europe, meanwhile, there were also two AIDS epidemics, one linked to Africa and a later-starting scourge among gay men who had visited the United States. All Belgian AIDS cases at this time, for example, were among Central Africans, largely Zairians, or people who had recently visited that continent. All forty-four cases of AIDS reported in West Germany as of March 31, 1983, were either among people who had traveled to Haiti or Africa, or among gay men who recently had vacationed in Florida, California, or most commonly, New York.

As for the United States, by March 31, the Centers for Disease Control had received reports of 1,279 cases of Acquired Immune Deficiency Syndrome. Of these, 485 had died.

April 4
VANCOUVER, BRITISH COLUMBIA

Legally, their hands were tied.

The board of directors of AIDS Vancouver had agreed on that. Everybody was talking about the "Orange County connection" who was still going to the bars. Legally, they decided there was nothing they could do about Gaetan Dugas, though ultimately the board dispatched a physician-member to talk to him. After the board meeting, members wondered privately to each other: Why would anyone do what Gaetan was doing?

27 TURNING POINTS

April 1983

PITIE-SALPETRIERE HOSPITAL,
PARIS

Dr. Willy Rozenbaum did not get into medicine so he could watch people die. He was not suited for it. Rozenbaum long had noted that oncologists, or cancer specialists, seemed to have a fatalistic temperament that enabled them to accomodate themselves to death. Resignation just was not in the vocabulary of an infectious disease specialist, particularly in the latter quarter of the twentieth century. Rozenbaum was optimistic and active, the way he thought infectious disease experts tended to be. They dug right in and saved peoples' lives. So many battles against disease had been won in the past century that this did not seem an untenable posture to take, and besides, Rozenbaum felt that the medical specialties tended to attract their practitioners less through intellectual intrigue than through personal temperament. His incorrigible optimism was why he was nagging Dr. Jean-Claude Chermann over at the Pasteur Institute.

"My patients are dying," Rozenbaum complained. "I need a treatment."

Dr. Francoise Barre was already working to culture a second isolate of the retrovirus she had discovered in late January, this time from the blood of a hemophiliac. Dr. Luc Montagnier, as the senior researcher, was reluctant to come out and say they had found the cause of AIDS, because they still had to prove that the new virus was not merely a new opportunistic infection that had taken advantage of the lymphadenopathy patient's weakened immune system.

Willy Rozenbaum, however, was convinced. You don't find a new human virus that often; it was beyond coincidence. And his priority was to save lives. He was tired of treating the various opportunistic infections associated with AIDS. It was like putting a brick in one bank of the dam only to know the other side would collapse in minutes. He wanted an anti-viral drug, maybe a substance that could interfere with the chemical with which any retrovirus multiplied, reverse transcriptase.

One afternoon, Willy Rozenbaum was as excitable and eager as ever while Dr. Jean-Claude Chermann talked about a drug he had helped develop in the early 1970s. Its scientific name was antimoniotungstate, but Chermann called it HPA-23. During his long experiments with retrovirus in mice, he had found that the drug was effective in short-circuiting the reverse transcriptase process of the Murane Leukemia retrovirus. Other experiments had already determined the safe dosage levels humans could tolerate.

A new protocol would have to be worked out for AIDS patients, of course, but it could be tried, Chermann said.

People with AIDS, Rozenbaum reminded him, had nothing to lose.

⸺

At the Pasteur Institute, Dr. Luc Montagnier was polishing the scientific paper on the retrovirus discovery for its publication next month in *Science* magazine. Even though, oddly, his reagents had been almost dead when they arrived from Dr. Robert Gallo at the National Cancer Institute, Montagnier had avoided delays, and he again ran tests to see whether his virus was the same as Gallo's HTLV. There was some reaction, but it did not appear to be the same virus. Montagnier determined that he would not call his virus HTLV. Instead, he decided to call it RUB, a rearranging of the initials of the flight steward from whose lymph node the virus was cultured.

As part of the review process for the paper's publication, Montagnier's manuscript had been sent to Dr. Gallo in Bethesda, Maryland. Montagnier and Gallo were as dissimilar as two human beings can be, and each made the other vaguely uncomfortable. While Gallo was chummy, aggressive, and charismatic, Montagnier held himself aloof and was frequently described as doughty and patrician. Still, Montagnier recognized Gallo as a leader in human retrovirology. Moreover, Gallo carried enough weight in scientific circles to thwart any attempts the French might make to have their discoveries recognized in the United States, the only arena that really mattered.

According to Gallo, a *Science* editor thought RUB was a disgusting acronym for a virus relating to this particular disease. Gallo managed to persuade Montagnier to say his retrovirus was from the HTLV family that, coincidentally, Gallo had originally discovered.

Montagnier later marked the name change as one of the greater mistakes of his scientific career, the first step in the "long tunnel of darkness" that lay ahead.

April 10
SAN FRANCISCO

Ice.

The call came when Bill Kraus was in the shower.

Drifting snow.

The aide to Congressman Phillip Burton was crying. She could barely get her words out. The congressman, she sobbed, had collapsed early this morning. Remember? He'd complained all week about not feeling well.

The casket being lowered into the frozen ground. . . .

"He's dead, Bill," she sobbed. "Phil is dead."

Within days it was clear that Bill Kraus still had his job as congressional aide.

Phil Burton's widow, Sala, would run in the special election next month to fill the seat, and she would undoubtedly win. She had told Bill privately that he could continue his work on AIDS and gay rights. It would not be the same, however, and Bill knew it. At best, Sala Burton would be a freshman congress-woman in a chamber where seniority was three-quarters of the game and artful arm-twisting was the other quarter.

In the weeks that followed, Bill couldn't get over Phil's death. It wasn't just the practical considerations of working with Representative Sala Burton rather than Phil. Only a handful of friends understood Bill's anguish, recalling his infrequent allusions to a winter in 1958 when his father had died and left him abandoned.

That Afternoon
LENOX HILL HOSPITAL,
NEW YORK CITY

The rain pelted him, but Larry Kramer was ecstatic that, at last, his crusade to get New York Mayor Ed Koch to face up to AIDS was gathering some momentum. All morning, he and a small band of protestors had stood in the downpour waiting for Koch's appearance at a symposium on AIDS. For a year and a half, the mayor had successfully avoided any meetings with community leaders to discuss the epidemic. By the time Koch arrived, Larry was worked into a lather and shouted at the mayor: "When are you going to do something about AIDS? How many people have to die?" All this was duly recorded on the television cameras.

Conference organizers had been terrified that the protestors would sabotage their long-fought effort to get Mayor Koch to show up and speak some long-awaited words on the epidemic. Indeed, Koch had shown little enthusiasm for the conference, but it was so immaculately orchestrated, he had little political choice but to attend.

The unlikely conference organizer was Dr. Kevin Cahill, a giant in New York City's Irish community and one of the most prominent physicians in the United States. When the pope was shot in 1981, Kevin Cahill flew from New York to Rome to attend to him. When Daniel Ortega, the Sandinista president of Nicaragua, needed special medical attention, he called Kevin Cahill. And Cahill was New York State's public health commissioner under former Governor Hugh Carey. His integrity was above reproach and his credentials as a God-fearing Catholic Irishman could not be matched. Observers credited his interest in AIDS to a certain ethical posture derived from his serious commitment to Catholicism. In his office on Fifth Avenue, he was beginning to see the ravages of the epidemic; he couldn't believe nobody was shouting about it.

Kevin Cahill decided to hold a conference that would attract all the big-name AIDS researchers who could deliver state-of-the-art information on the epidemic. He quickly put together a book deal, which guaranteed virtually immediate publication of the papers that were to be presented at the conference.

Once published, Senators Edward Kennedy and Daniel Moynihan had promised to use the information as background for the first Senate hearings on the syndrome.

Cahill created another powerful inducement for the august doctors' participation: Anyone who presented at the conference would be invited to a private cocktail party with Leonard Bernstein at the composer's apartment. The experts themselves might not want to attend still another AIDS conference, organizers figured, but surely their spouses would not permit them to pass up a dinner with Leonard Bernstein.

The pieces fell together perfectly. Cahill was able to enlist a star lineup of speakers that included Dr. Don Francis from the CDC AIDS Task Force; CDC director Dr. William Foege; the specialist on Haitian AIDS, Dr. Sheldon Landesman; New York City Health Commissioner David Sencer; and, to sum up the government's response, Manhattan Congressman Ted Weiss. At Cahill's urging, Terence Cardinal Cook agreed to deliver the invocation, much to the horror of the archdiocesan staff.

The presence of Cardinal Cook made it virtually impossible for Ed Koch to turn down the group's request for a mayoral welcome. Koch reportedly called Cardinal Cook's offices repeatedly in the days before the conference to make sure that the cardinal actually would show up. The mayor's nervous aides even refused to list the event in the standard schedule of mayoral public appearances routinely issued to the media.

Dr. Cahill opened the conference with an indictment of the medical and governmental response to the epidemic, a theme picked up by Don Francis.

"AIDS occurred at a most inopportune time," Francis said, citing the "ravages" of budget cuts, the "cloud of reductions in force" over the CDC, and the "severe restrictions" on supply purchase and travel money. Hardly a minute in Francis's speech went by without some allusion to "lack of resources."

Don Francis was hoping that somebody would fashion his comments into the questions that needed to be asked of the federal government. He was handing the ammunition to them on a platter. Instead, the doctors applauded politely.

⬭

That night, organizers and presenters gathered for a post-conference cocktail party in Leonard Bernstein's sumptuous Dakota apartment. Within a few hours, there was that predictable moment when all the heterosexual guests had left, mentioning children that needed to be tucked in and schedules that needed to be met. And, as tends to happen at chic Manhattan parties, the only people left were gay men. And Don Francis.

Don Francis so rarely got to relax anymore. Recently, CDC brass had persuaded him to move to Atlanta, where he would finally get the formal title of lab director for the AIDS Activities Office, formerly called the AIDS Task Force. The decision had spurred Francis's determination for a CDC retrovirus lab. The morning Francis had left for the conference, he fired off another memo to Dr. Walt Dowdle, director of the Center for Infectious Diseases, insisting that "as part of CDC's continuing pursuit of the cause of AIDS, a laboratory with retrovirus diagnostic capabilities is necessary at CDC." The lab needed to be able to grow viruses, develop an antibody test for the presence of AIDS virus, determine the role of possible causative viruses in the syndrome, and next determine the prevalence of the virus's infection among the various AIDS risk groups. Only then, Francis felt, could serious control efforts begin to stop the spread of the disease. According to the current plan, Don Francis and Jim Curran would serve as co-leaders of the CDC's AIDS efforts, although CDC insiders knew that Curran held Francis in awe, given Francis's international reputation for smallpox control. They predicted that Don Francis either would emerge naturally as the leader or a power struggle would ensue.

On this night, however, Don Francis was able to let his thoughts drift as he listened to Bernstein play Chopin melodies on the piano. The other guests tried to figure out whether Francis was gay. He kept in good shape for a forty-one-year-old, they noted, and he didn't seem shocked or taken aback by any aspect of gay life. However, his appearance also counted against his gay quotient. His hair was just a bit too long, as if he yearned for his hippie days in his native northern California.

Larry Kramer, still delighted that the media had covered his protest, couldn't help but develop a minor crush on Don Francis. He was awfully cute. Besides, their thinking seemed to flow on parallel lines. The disease had to be stopped, to be controlled, they agreed, not just studied in some microscope. Larry also got the feeling that although Don Francis wanted to do more, his hands were tied by the bureaucrats who would fire him if he said any more than he already had, which still was more than anyone else was saying.

The music drifted around them while rain splattered on the windows, and Don Francis felt at home. He had found a group of people who cared about this epidemic, people who would get something done. With celebrities like Leonard Bernstein signing on, people would start listening, he thought. Finally, he would be able to start undertaking the work that needed to be done.

Monday, April 11

The AIDS epidemic earned its most important emblem of newsworthiness with the bundles of *Newsweek* magazine that appeared across the nation that day, featuring a cover on which a disembodied hand held a tube of blood. "Caution KS/AIDS," read the sticker on the tube. The cover line stated: "EPIDEMIC: The Mysterious and Deadly Disease Called AIDS May Be the Public-Health Threat of the Century. How Did It Start? Can It Be Stopped?" As usual, the magazine cover was better at posing questions than the story would be at answering them, but with AIDS finally ensconced as a legitimate news story, an avalanche of coverage began. The revelations about transfusion AIDS in late December had started it all. In the first three months of 1983, 169 stories about the epidemic had run in the nation's major newspapers and newsmagazines, more than four times the number of the last three months of 1982. Moreover, from April through June, these major news organs published an astonishing 680 stories. The media blitz on AIDS lasted into the summer and provided an unprecedented, albeit brief, degree of attention to the epidemic.

Every newspaper found its own angle to the story, although most papers, like the newsmagazines, handed it to their science writers, who preferred penning yarns about the people in the white coats. Occasionally, there was coverage of the trials of an AIDS patient, told in sudsy, soap opera–style journalism. In San Francisco, New York, and Los Angeles, these stories included polite homosexuals who went by their real names; in less cosmopolitan locales, the character of such stories invariably became let's-call-him-Bob. Even the supermarket tabloids got into the act. The *Globe*, for one, ran a lengthy cover story saying that AIDS actually was part of King Tut's curse, having followed the tour of the Tut treasures to the United States in the late 1970s. "Either Tutankhamen died from the disease or it was placed in the tomb to punish those who might later defile his grave," said a former San Diego coroner who dabbled in archeology.

Two trends were most pronounced in the coverage. First was the complete lack of any story concerning the shortfalls of resources for AIDS research. Usually, there was a complaint about the lack of funds from a gay doctor and a heated denial from somebody at the Centers for Disease Control or the National Institutes of Health. That would be that. No more digging. No more research beyond perusing the government press releases. The profession that had toppled a president over a burglary less than a decade before had returned to the fold of official-statement journalism. This, of course, was not the case with other perils to the public health; other issues, such as toxic waste or even Tylenol, called for huge investigative teams and filing Freedom of Information Act requests. But there was something embarrassing about this whole story; you could tell by the cursory coverage and all the talk of "bodily fluids" instead of semen and anal intercourse. *Newsweek* called AIDS the "public health threat of the century" on its cover, but it never treated the epidemic as such in its newsroom. Nor did any other news organization outside San Francisco.

The media watchdogs had gone to sleep on this story. Because of it, government agencies on both the federal and local levels were left to deal—and to not deal—with the AIDS epidemic as they saw fit. This would not be obvious at first, for the government appeared to spring into action at the sight of this first media blitz. Later, however, the real quality of AIDS journalism was clear: Reportage would be like the Mississippi River that year, with much breadth but little depth.

The second trend was fascination with how San Francisco homosexuals were reacting to the AIDS crisis. By mid-spring, news crews were endlessly trooping up and down Castro Street for such stories. Of course, New York City had three times the AIDS cases and nearly one-half of the nation's AIDS caseload. But there, you wouldn't be able to get the mayor to say anything for your story because his office referred calls on AIDS to the health commissioner, and you wouldn't find city programs to write about because there were no city programs, and you didn't have the flurry of civic attention to AIDS because New York City officials seemed largely impervious to the fact that an epidemic existed. As the months wore on, San Francisco became AIDS City, U.S.A., not only in the popular imagination but in its own. The city's gay men were as intently watched and studied as a newly discovered tribe of cave dwellers in an exotic tropical paradise.

Late Afternoon
NATIONAL CANCER INSTITUTE,
BETHESDA

Francis Anton Gallo was the son of immigrants from Turin, Italy, and he shared the northern Italians' cool, intellectual disposition even after he forged an immigrant's success story in Connecticut, rising from welder to metallurgist to president of the company where he once was among the proletarians. His wife's family hailed from the warmer climes of Italy, and she luxuriated in that region's warm, extroverted, and clannish qualities. The couple's son, Robert, expressed both the charisma of his mother and the workaholism of his father.

The latter aspects of his personality were not evident in Robert Gallo's early life in Waterbury, Connecticut. But the turning point of his life was in 1949, when he was thirteen and his younger sister contracted leukemia. This took Bob Gallo to Harvard University for hospital visits. There, he met a famous cancer expert named Sydney Faber, and he saw scientists in their laboratories struggling to save the lives of ailing children. His sister died from leukemia, but Bob Gallo's fascination with research biology continued. Encouraged by an uncle who taught zoology at the University of Connecticut, Gallo found himself trailing after a research pathologist at a local Catholic hospital. The pathologist was the first cynic Gallo had ever met. Young Gallo tended more toward melodramatic flourishes than contemplation, but he slowly learned what critical thinking was. By his teen years, he was allowed to perform his own autopsies, as he dove passionately into his preoccupation; by the time he was eighteen, Bob Gallo knew he would spend his life at the bench, doing medical research.

Still, Gallo's teen years were trying times. He was not an excellent student. He spent less time on homework than on the basketball court and was out late every night dating. Had he not broken his back during a basketball game and been confined to bed for nearly a year, he might never have blossomed from mediocrity. During his difficult recuperation, however, he read everything he could on biology. While in college, he slew scores of mice in a makeshift laboratory above his mother's garage. After his residency at the University of Chicago, Gallo's determination to stick to the research bench was hardened by his first assignment at the National Cancer Institute. By some macabre chance, he was assigned to work in the acute children's leukemia ward at the National Institutes of Health hospital. From then on, he told himself, he would never work with patients again.

Gallo started to do research in 1966, and by 1970 he had embarked on the work that would earn him fame. At that time, substantial controversy had enveloped the theory that viruses might cause leukemia and even some forms of cancer. Gallo focused on retroviruses and by the mid-1970s was among the scientists to characterize the enzyme reverse transcriptase, the chemical that retroviruses secreted to replicate themselves in their victim cells. The work gave science the marker, a chemical footprint, that could aid in detecting retroviral infection. This alone represented a significant advance for retrovirology, yet few scientists appeared particularly impressed. After all, retroviruses were largely viewed as bugs of chickens, mice, and cats. What relevance did this have to humans?

Bob Gallo thought science was merely looking toward the obvious. When these animals were infected with a retrovirus, they shed virus like there was no tomorrow. It was easy to detect because there was so much of it. In humans, although the virus might be there, it was just not as easily detectable. What Gallo needed was a way to grow blood cells in such quantities that he could prospect for retrovirus in a rich vein. That was the logic that led to Gallo's discovery of the first permanent cell line for blood cells. He figured out how to keep permanent cultures of T-cells alive and, in the process, discovered interleukin-2, a culture that would later show immense promise in the fight against cancer.

With these discoveries, Bob Gallo's career advanced smoothly—until the false alarm of 1976. It appeared that he had discovered a new virus, and proudly, Gallo announced that to the world. When it turned out that an animal germ had contaminated his cell line, and there was no new virus, Gallo's reputation plummeted. It seemed that his life always swung to such extremes, so the researcher pushed on. In 1978, he discovered a new retrovirus, HTLV, but, fearing that his latest work would be dismissed because of his earlier problems, he labored until he could prove his case perfectly. This time he definitively showed that he had a microbe that caused leukemia. After publication of his findings in 1980, Gallo was a star again, receiving the coveted Albert Lasker Award. He became a recognized patriarch in the field of retrovirology. By the spring of 1983, a second variant of HTLV had been discovered by another scientist, who dubbed it HTLV-II.

For all his accolades, Bob Gallo remained a controversial figure in science. Detractors considered him pompous and arrogant. In scientific politics, he could be ruthless, they said, often pointing back to the 1976 embroglio as proof that Gallo was not always reliable. Gallo himself saw the criticism as reflecting the shadow side of his character. Yes, he was arrogant and proud, but that was what was required from the few brave scientists who challenged nature to yield its secrets to them. Still, he knew that his strength was his destroyer; it would be a theme in the coming years.

On this Monday afternoon in Bethesda, Dr. Robert Gallo was restless, drawn back to the disease that had frustrated him the year before in the first scans for a retrovirus in AIDS blood. Jim Curran was trying to embarrass Gallo into working on the disease. Jacques Leibowitch was prodding him with constant phone calls from Paris. Despite his distaste for the whole subject of AIDS, he could see that the stakes were being redefined. One needed to look no further than the new cover of *Newsweek* to see that.

Officials at the National Cancer Institute were restless as well. With the imminent publication of the French research and the HTLV studies of Max Essex at Harvard, the institute knew it was time to get serious about AIDS. Deputy Director Peter Fishinger called a meeting for 4:30 P.M. in the conference room of the NCI director. Fishinger now grasped that the NCI response to the epidemic had been less than ideal, but he saw the problem as partly the result of the way the system was constructed. Health agencies did not have the budgets to fire off large sums to the brash young doctors who were virtually the only scientists involved in the epidemic up to that point. Just to get the first round of grants out, the NCI had dropped its standards below what it considered acceptable quality for research projects. With the media now starting to focus on the problem, however, all this was going to have to change.

This meeting marked the first gathering of the NCI Task Force on AIDS, said Fishinger, scanning the room. Dr. Bill Blattner from the family section of NCI's cancer epidemiology unit was there, as were James Goedert and Bob Biggar, who were among the lonely NCI doctors who had worked on AIDS from the start. Anthony Fauci, who coordinated AIDS for the National Institute for Allergy and Infectious Diseases, also had sent a representative.

Robert Gallo spoke forcefully. The French claimed they had something, he noted. Somebody had even delivered a lymph node all the way from Paris for him to study.

"I believe a retrovirus is involved, and we're going to prove it or disprove it within a year," said Gallo. "We're going to spend a year and nail this down one way or another."

Fishinger promised Gallo that he could have the full resources of the NCI's elite laboratory in Frederick, Maryland. He would make sure everybody worked with the retrovirologist. Dr. Sam Broder, who was the NCI's clinical director, promised that Gallo would have "absolute priority" for tissue specimens from AIDS patients at the sprawling NIH hospital. Finally, the battle would be joined.

This date, April 11, 1983, was later cited by the officials of the National Cancer Institute as the turning point, the time that the institute became firmly committed to finding the cause of Acquired Immune Deficiency Syndrome. It was precisely one year, ten months, and seven days after the *MMWR* had announced the first twenty-six cases of Kaposi's sarcoma in gay men, as well as the eighteen other mysterious cases of *Pneumocystis* and other unexplained opportunistic infections. Between the time of that announcement and the date of the NCI's commitment to finding the cause of the disease, 1,295 Americans had contracted AIDS and 492 had died. Later, the Centers for Disease Control calculated that the numbers infected with the strange new virus behind the epidemic had grown by the tens of thousands, if not hundreds of thousands, during those twenty-two months.

Although the commitment proved to be a boon to Robert Gallo's lab, other AIDS research at the National Institutes of Health foundered for lack of money. When Jim Goedert and Bob Biggar had started their research on cohorts of Washington and New York City gay men in 1982, they had hoped they could learn what factors might lead some gay men to come down with AIDS while others remained healthy. Such a long-term study was essential to understanding not only the cause or causes of the syndrome but the natural history of the disease. By 1983, however, Goedert still did not have the funds to hire even a nurse to do the most basic tasks. The researcher had to drop plans to follow his Washington group. Just drawing blood and conducting physical exams on the New York cohort took six weeks. This left Goedert with mountains of data that could not be analyzed because he did not have adequate staffing.

Meanwhile, Jim Goedert's conversations with Jim Curran thoroughly committed him to the idea that a new infectious agent was causing the syndrome. Moreover, his physical exams in New York had convinced him that the disease was wearing many faces, appearing as full-blown AIDS in some, lymphadenopathy in others, and even a vaguer malaise in many more.

Belatedly, Goedert discovered that the NCI lab where he sent his blood samples for AIDS did not have the capabilities to look for reverse transcriptase, the sure marker of retroviral infection. The tests were never run. Life as an AIDS researcher at the National Cancer Institute, he later remarked, meant "chronic frustration."

At the National Institute for Allergy and Infectious Diseases, Dr. Anthony Fauci shared Goedert's discontent. You needed a pot of gold to draw researchers, and such money was not forthcoming from an administration that was nickel and diming its way through an epidemic. Unlike the NCI, the NIAID saw no pressing need to accelerate its AIDS research. NIAID Director Richard Krause was dumbfounded at criticism leveled at his institute. It was the clinicians who were making the most noise, he noted, the doctors in the field with the patients. Sending money to them, Krause felt, would be like pouring funds down the drain; most had no experience in research. But the NIAID had a balanced portfolio of research on the immune system. In the field of battle, a wise general did not send troops scurrying every which way at whim. They were placed strategically, according to a plan. "How," Krause wondered, "could it move any faster?"

Besides, he thought, there were plenty of centrifuges and culture disks in labs across the United States. The resources were there if the doctors wanted to use them.

CENTER FOR HUMAN TUMOR VIRUS RESEARCH, UNIVERSITY OF CALIFORNIA, SAN FRANCISCO

The talk about the French and American publications on HTLV made Dr. Jay Levy even more enthusiastic about looking for a retrovirus. All the publicity about AIDS, however, had created another obstacle. No lab would let Levy use its ultracentrifuge to experiment with blood from AIDS patients. Scientists were growing antsier about picking this horrible thing up in the lab. Levy, who only recently had experienced a six-month delay in getting a flow hood for the most basic lab research, found his AIDS research delayed once again, this time for lack of an ultracentrifuge.

April 12
Capitol Building,
Washington, D.C.

"In terms of AIDS, the Department [of Health and Human Services] has made a very strong commitment," Secretary Margaret Heckler told a House appropriations subcommittee. "In fact, I have spoken to the head of the CDC personally on a number of occasions on the subject and there is no stone being left unturned to pursue an answer. This is a serious, very serious problem and every single research avenue of the Department is being directed toward the resolution of this problem. . . . The Public Health Service is going to use every dollar necessary to try to find an answer because the fatality rate of this disease is so staggering and so high that it threatens this whole society. . . . I have to say that, in the AIDS situation, I really don't think there is another dollar that would make a difference, because the attempt is all out to find the answer."

That afternoon in Atlanta, Don Francis again wrote a memo to Dr. Walt Dowdle, offering a far different assessment of the federal government's response to the AIDS epidemic.

"Our government's response to this disaster has been far too little," wrote Francis. "Much of this is because the slope of the epidemic curve has been gradual, lasting years instead of days. We are not accustomed to dealing with outbreaks having long latent periods. But these situations require even greater speed because even after discovery of the cause, we will be so far behind and control will be even more difficult. . . .

"The inadequate funding to date has seriously restricted our work and has presumably deepened the invasion of this disease into the American population. . . . Because of the slow and inadequate funding process, it seems that after we get funds and recruit staff, we are always too late—the disease has passed us up again and we are again understaffed and underfunded.

"There must be some way to do it right. . . . In this vast and wealthy country there must be a way to get $10 to $20 million immediately for this disease. I stress speed because the usual government funding *and* spending processes are so slow as to be unacceptable in such an emergency situation.

"For the good of the people of this country and the world, we should no longer accept the claims of inadequate funding and we should no longer be content with the trivial resources offered. Our past and present efforts have been and are far too small and we can't be proud. It is time to do more. It is time to do what is right."

San Francisco

Gary Walsh's idea for a candlelight march had spread nationally by mid-April. AIDS sufferers in dozens of cities took the lead in putting together observances under the glare of newfound media attention. The San Francisco planning sessions for the protest, which had been named "Fighting for Our Lives," were a scream. Gary traded the latest AIDS jokes with the other AIDS casualties. Should they play connect-a-dot with their lesions? How does Anita Bryant spell relief? Gary asked. A-I-D-S. One Kaposi's sarcoma patient went to a meeting with a hankie marked with purple spots to signify his interest in "victim's sex." The latest quip on Castro Street concerned the news that the CDC finally had discovered the cause of AIDS to be track lighting on industrial gray carpeting.

Gary did hilarious imitations of himself lobbying the legislature in Sacramento for a bill to establish a panel that could assess the needs for AIDS funding in the state. "I'm dying of this disease," he'd say. "How can you vote against it?" It was shamefully melodramatic, which only made Gary love it more.

They shared stories about acquaintances who tried discreetly to eye their lesions. Gary had called attention to those doing so, much to the chagrin of people who thought they were being ever-so-subtle.

They also shared their anger. They were sick of being called AIDS victims, because the semantics implied that they were passive and helpless at a time when they wanted to fight actively to regain their health. They were tired of being called AIDS patients because most of them weren't in the hospital, the normal criterion for defining a patient. They wanted to be people with AIDS or, in the acronym-loving gay community, just PWAs. A nasty fight over such issues had broken out between the PWAs and the *Bay Area Reporter,* the idiosyncratic weekly that boasted the largest circulation of any local gay newspaper. Editor Paul Lorch had begun criticizing the various AIDS programs, such as the Shanti Project and the KS Foundation, as gravy trains for gay radicals, "wolves" and "AIDS pimps" out to leech a stricken gay community.

In a letter signed by a number of PWAs, including Gary Walsh, Paul Lorch was accused of a "sensational approach to reporting [that] only fuels the fire of fear, guilt, homophobia and adds to the everyday stresses of PWAs." The letter asked that *Reporter* publisher Bob Ross either fire Lorch or resign from the KS Foundation's board of directors. Ross was not impressed, and Lorch wrote a rather ungentlemanlike response.

"Had I from the first spoken louder—even more shrill—some of you might not be the marked men you are today," wrote Lorch. "What's more, I sense that your experiences have failed in making you bigger men. The letter reveals a reverse trend, a trend toward peevishness. What a time in your lives to be without honor. Taken to tattling. Exiting with a whimper. . . . For most of the names on your list, the only thing you have given to this gay life is your calamity."

This rejoinder stirred more controversy.

Paul Lorch decided to exact his own revenge. He took the letter demanding his termination and the list of all the people who signed it, and set it aside. One by one, as they died, he crossed their names off the list, getting the last laugh, so to speak.

April 14
NEW YORK CITY

Larry Kramer arrived late for the meeting of the New York AIDS Network, but he didn't think it would matter. Within days of Larry's protest at the AIDS conference, Mayor Ed Koch had agreed to a meeting on April 20 with a maximum of ten people. Each organization in the network would send two. Larry figured that he and Paul Popham would represent the Gay Men's Health Crisis. By the time Larry arrived, however, the ten representatives were chosen, including two from GMHC. Larry was not among them. Instead, Paul Popham and the executive director, Mel Rosen, would represent GMHC.

Larry Kramer was stunned and then he became angry. The meeting was all his work, he complained. He had organized the protest that pressured Mayor Koch into having the conference in the first place, not to mention the past eighteen months of *kvetching* on top of that. How could they leave him out? GMHC was organized in his own living room.

Paul said that his choice of Mel Rosen only made sense. The president and the executive director should be the two people who represent the organization. Privately, Paul shuddered at the notion of taking the easily incited Larry Kramer into a meeting with Koch. There was no telling when Larry would start screaming, and once the mayor was put on the defensive, he would dig in his heels.

Larry upped the ante. If he did not go to the meeting with Mayor Koch, he would resign from the board of directors.

Paul said that would be fine. Later that night, Paul polled the board of directors and found unanimous support for his position. Everybody was tired of the fighting, and that's what being with Larry Kramer meant—fighting.

Larry was in shock. GMHC had been his family. It was all he had been doing for the past year, and now they were rejecting him. The fact that he always was half in love with Paul Popham made the rebuff all the more stinging. He hated them; he loved them. They had betrayed him. He was alone.

April 19
CENTERS FOR DISEASE CONTROL
HEPATITIS LABORATORIES, PHOENIX

Don Francis had typed up the speech he had given in New York and sent it off on April 12 to Kevin Cahill for inclusion in the AIDS conference book. As per CDC policy, however, the paper needed to be cleared by CDC higher-ups. Jim Curran sent it back to Don Francis with his handwritten notes.

"I would suggest omitting p. 10, and parts of pp. 9, 11, 15, 16 re: the 'lack of resources' available at CDC—Although I believe Don is correct, *in part,* there is little benefit to publishing this, esp. in a 'political' book."

The censored comments included every remark Don Francis had made about the "ravages of budget cuts" and the problems of fighting an epidemic under an administration committed to reducing health spending. Making such extensive cuts in the manuscript would be difficult, Jim Curran noted, advising that "since this ms has been sent to Cahill, the revision may need an excuse."

April 20
MAYOR'S OFFICE,
NEW YORK CITY HALL

There were two types of requests the New York AIDS Network took with them to their first and only meeting with Mayor Ed Koch at City Hall—the kind that cost money and the kind that didn't. Mayor Koch warmly embraced the requests that cost the city nothing. Yes, he would declare a "state of concern" about AIDS for the week of the GMHC circus fund-raiser and the candlelight march. Of course, he would join Dianne Feinstein's AIDS Task Force of the U.S. Conference of Mayors. He also supported confidentiality for AIDS patients and agreed that the federal government should be spending more money on AIDS research. He'd talk to the city's lobbyist about pushing for more federal funds.

Then, there were the other, peskier requests. No, the city would not provide housing or hospice space for AIDS patients kicked out onto the street. That would be perceived as being "special treatment" for gays. New York, Mayor Koch noted, had a gargantuan homeless problem. How could he single out one group for help? As for gay requests for a health center in Greenwich Village, that was impossible. On a general level, Koch said he would match San Francisco's spending on AIDS, "dollar for dollar," but he never indicated where that money would be spent.

After the meeting, the AIDS Network issued a press release discussing only the points that Koch agreed to and not alluding to the mission's failures. It wouldn't do to offend the mayor just when gays finally had a foot in his door. Yet even the ever-optimistic Paul Popham was disheartened by the visit. The mayor did not seem vaguely concerned about the epidemic. Every answer came too quickly, almost flippantly, Paul thought. And he could see that Health Commissioner David Sencer was not going to push the mayor on this issue. Sencer clearly was full of good intentions on the AIDS issue, but he appeared to have little authority with a mayor who relied on his own staff for health policy. There was nobody in city government who had responsibility for the AIDS epidemic, Paul could see now; there was nobody in city government who really cared.

      ⬭

It was during this month of April 1983 that the momentum of movement on the AIDS epidemic shifted from New York City to San Francisco, typified, as much as anything else, by that meeting in New York City Hall. For the next two years, AIDS policy in New York would be little more than a laundry list of unmet challenges, unheeded pleas, and programs not undertaken. The shift was ironic, considering that New York City was the epicenter for the epidemic, both biologically and, at first, psychologically. Because of the extraordinary reporting of the *New York Native,* the city's gay community had been exposed to far more information about AIDS than San Francisco's in 1981 and 1982. All the ingredients for a successful battle against the epidemic existed in New York City, except for one: leadership. In San Francisco, the plethora of gay leaders created an environment in which questions of AIDS policy were debated, albeit brutally. Larry Kramer's resignation left New York City without a leader willing to take unpopular positions, whether they were favoring bathhouse closures or opposing a popular mayor. Instead, the city's gay leadership pursued its timid policy of constructive engagement with a mayor who seemed petrified of being highly identified with any gay issue, perhaps because of his status as a perennial bachelor. The New York fight against AIDS would be left to a handful of doctors and overtaxed gay organizations, and many would die there, while AIDS came to be seen as a San Francisco phenomenon because that's where the action was.

April 23

The search for the beginnings of AIDS had taken scientists back to Africa, and the medical journals of spring 1983 were crowded with letters and notations of early, Africa-linked AIDS cases. The Belgians published notes in the *New England Journal of Medicine* about the Zairian cases that appeared in their country as early as 1977. Meanwhile, other Belgian tropical-disease specialists had ventured to Rwanda and Kinshasa, where they reported current outbreaks of AIDS, apparently among heterosexuals. The earliest documented AIDS case was reported in the letters section of *Lancet* on April 23. A brief letter from a Danish communicable-disease doctor named Ib Bygbjerg told of a previously healthy Danish woman who worked as a surgeon in a primitive hospital in northern Zaire from 1972 to 1975. She had died from *Pneumocystis* in December 1977, Bygbjerg wrote, noting, "She could recall coming across at least one case of KS while working in northern Zaire, and while working as a surgeon under primitive conditions she must have been heavily exposed to blood and excretions of African patients."

During his stay in Zaire, Bygbjerg concluded, he had been impressed by the CDC teams from the United States, who so quickly identified the Ebola Fever virus. "Perhaps such teams should search for another African virus," he suggested.

28 ONLY THE GOOD

April 26, 1983
SAN FRANCISCO CITY HALL

In the beginning, there were two major figures in San Francisco gay politics, Jim Foster and Harvey Milk. Jim Foster had worked since 1964 to lay the foundations of gay political power. His most lasting achievement was the founding of the Alice B. Toklas Memorial Democratic Club in 1972, the year that Harvey Milk moved to San Francisco. Within months of his migration, Harvey Milk decided there needed to be a gay member of the San Francisco Board of Supervisors instead of the polite liberal heterosexuals whom the Toklas Club preferred. The Toklas leaders worried about pushing too hard—that if they were overweening, gays might lose everything they had won. Harvey Milk considered this obsequious and figured homosexuals hadn't won that much if they couldn't even stake claim to their own elected officials.

When Harvey Milk asked Jim Foster for his support in his 1973 campaign for supervisor, however, Foster was aghast. Who was this Johnny-come-lately to run for supervisor? he wondered. "We're like the Catholic Church," Foster told Milk. "We take converts, but we don't make them pope on the same day."

That comment made Harvey Milk hate Jim Foster, more for the personal rebuff than for the loftier philosophical differences. The Toklas Club never endorsed Harvey Milk for anything. By 1976, Milk had organized his own club, the San Francisco Gay Democratic Club, based on his own style of pragmatic power politics. The club's clout grew with Milk's election in 1977 and renamed itself the Harvey Milk Gay Democratic Club days after its mentor's assassination in November 1978. Five years later, both Harvey Milk and Jim Foster were absent from the political scene, the latter nursing a lover stricken with AIDS. Nevertheless, their feud lingered and defined San Francisco gay politics. The Toklas and Milk clubs still hated each other passionately, with the Toklas faction probably fostering the bigger resentment because it had been eclipsed by the Milk Club in recent years.

Tonight all that was changing.

Reporters, pundits, and various political hangers-on listened in astonishment as the registrar of voters methodically announced the returns from the recall vote on Mayor Dianne Feinstein. Not only had San Francisco's first female chief executive won, she had seized the election with a majority rarely observed in democracies west of the Soviet Union, tallying 81 percent of the vote in her favor. Her weakest precincts were, predictably, in the Castro area, where she won only 58 percent of the vote.

Rather than being an indictment of Feinstein's four-year-old administration, the recall vote had proved to be a major triumph. Already, her critics were finding that no credible politician would oppose her reelection in the fall. Her only announced opponent was a disciple of some political wacko named Lyndon LaRouche who talked about "curing" homosexuals. Moreover, just days before, Feinstein had secured the biggest plum of her mayoral career when the Democratic Party announced that it would hold its 1984 national convention in San Francisco. This raised the hackles of conservative Democrats, who fretted that a party meeting by the Golden Gate would hopelessly identify the party with fringe faggotry, but the Democratic national chairman was a Californian who preferred the mediterranean city for sentimental reasons. Already, there was speculation that Feinstein might be chosen as the Democratic vice-presidential candidate in 1984.

Most of this would be a mere embellishment to our tale except that the recall election set in motion an unfortunate political mechanism that would have a profound effect on the city's battle against an encroaching viral invader. The battle lines drawn between recall opponents and supporters in the gay community roughly paralleled the divisions among gay leaders on how to handle the AIDS epidemic. On one side were Bill Kraus and the Harvey Milk Gay Democratic Club, who favored an aggressive campaign to alert gays to the dangers of the disease. The biological survival of the gay community was at stake. The Harvey Milk Gay Democratic Club was one of the few major political organizations in the city to support recall, largely out of anger over the domestic partners' ordinance. On the other side were leaders of the Alice B. Toklas Memorial Democratic Club and such groups as the Coalition for Human Rights, who favored a low-key approach to the epidemic, fearing that panic could spread to heterosexuals who might resort to such unsavory actions as mass quarantines of gays. For them, the political survival of the gay community was at stake. Toklas Club members became Feinstein's staunchest supporters in the recall election.

Politics knows only two principles: loyalty and revenge. As of this night, these two principles dictated who would wield the most influence in municipal politics and policies. The Milk Club might curry more favor among the city's two congressional representatives and sundry state legislators, but the Toklas Club carried the weight in matters pertaining to the city and county of San Francisco, including health policy. It was an ironic state of affairs, given the fact that Mayor Feinstein's status as a doctor's daughter and her own instincts always favored the more assertive stance of the Milk Club. Nevertheless, a good politician must listen to her allies, and the mayor was nothing if not an artful politician. Her allegiance to the Toklas Club would have an effect on public policy for the next crucial year. San Francisco remained the most highly politicized city west of

Chicago, and everyone knew whose advice pulled the most political leverage, whose counsel could be heeded and whose could be ignored.

All this would become more obvious, but it was even apparent on that Tuesday in April in the memo Supervisor Harry Britt wrote to Public Health Director Dr. Mervyn Silverman. At this point, Britt was still in the phase of politely pressuring Silverman to issue risk-reduction guidelines to gay men. The San Francisco Department of Public Health had yet to put out so much as one brochure on the epidemic. The supervisor had personally ushered appropriations for such publication through the city government. Bill Kraus and Dana Van Gorder, Harry Britt's aide, then sat down and wrote specific language for a pamphlet. "It was great to hear the department will have money to print this piece," Britt wrote in his memo to Silverman that day. Just in case the department was having trouble coming up with guidelines, Britt wrote, some suggested language was enclosed.

The recommendations, of course, were ignored; Harry Britt had had an unfortunate association with the Harvey Milk Club, having been its president when tapped to succeed the slain Milk as supervisor.

Things would become far less polite later, but by that night, the battle lines were drawn and probable victors could be predicted. It would be problematical to calculate how many San Franciscans would be infected with a deadly microbe and ultimately die because of political loyalty and because in 1973 Jim Foster and Harvey Milk decided they hated each other.

April 29
LOS ANGELES, CALIFORNIA

Michael Gottlieb knew he was taking a chance when he joined other University of California AIDS researchers in the Los Angeles office of California Assembly Speaker Willie Brown. But it was worth the risk. Gottlieb could see the need in the gaunt faces of the men he was treating at UCLA. They were dying and the system wasn't working. The first federal AIDS grants for nongovernmental research were due to be released in a few days, but they would scarcely cover money already diverted from other sources to pay for the past two years of AIDS studies, much less the work that needed to be done in the months ahead. Traditional university channels weren't responding to the crisis either. The epidemic demanded that its researchers wear many hats, Gottlieb saw. He was spending free nights on the board of directors of the AIDS Project–Los Angeles. Now he would enter a realm even more unfamiliar to a scientist—partisan politics.

As Gottlieb scanned the room, he knew that the assembly of twenty-eight AIDS researchers from the various campuses of the University of California system shared his fears. They were about to make an end run around the university's hierarchy and plead directly to the legislature for money for AIDS research. As it was, UC officials tolerated the legislature's involvement in its funding as a disdainful necessity born from the peculiarities of democracy and the role of state tax dollars in underwriting the institution. But university officials routinely repelled attempts by legislators to insert their own agenda into university priorities. Few UC instructors dared to circumvent their administrators by going directly to the legislature, much less mere assistant professors like Michael Gottlieb or Paul Volberding. Gottlieb understood that the penalties for breaking this unwritten university code could be far more severe than the revenge meted out even in the political arena. In politics, the players jockey for power; in academia, they play for vanity, a far more compelling instinct that could conjure far more vindictive punishment.

Marc Conant, who was wearing many hats himself as he tried to organize a national foundation to raise funds for AIDS research, had called the meeting on a few days' notice. The meeting was designed to put together a coordinated proposal for all the projects the UC researchers were undertaking on AIDS. The San Francisco doctors had come with a neatly organized plan. The southern California researchers tended to be more competitive, fractiously bickering about turf. However, agreement was worked out by the end of the day. Essentially, the group devised a wish list for the budding AIDS experts, although, given the dearth of interest among university researchers, the funding amounted only to $2.9 million. The idea was to channel money quickly to the impoverished AIDS labs, they agreed. Time was the enemy; they needed speed.

With Willie Brown, they knew they had an effective champion. He was generally regarded as the second most powerful official in the state, after conservative Republican Governor George Deukmejian. His sponsorship of the appropriation virtually assured its passage. Within days of the meeting, Brown introduced the measure into the legislature and started speeding it through committees as emergency legislation. The cavalry was at hand.

$$\bigcirc$$

Days after the Los Angeles meeting, Marc Conant got a taste of the problems that lay ahead when he received a call from a prominent UCLA retrovirologist. The scientist had not tempted fate by attending the meeting but, instead, had sent an assistant, who observed the proceedings and secured a modest sum for the researcher's lab. Now that a proposal was actually going to the legislature, however, the doctor wanted a bigger piece of the action. He was particularly peeved that his laboratory was to receive less money than Dr. Jay Levy for retrovirology research.

"I'm going to sabotage the whole thing if I don't get as much as Jay Levy," said the eminent scientist.

Conant knew the man carried a lot of weight with university administrators. The active opposition might doom the proposal. Still, Conant was irritated that the professor would demand a certain sum of money even though he had no proposal for how he would spend it. Until this point, there had been little evidence that the man had harbored much interest in AIDS.

"We're talking about science, not whether you have parity," Conant argued.

The researcher repeated his threat, and Conant ultimately figured out an agreeable allotment of funds. It was only the beginning of the problems AIDS research would face in the UC system that year. Later, the University of California boasted of doing more than any other university system in the nation on the AIDS epidemic. And the claims were truthful; that was precisely the problem.

Saturday, April 30
MADISON SQUARE GARDEN,
NEW YORK CITY

All day Paul Popham worried, although not about whether the circus would succeed; that already was assured. All 17,000 seats had sold out a week ago, the first time a charity benefit sold out Madison Square Garden in advance. Aside from gay parades, the night was shaping up as the biggest gay event of all time and had put $250,000 into the treasury of Gay Men's Health Crisis. This was terrific, but Paul was still anxious about whether his face would be on television and his name in the newspapers as president of the Gay Men's Health Crisis. The title said it: gay. Paul really didn't want it to get back to work. Not that he was ashamed, he'd tell you. He just felt it would create problems. How would people react? He didn't feel anybody had an obligation to come out openly as gay and had argued endlessly about it with Larry Kramer. Now, Larry was gone and Paul had only himself to argue with.

By the 6:30 P.M. press conference before the circus, Paul could see that his fears were unfounded. He should have known. The straight media in New York didn't cover AIDS or gays, and they weren't about to cover some queer circus for AIDS, no matter how big it was or how worthy the cause. Paul was relieved that his secret was safe. He let himself fall into exultation at the scope of how far the gay community had come.

The entire spectrum of Manhattan gay life was at the Madison Square Garden circus. Wealthy and perfectly coiffed men sauntered to their seats with leather queens and drag queens and lesbians in fashionable attire. Enno Poersch had designed a program for the event that listed the impressive accomplishments the Gay Men's Health Crisis had made in its twenty months of existence. The group had distributed a quarter-million copies of its "health recommendations" brochure and put hundreds of volunteers to work as "Buddies," doing chores and providing a sympathetic ear to AIDS-stricken men. Over 100 volunteers had been trained for work on the group's crisis line. In San Francisco, the various services of education, counseling, and support were being handled by different groups with diverse emphases, but New York did not have such luxuries. GMHC was doing it all and had become the largest gay organization in the country.

The program also contained the official proclamation of "Aid AIDS Week" by Mayor Koch. Most poignantly, on page after page, were memorial notices of the people who had died. These were the names and faces behind the numbers the CDC released every week.

"I think the most impressive thing I've seen over the last year and a half is how affectionate men have grown," Paul Popham wrote in the program's introduction. "We are finding out who we are, what we can do under pressure. And that we're not alone. We're not alone now; we're very much together. We'll get through this somehow. And although we're paying a terrible price, we're finding in ourselves much greater strength than we dreamed we had."

$\bigcirc$

As he watched Leonard Bernstein conduct the circus symphony in the national anthem, Larry Kramer felt torn between pride at the event's success and the sadness of being strangely on the outside. The days after his departure from GMHC were filled with such bitterness he sometimes thought he could not contain it. He was genuinely surprised when Paul Popham, ever the gentleman, asked him to stand and be recognized as a GMHC founder. The resignation was intemperate, Larry could see, though the idea was forming that he had not resigned but been forced out. If they really cared, they would not have let him resign; they had forced him out. Ultimately, however, they would let him back on the board, Larry thought; of course they would.

$\bigcirc$

Enno Poersch would remember the circus as the time Bob, Rick Wellikoff's lover, was diagnosed with AIDS, adding still another member of the Ocean Walk household on Fire Island to the list of the epidemic's casualties. The diagnosis was almost simultaneous with the death of Wes, who also had spent the summer of 1980 in that ill-fated house with Nick and Rick and Paul Popham's dead boyfriend Jack Nau. Of the household, only Enno, Paul, and one other were not dead or dying.

May 1
WARD 86,
SAN FRANCISCO GENERAL HOSPITAL

When Paul Volberding received the official notification of his $419,463 grant for AIDS research, he knew he was supposed to be happy. It was the largest single grant doled out by the National Cancer Institute for the epidemic. Michael Gottlieb at UCLA had received only $200,000, and for all practical purposes it was Gottlieb who had discovered the epidemic. At this point, no institute of the NIH had announced any intention of releasing any more money for AIDS.

Volberding was less cheered than depressed, however, when he saw the grant notice. The modest bequest underscored less what he could do than what he would not be able to do.

Jay Levy's share of the grant, for example, was $80,000. Since only $13,000 went to supplies, Levy still would not have enough money to buy the ultracentrifuge that was essential to his future research. He'd have to wait on the state legislature. Similar stories came from every lab at UCSF doing AIDS studies.

Volberding was the first to admit that he was better off than any of his colleagues in AIDS research. Unlike most, he was free to comment when the television crews rolled in. Although hospital administrators had toyed with the idea of delaying the opening of the AIDS ward, the shower of media attention on the epidemic had moved up the planned opening to mid-July.

Paul Volberding knew he was in the best of all possible worlds as a clinician in the AIDS epidemic; from a more global perspective, this showed Paul how bad things were.

Early Evening, May 2
CASTRO STREET, SAN FRANCISCO

Most Americans believe that bad people do not die young.

There is something tragically romantic about untimely death. Ultimately, it was this emotional factor, more than any other, that shielded gays from the horrible backlash they so dreaded. This kinder side of the nation's psyche would prevail over the demagogues who talked of God's wrath. Moreover, gays themselves were by now in the business of romanticizing premature death. At the Shanti Project, where scores of gay men were signing up as grief counselors, the more experienced gurus of mourning talked of "going to the other side," as though AIDS were a train ticket to some Xanadu of peace and serenity. Such sentimental notions guaranteed success for the candlelight marches assembling all over the United States that night.

From the moment Gary Walsh walked down the hill into the small valley where the Castro neighborhood was nestled, he knew the procession was going to be a hit. Gay marches in San Francisco had become so routine as to usually have the ambience of cheerful cocktail parties. This was different. Some of the gathering thousands had brought snapshots of friends who had died and others carried signs: "In memory with love for Jim Daye. July 2, 1982." Some read like gravestones:

> Ken Horne
> Born July 20, 1943
> Died November 30, 1981

The mood was somber. Gary felt uplifted. For all these months, he had felt so alone. But all these people cared.

Gary's nephew Rick Walsh had driven up from the suburbs with his wife. Angie Walsh had never seen anything like this—men dressed as nuns and guys holding each others' hands. Right in public. Angie gripped Rick's hand tightly. Already in the copy center where Angie worked, some people were talking darkly about how AIDS might be God's curse on homosexuals.

Matthew Krieger met Gary Walsh on the corner of Market and Castro streets and handed his former lover the flowers he had purchased. Thousands now milled around the intersection with their candles and signs. Matt had never felt so proud of Gary, of how he brought people together like this.

As the group stepped onto the broad swath of Market Street to make the familiar eleven-block walk to City Hall, television crews swarmed to record the dozen AIDS sufferers carrying the banner: "Fighting for Our Lives." The media-minded Cleve Jones had taken the job of preserving clear camera lines for the front banner, of ushering to the side sundry politicians, would-be gay leaders, and camera-hungry drag queens who kept trying to edge their way into the media limelight. Cleve knew the picture he wanted to go out around the world; it was these flesh-and-blood human AIDS patients.

The march had turned into such a wonderful media opportunity that Cleve was embarrassed he had not thought of it himself. Events, of course, had conspired to assure the night's success. Media tended to act as a machine of perpetual motion, fueling itself. The legitimacy lent by newsmagazines had created still more cover stories and more official interest, which gave fresh news pegs for still more coverage. The morning paper had carried a front-page story on changing gay life-styles. That day, the health department had announced it was expanding its AIDS screening in public health centers. That afternoon, Mayor Dianne Feinstein had welcomed a contingent of AIDS sufferers into her office, with hugs and eloquence, for her proclamation of AIDS Awareness Week. She also had pleaded for more congressional spending on the epidemic.

In a way, the television cameras and print journeymen had come to need events such as the candlelight march as much as the marchers needed the reporters. Much of modern news is shamelessly artificial, coming from press conferences hyped by press releases written by legions of public relations people; the march lent an authenticity to the epidemic, even if it truly was designed to generate media coverage. There was the fragrance of sincerity to it.

Candles flickered for a mile now, as the group neared City Hall, a ribbon of light and people in the twilight. The sight made Cleve Jones remember the year he had spent struggling to make gay people care about AIDS. He had done his job. The KS Foundation was changing its name to the AIDS Foundation, and it didn't need him anymore. It was becoming a realm of process-minded bureaucrats, not rabble-rousers. Cleve knew he should feel inspired by the long procession, but it made him sad. More friends were being diagnosed. Just the word "diagnose" was a mark of how much Cleve's life had changed. People now said so-and-so was "diagnosed" and you didn't have to ask what with; for gay men, it had become a verb that needed no object. Beyond this, Cleve had spent a lot of time with all the Bobs, Davids, Kevins, and Jeffs who had stopped into the foundation's office in the past year; it was hard to feel uplifted about anything. He was tired. Maybe he needed to leave town altogether, he thought.

◯

Six thousand people stood in United Nations Plaza, near the dome of City Hall, listening to speeches by people with AIDS. Most of the speakers were losing weight so rapidly that their clothes fit loosely. Months ago, they had been strong and vital, but now they leaned heavily as they walked. They stood with painful stiff joints, staring out like scarecrow men.

Gary Walsh held the banner between Bobbi Campbell, the nurse who had proclaimed himself the "KS Poster Boy," and Mark Feldman, an old boyfriend who was looking particularly gray and wasted that night.

"Our president doesn't seem to know AIDS exists," Mark Feldman told the crowd. "He is spending more money on the paints to put the American flag on his nuclear missiles than on spending on AIDS. That is sick."

The concern was nearly tangible, Gary thought, as he looked across the crowd from the stage. He thought he could almost feel his lesions fading.

○

Bill Kraus was exuberant when he left Civic Center. The community was waking up to AIDS. Journalists finally were paying attention to the epidemic. Certainly deeper news investigations would force the Reagan administration to start funding research adequately, he thought. Everything was going to change now.

○

As Cleve had wanted, the unobstructed picture of Gary Walsh and the other AIDS sufferers holding the "Fighting for Our Lives" banner had flashed all over the world. Marches in Houston, Chicago, Dallas, Boston, and other cities sparked some of the first local coverage of the epidemic. In New York, of course, the media, most notably *The New York Times,* was recalcitrant. Not an institution to get swept away by cheap sentiment, *The Times* relegated its coverage to a few buried paragraphs and did not make any reference to the fact that the outpouring of concern came largely from homosexuals. Instead, it called the crowd "mostly male" and left it at that.

○

It was four months since Gary Walsh had been diagnosed, when the nation's AIDS caseload first exceeded 1,000 cases. According to figures released by the Centers for Disease Control on May 2, 1983, the day of the candlelight march, the number of new AIDS diagnoses in the United States had increased by 36 percent to 1,366 cases. About 38 percent of them, or 520, already were dead. This mortality rate belied the true prospective of death from AIDS. At least 75 percent of those who had the disease for two years were dead. Nearly half of the AIDS casualties were men between the ages of 30 and 39. Another 22 percent were men in their twenties. Of all the cases, 27 percent of these people had Kaposi's sarcoma, 51 percent had *Pneumocystis carinii* pneumonia, 8 percent had both KS and PCP, while another 14 percent had different opportunistic infections, such as cryptococcus, toxoplasmosis, or cryptosporidium. About 44 percent of the country's AIDS patients lived in New York City, largely in Manhattan. In San Francisco, 169 people had contracted AIDS, including 47 who had died. Los Angeles, Miami, and Newark had the next highest numbers of AIDS cases.

Many mysteries remained with the epidemic. Gay men, who composed 71 percent of the AIDS victims, were virtually the only people who got Kaposi's sarcoma, while the intravenous drug users rarely contracted anything but *Pneumocystis.* CDC speculators tended toward the idea that poppers might play a role in the development of KS, although there was no evidence for this because the CDC had not been able to conduct any further epidemiological studies due to lack of funds.

In fact, the CDC even had been forced to stop interviewing new AIDS cases because there weren't enough staffers. They had been hearing from local public health agencies that more recently detected cases tended not to be drawn from the promiscuous, drug-using fast lane that characterized previous cases. This made sense because the contagion was so much more widespread now; a guy didn't need 1,100 sexual contacts to run into somebody who carried the virus. In New York City and San Francisco, just a few partners could do the trick. The CDC could not launch educational campaigns to warn gay men about this, however, because it did not have the money.

Like Bill Kraus, many in the CDC AIDS Activities Office hoped all the media attention would change this. And like Bill, they would be disappointed.

○

"AIDS à la Americaine," Dr. Jacques Leibowitch thought when he watched the television coverage of the AIDS patients behind their banner in San Francisco. Parisian media was filled with talk of AIDS now too, largely because so much of the blood used in French transfusions came from the United States. It was so like Americans to expose themselves and march in big, dramatic parades. You'd never see anything like this in Paris, Leibowitch thought. This was distinctly American, like the Phil Donahue show, so naive and so distasteful.

○

Gary Walsh drifted through the first days after the candlelight march on a pink cloud of elation, but that faded as he found himself burdened by fatigue and depression. His friend Mark Feldman was back in the hospital with *Pneumocystis,* and people were saying he might not come out again. A week after the march, Marc Conant had found three new lesions on Gary. He was also losing weight.

On the rare occasions Gary felt up to making the short trek to Castro Street, strangers stopped him on the street to tell him how wonderful, brave, and courageous he was. Gary didn't feel he was any more holy because he might die young. Having AIDS had not imbued him with any more wisdom than he had had before. Having AIDS was not beautiful; it was painful, miserable, and depressing. It was like being told you were going to die in a car accident at some point in the next year. Nobody told where or when you were going to die, just that you would perish. A mixture of anticipation and dread filled Gary's spare moments. When he experienced a shortness of breath a day or so after seeing Dr. Conant, he wondered whether it was his mind playing tricks on him again.

29 PRIORITIES

May 1983
CENTERS FOR DISEASE CONTROL,
ATLANTA

Everybody had told Don Francis that Atlanta wasn't really so bad, but it was. Don attended meetings around the clock; his wife Karen and their two children stayed in a motel until Karen found a house. For the first time since the Atlanta–Phoenix commuting began, Don felt he had a home again. However, he rarely had a chance to enjoy it.

Battle lines were drawn between the CDC brass and the administration's budget people on whether money for AIDS research should come from new funds or be redirected from other projects. The party line that health officials were forced to follow publicly was that the agencies had all the money they needed to fight AIDS, since they could divert money from other programs' budgets for it. As far as the Office of Management and Budget was concerned, the $8 billion spent in the Public Health Service was generous enough to allow such diversions. At the CDC, where Don Francis was trying to put together the agency's first AIDS lab, it meant chaos.

He couldn't believe the laboratories he needed to remodel; they were like something out of a Louis Pasteur movie, with copper and asbestos incubators. Researchers so far had improvised their labs. To pipe carbon dioxide into a room with viral cultures, for example, one virologist had indelicately used a screwdriver to smash a hole in the drywall so he could pull a rubber tube from the room with a carbon tank into the lab with the cultures. This is modern science? Francis wondered.

Within a few weeks, Don Francis suggested that the CDC simply start spending money, even if it were not allocated to them. Congress would bail the CDC out; the agency should put itself in the red now, he argued. The more bureaucratically minded people shuddered at Francis's brash strategy.

Other AIDS researchers faced similar problems. The AIDS Activities Office ran wholly on a crisis mentality, jumping from one emergency to the other. There was never enough time to write up findings for publication. There were never enough lab people to study tissue specimens. There was never the opportunity to look at the subtler nuances of the epidemic, such as the role of possible co-factors. The CDC had yet to do a complete study on which sexual behaviors were responsible for spreading AIDS and which weren't. At one point, Don Francis ordered a basic textbook on retroviruses, only to have the requisition refused. The CDC could not afford even $150 for a textbook.

The announcement about the links between Human T-cell Leukemia virus and AIDS would be published within days in the *Morbidity and Mortality Weekly Report*, CDC Director Dr. William Foege knew. The data, from Drs. Robert Gallo, Max Essex, and Luc Montagnier, represented the first hard evidence pointing toward a specific virus. Gallo was actively promoting HTLV-I, while the French in recent weeks had become more outspoken in advancing their isolate as an entirely new virus. No matter which, Foege could no longer justify the delays in CDC funding. On May 6, he started writing a long memo to his boss, Assistant Secretary for Health Edward Brandt, to lay out his requests.

"CDC is being pressed from many different sides for information about its resource needs related to the AIDS problems. The questions are coming in from gay groups, Congressional committees, individual Congressmen's staffs, and even the Library of Congress. This heightened interest and concern has been stimulated by recently held appropriations committee hearings, media coverage of the HTLV lead, and demonstrations by interested groups.

"We understand that various proposals to increase both the 1983 and 1984 funding for AIDS are being considered in Congress. This puts both PHS and CDC in the frustrating position of once again playing 'catch up' in regards to AIDS funding.

"Clearly, we can effectively use additional funds and positions this year and we definitely should be expanding our efforts around in 1984. In fairness, I must point out that our plans and our resource estimates are based on what we *now* know about AIDS. We have *not* included estimates of resource needs beyond the first phase of the investigation. I anticipate that once we have identified an agent, our efforts will change direction, intensify, and our needs will escalate."

Attached to William Foege's memo were fourteen pages crammed with studies the CDC would undertake if it had adequate AIDS funding, and the projects that would be cut if the administration provided no further money for AIDS and forced CDC administrators to gut other projects for bucks. The requests included the laboratory for which Don Francis was agitating, studies of Haitians and blood donors, an international AIDS conference, and expansion of field surveillance of the disease in New York, Los Angeles, and San Francisco. Altogether, the memorandum marked a new step for the epidemic, as its funding concerns now were being advanced to the level of agency chief.

It wasn't going to make a lot of difference. When the memorandum was released as part of a Freedom of Information Act request, a pen had slashed a black mark across its first page, underlining the word "withdrawn."

Monday, May 9
HEARING OF THE HOUSE SUBCOMMITTEE
ON HEALTH AND THE ENVIRONMENT,
CAPITOL,
WASHINGTON, D.C.

MR. HENRY WAXMAN: I would like to take a few more minutes to go over with you the response of our government to the AIDS crisis. . . . Now, the first crisis was dealt with by the Centers for Disease Control, and the CDC had to divert some of its activities that it ordinarily undertakes for hepatitis, venereal disease, and other public health problems in order to meet the pressures of the AIDS epidemic suddenly staring them in the face.

Congress came along and said, we realize you have a very difficult job to do; we are appropriating $2 million more. The Centers for Disease Control has spent $4.5 million last year on AIDS; is that a fair statement?

DR. EDWARD BRANDT: Yes, sir, that is a fair statement.

MR. WAXMAN: Now, when the Reagan administration has submitted its budget for 1984, the request is not for $4.5 million or more to deal with an ongoing public health crisis; the request is for only $2 million.

A few minutes ago, you said that this is a complex medical problem; it is an epidemic that we must deal with; it is a problem that must be solved. Your rhetoric was one of resolve. But the actions of this administration are one of neglect. How can you justify reducing the amounts of funds for the CDC to deal with this public health crisis when we are in the middle of this public health crisis, not the end of it?

DR. BRANDT: Well, you know obviously one can always go back and look at one's actions earlier and try to determine whether you would have done things differently, and I think in most instances everything would have been done.

I think we followed leads as they developed, Mr. Chairman. This looked like a drug problem early on, and great attention was paid in trying to determine whether or not the use of certain drugs—I am not talking about illicit drugs—could, in fact, lead to immune suppression. . . . That is why the early efforts of the NIH were aimed in that direction.

As that concept was rejected—largely on the basis of both animal studies at the NIH as well—we then moved toward the transmissible disease concept. That is why I think it is in the last few months that we have begun to more fully understand the complexity of the illness.

MR. WAXMAN: Now that you understand the complexity of the illness, why are you asking for funds to be reduced for the Centers for Disease Control?

DR. BRANDT: I will have to go back and look at that. I heard you say that earlier. I was not aware that we had done that, and indeed information I was just handed is that the money will probably go up in 1984. . . .

MR. WAXMAN: I want to just conclude my comments with you to say that I am very disappointed with the administration's response to the AIDS issue. In April

1982, we held a hearing in Los Angeles to look at the problem, and one of the leading CDC researchers told our subcommittee that the 300 cases were the tip of the iceberg. I am sure if he was telling us that information, he was telling the Reagan administration as well.

That was April 1982.

Not until a year later have we seen any funds go out from the NIH to do research in this area, specifically directed to AIDS; and at least it is our information that the CDC is going to be cut in its own activities; and now with the Congress coming in saying to the administration, let's set up a fund for you to deal with this crisis and other crises in the future, rather than saying to us, that is a constructive approach, you say you don't mind the concept; you are not sure about the money, but you have the authority already to do it, but you are not doing it.

I just think this is a very disappointing way to respond to the Congress in trying to deal with the problems. . . .

⬭

Privately, Edward Brandt's own opinions were not that distant from Henry Waxman's; moreover, Brandt knew that Waxman knew this; and Waxman knew that Brandt knew that he knew. Waxman personally respected Brandt, who was both a tough spokesman for the administration and a committed doctor as well. Brandt's job was to stand behind his boss, President Reagan; Waxman's job was to oppose him and try to protect the public health. All these components were in evidence when Waxman dismissed Brandt as a witness. "I know that you have a deep personal feeling and commitment to having the government do all it can," said Waxman. "I know you don't make all the policies for the Reagan administration. But, unfortunately, those who make the policies sent you down to talk to us and to take the sting of some of our unhappiness."

⬭

After the hearing, Waxman aide Tim Westmoreland, Representative Ted Weiss aide Susan Steinmetz, and Michael Housh, an aide to San Francisco Congresswoman Barbara Boxer, walked to Susan's office, where they munched on sandwiches and plotted strategy. The hearing had confirmed precisely what they feared. Rather than admit to past deficiencies and try to reconcile itself to AIDS funding needs, the administration would make its health officials lie about AIDS resource problems. The aides needed to get together some kind of numbers to present as the funds needed for AIDS research, and they needed to do it fast. In order to appropriate supplemental funds for the 1983 fiscal year ending in October, they had to get the money passed by Congress within the next three weeks. To do that, they needed proof that AIDS research was being shortchanged.

For her part, Susan Steinmetz was going to Atlanta the next day to study CDC files on orders from Weiss's oversight committee on intergovernmental relations. Her private sources within the CDC told her there were some dandy memos from frustrated staffers to CDC brass.

The Next Day
CENTERS FOR DISEASE CONTROL, ATLANTA

CDC Director William Foege wanted to make two points clear from the start. Susan Steinmetz could do whatever she wanted, but she would not have access to any CDC files, and she could not talk to any CDC researchers without having management personnel in the room to monitor the conversations. The agency also needed a written, detailed list of specific documents and files Steinmetz wanted to see.

Susan Steinmetz was flabbergasted. What did they think oversight committees did? Their work routinely involved poring through government files to determine the truth of what the high-muck-a-mucks denied, and then privately talking to employees who, without the prying eyes of their bosses, could tell the truth. This was understood, she thought. She already had made a number of appointments for discussions with people like Jim Curran, Harold Jaffe, and Don Francis. She wanted to talk to them. Alone. And she wanted to see if CDC files yielded memoranda that proved what she suspected: that, contrary to government claims, AIDS researchers did not have all the funds they could use to battle this scourge. She couldn't provide a list of memos when she had yet to establish their existence.

To counter this, William Foege advanced a unique argument. All files contained the names of AIDS patients, he said. Therefore, if the CDC showed Susan Steinmetz the files, they would be violating the confidentiality of patients.

Steinmetz explained again that she was interested in the policy aspects of the epidemic, things like planning, resources, and budgets. She wondered why an agency truly dedicated to confidentiality would be sticking peoples' names into such files where they so clearly could be irrelevant.

Complicated negotiations marked the next two days, with Susan Steinmetz filing frequent advisories to Washington, where Representative Ted Weiss had angrily staked out the obstructionism. CDC personnel, who struck Steinmetz as peculiarly contentious, wanted to conduct their own review of files before letting Steinmetz see them, but Weiss wouldn't budge. They might throw away revealing memoranda, he figured. Ultimately, Steinmetz and the CDC hierarchy negotiated a fifteen-point process whereby they would pull files and delete names, although she could see the document, without the name, to ensure that the CDC wasn't merely sanitizing their records.

As another demand, the CDC insisted that before any interviews with CDC staff took place, the agency would screen questions that Susan Steinmetz put to scientists.

This is getting pretty strange, Steinmetz thought. On the phone, other oversight committee staffers in Washington confided that they had never heard of an agency being so recalcitrant to Congress, particularly in a case such as this where the oversight would result only in the release of more funds.

Finally, on the second day of Susan's visit, Elvin Hilyer, the CDC manager coordinating her visit, abruptly announced that Steinmetz's presence would no longer be permitted in the CDC building and that no agency personnel would be allowed to speak to her.

Susan Steinmetz was crestfallen. Ted Weiss was furious. He fired off a letter to Health and Human Services Secretary Margaret Heckler, demanding immediate cooperation. Heckler said Weiss should proceed in a more "orderly" fashion and said she would have HHS officials help him once he outlined specific questions and areas of research. Weiss had no choice but to call Steinmetz back to Washington.

In Bethesda, Steinmetz encountered many of the same problems at the National Institutes of Health. The National Cancer Institute officials issued a memo demanding that all interviews with researchers be monitored by the agency's congressional liaison. At first, the National Institute for Allergy and Infectious Diseases was cooperative, but then, in an apparent NIH-wide clampdown, information became difficult to excavate there as well.

May 12
CAPITOL,
WASHINGTON, D.C.

The hearing before the House Appropriations Subcommittee on Labor, Health and Human Services brought out the panoply of the nation's top health officials, including the directors of the NIH, CDC, NCI, and NIAID. A month before, Secretary Margaret Heckler had set the tone for testimony when she told Congress that "I don't think there is another dollar that would make a difference because the attempt is all out to find an answer." That was the policy of the Department of Health and Human Services and of these health officials. They would not have the luxury of partaking in "budget-busting" with these congressional representatives. Thus, when the ranking Republican on the subcommittee, Representative Silvio Conte of Massachusetts, pressed each agency director about the adequacy of resources, he was assured repeatedly that researchers had adequate funds and that if agency chiefs needed more money, they'd be sure to ask for it.

"Are you equipped now to go ahead with your work on this?" Conte asked of William Foege.

"As we have in the past, when we have a health emergency, we simply mobilize other resources from other parts of the centers. . . . If we reach a point where we cannot do that, of course, then we will come back and ask for additional funds, but at the moment that is the way we intend to handle it," said Foege, who just six days before had privately written Edward Brandt that the CDC "clearly" needed more money.

Dr. James Wyngaarden, director of the NIH, similarly stated that everything was going smoothly with AIDS research: "We have been investigating this problem of acquired immune deficiency for some time."

"Do you have enough flexibility within your existing resources, Doctor, to be able to respond adequately and quickly to this emerging health problem?" Conte asked Dr. Vincent Devita, director of the NCI.

". . . We have been able to respond quickly and I think cover every lead that we now have in this particular syndrome," said Devita, who had written a memo to Wyngaarden just five weeks before, pleading for extra NIH funds for AIDS grants. "I think we do have a great deal of flexibility."

Dr. Richard Krause of the National Institute for Allergy and Infectious Diseases agreed that NIAID was "doing all within our power to learn how to treat this terrible disease."

⊂⊃

Tim Westmoreland watched the hearing, thinking this was Washington at its worst. The witnesses were treading one step shy of perjury. Nor was that much of a secret. The Reagan administration wrote its policy on calculators in the Office of Management and Budget. Members of Congress and the scientists lying to them understood it. Later, some admitted privately that they knew they were making a mistake by lying, but they comforted themselves with the idea that they needed to keep their jobs to prevent their replacement by people who would make bigger mistakes. "If I were to leave, who would take my place?" they'd ask aloud. "With this White House . . ."

Westmoreland was also surprised at the gullibility of the press. It was as if the initials M.D. or M.P.H. after these officials' names had conferred upon them the credibility of Moses. Didn't reporters know how to ask that tough second question? Or was it the more likely scenario, that they simply did not care?

The Next Day
HUBERT H. HUMPHREY BUILDING,
DEPARTMENT OF HEALTH AND HUMAN SERVICES,
WASHINGTON, D.C.

Ed Brandt would have preferred not to be in his office that day. The Oklahoma City native had planned to stay only two years on the job, after being pulled from his post as assistant chancellor for health affairs at the University of Texas to join the Reagan administration. He figured he owed it to himself and his country to put to work finally all those less-government-is-better ideas he'd been espousing his whole career. He had talked about leaving when Reagan's first HHS secretary, Richard Schweiker, resigned last year, but Schweiker had persuaded him to stay on and help the transition.

At the start, Brandt had viewed AIDS as a minor problem. It would be poppers, the experts told him, so he hadn't cared much. Now, the blood transfusion cases had instructed Brandt otherwise, and he figured it was his job to hold a steady course.

Although a Baptist Sunday School teacher, Brandt wasn't big on proselytizing other peoples' morality, and he was too much a doctor to see AIDS as some curse from the Almighty. Already, however, some of the more conservative doctors in the administration, the religious ones who came on board with Reagan, were alluding to the God's-curse theory and wondering whether too much money wasn't going into AIDS research. There were letters too, like the one from the second-grade teacher who said her mom suffered from multiple sclerosis. "Why are these homosexuals getting all the research money and my mom with MS isn't? Are they something special?"

Ed Brandt saw it as his job to keep rational about this. Some mid-level White House types had tried to jump the AIDS bandwagon by writing legislation that would make it a crime for a person with AIDS to donate blood. Dr. Brandt had squashed that fast. There was no evidence that AIDS patients were streaming into blood banks, he noted. There was an element of meanness to the proposal that bruised the doctor's midwestern sensibilities—like the White House guys enjoyed kicking a guy when he was down. That wasn't American.

Brandt was, however, a loyal follower of President Reagan, whom he truly respected. He had played the role for months now, holding back the line on health spending, the way he believed it should be held.

Today, that was going to have to change. Brandt didn't believe in throwing money at a problem, but he didn't believe in starving science either, especially when Americans were dying. AIDS, he now saw, was simply too important to have its funding scuttled from this or that program. He started writing his memo to the Assistant HHS Secretary of Management and Budget.

"It has now reached the point where important AIDS work cannot be undertaken because of the lack of available resources," he wrote. The CDC needed new money, not just the money that they were pirating from other budgets. He listed the "important prevention programs" that had been "postponed, delayed or severely curtailed" by the funding diversions. ". . . 1984 will represent the third year in a row that we will be faced with major reallocation of resources to the AIDS program," Brandt wrote. "Such long-term diversion of resources will have a detrimental effect on CDC's important prevention programs."

The memo was written just four days after Dr. Brandt told a House subcommittee that a Public Health Emergency Fund was "unnecessary" because "existing budget and appropriations processes are effective in funding these [AIDS] activities."

May 18
CAPITOL,
WASHINGTON, D.C.

The letter from Dr. Brandt arrived minutes before the full House Appropriations Committee was to hold its final session on the last major supplemental appropriations bill for the current fiscal year. Even before the letter arrived, everybody on Capitol Hill knew that the committee would vote some increase for AIDS money. The question was how much they would approve. Proponents of more research were pulling numbers from the air. Brandt solved that problem.

"You also asked whether additional resources could effectively be used in the current fiscal year," Brandt wrote. "As with any situation as dynamic and critical as that of AIDS, funding requirements can change rapidly. Enclose 2 is a description of additional efforts which could be accomplished now and in future months.

"While we are not requesting additional budget authority for these items, we would not oppose Congress giving the Secretary of Health and Human Services discretionary authority to transfer up to $12 million for AIDS activities across appropriations lines of HHS."

The words stunned administration supporters who had taken the health officials at their word when they said they had all the funds they needed for research. Although Brandt had tried to step delicately around the issue, even the administration's most fervent supporters did not believe that the request stemmed from any "dynamic or critical" new developments in AIDS. No matter how "rapidly" the situation changed, no dramatic breakthroughs had occurred in the days since Brandt, Foege, Devita, and Krause testified against more funds.

The Appropriations Committee refused Brandt's request that money be diverted from other programs and quickly approved a bill for $12 million in new funds for the NIH and CDC. Word spread through the Hill that a number of congressional members, including some Republicans, were royally pissed at the dishonesty to which they had been subjected. This thing wasn't over yet. The House would vote on the package the next week, and aides were betting that the whole sorry story would make it to the House floor.

In the Senate, AIDS posed a different problem, requiring maneuvers to deny that body's cadre of ultra-right-wing members, elected during the Reagan landslide of 1980, an opportunity to expound on AIDS. Although he was a conservative Mormon from Utah, Senator Orrin Hatch, chair of the Senate Committee on Labor and Human Resources, was committed to not letting health become a partisan issue, particularly in regard to AIDS. Hatch's committee, however, included some of the looniest, raving New Right homophobes in the Senate— Jeremiah Denton from Alabama and John East from North Carolina. Thus, when Henry Waxman's Public Health Emergency Act went to Hatch's committee, he made the unusual parliamentary move of holding the bill at his desk and allowing it to go straight to the Senate floor without a hearing. Hatch figured that it was better to have no hearing, than one in which health issues would get mixed up with the fringe Moral Majority politics.

These were the legislative acrobatics that AIDS would routinely demand on the Hill for years to come.

May 20

The National Cancer Institute and National Institute for Allergy and Infectious Diseases issued a request for scientists to apply for the $2 million in grant money that Bill Kraus and Tim Westmoreland had maneuvered through Congress last fall. The application deadline was August 1. Under new, expedited processes, the money might be available by the end of the year, although, privately, most scientists figured that the money would not actually get to research institutions until 1984. This $2 million in awards marked only the second call for research proposals issued by the NIH during the epidemic.

May 24

With the full House vote on AIDS funding due the next day, Dr. Edward Brandt assembled the top officials from the CDC and NIH for a news conference. There was much said about the promise of the HTLV lead and about people not panicking over blood transfusions, but only one sentence mattered.

"It's our number-one priority," Brandt said. "I feel a great sense of urgency about AIDS.

"I am aware of the fact that a number of people feel we have not been sensitive enough to the problem," said Brandt. "Our response has had nothing to do with the membership of any high-risk group involved. These people are victims of an illness and we are going to do whatever we can to stop that problem."

With those words, Brandt stole the thunder that the House of Representatives had planned to unleash a day later and elevated AIDS to a new dimension of importance, even if the administration was not willing to spend any more money on the problem. From now on, whenever administration officials were pressed on the federal response to AIDS, they would reply: "This is the administration's number-one health priority." It certainly sounded sincere enough.

◯

By the day that Dr. Edward Brandt declared AIDS to be the administration's top health priority, 1,450 Americans had contracted the disease and 558 had died.

The Next Day
U.S. HOUSE OF REPRESENTATIVES,
CAPITOL

Congressman William Natcher needed unanimous consent of the House to introduce his last-minute amendment for an additional $12 million for AIDS research. Congressional aides Tim Westmoreland and Michael Housh held their breath in the gallery, hoping no redneck would object and wreck everything. Nobody did. Natcher and Silvio Conte co-sponsored the measure. Upon its introduction, Natcher asked that the earlier testimony of Margaret Heckler and Ed Brandt against new AIDS funding be introduced into the record. The remarks, he felt, spoke for themselves.

Congressman Conte was obviously angry as he rose to recall how he grilled the various chiefs of the CDC, NCI, and NIAID about the adequacy of funding. To make sure their duplicity was accurately recorded, Conte inserted the interrogations word for word into the *Congressional Record.*

The House of Representatives passed the funds unanimously.

◯

Congressman Henry Waxman shuddered as he read all the news stories about the nation's number-one health priority. If this was how they treated their number-one health priority, he wondered, what do they do with number two or three?

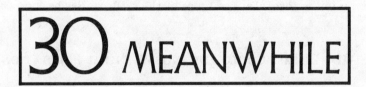

30 MEANWHILE

AMA News Release
FOR RELEASE FRIDAY, MAY 6, 1983

EVIDENCE SUGGESTS HOUSEHOLD CONTACT MAY TRANSMIT AIDS

CHICAGO—Evidence suggesting that Acquired Immune Deficiency Syndrome (AIDS) can be transmitted by routine household contact is presented in this week's *Journal of the American Medical Association.*

James Oleske, MD, MPH, and colleagues report eight cases of otherwise unexplained immune deficiency syndrome among children from the Newark, N.J., metropolitan area born into families with recognized risks for AIDS.

"Four of these children have died," the authors report. "Our experience suggests that children living in high-risk households are susceptible to AIDS and that sexual contact, drug abuse or exposure to blood products is not necessary for disease transmission."

Related articles by Arye Rubinstein, MD, and others, and Joseph Sonnabend, NB, MRCP, and colleagues suggest that AIDS can be transmitted to fetuses in the mother's womb, and that the syndrome is acquired by male homosexuals as a result of life-style behavior that apparently overworks and ultimately virtually destroys the immune system. . . .

Commenting on the study in an accompanying editorial, Anthony S. Fauci, MD, of the National Institutes of Health, points out, "We are witnessing at the present time the evolution of a new disease process of unknown etiology with a mortality of at least 50 percent and possibly as high as 75 percent to 100 percent with a doubling of the number of patients afflicted every six months."

At first the disease appeared to be confined only to male homosexuals, he adds. Then it became clear that IV drug users also were susceptible, and after that the disease was found among Haitians and hemophiliacs, the latter apparently exposed through transfusion of blood products.

"The finding of AIDS in infants and children who are household contacts of patients with AIDS or persons with risks for AIDS has enormous implications with regard to ultimate transmissibility of this syndrome," Fauci says. "If routine close contact can spread the disease, AIDS takes on an entirely new dimension," he adds.

"Given the fact that incubation period for adults is believed to be longer than one year, the full impact of the syndrome among sexual contacts and recipients of potentially infective transfusions is uncertain at present. If we add to this the possibility that nonsexual, non-blood-borne transmission is possible, the scope of the syndrome may be enormous."

◯

AIDS Disease Could Endanger General Population

CHICAGO (AP)—A study showing children may catch the deadly immune deficiency disease AIDS from their families could mean the general population is at greater risk from the illness than previously believed, a medical journal reported today.

If "routine" personal contact among family members in a household is enough to spread the illness, "then AIDS takes on an entirely new dimension," said Dr. Anthony Fauci of the National Institutes of Health in Bethesda, Maryland.

◯

Arye Rubinstein was astounded that Anthony Fauci could so much as even imply that household contact might have anything to do with spreading AIDS. Rubinstein had never been a great admirer of New Jersey's Dr. Oleske; they had antithetical views of AIDS in children. To Rubinstein, the mode of transmission was fairly obvious and fit quite well with existing epidemiological data on AIDS. The mother obviously infected the child in her womb. The fetus and parent shared blood as surely as an intravenous drug user, hemophiliac, or blood transfusion recipient. The fact that none of the infants in Oleske's study were over one year old reinforced this notion. In order to interpret this data to mean that "routine household contact" might spread AIDS, an entirely new paradigm for AIDS transmission was needed. Rubinstein's paper explained it all very easily, though the *Journal of the American Medical Association* seemed more enamored with Oleske's specious analysis. In fact, the journal at first returned Rubinstein's paper with the section on intrauterine transmission crossed out. The paragraphs had only appeared because Rubinstein had insisted that they be retained.

What was Fauci's problem?

Upon investigation, it turned out that Anthony Fauci had not been sent Rubinstein's paper before writing the *JAMA* editorial. Instead, he read only Oleske's conclusions before writing his editorial.

◯

As an AIDS clinician at the National Institutes of Health Hospital, Anthony Fauci was noted for his heroic efforts to save lives early in the epidemic. He had risen rapidly in the NIAID hierarchy and was deemed a major NIH expert on AIDS at the time the infamous *JAMA* editorial was published. Fauci quickly cast blame on a hysterical media for taking his comments "out of context." After all, he had said only that the *possibility* of household transmission *might* raise all these scientific implications. The lay public did not understand the language of science, he pleaded. Science always dealt with hypotheticals; this did not mean he was saying that AIDS actually *was* spread through household contact. Moreover, the chief villain, he would accurately note, was the press office of the American Medical Association, which had so shamefully sensationalized the medical journal articles in an effort to draw attention to a journal that always found itself playing second fiddle to *Science* and the *New England Journal of Medicine.*

No matter who was to blame, the coverage afforded to the "routine household contact" press release set in motion a wave of hysteria that no disclaimer would prevent. At the *San Francisco Chronicle,* science editor David Perlman rewrote the story, focusing instead on Rubinstein's interpretation of the data. After completing his revisions, Perlman proceeded to call the *JAMA* press office and deliver a loud dressing-down to the public relations director who had unleashed this mischief. Few other newspapers had writers as sensitive to the social fallout of AIDS stories. *The New York Times* and *USA Today* ran the flawed AP version of the press release, as did most newspapers in the United States.

As it was, nervous health officials and reporters had spent months talking about AIDS being spread through "bodily fluids." What they meant to say was semen and blood, but the term "semen" is one that polite people don't use in conversation, and blood banks still objected to the use of the term "blood." The media's circumlocution salved sensibilities but not public fears. Saliva was a bodily fluid. Could AIDS be spread through coughing? It was a question already being asked of Selma Dritz with greater frequency. Moreover, the report created a lasting impression on the public that would raise the hysteria level around AIDS for years to come. Scientists just aren't sure how AIDS is spread, the thinking went. Because of the long incubation period, possible transmission routes existed that might not reveal themselves until later—until it was too late. Anthony Fauci had said as much in his ill-considered editorial.

Indeed, transmission routes may have seemed mysterious in 1982, but by 1983 the mysteries were solved. All the ways to get AIDS were established by then, and scientists, at least at the CDC, understood precisely how AIDS was spread. Nevertheless, the report of routine household contact lent scientific credibility to ungrounded fears; the social damage would linger for years. The fear inspired by this one story defined the context within which AIDS was discussed for the next crucial months.

⬭

The pictures on the front page of the morning paper a week after the *JAMA* story marked the first tangible fallout. For weeks, San Francisco police officers had been sending memos through their union, posing fears about what they should do with bloodstained clothes of a crime victim who might be gay. Some union officials advised officers to write a special report every time they had contact with a possible AIDS sufferer. The report could be used at a disability hearing if the policeman got AIDS. The household contact study ignited similar fears among firefighters. Within days of the article, San Francisco officials had to act. By the next Friday, face masks, rubber gloves, and ten-minute education tapes on AIDS were being passed out in every firehouse and police station in the city. The photo of an officer trying on one of the resuscitation masks started cropping up in dailies and newsmagazines across the country in the fearful weeks that followed, a virtual emblem of the AIDS hysteria that enveloped the nation because of the household contact "findings." The second epidemic had commenced—the epidemic of fear.

The same day that masks were handed out in San Francisco, prisoners at a New York State prison in Auburn started a hunger strike because the cafeteria's eating utensils had been used by an inmate who had died of AIDS a week earlier. Days later, California dentists were advised to don gloves, masks, and glasses to protect themselves from AIDS-infected patients. New York City morticians began rumblings about whether they should be forced to embalm AIDS victims, and police departments across the country started agitating for face masks, like those in San Francisco.

May 16
LUNDYS LANE, SAN FRANCISCO

Matt Krieger was in his office at his cottage in Bernal Heights when Gary Walsh called.

"I'm in the hospital," Gary said. *"Pneumocystis."*

Matt started to cry.

"I'm going to beat it," Gary said. "I'm just tired a little, but I'm going to survive."

When Matt hung up, he called his best friend Liz over to his home and explained the situation. He and Gary had been drawing closer in recent weeks, but Matt had been more distant than he would have preferred, trying to respect Gary's apparent need to be alone. With Gary in the hospital for the first time, Matt now wanted a complete rapprochement. He wanted to be back in Gary's life full time. It was what he had wanted since moving to San Francisco: a lifelong commitment in which you shared everything, the good and the bad, the joy and the pain.

"I want to be with him," Matt said.

Liz put her hand on Matt's tear-stained face and smiled: "Well, you certainly can't go looking like this."

Matt arrived at Davies Medical Center on Castro Street with a bouquet of helium balloons, all in the bright colors Gary fancied. When Matt walked into Gary's room, Gary smiled weakly and Matt knew he was exactly where he was supposed to be. The couple picked up almost where they had left off, and from then on, Matt and Gary were closer than ever.

The next days were tough on both of them. The strong antibiotics the doctors used to purge Gary's lungs of *Pneumocystis* kept him sleeping most of the time. When he woke up, Gary chatted with Matt or jotted down notes for his friend Mark Feldman who was in another wing of the hospital, also suffering from the virulent AIDS pneumonia. "Keep fighting," Gary wrote.

Struggling for breath was the hardest, most frightening part, Gary confided.

"When you've got this, you don't think you're going to live," he told Matt, "and sometimes you hope you won't."

Within a few days, his energy started rebounding and he started talking enthusiastically about leaving the hospital. Maybe he'd get back to Sacramento and lobby the legislature more for a governor's task force on AIDS, and money for AIDS education. He was so angry that people weren't taking AIDS more seriously. Maybe that anger, Matt thought, was keeping Gary alive.

The nurses enjoyed Gary's spunk and were amazed when he walked them through an informal therapy session if they seemed down on a particular morning. "This guy's in the hospital with AIDS and he's worried about *my* problems?" they'd whisper to Gary's doctor.

Matt was relieved he'd have the next months with Gary. Now that they were reunited, Matt decided he would keep a journal of every day they spent together. This would be a special part of his life, he knew, and he wanted to be able to remember it precisely and not let later years fuzz the images and feelings. As Gary recovered, Matt wrote, "It has been hell, and I thought I would not survive."

When it came time to go home, Gary felt he was abandoning his longtime friend Mark Feldman, somehow, even though Mark had a devoted lover and many friends to keep vigil near him. Mark was wasting away to nothing when Gary visited him before checking out. And it was the last time Gary saw him.

May 17
LONDON

In the first official report on the spread of Acquired Immune Deficiency Syndrome to the United Kingdom, London health authorities reported that three Englishmen had died of AIDS as of mid-March and six more cases were being monitored nationwide.

The report, combined with troubling news from the United States about the epidemic being spread in households, sparked a wave of AIDS panic in the always-hysterical British press. Health authorities began to debate whether to ban the import of American plasma, which made up half of the blood products used in Britain.

May 19
METROPOLITAN COMMUNITY CHURCH,
CASTRO DISTRICT, SAN FRANCISCO

The Reverend Jim Sandmire was a tall, sturdy man with unquestioned integrity, a deep booming voice, and a thick shock of white hair. On Sunday afternoons, when he would shake hands with the parishioners of his largely gay congregation, somebody inevitably commented that Jim Sandmire looked the way a minister should. Somebody else would then wink at Sandmire, because he had seen the reverend hunkering down Folsom Street in full black leather regalia the night before. Sandmire believed that the houses of God were to be found on many streets; he felt equally comfortable in all the various milieus to be found in the gay community. That was why Dana Van Gorder had called him for a meeting between gay political leaders, AIDS educators, and the bathhouse owners. Van Gorder wanted Sandmire to be moderator.

"You're the only one everybody trusts," said Dana.

Jim was in bed, with a severe case of shingles. It was not the first time he had been called upon to moderate some dispute among the always-cantankerous gay factions, but he wanted to beg out of it. Any movement caused him ferocious pain. When he achingly eased himself into the conference room of the Metropolitan Community Church off Castro Street, he wished again he had said no. This discussion, he could see, was going to need some serious moderation.

The invitations had gone out from Harry Britt's office a week before, signed by a remarkably broad array of gay leaders such as Cleve Jones, Catherine Cusic, two MCC ministers, and leaders of all the gay Democratic and Republican clubs, as well as the normally timorous Bay Area Physicians for Human Rights (BAPHR). An attorney for the police department, Lawrence Wilson, who served on the Toklas executive committee, also signed the letter.

"At this meeting we will suggest several steps which we believe are particularly important in light of the large number of gay males who regularly visit San Francisco, particularly during Lesbian/Gay Freedom Week, and who may become infected with AIDS and could spread it to their hometowns upon departure," the letter read. "We believe that men should be informed of ways to engage in sexual conduct in a fashion that minimizes their risk of becoming infected or spreading infection. Information on this topic is not generally available to visitors coming to San Francisco who may patronize your establishment."

The letter said the group would discuss ways to make sure bathhouses were clean, that each patron was provided AIDS information, and that notices were prominently posted warning of AIDS. The BAPHR safe-sex guidelines were enclosed as suggested brochure material.

Before the meeting started, Toklas Club president Randy Stallings had spread word among the bathhouse owners that Bill Kraus and his Milk Club allies wanted to shut the places down. It was the next logical step in their rhetoric about changing life-styles. The incitement proved unnecessary. A number of bathhouse owners were incensed that such a meeting would even be called. The owners of one South-of-Market sleazy leather den, Animals, handed out a flier stating, "We do not intend to be singled out, subjected to an inquisition-like atmosphere. We find no evidence either from the medical community or health department which indicates that bathhouses are either the source of or a primary contributing factor to the AIDS threat."

When a reporter for a gay newspaper walked in, Rick Crane, the director of the KS Foundation, ordered him out. It wouldn't do to have public discussions of bathhouses. No, this needed to be decided in an . . . appropriate way.

Some of the entrepreneurs were open to suggestions. The owner of one private sex club, The Caldron, conceded that the sex business was soft lately.

He already had published his own "health hints" guide and had oriented his business toward jack-off nights, promoted as rollicks during which gay men could give each other a "helping hand." The city's only bisexual bathhouse, Sutro Baths, also had put out its own safe-sex guides, though this did little to calm the heterosexual clients' fears; they were staying away in droves.

Other bath owners were querulous that anyone should think they owed it to their clients to post warnings. The owner of the Jaguar Bookstore, for whose license Bill Kraus had worked so hard, was on record as telling the *Bay Area Reporter,* "I don't want that [passing out brochures] going on. People come here to forget what's going on." The owner of the Liberty Baths best summed up the sex business's sentiments on AIDS: "I wish the whole problem will go away."

The problem was not going away, Bill Kraus knew; it was gay men who were going away, dying, while the bathhouse owners did nothing. As soon as Bill walked in with Catherine Cusic, he could see there were problems. Stallings's allies quickly took up the call against "sexual fascists" who would "stifle sexuality." And what for? Nobody really knew how AIDS was spread, they argued. Nobody could prove it really was a virus. You were as likely to get this from somebody you pick up in a bar as at the baths.

Nobody lies facedown in a bar with a can of Crisco and takes on all comers, thought Catherine Cusic as she watched the tide of denial wash over the meeting. These politicos are acting as though they don't know what goes on in a bathhouse, she thought. Cusic was surprised at how quickly the rhetoric turned harsh. She figured that the bathhouses would be smart enough to cut a deal. Nobody would come out for closure if they took these steps in time for the parade.

As the talk got more belligerent, a San Jose bathhouse owner announced that he was forming the Northern California Bathhouse Owners Association. In the end, the group reached no consensus, although they put out a press release saying they had met.

"They should be shut down," Bill Kraus said calmly to Catherine Cusic on the way out. "They don't care that they might be killing people, they are so greedy. Every one of them should be shut down."

Shortly after the meeting, the owner of Sutro Baths appeared in Selma Dritz's office. He had heard that the communicable disease specialist had made no secret of her view that bathhouses were a cesspool of AIDS contagion.

"If you try to shut them down, I'll have you in court a day later with a temporary restraining order," he shouted.

Dritz feared he would stick to his word. She already had asked for an opinion on the legality of closure from the city attorney's office. It had not come through, but she knew that a closure order might be difficult to get because doctors had not yet isolated an AIDS virus. Epidemiology was at best inferential data. Would it stand up in court?

Still, Selma Dritz had no doubts about the role that bathhouses played in the epidemic. Going to a bathhouse was not like picking someone up in a gay bar or even a park. Picking up in a bar only gave somebody one shot at the virus. It was haphazard. Parks were more iffy; the weather did not always cooperate and shrubs did not provide a good ambience for anal intercourse, the riskiest sexual behavior. On the other hand, bathhouses were havens for anal intercourse. The only limit to promiscuity was stamina. The institutions were designed to expedite many partners, thus ensuring that everyone there had a higher chance of being infected because they were exposed to many others.

For this reason, Don Francis had called "commercialized gay sex" an "amplification system" for the disease. Virtually every study on sexually transmitted diseases had shown for years that gay men who went to bathhouses were far more likely than others to be infected with whatever venereal disease was going around, whether it was gonorrhea or syphilis, hepatitis B or AIDS. Bathhouses guaranteed the rapid spread of AIDS among gay men. To be sure, the disease would have crept through the United States without bathhouses, but these foci of sexual activity fueled the brushfire propagation of the infection more than any other single element of American society.

Common sense dictated that bathhouses be closed down. Common sense, however, rarely carried much weight in regard to AIDS policy. Indeed, the debates that simmered around the country over bathhouses in the next two years emerged as paradigms of how politics and public health could conspire to foster catastrophe.

In other parts of the United States, the bathhouse issue was becoming troublesome as well. A week after the San Francisco meeting, a Washington, D.C., gay bathhouse canceled an AIDS fund-raiser because a local organization issued a brochure advising gay men to "eliminate or decrease sexual activity in places where multiple sexual contact is frequent, such as the baths, the bookstores, the bushes, and backrooms of bars."

The bathhouse owner complained that the advice linked bathhouses to AIDS. The city's gay leaders came rushing to his defense with the chorus that gay businesses should not be singled out for harassment during this crisis.

In Miami, Jack Campbell, owner of the Club Baths chain of forty-two bathhouses, brushed off questions about the baths' role in the epidemic by insisting that most of Florida's AIDS cases were Haitians, and it wasn't a problem for gays. This was not accurate. Campbell's role in the gay community, however, illuminated one reason the gay political leadership would be reluctant to get stern with bathhouses. Campbell, for example, served on the boards of five major national gay organizations. Without dispute, he was the most powerful gay leader in Florida. No Miami gay leader and no liberal politician out to curry favor with Florida's sizable gay community would drop a word about bathhouse closure.

A similar scenario shaped up in Los Angeles, where the godfather of local gay politics was Sheldon Andelson, the owner of the property where that city's most popular bathhouse, the 8709 Club, was housed. He had been listed as an owner of the bathhouse, but another person's name suddenly appeared on city permits once Governor Brown appointed Andelson to the prestigious University of California Board of Regents. In Chicago, bathhouse owner Chuck Renslow published the local gay paper and carried substantial weight in gay Democratic politics. The owner of the St. Mark's Baths in New York City had made himself invaluable by providing his popular disco, The Saint, as a site for gay community fund-raisers.

Moreover, most of the nation's gay newspapers received substantial advertising revenues from the bathhouses and sex businesses. This business and political clout assured that not only would few gay leaders support moving against the baths, but that the gay newspapers would unanimously support their advertisers. Potential bathhouse closure was not even to be discussed as an alternative.

In the aftermath of the San Francisco meeting, local bathhouse owners launched a counterattack. "If AIDS is indeed sexually transmitted, why have there been so FEW cases?" asked an advertisement from Liberty Baths. "Yes, I say few because if an estimated 20,000,000 gays have an estimated 200 contacts per year this means that in 4½ years we have seen 1,279 cases of AIDS in 4,000,000,000 contacts, or odds of 3,127,443 to 1 against getting AIDS during a given contact. With all this gay play going on, why aren't we all getting AIDS instead of only 1,279 of us?"

STANFORD UNIVERSITY BLOOD BANK

One-in-a-million chance.

It had become the cliché for blood bankers to talk about how a transfusion recipient's chances of getting AIDS from blood products was one in a million.

In his office at the Stanford campus, Dr. Edgar Engleman viewed the estimates as a cruel hoax on the American people. The tall, lanky Engleman—who bore a striking resemblance to comedian Chevy Chase—had served for five years as medical director of the blood bank for Stanford University Hospital, the biggest hospital blood user in the country. As an immunologist, he had closely followed the epidemic. Not long after the first cases of AIDS were reported among hemophiliacs in mid-1982, he added two and two, and figured the disease could be spread in blood transfusions as well. By early 1983, three AIDS cases were lying in Stanford University Hospital wards; for all three, their only "risk behavior" was having a blood transfusion in San Francisco.

The blood banking industry was insisting that because only one or two blood-transfusion recipients with AIDS could be linked to donors who had full-blown AIDS, the chance of contracting AIDS from a blood transfusion was one in a million. After all, three million Americans are transfused with blood each year, they said. But Dr. Engleman calculated the odds differently. First, the blood bankers weren't counting the growing number of transfusion recipients who came down with AIDS from blood donated by someone with lymphadenopathy or pre-AIDS symptoms. Clearly, these people were also infected with the virus; the blood banks were playing semantics by not including them in the calculations. Moreover, there may be three million blood units donated every year, but a typical patient is transfused with three, not one unit, increasing the odds further. Nor was it fair to figure in the transfusions of areas with no incidence of AIDS. The honest way to figure the odds was to use numbers from the major urban areas where the AIDS virus was prevalent. At San Francisco's Irwin Memorial Blood Bank, for example, officials figured they were losing between 7 and 15 percent of their blood for the lack of gay donors. If these people were donating in 1981 and 1982, this translates into a lot of blood potentially infected with AIDS years before anybody even knew the epidemic existed.

No, this one-in-a-million rhetoric was bullshit, Engleman thought. Instead, he figured that a person's chance of contracting AIDS from a San Francisco transfusion was more on the order of 1 in 10,000, maybe 1 in 5,000.

People play the California lottery with hopes of winning $100 on precisely those odds, which weren't a good enough margin of safety for Engleman.

From the start, Engleman had thought that the federal government's guidelines requiring only the questioning of donors were inadequate. Nearly three months after they went into effect, he could see that some people in high-risk groups still were donating blood. Not everybody bothered to read the little pamphlets handed out at the desk for self-deferral. For some, it appeared that donating blood was an act that could overcome their personal fears about having AIDS. Thus, blood banks occasionally became the stages for gay men living out the psychodramas of denial.

Stanford needed a blood test, Engleman decided. As a specialist in the new field of helper and suppressor lymphocytes, Engleman quickly opted for putting each blood donation through the university's new Flourescent Activated Cell Sorter machine to run helper-suppressor ratios. The tests were expensive, increasing the price of each blood unit by $6, or about 10 percent. But how do you define "expensive" when you're talking about saving lives?

By the end of May, Stanford University Hospital became the only major medical center in the United States to decide to start testing blood for evidence of AIDS infection. The rest of the blood industry was stunned that Engleman would conduct tests that the industry had rebuffed. Some said it was a gimmick to draw AIDS-hysteric patients to Stanford from San Francisco hospitals.

The anger ran deeper, Engleman noted even then. It was as if the blood bankers themselves were caught in the psychological web of denial. They wanted proof of the existence of an AIDS virus; they wanted extraordinary evidence that transfusion AIDS existed; they fundamentally wanted to deny that they could be part of something so horrible. Engleman had broken rank just when it was time to pull the wagons together.

Engleman could comprehend the psychological processes at work. Blood bankers were good people, he knew; they just weren't using their full intellectual facilities on this issue. Stanford made no great fanfare when the testing began and issued no press releases. Engleman, however, was firm on one point. He didn't want any nontested blood in his hospital. In a tense meeting with officials of the Peninsula Blood Bank, which supplied additional blood to the Stanford Medical Center, Engleman ordered them to begin having their blood tested within thirty days or Stanford would stop buying from them. Reluctantly, the blood bankers complied. San Francisco's Irwin Memorial Blood Bank did not follow suit, however, telling the press that testing was unnecessary. They had self-deferral guidelines, they said, and there was only a one-in-a-million chance that somebody would get AIDS from a blood transfusion.

CENTERS FOR DISEASE CONTROL, ATLANTA

Dale Lawrence met with blood bankers again in early May to present ten more cases of transfusion-associated AIDS. His job was to convince them that this was real, a problem they should be *doing* something about. And he was failing. The blood bankers wanted to pick apart each case study and talk about this or that detail, rather than what, taken together, the whole phenomenon meant: AIDS still was spreading, unabated, in blood.

Blood issues continued to dominate the AIDS Activities Office's concerns. Dr. James Allen had taken over transfusion work and had become increasingly convinced that donor-deferral guidelines would bring disaster. The questions would have to be asked by blood bank volunteers, Allen knew, who tended to be sweet retired ladies out to do something civic minded. Asking about homosexuality and intravenous drugs was not the same as asking for an address and social security number. CDC anxieties were not calmed when one sociopathic gay rights attorney in Texas suggested gays should threaten "blood terrorism" and say they would donate blood en masse if the government didn't launch serious AIDS research programs. The issue had international ramifications as well. France had banned the import of American blood in mid-May. Dutch and British health authorities were considering similar proposals.

Ideally, the CDC could nail down the blood question by tracking down every recipient of a transfusion donated by someone who later came down with AIDS. Dale Lawrence had proposed such a project, but there wasn't enough money to support it.

May 23
UNCLE CHARLIE'S BAR, NEW YORK CITY

"Has he finally gone completely and utterly crazy?" wondered Paul Popham as he watched Larry Kramer barge into the deejay's booth at the popular bar. Paul had been hosting the party for the new volunteers of Gay Men's Health Crisis. Everybody still was gossiping about how angry Larry remained at his departure from the board, but Paul had never expected this. He wasn't sure whether he should shout or laugh.

"This is Larry Kramer," Larry yelled into the microphone to the stunned volunteers and GMHC staff. "We're poised at a crucial point. I think this organization was founded to fight. I think the board of directors is very, very timid."

He's really gone off the deep end this time, thought Paul.

Larry felt he had been driven to this. In the weeks since the meeting with the mayor, nothing had changed. At a recent AIDS hearing, New York City Health Commissioner Dr. David Sencer had blandly stated that AIDS was not "an emergency" in New York City. The city needed no education programs because gays were doing such a good job of educating themselves. There needed to be no planning for even the most basic health needs, such as hospital beds. The city's gay health coordinator, Dr. Roger Enlow, also had turned aside the idea that the city begin education programs with the libertarian argument that the "city should not tell people how to have sex."

Both city and state officials were responding to growing alarm by having meetings. Indeed, David Sencer frequently joked that the epidemic of AIDS had spawned an epidemic of conferences. A week before, Governor Mario Cuomo had announced at a political gay fund-raising dinner at the Plaza hotel that he would establish an AIDS task force. The next day, the state government announced a $100,000 grant to GMHC for education. It would never be clear whether the grant reflected genuine concern on the part of the state or the resumption of the longtime feuding between the governor and the mayor. Mario Cuomo rarely let pass an opportunity to embarrass his nemesis, Ed Koch, and the release of this token amount of money did little but highlight the city's own inaction on the issue.

The city also had its own Interagency AIDS Task Force, meeting under the authority of David Sencer. At virtually every meeting, representatives from various AIDS groups talked about the need for education programs, hospice beds, home health-care nurses, and planning for future hospital needs. This or that city bureaucrat would promise to look into the problem. The task force would meet again, and the city officials would talk of this or that obstacle. They'd have more reports at the next task force meeting. And the next meeting brought still new obstacles and rarely any resolution. Every task force meeting became a recitation of problems and official procrastination. Everybody got to vent steam but little was actually accomplished. The city of New York had yet to devote one penny to any AIDS education or services, despite being home to 45 percent of the nation's AIDS victims.

Nothing was happening, Larry Kramer thought.

"We need fighters," he exhorted the crowd at Uncle Charlie's. "We need a board of directors that will get confrontational and slug things out."

Paul Popham watched Larry Kramer as he joined the volunteers after his impromptu stump. You can't go around telling people how to have sex, Paul thought, which is what Larry wanted GMHC to do. You gave them the information. You didn't scold and you didn't act moralistic. And Paul was tired of hearing Larry bitch about Mayor Koch and *The New York Times.* There were problems, but you worked within the system to solve them. If Larry didn't like the way GMHC was doing things, Paul thought, why didn't he go off and form his own organization? He's out of step with the way New York gay men are,

Paul figured, or they'd be out joining a Larry Kramer Club. Instead, they're here.

Enno Poersch's assessment was more succinct. "The guy has gone absolutely bonkers," he said.

Larry was pleased that his speech had generated some applause. A number of volunteers came over and told him they had volunteered because of "1,112 and Counting." Larry saw Paul across the dance floor and wished Paul would come up and ask him to be on the board again. But Paul stayed put.

◯

On the night that Larry Kramer lectured GMHC about confronting the city government over the lack of AIDS services, the San Francisco Board of Supervisors passed $2.1 million for the city's growing AIDS programs. Of the funds, $1 million went toward equipping the outpatient clinic and planned inpatient ward designed specifically for AIDS patients at San Francisco General Hospital. The board also gave enough money to establish residences to house forty-eight homeless AIDS patients under the auspices of the Shanti Project. Funds also were released to fund the support staff from the vast network of volunteers at the Shanti Project and KS Foundation. With the $1 million enacted for AIDS in 1982, the level of city spending on AIDS in San Francisco now exceeded the funds released to the entire country by the National Institutes of Health for extramural AIDS research.

May 24

"The sexual revolution has begun to devour its children. And among the revolutionary vanguard, the Gay Rights activists, the mortality rate is highest and climbing."

The commentary that appeared in newspapers across the United States that day was the dropped shoe so many gay politicians had awaited. A speech writer for former President Nixon, Patrick J. Buchanan had served in recent years, as a right-winger without portfolio, making his most dashing appearances on editorial pages where editors were constantly searching for conservative columnists to compensate for the media's liberal bias. Buchanan was said to hold much favor with the more conservative of White House aides, and so his first column on AIDS was viewed with much interest. Where would President Reagan, who had somehow managed to make it through two years of the epidemic without whispering a word about it, end up on AIDS? Conservatives thus far had stayed away from talk of the disease; even Jerry Falwell wasn't saying much. Now, with AIDS in the headlines, those days were coming to an end and the first signs of potential backlash came with this column.

"The poor homosexuals—they have declared war upon nature, and now nature is exacting an awful retribution," Buchanan wrote.

Like most extremists, Buchanan did not strive for any particular consistency in his arguments. He drew on Kevin Cahill's assertion of a "conspiracy of silence" about AIDS among doctors to support the contention that liberals were covering up the horrible threat to Americans posed by AIDS-carrying homosexuals. He conjured the image of San Francisco's police officers putting on their masks and gloves to establish the danger of AIDS. After citing many irrelevant medical statistics, Buchanan concluded by saying no homosexual should be permitted to handle food and that the Democratic party's decision to hold their next convention in San Francisco would leave delegates' spouses and children at the mercy of "homosexuals who belong to a community that is a common carrier of dangerous, communicable and sometimes fatal diseases."

Days later, Buchanan followed this with a second column quoting from *The New York Times'* unfortunate coverage of the "routine close contact" study. Gays not only were slaughtering hemophiliacs and blood-transfusion recipients, Buchanan said, but now they threatened to kill children by working as pediatricians and custodians in day-care centers. "It has long been the defiant slogan of the gay rights movement that, so long as we don't injure anyone, what we do is our own business," he concluded. "If promiscuous homosexuals in the urban centers of New York and San Francisco are capable of transmitting death with a casual sexual contact, their slogan, to put it mildly, would no longer seem to apply."

May 26
CASTRO STREET, SAN FRANCISCO

"You're a sexual Nazi."

Bill Kraus heard variations on this theme from the moment he stepped onto Castro Street that afternoon. His essay calling on gay men to change their life-styles and redefine gay liberation had been printed in the *Bay Area Reporter* that hit the streets that afternoon. Bill had tried to be positive in the article, advancing the idea that "we gay men can transform this epidemic into our finest hour." Nevertheless, the reaction was swift and nasty. Bill was called an "anti-sex" brownshirt, out to destroy the gay community with his talk about not going to bathhouses. Bill's critics in the Toklas Club were ecstatic that he had handed them such explosive ammunition to use against the Milk Club.

The right wing was beginning to draw battle lines around issues of promiscuity and bathhouses. Rather than define their own battle lines, many gays adopted these issues as their front line of defense. By acknowledging defects in the old gay life-style, Bill had strayed to the enemy camp, as far as many of his critics were concerned. They started whispering the ultimate psychological insult, that he hated himself because he was gay, that he suffered from "internalized homophobia."

Bill Kraus was crushed at the criticism, especially coming at a time when his own work on AIDS had accelerated into hyperdrive. He was working sixty-hour weeks at the congressional office, monitoring national AIDS legislation and funding. Days before, he had been elected to the board of directors of the National KS/AIDS Foundation that Marc Conant was organizing as an American Cancer Society–type group for AIDS. Bill was also working with Dana Van

Gorder to devise a local public education campaign for AIDS risk reduction to try to bolster the long-stalled efforts of the San Francisco Department of Public Health.

"Don't they see I want to save their lives?" Bill moaned to Kico Govantes.

Although the two weren't lovers, Kico remained Bill's confidant. Kico ran his fingers through Bill's thick curly hair and hugged him. He couldn't understand how gay politicians, people who said their cause was to promote love, could be so cruel to each other. He could also see that the rejection stung Bill deeply, far more acutely than something merely political should.

"If I get AIDS," Bill said, "it's going to be those people's fault."

31 AIDSPEAK SPOKEN HERE

In San Francisco, plague met politics. Instead of being confronted by a united authority with intelligent plans for defense, it found divided forces among which the question of its presence became the subject of factional dispute. There was open popular hostility to the work of the sanitarians, and war among the City, State and Federal Health authorities . . . For a while the people were in the gravest danger and it seemed impossible to convey any adequate warnings to them.

—Eradicating Bubonic Plague from San Francisco, 1907,
The Report of the Citizens' Health Committee

June 2, 1983
SAN FRANCISCO DEPARTMENT OF PUBLIC HEALTH

"Dr. Silverman, this poster says people should have fewer sexual partners. Does that mean that if somebody had ten sexual partners a week last year that they can cut down to five sexual partners a week now and they won't get AIDS?"

Merv Silverman looked uncomfortable. He had taken Barbara Taylor, a no-nonsense reporter for the all-news KCBS radio, and a *Chronicle* newsman to proudly unveil the health department's AIDS poster, the one everybody was talking about.

"We're trying to give a message that people will pay attention to," said Silverman.

For five years Merv Silverman had served as a popular public health director. The media loved him; the gay community adored him. He wasn't accustomed to such sharp questioning. Barbara Taylor, who had spent the last seven years listening to politicians, pressed on.

"Dr. Silverman, it says on this poster that people should limit their use of recreational drugs. Does that mean that if somebody was shooting up, say, three times a week, that they'd be safe from AIDS if they shot up just once a month? You're not saying not to use recreational drugs; you say limit your use of drugs."

"We're trying not to lecture people," answered Silverman. "It doesn't do any good if you give people a message they don't listen to."

"I thought we were trying to tell people how not to get AIDS," said Taylor. "Why aren't we telling them that?"

Merv Silverman thought Barbara Taylor was taking an old-fashioned, text-book kind of approach to public health. The health director understood this approach; after all, his master's in public health came from Harvard. The silver-haired forty-five-year-old had spent his life in the field. But AIDS was not a classical public health problem. It was sensitive. It required messages that were . . . appropriate.

Taylor thought the poster was a lot of bullshit and that Silverman was soft-peddling AIDS prevention so he wouldn't have a lot of angry gay activists yelling at him for being homophobic. There'd been a lot of that in the past few days.

The reality was a mix of both Silverman's good intentions and Taylor's more cynical political analysis. The result was the first major public demonstration of AIDSpeak, a new language forged by public health officials, anxious gay politicians, and the burgeoning ranks of "AIDS activists." The linguistic roots of AIDSpeak sprouted not so much from the truth as from what was politically facile and psychologically reassuring. Semantics was the major denominator of AIDSpeak jargon, because the language went to great lengths never to offend.

A new lexicon was evolving. Under the rules of AIDSpeak, for example, AIDS victims could not be called victims. Instead, they were to be called People With AIDS, or PWAs, as if contracting this uniquely brutal disease was not a victimizing experience. "Promiscuous" became "sexually active," because gay politicians declared "promiscuous" to be "judgmental," a major cuss word in AIDSpeak. The most-used circumlocution in AIDSpeak was "bodily fluids," an expression that avoided troublesome words like "semen."

Most importantly, however, the new syntax allowed gay political leaders to address and largely determine public health policy in the coming years, because public health officials quickly mastered AIDSpeak, and it was fundamentally a political tongue. With politicians talking like public health officials, and public health officials behaving like politicians, the new vernacular allowed virtually everyone to avoid challenging the encroaching epidemic in medical terms.

Thus, the verbiage tended toward the intransitive. AIDSpeak was rarely employed to motivate action; rather, it was most articulately pronounced when justifying inertia. Nobody meant any harm by this; quite to the contrary, AID-Speak was the tongue designed to make everyone content. AIDSpeak was the language of good intentions in the AIDS epidemic; AIDSpeak was a language of death.

As public health director for the only city in the United States that was paying much attention to the epidemic, Mervyn Silverman became the chief translator of AIDSpeak for the general population. The former Peace Corps administrator was well-qualified for the role since he was a virtual warehouse of good intentions for the gay community. The past few days had demonstrated this amply.

The brouhaha had started on page two of the *Chronicle* a few days before in a story concerning the lack of any AIDS information in the city's bathhouses and sex emporiums. At least 200,000 gay tourists were about to descend on the city for the Gay Freedom Day Parade, the story noted. Many gay men came, in part, to make use of San Francisco's fabled sex emporiums; most still regarded AIDS as strange media hype. The scenario was one in which epidemics thrived.

Bill Kraus had quietly leaked an account of the ill-fated meeting with bathhouse owners. A public health official, who was not Mervyn Silverman but who asked not to be identified, told the paper about how it would be best to close the joints down; but barring that, they should be required to post some kind of warning.

"I don't have the power to force the bathhouses to post anything," Silverman initially told an inquiring reporter.

Technically, he was telling the truth. The only power Silverman had was to use his broad authority to close anything that was a threat to public health. He wasn't about to do that. In a letter to a citizen in May, Silverman had denied even having this power, saying it would be "illegal for me to close down all bathhouses and other such places that are used for anonymous and multiple sex contacts. It is my belief that we would insult the intelligence of many of our citizens and it would be an invasion of privacy to take such an action."

Silverman also was not inclined to force the gay businesses to alert customers about the death potential inherent in the use of their facilities. "The government can only play a certain role in this," he said. "The real validity comes with information from peers. The information that will get across will come from the gay community itself."

Like all AIDSpeak, the explanation sounded sensible, although it evaded the question of why public health officials exist. If preventing disease in a community was best done by the community itself, why bother to have a public health department?

Dr. Silverman was well-tutored by gay political leaders on the question of why the bathhouses shouldn't be shut down. "If you close the bathhouses, people will simply go elsewhere to have unsafe sex," he said.

For the past decade, spokespeople of the gay rights movement had held endless press conferences to argue against the stereotype that gay men were sex fiends wholly preoccupied with getting their rocks off. With AIDSpeak, however, many of these same spokespeople were now arguing that bathhouses must stay open because gay men were such sex fiends that they would be screwing behind every bush if they didn't have their sex clubs.

After the initial *Chronicle* story on the sex managers' refusal to post warnings, Mayor Dianne Feinstein inveighed: "Within the language of the health code, I think Dr. Silverman can write to them and tell them to post whatever warnings are necessary. I do think it is advisable." A majority of the board of supervisors also said that the public health director should order the obdurate bathhouse owners to post warnings. A day later, Dr. Silverman announced he would require warnings in the bathhouses. If the proprietors didn't cooperate, he would shut them down. "We would have done this anyway," he said.

By Thursday morning, June 2, Silverman was meeting with the bathhouse owners who suddenly said they were "looking forward" to putting up the posters. The public health director pledged the most "intensive" public health education campaign in city history. After that press conference, Silverman showed Barbara Taylor the AIDS poster. It gave four pieces of advice: "use condoms," "avoid any exchange of bodily fluids," "limit your use of recreational drugs," and "enjoy more time with fewer partners." The poster did inform gay men that there was a nasty disease out there that could kill you; but in saying to only "reduce" the number of partners and "limit" drugs, it did not get to the blunt fact that just one partner or bad needle could bring death.

○

The leadership of the Alice B. Toklas Democratic Club figured from the start that the bathhouse controversy had been raised by Bill Kraus and his Milk Club allies. Randy Stallings, the Toklas Club president, quickly launched a vitriolic counterattack. Kraus had violated the unwritten agreement that bathhouses were something that should not even be discussed publicly. The official Toklas policy was released the day after Silverman's meeting with the bathhouse owners.

The order requiring health warnings was a "direct attack on the social and economic viability of our community," the Toklas Club complained. "There is no evidence that the bathhouses or private clubs are the cause of this illness. To single out one type of gay business as somehow 'responsible' for this epidemic is to begin the process of destroying our community."

As for Kraus's essay in the *Bay Area Reporter,* the Toklas Club editorialized, "It is the height of arrogance to assume that only a small group of 'concerned individuals' are aware of this epidemic and are capable of dictating sexual behavior for the rest of us. There is a trend among some elements of our community to be anti-sexual and panic prone at a time when we should be banding together to defend a way of life that is precious and hard-won."

Now they were convinced Bill Kraus suffered from "internalized homophobia"; otherwise he would say that gay men were sex fiends and needed their bathhouses.

The most rabid supporter of sexual liberation was Konstantin Berlandt, the co-chair of the gay parade board of directors. "I didn't become a homosexual so I could use condoms," said Berlandt. "Of course, we're concerned about spreading a disease. But what should we do? Take our bodily fluids and put them in barrels off the Farallons?"

Kraus thought it was strange that anybody would reduce the aspirations of the gay movement to a disinclination for rubbers.

○

Like so many public policy issues in the epidemic, the bathhouse altercation of early June 1983 demonstrated the complex interrelationship that had grown between media and government. The matter arose only because a newspaper wrote a story about it, forcing public officials to take some rather obvious positions. In Los Angeles and New York, the newspapers didn't write about such distasteful subjects and the issues were not raised.

Moreover, public health officials in those two cities had already issued blanket assurances to anxious gay leaders that they would never close the bathhouses under any circumstances. In San Francisco, it was only the threat of closure that secured the agreement of bathhouse owners to the notices and brochures. Bathhouse owners in New York and Los Angeles, guaranteed that no such action would happen in their cities, had no similar incentive to provide education on AIDS. The handful of gay leaders who prodded for such materials found they had no leverage with the businessmen.

Selma Dritz thought the posting of signs was a cop-out. The U.S. Constitution might be construed to allow the right to commit suicide, but the ramifications of bathhouses did not end with the patron. These people went to other places, picked up and infected others. The Constitution did not grant the right to take other people with you. The day of Silverman's announcement, the city attorney issued an opinion telling the public health director that under the state health code "you may . . . order the public bathhouses closed immediately."

In the weeks after Dr. Silverman's press conference, the posters and brochures were distributed to bathhouses. A few honest bathhouse owners posted the notices prominently, but most put them in the darkest corners, if they bothered to post them at all. The syntax of AIDSpeak was in word not deed. Dr. Silverman did not dispatch anyone to see whether his orders were executed. By the thousands, gay men continued to go to the baths, and by the thousands they would later die.

June 3

There was venality, and there was also courage.

Gary Walsh's friend Mark Feldman died one month after he joined other AIDS patients in the candlelight march. Gary took his friend Lu Chaikin with him to the memorial service. Mark was the first to die among those early AIDS victims who had gone public with their plight. Though near death, they had braved social hysteria and personal rejection from friends so they could make people understand, so they could make people care.

Mark had died a particularly gruesome death. For weeks, his mouth was so engulfed in excruciating herpes sores that he could not eat. He was fed intravenously while the Kaposi's sarcoma lesions covered his insides and *Pneumocystis* protozoa filled his lungs.

Gary was grim at the service. Lu wasn't particularly cheerful herself, because she couldn't put aside the thought that one day she would have to sit through a similar service for Gary.

Gary scanned the room. He saw the faces of those who would die; he saw the faces of those who had died; he saw himself.

Despair overwhelmed Gary Walsh in the days after the service. He started lodging calls to Secretary Margaret Heckler's office. She should talk to him before she goes around saying that the government is spending all it needs to on AIDS research. She should talk to somebody who has had a friend die, he said. Gary tried to get an appointment with Governor Deukmejian, who had yet to utter one word of concern about the epidemic. He even wrote Ann Landers. For once, fighting didn't salve the anger, the depression, or the fear.

A few weeks later, Gary mentioned to Lu that he didn't think he would be going to any more memorial services.

The service also marked the first such ceremony for Bill Kraus. Bill had gone with his friend Ron Huberman, who had dated Mark Feldman before his illness. Afterward, Ron noticed that Bill was unusually somber. Ron thought it was because Mark's death battered any remnants of denial they could have about the severity of what the community was facing. This wasn't just hitting those other people—the fist-fuckers on Folsom Street—it was affecting respectable middle-class gays like themselves. Bill had a broader concern as well.

"Anita Bryant couldn't destroy our community. The FBI could never destroy our community; the police couldn't; Dan White couldn't; the government couldn't do it," confided Bill. "But AIDS might. We've made all this progress only to be undone by some virus."

Mark Feldman was one of the people with AIDS who had signed the letter asking the *Bay Area Reporter* publisher to fire editor Paul Lorch. When Lorch learned that Feldman had died, he pulled out the list of AIDS patients and crossed off Feldman's name.

PASTEUR INSTITUTE, PARIS

Luc Montagnier now knew that the new AIDS-related retrovirus was not a leukemia virus. He no longer called it RUB or HTLV. He had devised a new name, stemming from its retrieval from the lymph node of a lymphadenopathy patient. It was now called LAV, or lymphadenopathy-associated virus. Montagnier was surprised that there wasn't more enthusiasm about the Pasteur Institute's announcement of a new retrovirus. Most scientists wanted to defer final judgment until more research came from Robert Gallo's lab at the National Cancer Institute. Gallo was, after all, a far more famed retrovirologist, and he was talking HTLV. Montagnier, however, felt his group was more on target. In recent weeks, Pasteur researchers had isolated LAV in the blood of some hemophiliacs. Montagnier was gaining more confidence that the Pasteur Institute had indeed discovered the virus that caused AIDS. Still, he was stumped as to which family of viruses LAV belonged. If not HTLV, then what?

The chance encounter with another virologist on the Pasteur campus gave Montagnier the final piece to the puzzle. The associate mentioned a family of viruses, primarily found in animals, called lentiviruses. Lenti means slow. These viruses go into the cells, lie dormant for a while, and then burst into frenzied activity. Montagnier had never heard of the family before. He spent the night reading about equine viruses and was amazed at the similarities. LAV had the same morphology, the same proteins, and even looked the same in the electron microscope pictures. At the regular Saturday meeting of the doctors working on AIDS, Montagnier confidently announced that they had indeed discovered a new virus and it was not HTLV.

This proved to be a turning point in the scientific understanding of the epidemic. In the lives of the French researchers, it was noted as the beginning of the great frustration. They had taken the mystery out of the mystery disease but nobody was going to believe them.

June 13
NEW YORK CITY

The headline screamed from every newsstand in the New York metropolitan area. The *New York Post* had struck pay dirt: "L.I. Grandma Dead of AIDS," read the bold headline. The blood bank wouldn't admit it, of course, because blood banks still weren't admitting that transfusion-associated AIDS even existed. The Mineola grandmother, however, appeared to have no other risk for AIDS than the blood transfusion she had received three years before during heart surgery. Like most transfusion-AIDS cases diagnosed in 1983, Lorraine DeSantis had received the blood in 1980, long before the epidemic was even detected.

Suddenly, again, AIDS seemed a threat to everybody, and the wave of hysteria that had started building months before reached its crescendo in the final weeks of June and the first weeks of July. No part of the country seemed immune.

Each anecdote had the same premise spoken in the rarely heard dialect of AIDSpeak whispered outside the gay community. "Scientists don't really know . . ." In gay AIDSpeak, that meant that scientists couldn't prove AIDS was spread by sex, so people shouldn't take measures to protect themselves. When those same words were spoken with a heterosexual accent, however, they meant that scientists couldn't prove that AIDS was not spread by casual contagion, therefore people should take any measure possible to protect themselves and society. Both dialects were rooted in the same language of paranoia, one political and the other medical, although they implied drastically different solutions.

During this wave of AIDS hysteria in 1983, the heterosexuals got the most press. Every corner of the country seemed to have its own twist on AIDS fright. Because the *New York Post* had mastered the art of fashioning exaggerated fear and paranoia into headline copy, it seemed the best stories were happening in the five boroughs.

The day after the Long Island grandma headline, the *Post* ran another frightening story: "Junkie AIDS Victim Was Housekeeper at Bellevue." The story, strategically placed next to "A real-life Bambi finds a home in Westchester," told of how a thirty-one-year-old drug addict had been toting sheets and changing beds at Bellevue. When police officers delivered him to court for an arraignment, they wore rubber gloves and surgical masks.

A day after that, jail guards showed up at suburban Westchester County Jail in protective suits and surgical masks. The county jail did have one AIDS sufferer, but he was housed a quarter mile away from the main prison building where the guards wore padded nylon coveralls with hoods. "Grim future is here as guards model garb for handling AIDS inmates at Westchester County Jail," read the caption.

The news that a jail cook at the Queens House of Detention had died of AIDS complications sent officials of the prison guards' union scurrying in protest. When a Department of Corrections official told guards that they had nothing to fear from AIDS patients as food handlers, the president of the Correction Officers Benevolent Association said he would buy a steak and lobster dinner for the entire Department of Corrections executive staff if the food could be prepared and served by AIDS patients.

San Francisco was suffering a simultaneous case of the AIDS jitters. The day after the *Post*'s classic grandmother headline, two AIDS sufferers were scheduled to be part of an "A.M. San Francisco" segment whose goal was to "demystify" AIDS and calm the fears. However, the two patients couldn't appear on the show because studio technicians refused to mike them. Then, cameramen said they would not shoot the show if they had to walk onto the same sound stage as the two gay men. The two patients instead talked through a telephone in a separate room; only their disembodied voices appeared in the "demystification" show.

While this drama unfolded in the ABC studios, a Superior Court judge at San Francisco City Hall was handed a piece of paper torn from a pocket-sized spiral notebook. "We the undersigned protest having to sit in a confined space with an admitted victim of a fatal disease which has baffled science and methods of transmitting are still not fully known," it read.

Andrew Small, the thirty-year-old "admitted victim," was stunned. He knew he could have pleaded his health to get out of jury duty altogether, but he still felt such service was a civic responsibility. When word had spread among jurors, one woman's husband demanded that she leave the jury. The others were upset as well. After the judge received the note, she called in the presiding Superior Court judge and Dr. Marcus Conant for consultation. Conant advised her that AIDS was not easily spread, and the judge was not inclined to let this crazy fear interfere with her courtroom. Andrew Small ended up resigning from the panel, however, deciding it was unfair to the litigants to have a splintered jury bickering over the hepatitis B model.

On the same day, the papers featured the story of two San Jose nurses who quit their jobs after refusing to treat an AIDS patient. "There really isn't anyone who wants to go in the room," said one nurse. Among AIDS groups in Manhattan, word spread that nurses were similarly refusing to treat some people with AIDS, although New York hospitals did not see the problem as serious enough to warrant dismissal.

Even in death, AIDS sufferers would not find respite from the fear and ostracism. The New York State Funeral Directors Association that week recommended that its 11,000 members refuse to embalm anyone who appeared to have succumbed to the epidemic.

Doctors harbored no protective antibodies to hysteria. At the AIDS clinic at San Francisco General Hospital, clinic director Dr. Paul Volberding noticed that colleagues were less likely to shake his hand. Many seemed standoffish around him. Television news crews were similarly nervous about any physical contact.

In San Antonio, paramedics demanded their own protective suits—consisting of a hospital gown, pullover hood, surgical mask, and shoe covers—for use when they neared a suspected AIDS patient. In a suburb of San Diego, authorities canceled a class in resuscitation techniques because nobody wanted to share the dummy used for demonstrations, fearing they might get AIDS. Haitian Americans suffered multiple indignities in the two cities where they were most concentrated, Miami and New York. Just trying on a pair of shoes in Florida sometimes became a traumatic experience, because salespeople declined to let anyone who looked Haitian near any merchandise. Haitian community leaders argued loudly that the Haitian category should be dropped from the CDC's list of risk groups because they were the only nationality so singled out for treatment. In New York, some Haitians reportedly reassured anxious prospective employers that they hailed not from Haiti but from Martinique, another Francophonic Caribbean isle.

Sociologists hypothesized that AIDS hysteria was more profound than the anxiety surrounding other diseases because AIDS was first identified in the gay community, a group that already suffered social stigma and inspired fear among many heterosexuals. The epidemic gave new fuel to old prejudices. Scientists themselves promoted the fear further with all the "ifs" and "buts" with which they compulsively qualified any statement about the disease. The pusillanimous talk about bodily fluids only made it worse.

Where there are old anti-gay prejudices given new life, the Moral Majority cannot be far behind. Although the organization was still in the process of forging its final policy statement about the epidemic in the last weeks of June, its leaders were running trial balloons on the nascent rhetoric. "We feel the deepest sympathy for AIDS victims, but I'm upset that the government is not spending more money to protect the general public from the gay plague," said Ronald Goodwin, executive vice-president of the group. "What I see is a commitment to spend our tax dollars on research to allow these diseased homosexuals to go back to their perverted practices without any standards of accountability." Another Moral Majority spokesman was more aggressive: "If homosexuals are not stopped," said the Reverend Greg Dixon, "they will in time infect the entire nation, and America will be destroyed."

In Houston, fundamentalist preachers called on health authorities to close gay bars. The Dallas Doctors Against AIDS started litigation to set aside a court ruling that decriminalized gay sexual activity between consenting adults in Texas.

When the newspapers weren't writing stories about AIDS hysteria, they were touting cures and breakthroughs. It seemed every edition of each daily paper in the country that year could not go to bed without some doctor somewhere announcing something that "was a first step in the long road to a cure/vaccine for AIDS." Papers around the country reprinted an excellent series by *Philadelphia Inquirer* science writer Donald Drake about Anthony Fauci's heroic effort at the National Institutes of Health hospital to save a gay man with interleukin-2 treatments and a transplant of lymphocyte-producing bone marrow from his healthy twin brother. Across the country, the series boasted headlines about how this could lead to an AIDS cure. Only at the end of the stories did the reader find out that the AIDS victim went blind and died. In June there also was much talk about using the thymus gland to create an AIDS breakthrough, while genetic engineering firms promoted cloning as a way out of the AIDS mess. At the KS/AIDS Foundation, the stories became known as the Cure-of-the-Week features.

Such stories kept the focus of coverage on research and researchers. By now, AIDS largely was anchored in the area of science writers. General-assignment reporters might write an occasional social impact story, but AIDS fell into the science beat at virtually every American newspaper. Because of this, AIDS stories often had the explanatory flavor of Mr. Wizard—in deft hands, a good whodunit. They were not exposés or explorations of public policy questions. Thus, for all the coverage of the epidemic, there were precious few paragraphs delving into the politics of AIDS. A brief interlude came in early June when a frustrated Representative Ted Weiss went public about the problems Susan Steinmetz encountered in her CDC investigation.

"It appears that we have something to hide," responded Elvin Hilyer of the CDC, "but we don't."

It was during this intense media interest in all things pertaining to AIDS that somebody at the CDC took a paper napkin from the downstairs cafeteria and wrote a historical marker for an office door. It read: "In this office in April 1981, Sandra Ford discovered the epidemic that would later be known as Acquired Immune Deficiency Syndrome."

32 STAR QUALITY

June 14, 1983
<u>DENVER</u>

Assistant Secretary for Health Ed Brandt thought the times demanded a forth-right speech from Secretary Margaret Heckler. The homophobic tenor in the fear of AIDS rankled him. Brandt's lifelong conservatism was deeply rooted in his straight-arrow sense of right and wrong. He wanted a clear statement that AIDS would not become a tool of discrimination against gays. He also thought gays deserved a pat on the back for having organized their own volunteer educational and service organizations to cope with the disease. It was, after all, what the Reagan revolution was all about: people doing for themselves, without government programs.

Secretary Heckler agreed, although she knew she was walking into a lions' den of critics in her scheduled speech before the U.S. Conference of Mayors. The mayors of the hardest-hit cities had called for $50 million in new federal AIDS research money and the promise of a presidential signature on the $12 million already passed by the House. Already, however, officials at the Office of Management and Budget (OMB) were saying that President Reagan would veto the $12 million; he wanted new AIDS research money to be diverted from other "wasteful" programs at the Department of Health and Human Services. An additional $50 million was an unbelievable sum to try to weasel out of the OMB. Heckler opted for the usual administration tact on such issues—say everything's fine and you don't need more money.

The resulting seventeen-page speech, delivered by Secretary Heckler at the closing session of the mayor's conference in Denver, marked the first official enunciation of AIDS policy by a cabinet official, and it dominated the day's headlines.

"Nothing I will say is more important than this: that the Department of Health and Human Services considers AIDS its number-one health priority," said Heckler. "Your fight against AIDS is not a solitary one. We are in the fight with you."

After much reassurance that AIDS was not spread through casual contact, Heckler praised the "immediate" response of the National Institutes of Health and the government's "non-stop pursuit to identify the cause of AIDS."

The most intriguing part of the speech was the section that was least quoted in the mainstream media. "Any reference to sharing information would not be complete without acknowledging the excellent work done by gay networks around the nation," said Heckler. "They have responded to the crisis by offering comprehensive support to AIDS victims, and by working to inform the gay communities of the risks of AIDS, and how to minimize them. I know many of you in this audience have worked extensively with these groups, and I applaud their compassion."

By coincidence, the mayor's meeting coincided with the second National AIDS Forum. In the highly charged atmosphere, virtually every issue sparked contentious debate; the AIDS Forum turned into a festival of AIDSpeak.

The most vitriolic debates centered on the AIDS-prevention brochures the San Francisco delegation brought to the conference. The San Francisco Department of Public Health had hurriedly assembled its literature, a black-and-white flyer typed out on some department typewriter. Bill Kraus thought it was disgustingly amateurish and timid. There was no mention of bodily fluids or of specific sexual acts to avoid, such as anal intercourse. Instead, the flyer advised gays to decrease their partners, choose healthy partners, and "avoid sexual activity that may cause bleeding." The flyer and the new poster were held up as models for other cities to follow. Indeed, they were the only AIDS prevention advisories that any public health agency in the entire country had issued.

Bill Kraus and Catherine Cusic, co-chair of the Harvey Milk Club's AIDS committee, had arrived at the forum with boxes of the Milk Club's frank three-color brochure, "Can We Talk?" In cartoons and witty captions, the brochure explicitly told gay men what was safe and not safe. The advice came under such candid headings as Sucking and Fucking, with the appropriate subcategories of being sucked and sucking, being fucked and fucking. Kraus could appreciate that the health department could not issue such controversial brochures, but he thought the department should be ashamed to put its name on the sophomoric paper it was handing out at the conference.

The New York contingent, largely from Gay Men's Health Crisis, had arrived with a management plan. The neatly collated documents included flow charts and formal job descriptions that, to president Paul Popham, were the stuff of a sound organization. The booklet reflected GMHC's dedication to nonpolitical service now that Larry Kramer was off the board of directors. Its education program consisted of symposiums on AIDS with eminent scientists and researchers. Unfortunately, though, the symposiums' audiences were all full of the same 500 well-informed people. The lectures did not reach the people who needed an education most—the gay men who didn't perceive AIDS as a threat to their own lives. To this accusation, GMHC AIDS activists came up with their own addition to the AIDSpeak vocabulary: "informed choice."

"You don't tell people how to have sex," the argument went. "You give people the information about how AIDS is transmitted and you let *them* make their own informed choice."

The strategy was consistent with the New Yorkers' concerns over civil liberties. Health policy that could not pass muster with civil liberties lawyers was simply not considered. "Informed choice" had become an article of faith, not only for GMHC but for the New York Health Department, which showed no inclination to spend the money that health education would require. Even the bashful efforts of the San Francisco Department of Public Health were far too bold for these New Yorkers. When Pat Norman presented the San Francisco bathhouse poster, some New Yorkers booed openly.

The concern that rallied New Yorkers was not education but confidentiality, the preferred word in the Manhattan AIDSpeak lexicon. The issue had exploded in New York not long before when the Centers for Disease Control contacted the New York Blood Center in hopes of nailing down more transfusion AIDS cases. The CDC had asked the blood bank for a list of its donors. Citing confidentiality procedures, the blood center refused this but said that if the CDC gave them a list of all the state's AIDS patients, blood bank officials would compare the names to its roster of donors. In a moment of sheer buffoonery, the CDC complied. Even before this foul-up, New York gay doctors were angry at the CDC for its conduct of the cluster study in 1982, when researchers read names of early AIDS cases to other patients to see if they had had sexual contact with each other. Such research had helped establish that AIDS was a communicable disease, but this did not calm criticism of the CDC. Now, many New York City gay physicians refused to report AIDS cases for fear the CDC would hand out names right and left.

Like most West Coast gay leaders, Bill Kraus didn't get excited about the confidentiality issue, viewing the matter as typical East Coast closetry. Although he thought the CDC officials were idiots to give their lists to anyone, he couldn't see spending much political capital on it. After all, the people on the lists were dying—it wasn't as though they would be around for years to suffer much ignominy. New York City health officials, however, moved confidentiality to the top of their agenda. Commissioner David Sencer spoke of the need to preserve confidentiality as the city's number-one priority. This pleased the Manhattan AIDS activists and took some of the sting out of the anger they felt about the lack of any city services or education programs. The city was very good on confidentiality, they assured each other. Only a handful of cynics pointed out that confidentiality, like the gay bathhouses, was a perfect issue for David Sencer to champion, because it did not require spending a dime. Symbolism nearly always triumphed over substance in the world of AIDSpeak.

$$\bigcirc$$

The final conference reports were perfect verses of AIDSpeak. The blood policy workshop, for example, issued a report that cast important public health issues in entirely political terms. Any blood screening, the report said, "must seriously weigh such issues as donor confidentiality, and the political and social effects of the method on donor groups. . . . In effect, direct or indirect questioning has excluded gay men as a class from donating blood. The quarantine of blood is an ominous first step towards further social, political, economic and even physical quarantine of a community already denied many basic civil rights protection.

Stigmatizing the blood of an already disenfranchised segment of society may permit homophobic and racist forces to accomplish in the name of 'science' what they thus far have been unable to fully accomplish politically."

The public policy committee voted to "reaffirm our support for individual rights and vigorously oppose any attempt to legislate morality. This means that we oppose any legislative attempts to restrict sexual activities or to close private clubs or bathhouses." In a final, glorious burst of immaterial rhetoric, the committee ended its report with the observation that, "We should never forget that we live in a homophobic society, or that homophobia is the major threat to our health. We must constantly struggle against internalized homophobia as we strive for gay and lesbian wellness."

With scientists increasingly leaning toward the theory that a single viral agent caused AIDS, the political strategies workshop concluded their report with a cautionary note. "We hasten to point out that the single virus theory is just that—a theory," the workshop decided. "We believe the premature endorsement of any one theory prior to scientific proof will be devastating to the civil rights of the gay and lesbian community."

The risk-reduction workshop, which became the "Making Positive Changes in Sexual Mores Workshop," had the opportunity to make the major contribution to the conference by agreeing on guidelines that might save lives. Instead, the workshop's final report conceded, "No consensus could be reached with regard to essential versus elaborations of current risk-reduction guidelines. It was concluded that further debate was necessary."

$$\bigcirc$$

"It was concluded that further debate was necessary." Bill Kraus read the line aloud to Catherine Cusic, then wadded the paper in his hand. "Everybody in the gay community will be dead except two of these political dinosaurs debating over whether it's politically correct to tell people to stop having anal sex."

$$\bigcirc$$

Mervyn Silverman had always known he would be a doctor. His father was a dentist, so it was natural to pursue medicine and attend college close to his Washington home at Washington and Lee University. His internship at a county hospital in Los Angeles, however, convinced Silverman that he didn't want to practice medicine, so he joined the Peace Corps and served two years in Thailand. As the Peace Corps medical director for Southeast Asia, Silverman learned the value of preventive medicine and found his calling. He then earned a master's degree in public health at Harvard, and joined the Food and Drug Administration, eventually serving as director of its division of Consumer Affairs. Seeking more direct authority, he took the job as Wichita, Kansas, public health director, where he was an unlikely public official with his longish hair and handlebar mustache.

When Mayor George Moscone tapped him to be San Francisco health director in 1977, Merv Silverman knew he was moving into a highly politicized job. Unlike homogeneous Wichita, San Francisco was teeming with various constituencies, most of which were highly vocal. No fewer than thirty-four advisory committees advanced various special interests there. In San Francisco more than anywhere else in the United States, he learned, there was no separating politics from public health.

This thought recurred to Silverman in Denver when Mayor Dianne Feinstein took him aside to talk about the bathhouses. The mayor had first broached the subject in late 1982. Both her father and her second husband were doctors, giving her some definite opinions on medical matters. "If you have a problem, you get rid of it," she said. Silverman hadn't considered promiscuity to be some isolated tumor that you could separate from the body; but with AIDS, the entire gay community was the patient, he argued. Scaring the patient away from the doctor wasn't the route toward a cure.

Feinstein's concerns weren't so easily allayed now that the epidemic had moved to the front pages. She still didn't understand why Merv Silverman didn't take action against the baths. Silverman went over his logic again: A more sweeping behavior change was needed in the community, he argued. Closing the baths might merely move the sexual activity elsewhere.

Feinstein remained unconvinced, but she did not press the point in Denver. She had no authority to order Silverman to do anything, she knew, since he reported not to her but to a city manager. For his part, Silverman thought Feinstein just wanted to clean up the town for the 1984 Democratic National Convention. It didn't seem likely that the issue would go away.

June 16
CAPITOL,
WASHINGTON, D.C.

The U.S. Senate passed the $12 million AIDS supplemental appropriations bill overwhelmingly and with little debate. Although the White House threatened a veto of the larger supplemental appropriations bill in which the AIDS money was included, overpowering bipartisan support for AIDS research money was enough to ensure that it would be allocated. The sums under consideration were, after all, barely nickels and dimes out of a federal budget approaching $1 trillion.

Nevertheless, religious conservatives began to come alive on the AIDS issue. The right-wing magazine *Human Events* denounced the Senate vote. "The [appropriations of $12 million] represents a response to a massive lobbying campaign by militant homosexuals," the magazine editorialized.

It was a truism for AIDS budgets in Washington that no sooner was one proposal run through the necessary channels than scientific breakthroughs rendered it obsolete. Already circulating in the Public Health Service was a confidential memorandum indicating that the $17.6 million the Reagan administration had proposed spending on AIDS for the fiscal year beginning October 1983 was woefully inadequate for the work the CDC, NIH, and FDA wanted to undertake. To seriously tackle the burgeoning AIDS problem, the Public Health Service would need to triple AIDS funding to $52.3 million, the agency directors believed. Despite these calculations from the agency chiefs of the federal research centers, the Reagan administration put forward no new initiatives for AIDS funding. The administration's course was firm: The scientists already had all the money for AIDS research they needed.

⊂⊃

As of June 20, 1983, AIDS had stricken 1,641 Americans, killing 644, according to a special update on AIDS that the Centers for Disease Control had prepared for the weekly *MMWR*. New York City reported 45 percent of the cases; 10 percent resided in San Francisco; and Los Angeles was home to 6 percent. With the first AIDS diagnoses reported from New Mexico and Alabama, the epidemic had spread to thirty-eight states, as well as the District of Columbia and Puerto Rico. The CDC reported that another twenty-one infants in the United States were suffering from what appeared to be AIDS, although they were not yet to be included as reported cases in the CDC statistics as long as the agency was investigating other possible causes of their immune suppression. The numbers stricken with the deadly disease had precisely doubled over the last six months, and the CDC predicted that the numbers of dead and dying would double again in the last six months of 1983, and double again after that.

June 21
WASHINGTON, D.C.

Marc Conant stared across the big elliptical oak desk in the Hubert H. Humphrey Building, where the U.S. Department of Health and Human Services was headquartered. Conant had chosen his seat so he could look Thomas Donnelly in the eye. Donnelly was the Assistant HHS Secretary for Legislative Affairs. He was the man to whom agency chiefs pled their cases for more AIDS funding; he was the man telling them they could not expect the administration to approve new money for AIDS, and that they should pay for AIDS studies by looting other programs. Judi Buckalew from the White House was there too, but she was merely a special assistant to the Office of Public Liaison, a rather meaningless agency whose job it was to have meetings with people the White House didn't really want to talk to. Already the White House had distanced itself from this meeting by ordering its site changed from the Old Executive Office Building, located next to the White House, to the HHS headquarters. At the last minute, Buckalew had almost backed out of the conference altogether when National Gay Task Force leaders, who had organized the meeting, mentioned they would bring Marc Conant as well as Michael Callen, the leader of the New York People With AIDS group.

To get some common agreement on the dimensions of the crisis, Conant had prepared a one-page introduction to the epidemic for the meeting. It lay now on the oak table with its prescient final paragraph: "Western Civilization has not confronted an epidemic of this magnitude in the twentieth century. Perhaps this is why our government has been slow to respond to this challenge. Fortunately we have the knowledge and the tools to conquer an infectious disease. Emergency action is desperately needed to put these tools to work immediately to slow the spread of this epidemic and prevent a calamity of incalculable magnitude."

Marc Conant had other reasons to think Thomas Donnelly might be personally sympathetic, but his hopes were quickly dashed when Judi Buckalew set the tone for the meeting.

AIDS would be like cancer, she said. It would take years to unravel. There would be no "quick fix."

AIDS is an infectious disease, argued Conant. It will be much easier to find the cause. Moreover, even today, programs could be begun to prevent its spread.

Donnelly's tone was not condescending, just officious, Conant thought, when Donnelly dismissed Conant's worries about hundreds of thousands dead in the future.

"Once gay men realize it's a fatal disease, they'll change their behavior and it will go away," Donnelly said.

Conant thought that Donnelly, of all people, should know better.

"People aren't changing their ways," said Conant, "and people are dying. The administration needs to move faster."

A number of congressmen had called for a federal AIDS coordinator. Conant agreed, saying the work of the NIH, CDC, and FDA had to be more carefully organized with goals set and priorities arranged. "The response of our government should be the same as to an outside invasion," he said. "Unless we respond, a solution will be five or ten years down the road."

Donnelly launched into a long recitation of what the administration had done so far, a speech that had been carefully prepared for the health officials streaming to congressional inquiries with greater frequency.

It was hysterical to suggest that the time-honored peer review system for distributing grants should be expedited, Donnelly said. He couldn't believe scientists were asking that this process be short-circuited for AIDS money.

The National Gay Task Force issued a press release after the meeting, saying Virginia Apuzzo was "encouraged by the administration's commitment to maintaining a dialogue with those most affected by AIDS."

As Marc Conant boarded his jet at Washington's National Airport, he was not encouraged by anything. On the flight back to San Francisco, he wrote a letter to President Reagan. The country needed to organize experts for an expedited peer review of research and appoint an AIDS coordinator who could draft a national plan, Conant wrote. Ultimately, this epidemic could overshadow all the ambitions the president had articulated for America's future. In history, Marc Conant warned, Ronald Reagan could go down as the president who did nothing while thousands died. And thousands and tens of thousands and perhaps hundreds of thousands would die, he wrote. Most of them needlessly.

Conant gazed blankly from his small window toward the Bay Area as the plane circled for landing. He saw the fog sweeping from the sea into the western half of San Francisco, its ghostly fingers creeping over the hillsides that guard Castro Street from the ocean breezes. At forty-seven, Conant felt too old for all this. He wondered when he would ever rest.

June 23

The fund-raiser for the National KS/AIDS Foundation had all the raciness of a true San Francisco event. When host Debbie Reynolds introduced the surprise guest, actress Shirley MacLaine, with the comment that MacLaine had great legs, MacLaine responded by pulling down the top of her long strapless gown, demonstrating that she had other equipment to match. The crowd cheered enthusiastically: "We love you, Shirley." Not to be outdone, Reynolds lifted the rear of her slitted gown to reveal her brief black underwear.

"Debbie's *Tammy* image is blown forever," sighed one realtor in the audience.

"Wait till I flash," joked singer Morgana King moments later. Instead, she played it safe and stuck to crooning "My Funny Valentine."

Eyebrows raised when news of the shenanigans spread to other parts of the country, but that long had been the reflex San Francisco inspired in the hinterlands. More noteworthy was the fact that the night brought out the first array of big names to work a crowd for an AIDS benefit. In fact, the participants, who also included television actor Robert "Benson" Guillaume, were about the only big names who would associate themselves with AIDS. Most other stars, including many who had built their careers on their gay followings, were not inclined to get involved with a disease that was not . . . fashionable.

As an issue, AIDS still lacked star quality. Even among gays, the epidemic had yet to gain the aura of a trendy cause. The foundation sold far fewer tickets than it had hoped. Although the fund-raiser came out in the black, organizers had to paper the house, giving away free tickets to make sure the symphony hall looked more crowded than ticket sales would indicate. In fact, in the Castro, there was new talk: "I'm tired of gay cancer," people said. The last few months of intense media scrutiny had been exhausting; people were beginning to wish it would go away. The lines at bathhouses, which had thinned during all the publicity about posting warnings, began to swell again.

The Next Day
SAN FRANCISCO MEDICAL SOCIETY

During the summer of 1983, Dr. James Curran had grown fond of citing the "Willie Sutton Law" as evidence that AIDS was caused by a retrovirus. The notorious bank bandit Willie Sutton was asked once why he robbed banks, to which he replied, "Because that's where the money is."

"Where should we [at the CDC] put our money?" Curran would ask. "Where would Willie Sutton go? He would go with retroviruses, I think, right now."

The explanation was always good for a laugh. Jim Curran had become the federal government's ambassador of AIDS, taking his iceberg slides and scary graphs all over the country. Today he was talking to the Bay Area Physicians for Human Rights, a polite group of gay doctors who seemed downright giddy in the presence of such an important man. Curran's standard pitch now included little stories that showed how seriously the Reagan administration was taking the epidemic.

"The other day, I got a call in my hotel room—they said it was the secretary," said Jim Curran, now two years into his tenure as AIDS coordinator for the CDC. "Who got on the line but *The* secretary. Secretary Heckler. I wasn't expecting that."

As the chuckles subsided, Curran continued, "But the Secretary does support us in our efforts."

The well-mannered physicians blanched when they saw a *Chronicle* reporter trail Curran out of the room and into the men's bathroom and right up to the urinal, asking impertinent questions about the adequacy of funding resources. The polite doctors had not asked such questions, perhaps as a matter of professional courtesy to a respected colleague.

"We have everything we need," insisted Curran.

It was the message he delivered across the country that summer.

Three years later, the same reporter who had dogged Jim Curran in the lavatory asked him about those comments. Freedom of Information Act requests had revealed that things weren't so rosy at the CDC, and Curran knew it. Even while he reassured gay doctors in San Francisco, he was writing memos to his superiors begging more money.

Curran chose his words carefully.

"It's hard to explain to people outside the system," he said. "It's two different things to work within the system for a goal and talking to the people outside the system for that goal," he said. "Should I have answered: 'I've been trying to get a statistician but can't?' I knew the assistant secretary was working on budget proposals to get that. It was not time to stand up in San Francisco and announce it. Listen, you have three options: you can exit in frustration; maybe you can take a second option, exit and then become an outside voice; or you can be loyal and work on the inside. People on the outside might think you're lying or covering up. That's not true."

Besides, there weren't many willing to listen to complaints. The news media were not doing public policy stories, Curran later noted. No newspaper or television network showed any interest in using such information even if Curran had provided it. "There were only two things keeping AIDS programs alive—inside pressure and pressure from the gay community," he said. "That was it."

In Atlanta, Dr. Bruce Evatt of the CDC's Division of Host Factors was worried about how hardened the battle lines had become between blood banks and the CDC. He frequently flew to Washington to advise blood industry leaders about the mounting evidence that AIDS had contaminated the blood supply. Rather than reaching agreement on some course of action, however, each side grew more entrenched. Meetings often degenerated to blood bankers questioning Evatt's credentials as a scientist and mocking the CDC's competence to guide policy matters. Bruce Evatt had never seen such nasty personal attacks in all his years at the CDC. Repeatedly, Evatt warned the bankers that they were opening the way for negligence suits. Under special protection granted by Congress, blood banks were immune from product liability claims. But negligence was an entirely different matter, he warned. It could be argued that by now the blood banks knew better than to dispense freely blood they suspected of being infected with AIDS without taking any precautions except the cursory screening of donors. The argument, Evatt could see, carried little weight with a blood industry that considered itself above any law because of its special congressional protection.

In late June, the American Red Cross, the American Association of Blood Banks, and the Council of Community Blood Centers issued a joint statement decrying the fears about poison blood and insisting again that, if the problem existed at all, there was only "one AIDS case per one million patients transfused." As he tried to forge a consensus policy on blood, Assistant Secretary for Health Edward Brandt—the official at whose desk the buck stopped for health policy—reiterated his support for guidelines that permitted screening donors but did not require any actual testing of blood itself.

June 25
NAPLES, ITALY

As far as AIDS conferences went, the first workshop of the European Study Group on the Epidemic of Acquired Immune Deficiency Syndrome and Kaposi's Sarcoma did not attract a stellar cast of scientists. However, the conference did feature a most romantic setting, in the grand Castel del Ovo, a fifteenth-century castle set on the Bay of Naples. Dr. Michael Gottlieb was there from Los Angeles to present his current theory on a two-virus model for Kaposi's sarcoma. The cancer had presented Gottlieb with the most intriguing mysteries of the epidemic, because its appearance seemed limited to gay men. In Africa, the disease had long been linked to the CMV herpes virus, leading Gottlieb to believe that, perhaps, a second virus worked in tandem with a still-undiscovered AIDS virus to cause KS. According to his two-step idea, a person first needed infection with a virus that clobbered lymphocytes, a lymphotrophic virus, while a second virus caused the specific outbreak of KS. The lymphotrophic virus alone would bring about AIDS, under this thinking, which explained why intravenous drug users and transfusion recipients rarely experienced the skin cancer. Gottlieb's likely candidate for the KS-specific virus was CMV; he still lacked a nominee for the lymphotrophic agent.

Michael Gottlieb had read the Pasteur Institute's *Science* article on their discovery of a new human retrovirus, but he hadn't thought much of the work. Like most scientists, he needed more evidence. When Dr. Jean-Claude Chermann from the Pasteur Institute started presenting the institute's latest discoveries on its virus, Gottlieb perked up. Their virus, LAV, was incredibly cytopathic, Chermann reported, devastating the cells it infected. Gottlieb matched the viral description to the wasted immune systems he had seen as a UCLA clinician. It made sense. He raised his hand during the question session.

"Is this virus HTLV-I?" Gottlieb asked.

"Ah," said Chermann, warming to the question. "If you ask me if it's an HTLV, I'll say yes. It is a human T-cell lymphotrophic virus. But if you ask me if it's HTLV-I, no, it is not."

The Frenchman explained the differences between the core proteins and other characteristics of the virus. Meanwhile, another Pasteur immunologist, David Klatzmann, presented blood work from a variety of AIDS patients that clearly implicated LAV.

Michael Gottlieb was convinced. The French had discovered the necessary lymphotrophic virus behind AIDS. He asked Chermann to breakfast the next morning and invited the researcher to a conference he was organizing for next February at a ski resort in Utah. Unlike other conferences that dealt with a variety of epidemiological and psychosocial issues, Gottlieb wanted his symposium to be a high-powered gathering of scientific minds, dealing only with the pure science of AIDS. He hoped the seminar might light a fire under an American scientific community that had been slow to respond to the challenge of the new epidemic.

⬭

Another American AIDS researcher who was impressed by Dr. Jean-Claude Chermann's presentation was Dr. Harry Haverkos from the Centers for Disease Control. Over dinner, Haverkos, his wife, Chermann, and other Pasteur scientists toasted each other over the discovery of the virus. Haverkos wanted to fly to Paris immediately to pick up some virus that he could take back to Atlanta to study. However, because of CDC funding shortages, Haverkos couldn't add the side trip to his itinerary. The Pasteur Institute had to mail the virus to CDC, in test tubes packed in dry ice. By the time the samples arrived in Atlanta, however, the virus had died, requiring the institute to ship the virus again and delaying CDC tests on LAV for months.

June 26
SAN FRANCISCO

A contingent of people with AIDS led the 1983 Gay Freedom Day Parade, but police had received so many death threats that plainclothes officers circulated among their ranks to provide extra protection. Some of the uniformed patrolmen diverting traffic around the parade wore rubber gloves. After the festivities, four of the city employees assigned to sweep up the trash showed up in surgical masks and disposable paper suits. They were afraid they might get AIDS from the litter strewn on the streets.

Gay Freedom Day fell on Bill Kraus's thirty-sixth birthday, and that evening his friends held a small birthday party for him at his home above the Castro. Bill was less than ebullient. The onslaught of criticism over his push for a redefinition of the gay movement had disheartened him. He had figured that once the gay community realized that the AIDS epidemic posed serious perils, everyone would rally around the life-style changes that needed to be made. Instead, they were yelling at the people who proposed them.

At the party, Cleve Jones told Bill Kraus that he was leaving the country for a while. The last year of organizing the KS/AIDS Foundation had taken its toll, and the past weeks of insults and haranguing because he had signed Bill's essay had been devastating. Old friends from his street radical days called him a sexual fascist and homophobe. Cleve considered himself a gay libber, not a homophobe; he didn't know how to handle the criticism. The fight against the disease itself was also exhausting. This wasn't some political campaign that could be confronted and won. Every day was a battle, and the disease was so relentless it was hard to cull any success from his efforts, much less victory. Cleve needed to get away.

Everybody was going crazy, Bill and Cleve agreed.

In New York City, Mayor Ed Koch also had assigned extra police officers to the gay parade, fearing some outbreak of violence. In the days before the march, columnist Patrick Buchanan had released a new anti-gay diatribe calling on Mayor Koch or Governor Mario Cuomo to cancel the parade. The column quoted liberally from Anthony Fauci's discredited "routine household contact" editorial in the previous month's *Journal of the American Medical Association.* Also citing *JAMA* fears were two doctors who held a press conference on the steps of the city's Health Department building to demand the cancelation of the parade and the closure of all gay bars and bathhouses. The pair, from a group calling itself the Morality Action Committee, proposed screening all food handlers for signs of disease, and requiring airtight seals on the coffins of AIDS victims.

As in San Francisco and New York, the gay parade in Washington drew the largest turnout in history. After a day of speeches, volleyball, and music, about 650 participants took candles and marched to Lafayette Square, across the street from the White House. A light rain fell as speakers denounced the president's silence on the epidemic and the federal government's sloth.

Gesturing toward the White House, AIDS sufferer Arthur Bennett said, "I think in the beginning of this whole syndrome, that they, over there, and a lot of other people said, 'Let the faggots die. They're expendable.' I wonder if it would have been 1,500 Boy Scouts, what would have been done."

The following day, the Centers for Disease Control reported that 1,676 people had been diagnosed with AIDS in the United States, of whom 750 had died.

PART VI

RITUALS
JULY–DECEMBER
1983

The evil that is in the world always comes of ignorance, and good intentions may do as much harm as malevolence, if they lack understanding. On the whole, men are more good than bad; that, however, isn't the real point, but they are more or less ignorant, and it is this that we call vice or virtue; the most incorrigible vice being that of an ignorance that fancies it knows everything and therefore claims for itself the right to kill. The soul of the murderer is blind; and there can be no true goodness nor true love without the utmost clear-sightedness.

—ALBERT CAMUS,
The Plague

33 MARATHONS

July 1983
ALBERT EINSTEIN COLLEGE OF MEDICINE, THE BRONX, NEW YORK CITY

The baby girl, Diana, was brought to Arye Rubinstein's pediatric immunology clinic with all the classic symptoms of infant AIDS. Although only a few months old, Diana had never experienced the growth typical of infants in their first weeks of life. The parental profile was familiar too. Both the mother and father were intravenous drug users; the mother suffered from immune abnormalities such as swollen lymph nodes. Diana had an older brother with the same wasting syndrome. Dr. Rubinstein hospitalized the child for tests in Jacobi Hospital.

At first, the mother visited Diana and her brother occasionally. Then she disappeared, abandoning her two children to the care of the nurses and doctors; the white brick hospital complex in the Bronx became Diana's new home.

The scenario was repeated in the early summer months of 1983. Although AIDS may have made its splashiest debut among gay men, the disease also had taken root among the junkies of the ghettos, where shared hypodermic needles proved a remarkably efficient transmission route. The epidemic was creating its new class of victims among the children of women who were infected either through their own drug use or sexual contact with the babies' addict fathers. Abandoned or orphaned, the children were left homeless, living in municipal hospitals.

Arye Rubinstein despaired over the babies but soon arrived at a plan that might give them the semblance of a home while avoiding immense and unnecessary hospital bills. Foster parents were available for the children, Rubinstein knew, but they tended to be working people who could not care for the babies during the day. With a small day-care center, however, Rubinstein figured he could monitor the infants' medical conditions while foster parents worked. The city would save nearly $500 per day per child in medical costs.

The plan seemed both humane and cost-efficient, so Rubinstein approached city officials. Everybody was very sympathetic and praised his efforts, but nobody was interested in putting money into Rubinstein's center. This was when Rubinstein learned what gay leaders had known for two years: New York City's government had every intention of getting through the epidemic spending the least amount of money that was politically possible. Rubinstein warned that, given the projected increases of AIDS cases, such babies would be in the wards of all the city's hospitals if some plan were not instituted now. Rubinstein was dismissed as a fabulist. The doctor was shuffled from agency to agency, official to official.

New York City's reaction toward the epidemic was marked by the utter absence of any policy at all. Both state and city officials minimized the importance of the epidemic, thereby justifying their inaction. In late June, City Health Commissioner Dr. David Sencer had reported a "leveling off of cases" and proposed that gay men might be "getting immune" to the disease and that AIDS was perhaps "not as infectious as we may have thought." The chairman of the city's Human Rights Commission, Isaiah Robinson, flatly told the *Daily News,* "There is no epidemic." His calculations stemmed from the fact that 1,600 AIDS cases in a nation of 200 million meant only 1 in 100,000 Americans had contracted the disease. "One ten-thousandth of one percent is not an epidemic," he said.

In Albany, Governor Mario Cuomo was proof that official disinterest in AIDS knew no party lines. On fiscal grounds, the liberal Democrat had taken a strong stand against the Republican-dominated state senate's push to appropriate $4.5 million for AIDS research and $700,000 for education and prevention programs. The state senate voted unanimously to allocate the funds, but Cuomo threatened a veto. "It's a very good bill if you have the $5 million," Cuomo said. "I don't have the $5 million." Before a legislative investigations committee on the epidemic, Cuomo's state Health Commissioner David Axelrod dismissed criticism by saying hypertension was a more important state health issue in New York.

The vastly different political mechanics of San Francisco and New York ensured that few eastern gay leaders would launch any attacks on the officialdom. On the West Coast, gay political power was a grass-roots movement with mainstream politicians aware that their positions rested in part with their ability to please gay voters. In New York, gay power tended toward a top-down paradigm. Little evidence of a grass-roots movement existed, and gay political leaders thrived more on the favors of public officials. Though Democrats were sensitive to gay concerns, they were not as beholden to gay leaders as much as gay leaders were beholden to them. The result was tepid gay protest against official inertia, when protest existed at all.

Had gay leaders wanted to protest, there was little evidence that they could find a credible forum for their concerns. In late June, gay organizers had met with the vice-chairman of *The New York Times* in an effort to gain coverage of the community and the epidemic. Though the newspaper followed medical developments in the AIDS story, mention of the epidemic rarely appeared in the Metro section or national news reporting. Even the *Times's* recalcitrant executive editor Abe Rosenthal had sent "my regrets" to the Gay Men's Health Crisis for not covering the Madison Square Garden circus, attributing the neglect to "human error"; still, in the meeting with gay politicos, the *Times* vice-chairman had insisted the newspaper would continue to use the word "homosexual" rather than "gay" in its news coverage. The word "gay" implied happy to most people, the executive had maintained, even as he used the word in its twentieth-century meaning throughout the negotiations. After the talking was over, the amiable homosexual leaders thought they had made progress and told gay papers so. This evaluation was rebuffed by the executive's later appraisal that, "I didn't say the *Times* is open to criticism. I said it is open to suggestions."

New York City's languor staggered Dr. Mathilde Krim when she started pushing for more city services in the epidemic. In June, Dr. Krim and a number of gay doctors had organized the AIDS Medical Foundation, a group designed to spur medical interest in the disease. Soon, Krim found herself lobbying on municipal health issues, if for no other reason than few other people seemed willing to do it.

The fifty-six-year-old cancer researcher was first drawn to AIDS work in 1981 because of her work at the Memorial Sloan-Kettering Cancer Center, where she was popularly known as the "interferon queen." She had been scouting for a skin cancer with which to measure interferon's effectiveness on cancer. The mysterious appearance of KS intrigued her; tumors on the skin could be measured, providing a far more accurate appraisal of interferon's performance as a cancer-fighting agent.

As Mathilde Krim stepped up her own AIDS research in early 1983, she was surprised at the lack of coordination of services in New York City. Hospitals shied away from a leading role in facilitating an orderly response to the epidemic. The city's hospitals were petrified of being identified as an "AIDS hospital," which would surely lose them patients in the atmosphere of AIDS hysteria, so no institution was developing any specialty in the disease. Individual gay doctors built their files and collected data, but there were no AIDS clinics or wards even on the drawing boards in New York. In San Francisco, where studies were coordinated through the UCSF and San Francisco General clinics, interferon was having some effect on KS patients; in New York, Krim saw much less improvement among her subjects. The difference, she realized, was that by the time KS patients found out about her research at Sloan-Kettering, their condition had so deteriorated that they could hardly offer an accurate measure of the drug's effectiveness. They were already half-dead by the time they walked into her office.

The long-term implications of the lack of much official interest in AIDS also occurred to the researcher. Because the city had no outpatient clinics for AIDS patients, they were being needlessly hospitalized for problems that could be handled in a specialized ambulatory care facility. Lack of any home care or hospice beds also would exacerbate the problem of unnecessary institutionalization of AIDS patients, Krim saw. The cost would bear down most heavily on the city; because many patients lose their health insurance after losing their jobs, they would be forced into public hospitals. Given the projections of the spread of AIDS cases, the city faced a terrible expense. And the lack of any education programs only guaranteed that the long-incubating virus was creating fat AIDS caseloads for years to come.

By now, Krim had heard about Larry Kramer's fights with the city and had decided Kramer was right. Indignation was an entirely justified response, she thought. The city of New York was completely irresponsible.

Fortunately, Mathilde Krim carried more credentials than Larry Kramer, the angry writer who had dropped from the scene after his split with the gay group. Born in Austria, Krim had a thick Germanic accent that made her sound like an eminent researcher. She was married to Arthur Krim, the board chairman for Orion Pictures and an all-around mover and shaker in the powerful New York–Los Angeles circuit of high finance. With social connections and scientific prominence, Krim seemed a godsend to epidemic-fighters, who still lacked anyone of star quality.

None of this, she quickly discovered, made much difference.

Krim called a number of personal friends who ran prestigious medical and scientific foundations.

"AIDS is a local problem," they told her. "We deal with the big picture here."

When she started contacting city officials about lack of services, she heard, "Let's wait and see how it develops."

"If one waits and sees, it's going to be too late," Krim argued. "It will be totally out of hand and you won't have the programs to deal with it."

When pleading with Health Commissioner David Sencer yielded no results, Dr. Krim sought an appointment with Mayor Koch. Given the doctor's social connections, that proved to be no problem. The problem still was Koch.

"What should I do?" he asked at first. "The gay community doesn't like me. Everybody says I'm gay, and I'm not. I don't know what they want me to do."

Krim outlined a coordinated program of ambulatory care clinics, a home-care program, and a hospice, stressing the fiscal benefits of the plan.

"We want to see a document with numbers and proof that what you say is correct," Koch said.

When Mathilde Krim said she could provide such a document, the mayor seemed to soften.

"Okay, Mathilde, I'll make you the head of my task force on AIDS," he said.

Krim left the office feeling she had accomplished something, at last.

She never heard from Mayor Koch again.

Later compilation of AIDS diagnoses showed that during the month of July 1983, the city's AIDS caseload topped 1,000 patients. By July 30, 1,003 New Yorkers were stricken with the deadly ailment, more than had existed in the entire nation just a few months before.

⬭

On July 8, the first Australian death from AIDS was recorded at Prince Henry Hospital in Melbourne. The forty-three-year-old man, who had been living in the United States, had fallen ill on a visit home in April, doctors said. Authorities had by now confirmed four other AIDS cases in Australia and were investigating fifteen more. All twenty men reported having sex with American men in recent years.

The death engendered the first wave of AIDS hysteria on that continent. In Sydney, hospital lab workers discussed whether they should seek a ban on blood analysis of reported AIDS cases, fearing that they would contract the disease at work. One conservative religious group proposed closing all the nation's gay bars and quarantining all gay men returning from the United States. The *Medical Journal of Australia* commented, "Perhaps we've needed a situation like this to show us what we have known all along—depravity kills."

The same day the first Australian died, health authorities in Cape Town announced that five gay men in South Africa were suffering from AIDS. With 160 cases diagnosed in western Europe, socialist leaders in the European Parliament called on health authorities to ban the importation of all U.S. blood products. In France, authorities followed the American lead and began screening blood bank donors for their sexual and drug-use histories. The increase of cases in Europe prompted the World Health Organization to call an international meeting on the epidemic for November.

In San Francisco, Dr. Selma Dritz announced that AIDS was now the leading cause of death among single men in their thirties and forties. Analysis of AIDS cases further indicated that they were moving from a concentration in the Castro neighborhood to a broader cross-section of gay men living throughout San Francisco.

July 17
MIAMI

It was true of the AIDS epidemic that whenever a new discovery occurred, marking a moment things might turn more hopeful or more dark, the new turn almost always was dark, and far darker than anyone suspected.

Worst-case scenarios had so often compounded worst-case scenarios that Dr. Dale Lawrence of the Centers for Disease Control was not shocked when he went to Miami to investigate what appeared to be the first incidence of AIDS in the wife of a hemophiliac AIDS sufferer.

The seventy-year-old woman was breathless, having just recovered from her first bout with *Pneumocystis carinii* pneumonia. Her husband had died just two months ago of *Pneumocystis.* Dale quizzed her on every possible risk factor. Had they peeled vegetables together? Was there possible rectal bleeding in the shared toilet? Did the couple use the same toothbrush? There was only one risk behavior, she said, and it was far more obvious. Because the pair rarely had intercourse, Dale could estimate when the wife was infected. From the dead man's medical records, Dale soon realized that the husband had been infected with the virus long before his elderly wife. However, both became sick at virtually the same time.

The disease's incubation period could be either very long or very short, depending on the victim's own constitution. Moreover, the average incubation period for the disease could run four years, Lawrence now figured, far longer than the six months to two years that most researchers speculated.

Lawrence had spent the past year studying AIDS among hemophiliacs and blood transfusion recipients. He had long worried about what might happen to the wives and sexual partners of hemophiliacs, but the CDC, still starved for resources, had not devoted any research to this subject.

As the implications of these two AIDS cases in Miami took shape, Lawrence began to sense that the AIDS epidemic was unfolding in separate waves, or more precisely, like different marathons begun at differing times. The first race was run by gay men with AIDS. Another race, run by the recipients of blood products, had started much later, but its first runners had made it over the finish line in 1982, not much behind the runners of the first race. The hemophiliac's wife who had moved from infection to disease so rapidly was like the runner of still another marathon, making it across the finish line with her husband, even though he had started much earlier than she. She simply needed less time to complete the course. The first cases in this or that remote state, and this or that country, were merely the leading edge of the first race, and the "winners" of the second race would be arriving soon, even though they were not yet visible. The bulk of the runners had yet to come within sight of the race's end.

Standing at the finish line, the CDC was only clocking the arrival times. With the blood cases, where an infection date could be objectively ascertained by transfusion records, the CDC saw only the average times of the swiftest runners, who came down with AIDS two, four, or six months after their transfusion. The people who already had withstood two, three, or four years of incubation were yet to come.

Back in Atlanta, Dale Lawrence noted in his back issues of *Lancet* a study that had been conducted in San Francisco on the infection rate of gastrointestinal parasites among gay men. The study included a chart marking the steep curve of parasitic infection through the late 1970s and early 1980s. They were the very curves that had worried Selma Dritz years before, when she fretted about what would happen if some new infectious agent got loose in this population. Lawrence charted the numbers of AIDS cases in San Francisco and compared this curve to the *Lancet* curve on parasitic infections. They were virtually identical—but about five years apart. The slope of AIDS, of course, had just begun. Given the incubation period he now predicted, Lawrence had no doubts that AIDS would increase as dramatically as the parasite pandemic.

Meanwhile, as the Centers for Disease Control continued to struggle against a blood banking industry that preferred not to believe in the existence of transfusion-associated AIDS, a pharmaceutical company was licensed to start manufacturing heat-treated Factor VIII. The product was introduced to end the threat of hepatitis transmission from the clotting factor, and the CDC doctors figured that the heat used to sterilize the product also would kill the viral agent that they assumed was the cause of AIDS. However, the pharmaceutical company planned to price the heat-treated Factor VIII at double the cost of the traditional injections. A year's worth of treatment for this sterilized material, therefore, would cost the typical hemophiliac between $16,000 and $24,000, according to the estimates of CDC hemophilia expert Dr. Bruce Evatt. Few hemophiliacs could afford the more expensive treatment. Evatt considered the heat-treated material to be outrageously priced but could not argue for greater availability of the formula on the grounds of AIDS prevention. The CDC had not yet definitively proved the existence of an AIDS virus, much less isolated the microbe responsible for the plague. The agency was in no position to make demands of major corporations.

Within the federal government or the public health establishment, the CDC found little support for its concern about the integrity of the nation's blood supply. The administration's top health officials, most notably Health and Human Services Secretary Margaret Heckler and Assistant Secretary for Health Dr. Edward Brandt, toed the blood banks' line that there was minimal if any chance of contracting the disease through blood.

"I want to assure the American people that the blood supply is 100 percent safe," said Secretary Heckler in early July, when she went to the Washington, D.C., Red Cross office to donate blood. As a model citizen, Heckler spent half an hour filling out the medical form for the self-deferral program, to demonstrate the effectiveness of donor deferral. "The blood supply is safe both for the hemophiliac who requires large transfusions and for the average citizen who might need it for surgery," Heckler said at a Red Cross press conference.

Like blood banks across the country, the Washington facility had suffered a dramatic drop in donations during the preceding weeks of intense publicity over AIDS. In June, donations fell by 16 percent; in July, the level of donations in many blood centers was off 30 percent from the previous year. Spot shortages of blood occurred in urban areas. Controversy raged about consumers across the country who clamored for "designated" donor programs in which persons looking ahead to surgery would have friends and relatives donate blood specifically for their use. All the major blood banking organizations urged their members not to permit directed donations, fearing that the designated donor route would cause havoc in the blood industry.

"We want to help curb the panic," said Dr. Herbert Perkins, medical director of San Francisco's Irwin Memorial Blood Bank, when he announced that his center would ban designated donors. "The risk of getting AIDS from a transfusion is about one in a million."

With the best of intentions, the establishment rallied to support the blood banks; after all, you couldn't let hysteria undermine an institution that, undeniably, was a cornerstone of American medicine. Local public health officials demonstrated their interest by minimizing the threat of transfusion AIDS. In Los Angeles, for example, the announcement that three infants had died of AIDS probably contracted through transfusions brought heated denials from hysteria-wary local officials. "Unless you can find a direct link between a person with AIDS who exposed the infant in some way, it is difficult to call it AIDS," said Dr. Shirley Fanin, associate deputy county health director. Fanin said the cases probably stemmed from congenital immune defects. The doctors argued that the immune profiles were those of AIDS patients, not the victims of genetic immune problems, but to little avail.

In Washington, Secretary Heckler and Assistant Secretary Brandt delivered familiar reassurances at another news conference to counter fear over the Los Angeles cases. "I think it is very important that the public have confidence in the safety of our blood supply," said Heckler. Even if the cases did turn out to be AIDS, Brandt said, the problem was that the transfusions were given before the donor-deferral guidelines were established. "We think the guidelines will help considerably" to reduce risk, he said.

As was so often the case, the media became an integral part of the story. Seeing themselves as the bastions of common sense, science writers and reporters covering the epidemic also wrote curb-the-panic stories and avoided asking the blood bankers tough questions. Although there was ample evidence that gay men were sexually transmitting the disease to each other long before they showed any overt symptoms, the media accepted the blood bankers' assertion that transfusion AIDS could only be proved when a diagnosed AIDS case had given blood to a person later diagnosed with the disease. This is why *only* those people showing overt symptoms of the disease were disallowed from donating blood under the deferral guidelines, which remained the only protection Americans had against transfusion AIDS.

Rancor grew between blood banks and CDC researchers, who continued to insist that the banks needed to test the blood itself for signs of past hepatitis infection, and that deferral guidelines needed to be much broader. By summer, Dr. Harry Haverkos, who was organizing all the transfusion cases into a formal report on the AIDS danger, found blood bankers were becoming openly hostile to the agency. He now had documented ten transfusion cases. With the third case, he was convinced of the danger and was astounded that the Food and Drug Administration remained so skeptical of the CDC's conclusions. To the disbelieving blood bankers, he finally asked in exasperation, "Tell us a number you need. If we have 20, 40, 100 cases—will you believe it then?"

◯

At Stanford University Hospital Blood Bank, Dr. Ed Engleman was less convinced than most of his colleagues that donor-deferral guidelines were effective. The Stanford blood bank remained one of the only blood centers in the country to screen blood. One in fifty donations was being discarded because of immune irregularities. In July 1983, one donor imparted his "gift of life" at a bloodmobile visiting his work site. The blood, however, was discarded after Stanford tests measured the ratio of T-helper to T-suppressor lymphocytes to be .29 to 1, far below the average ratio of 2 to 1. The ratio was either the result of a botched test or severe immune problems. As was routine, the blood bank asked the donor, a thirty-nine-year-old male, to return to the blood bank for a battery of follow-up tests.

The man made the appointments but never showed up. Eight months later he was diagnosed with Kaposi's sarcoma. By that time, he had donated blood at all the major Bay Area blood banks, including the two largest, Irwin Memorial Blood Bank in San Francisco and the San Jose Red Cross. In fact, between 1981 and 1984, the man had donated blood thirteen times in Bay Area blood banks. The man's blood had antibodies to the core of the hepatitis B virus, and would have been eliminated had blood banks instituted the test the CDC had sought in January 1983. But he did not display visible symptoms of AIDS in those years, nor did he fit into any of the categories covered by the FDA's deferral guidelines. (In San Francisco, in fact, the first five months of donor deferral had weeded out only 16 donors of the 50,000 screened.) After repeated questioning, the man had conceded that he had had three to five different male sexual contacts over the past several years.

Only at Stanford, where blood was tested, was this man's blood discarded; eleven recipients of blood transfusions provided by other blood centers were not so fortunate.

SAN FRANCISCO

The same day that Dr. Dale Lawrence went to Miami, Gary Walsh found himself staring into a television monitor at the face of Rev. Jerry Falwell, live via satellite hookup from his headquarters in Lynchburg, Virginia. The local ABC affiliate had put together an hour-long show called "AIDS: The Anatomy of a Crisis."

The fundamentalist minister had recently entered into the AIDS debate. He didn't hate homosexuals, he said, just their "perverted life-style." Gay bathhouses, the sites of "sub-animal behavior," should be shut down, Falwell said, and blood donors should be required to fill out questionnaires about their sexual orientation. "If the Reagan administration does not put its full weight against this," he said, "what is now a gay plague in this country, I feel that a year from now, President Ronald Reagan, personally, will be blamed for allowing this awful disease to break out among the innocent American public."

Falwell began his televised discussion with Dr. Merv Silverman and Gary Walsh by citing Galatians. "When you violate moral, health, and hygiene laws, you reap the whirlwind," he said. "You cannot shake your fist in God's face and get by with it."

"My God is not a vengeful God," Gary Walsh countered. "When those children died of polio in the fifties, they were not punished by God. One of the most perverted uses of religion is to use religion to justify hatred for your fellowman."

Falwell smiled benevolently. "Gary has nothing but my compassion, love, and prayers," he said.

"I appreciate your prayers," Gary responded. "I'm quite a sensitive person. I have a hard time feeling that you do have that compassion, that caring, and that love for me, given that I'm gay. That does not come across. What comes across is your anger, your hysteria, and your pointing a finger. That comes across, but your compassion doesn't."

"I do have compassion for you," Falwell replied, "but I'd be less than honest if I told you that I find the homosexual life-style acceptable."

Falwell went on to say that his church had seven psychiatrists and counselors on call to help cure homosexuals. Gary said that his homosexuality wasn't what he wanted cured.

"I would publicly and personally like to invite Jerry [Falwell] to fly to San Francisco and spend a day with me," Gary said. "I would like to open my heart to him. Maybe we could learn from each other. I'll pay your way even."

Falwell didn't bat an eyelash. "I'd love to do that," he said. "Gary wouldn't have to pay my way. I'd love to come to San Francisco, pray with him, and read the Gospel, and show that kind of love."

Falwell changed the subject to blood transfusions, but Gary interrupted.

"When are you coming?" Gary asked.

Falwell ignored him and kept talking about blood transfusions.

"I'd like to know when you could do this," said Gary. "Let's set up a time."

"Gary," Falwell said. "I'd like to do that. Just write me, Jerry Falwell, Lynchburg, Virginia. Mark it personal. I will get it. I will be in touch with you. I will do everything I can to help you in every way possible."

That ended the show. Gary wrote Falwell and reminded the pastor that he had promised on television to come and spend a day with him in San Francisco. He was not surprised, however, that Falwell never answered his letter.

VANCOUVER

Gaetan Dugas loved slipping back into his navy-blue flight attendant's uniform for Air Canada. Although he was growing weaker and his health appeared to be slipping, he needed to return to work to keep his travel benefits. Other attendants were enraged at being forced to work with an AIDS victim and complained to management. Air Canada, however, was a government airline and found itself to be in no position to discriminate. Gaetan was kept on short flights, usually from Vancouver, British Columbia, to Calgary, Alberta, where he wouldn't get worn out. Sometimes at night, terror stalked his thoughts and he would call up friends to spend the night on the couch, just so he wouldn't have to be alone.

One evening, another steward was over at Gaetan's watching the news when Jerry Falwell came on, bellowing about AIDS and God's wrath. Gaetan grew sullen. His friend was surprised he didn't have some smart-ass comment.

"Maybe Falwell is right," said Gaetan. "Maybe we are being punished."

34 JUST ANOTHER DAY

On July 26, 1983, the CDC reported that 1,922 Americans had been stricken with AIDS. The disease had spread to thirty-nine states and twenty nations. The average age of the typical AIDS victim was thirty-five. Although only 39 percent of the total caseload was dead, the new figures did not offer a hopeful prognosis. Of all the people diagnosed with AIDS on or before July 26, 1982, at least two-thirds were dead. Few survived among the people who had suffered from the disease two years before.

July 26, 1983, was a warm and sunny Tuesday in most parts of the country. It was a day of scientific jealousies, academic intrigue, and funding shortages roundly ignored by reporters. Brushfires of hysteria flared, died away, and flared again. New computers spit out death tolls, doctors wondered when people would start caring, and thousands of Americans watched their lives slip away. In the history of the AIDS epidemic, it was just another day.

CENTERS FOR DISEASE CONTROL, ATLANTA

Don Francis had heard of Robert Gallo's legendary temper, but the meeting that morning was the first time he had seen the famed scientist's churlishness in full force. The gathering had been called to try to coordinate the search for the retrovirus responsible for Acquired Immune Deficiency Syndrome. The CDC had spent the past two years gathering specimens from cases and controls in their various AIDS studies. The National Cancer Institute had the technology and expertise to explore the CDC specimens for an answer to the epidemic. At this point, however, neither agency was sure of what the other was doing; it was time they started working together.

Earlier, Don Francis had explained the status of CDC lab work to Robert Gallo as he drove the retrovirologist from the airport to the CDC's Clifton Road headquarters. Francis had been searching for more than a year for a major retrovirology lab for AIDS work. Given the problems he faced in setting up a

CDC retrovirus lab, Francis was relieved that, at last, the National Cancer Institute seemed genuinely interested in doing research on the epidemic of immune deficiency.

For the meeting, the key CDC people involved in AIDS studies assembled in Director Walter Dowdle's office at the Center for Infectious Diseases with Dowdle's assistant John Bennett, Jim Curran, and Bruce Evatt. Harvard researcher Dr. Max Essex and an associate, fresh from research on links between AIDS and HTLV-I, had flown in from Boston. The talks broke down when Dr. Essex's associate mentioned their work on cell line CT-1114. For some reason, this CDC cell line, which had been infected with blood from AIDS patients, had burst forth with viral activity. The CDC had sent it to Essex's lab so the Harvard doctor could perform tests to see whether HTLV-I or HTLV-II was present, perhaps giving an indication of whether the viruses caused AIDS. Essex was using monoclonal antibodies in the studies.

Gallo interrupted and asked sharply where the antibodies came from.

Essex's younger associate said that they had come from samples Gallo had previously sent to him. Gallo exploded.

"How can you collaborate with me and you're doing stuff behind my back?" he shouted. "If you're using my materials on anything, I need to know about it in advance. You need my approval."

Gallo spent the next forty-five minutes berating Essex and his colleague. The CDC doctors were aghast. This guy came all the way to Atlanta so he could spend all this time abusing some junior researcher? This was the ugly side of the National Cancer Institute that the CDC researchers sometimes talked to each other about. To the more socially conscious CDC staffers, the NCI was a repository for researchers concerned with little more than personal glory. For their part, the NCI scientists tended to view the CDC researchers as naive do-gooders who needed to move over for the "big boys" when a serious crisis evolved. The outburst confirmed the CDC's darkest suspicions about the NCI and left the CDC officials visibly embarrassed by Gallo when the meeting was over.

Robert Gallo seemed embarrassed himself as Don Francis drove him back to the airport after the conference.

"I got carried away," Gallo confided. "My Italian style."

Francis was forgiving. He understood what Gallo knew about himself: that his greatest strength was also his major fault. The temper and arrogance were what made Gallo a formidable enemy to disease.

<hr>

Momentum propelled news coverage of the AIDS epidemic, and six months of growing media movement peaked in late July, bringing camera crew after camera crew to a simulated lab in a corner of the CDC headquarter's gym. The bogus lab was used to minimize interruptions in the real CDC work going on in labs. Here sundry teams from all the Eyewitness News and Instant Eye shows enthused that the CDC was on the trail of the killer, and that this or that "breakthrough" heralded a possible end to the disease. In early July, *Time* magazine had done a CDC cover, entitled "Disease Detectives: Tracking the Killers," and by July 26, *Newsweek* reporters walked the CDC hallways in preparation for their cover story due out in two weeks. Between July and September, the nation's major print media churned out 726 stories on AIDS, more than would appear in any other single quarter for another two years. In Washington, the Public Health Service issued regular bulletins to the press, making specious claims that "large [NIH] awards have already been made" for AIDS studies and that the CDC had embarked on "intensive laboratory investigations to identify the infectious agent of AIDS." The CDC's efficient media relations staff also provided videotapes of CDC scientists actually performing real AIDS research for the various Ken-and-Barbie television news teams.

Despite the reporters' optimistic chatter, personnel at the CDC's AIDS Activities Office recall these months as the most frustrating in the course of the epidemic. A new computer surveillance system was set up to monitor national AIDS trends more efficiently. Two months before, the CDC had made AIDS a reportable disease, requiring state and territorial health officials to report all known cases to Atlanta. Most state health officials, by now, had issued similar requirements to their county health authorities. The earlier dark predictions segued to reality, with the numbers mounting quickly. During the first six months of 1983, there were as many new AIDS cases as had been reported in all of 1981 and 1982 combined. One in six of all the nation's AIDS cases had been reported in just the past six weeks. The rapid increases in AIDS cases, however, revealed no new trends among victims. AIDS was not breaking new ground in the United States; instead, it was on its way to wiping out the people who had been identified for more than a year as the high-risk groups.

Reporters were routinely given bloated numbers about how many CDC researchers were working on AIDS, but in truth, the AIDS disease detectives numbered only between twenty-five and thirty, and they were nearly always behind in their work. Every new lead meant an old lead could not be followed. That summer, the hottest new lead sprang from all the European medical journal reports on the Zairian connection with AIDS. A CDC team was dispatched to Zaire to investigate.

A staff harried by pressing new demands barely had time to analyze even the old research. Only in August, nearly two years after it was launched, was the original case-control study slated to be published in the *Annals of Internal Medicine*. Difficulties in getting computer time for statistical analysis, and the business-as-usual publication schedules of medical journals, conspired to stall the dissemination of this essential AIDS information.

It seemed the CDC doctors were always on the phone with one or another local health official, or delivering the same old reassurances to the reporters. Later, dispirited AIDS staffers at the CDC complained they spent more time in July 1983 controlling AIDS hysteria than controlling AIDS.

⬭

On July 26, 1983, in Reno, Nevada, the National Gay Rodeo was only days away from opening. The Pro-Family Christian Coalition had organized opposition to the annual rodeo, which routinely drew 50,000 gays, for fear that all those homosexuals would spread AIDS throughout Nevada. The group took out full-page ads in local papers, urging the county government to cancel the contract allowing the gay organization to use the Washoe County Fairgrounds for the event. To buttress their arguments, the group recruited Dr. Paul Cameron, a longtime homophobe from Nebraska, who described the gay community as a "living, breathing cesspool of pathogens." Cameron also said, "Here is a subclass of people, who, as a function of their sexuality, are consuming prodigious amounts, from a medical standpoint, of fecal material. Any community that allows thousands of these people to congregate will run a considerable risk, not only from AIDS but other disease such as viral hepatitis." Cameron cited the *Journal of the American Medical Association* on "routine household contacts" as ample evidence for his views.

The Reverend Walter Alexander of Reno's First Baptist Church went one step further by telling reporters that, "I think we should do what the Bible says and cut their [homosexuals'] throats." The man who ran the anti-rodeo ads in the local newspapers opined that he didn't want to see anybody actually murdered because of the ads, although he wouldn't criticize Alexander's comments directly because the minister clearly had authority to speak on matters "biblical."

Few regions were immune to the AIDS anxiety sweeping the United States. In New York City, a bank robber used that fear, handing tellers a note demanding cash. "I have AIDS," the note read, "and I have less than 30 days to live." The strategy worked. One bank employee later admitted she could have dropped behind her bandit barrier and called for help, but she said she was so worried that she might have contracted AIDS from touching the note that she handed the man all $2,500 in her till. At a Chemical Bank branch, a teller broke out laughing when she read the note, thinking it was a joke. She was showing the note to other tellers and was still laughing as the disgruntled bandit made his way out the door empty-handed. By the time police captured the robber in mid-August, he had used the tactic in robbing ten banks of $18,000. He did not have AIDS.

Rumors spread that this or that celebrity had AIDS, often fostered by gay activists convinced that the epidemic would not get serious government attention until it hit somebody famous. In New York, Calvin Klein gave an interview to deny the widespread rumors that he had AIDS. He was "ridiculously healthy," he maintained. Apparently, rumor-mongers confused Klein with designer Perry Ellis, who died of AIDS three years later.

The Alert Citizens of Texas inflamed local fears with their brochure "The Gay Plague," which provided detailed descriptions of bathhouses, rimming, and golden showers. A nationally distributed *Moral Majority Report* also explored every unsavory aspect of gay life in gory full-color detail. And Rev. Jerry Falwell now told concerned Americans that they could fight the spread of AIDS by giving money to him.

In Seattle, gay-bashing was less figurative that week, as gangs of youths roved Volunteer Park, a local gay cruising spot, and beat up gay men with baseball bats, shouting invectives about "plague-carrying faggots" and "diseased queers." One gang raped two men with a crowbar. Once arrested, one attacker told police, "If we don't kill these fags, they'll kill us with their fucking AIDS disease."

Nationally, the response was less severe, although the marked lack of hysteria among most Americans received very little press. A Gallup poll conducted in late June reported that 77 percent of Americans had heard or read about AIDS. A second survey of adults quizzed on July 20 and 21, found that 91 percent had been exposed to AIDS information. Of these, 25 percent thought there was a chance they could get AIDS from casual contact with an AIDS sufferer. Of the one-quarter of respondents who said they had gay friends, only 21 percent said they were less comfortable in a homosexual's company. Although gay activists across the country defended such institutions as bathhouses on the belief that Americans were ready to confine gays to concentration camps, the poll revealed that support of gay rights had grown in the past year, with 65 percent of Americans supporting equal job opportunities for gays. This represented a 6 percent increase in gay rights support since 1982.

Hysteria stories were juxtaposed with those peddling false hope. That summer various snake-oil salespeople, including Swami Shri Mataji Mirmala Devi from India, claimed to have the power to cure AIDS. One San Francisco diet therapist lectured eager gay men on "Cum as an Indicator of Health." According to this dietician, men could monitor their health by examining the consistency of their semen. A press release boasted that he also could "talk about foods that are cum enhancers." Federal postal inspectors cracked down on a company that, for $1,900, would send AIDS victims an injection treatment that would cure the deadly syndrome.

The response of the U.S. Department of Health and Human Services to the mounting hysteria and misinformation was its toll-free hotline, which took between 10,000 and 13,000 callers a day. This was no small feat because the service, with its six operators, was designed with neither urgency nor a national perspective in mind. Indeed, more than 90,000 calls that came in to the hotline went unanswered just in the month of July.

Like most of the summer's hysterical episodes, the flare-up over the Reno Gay Rodeo produced more heat than light. On the night of July 26, the county commission's gallery was crowded with reporters, fundamentalists, and anxious gays from San Francisco, who had come to make sure boxcars weren't being readied in the hinterlands. The Washoe County Commission listened to the fundamentalists' fears and the researchers' reassurances, and determined that it could not legally break its contract with the National Gay Rodeo Association. Some 45,000 people bought tickets for the rodeo days, and there was no later appreciable increase in the number of AIDS or hepatitis casualties.

The last word on the controversy, however, came from Action for Animals, an animal rights group based in Berkeley, California, which expressed its indignation in letters to San Francisco's gay papers. Gays should be ashamed of any sport, the group wrote, that is based on the "exploitation and abuse of non-humans."

The day that Robert Gallo met with CDC officials in Atlanta, Assistant Secretary for Health Edward Brandt put together a new request for $35 million worth of further AIDS research at the Public Health Service. Brandt originally had requested the money for fiscal year 1984, which was due to begin in three months. Now, however, he asked Secretary Margaret Heckler for permission to go to the Office of Management and Budget for approval of the funds "on an accelerated business."

Brandt understood the dangers of his request. Congress had only recently approved the $12 million supplemental AIDS funds; another appeal so soon was guaranteed to generate a hard look by the cost-conscious OMB. Nevertheless, Brandt wrote, "Each of these proposals addresses a critical health need which is receiving increased public attention and congressional scrutiny. At the same time, these three items are appropriate areas of federal involvement in which the department should continue its leadership role." Brandt attached a six-page, single-spaced breakdown of how the FDA, CDC, and NIH would spend the money.

"The request for each of these agencies assumes that by FY [fiscal year] 1984 [October] a causative agent will have been isolated and a reliable screening test will have been developed," Brandt concluded.

Without such a breakthrough, the agencies would need even more money.

The next day, Secretary Heckler announced that, in keeping with the administration's commitment to AIDS as its "number-one health priority," the government would step up its AIDS education efforts by adding new staff to its toll-free AIDS hotline. She made no comment about added funds for AIDS research.

On Capitol Hill, Representative Ted Weiss prepared for the subcommittee hearing on federal AIDS funding to be held in a few days. He still struggled with the Department of Health and Human Services for permission to allow congressional investigators to review CDC budget records. However, the agency had turned over many of the relevant internal memoranda, two of which were of particular interest to Weiss. One, which came through less-than-formal channels, was from the National Cancer Institute, ordering that before any interviews with congressional investigators, NCI researchers should advise agency officials and "invite" a top administrator to attend. So much for an independent inquiry, Weiss thought.

A second memo, dispatched by CDC Director William Foege, simply told federal agency heads that, "All material submitted to the Congress must evidence the Department's support of the administration's stated policies."

At about the same time that Don Francis dropped Robert Gallo off at the Atlanta airport, reporters in San Francisco were being led through the cheerful yellow and orange hallways of a newly redecorated hospital ward that, until recently, was used by interns for naps between shifts. Now, San Francisco General Hospital's Ward 5B was the AIDS Ward.

All the nurses were volunteers. About half were gay men and the other half were women. All had undergone extensive encounter sessions to examine their sentiments about death and dying. Cliff Morrison, a gay clinical nurse specialist, organized and designed the ward as he saw fit, because the more important hospital administrators all seemed rather embarrassed by the ward and the disease. The thirty-two-year-old Morrison was a dedicated idealist who disliked the hierarchical doctor-nurse-patient model that dominated hospitals. Doctors would not run this ward; he would, and he wouldn't even call himself head nurse, preferring instead the less authoritative moniker of "nursing coordinator." Patients would have a louder voice in their own care, which only made sense, Morrison noted, because they usually knew more about the intricacies of their often-experimental medications than their doctors.

Community groups, such as the Shanti Project, which recently had opened its first city-funded residences for homeless AIDS patients, had free rein in Ward 5B. Volunteers from a number of AIDS organizations and gay religious groups bustled from room to room. The day that patients went in, a social services worker began developing a plan for their life after they left. Morrison also rejected the idea of visiting hours as a concept designed for the convenience of nurses rather than patients, and he instituted policies to permit visitors to stay overnight if they wished.

There were also conversations with every patient about code status. Upon respiratory failure from, say, *Pneumocystis* pneumonia, a patient could ask for code-blue status, a request that hospital staff use all necessary means to preserve his life. Usually that meant a respirator. After two years of experience with AIDS patients, however, doctors found that 85 percent of *Pneumocystis* sufferers who went on a ventilator never came off the contraption. They died a miserable and silent death, with a tube stuck down their throats. In Ward 5B, most patients opted to go without the blue code, asking that no extraordinary measures be used to preserve their lives. In the months to come, more patients in Ward 5B made that choice than in all the other hospital wards combined.

When Cliff Morrison and Dr. Paul Volberding, the AIDS Clinic director, cut the ribbon for the opening of Ward 5B on that Tuesday afternoon, Volberding was amazed that hospitals elsewhere, particularly in New York City, weren't planning similar wards; the facilities clearly would benefit both patients and doctors, who were still struggling to understand the grisly array of AIDS complications. It seemed that every new *MMWR* reported some new disease associated with the syndrome, some of which were maladies that most typically strike animals.

New research indicated that whatever virus killed the T-lymphocytes of AIDS patients also caused malfunctions of B-lymphocytes, another key component of the immune system. Neurological symptoms were becoming more common. Cases of lymphadenopathy were now so common that the CDC had recently defined a new phenomenon called AIDS-Related Complex, or ARC.

In a conference call with a number of AIDS researchers, including Dr. Don Abrams, assistant director of the AIDS Clinic, the CDC arrived at what Abrams called a "Chinese menu" approach for its definition. A person had ARC if he or she had two clinical conditions or certain lab test results on the CDC list. Two from column A and two from column B constituted ARC. The most pressing question was whether ARC was always a precursor to AIDS or simply a milder infection. In his two-year-old study of 300 lymphadenopathy patients, Don Abrams hoped to show that ARC was a healthy reaction to infection with an AIDS virus. Patients got swollen lymph nodes and a few mild infections like thrush, Abrams hypothesized, while their bodies kept enough lymphocytes to fight off one of the deadlier diseases associated with AIDS. Abrams's optimism was fueled by the observation that only a handful of the lymphadenopathy cohort had actually come down with AIDS—so far. However, Abrams wasn't sure what to make of the strange disorders of the central nervous system that he was beginning to see among these patients.

Each day of work resulted in a new level of despair for Don Abrams, Paul Volberding, and the other staffers at the AIDS Clinic. Volberding prided himself in patient involvement. He came to know the lover, helped bridge any problems with the family, and then watched the patient make that last, desperate gasp for breath before dying. As the number of new cases mounted in San Francisco, and scores of worried men in the early stages of AIDS infection filled the waiting room of the AIDS Clinic, Volberding considered the national funding problems surrounding AIDS research.

Like most AIDS clinicians, Paul Volberding had been forced into the unfamiliar realm of politics to scare up more money and attention for the epidemic. In the board of directors meetings at the National KS/AIDS Foundation, Volberding often was the only heterosexual in the room. He had always seen the gay community as a monolithic bloc and was surprised at its various factions and political divisions. Rather than unite them, AIDS divided them further.

Still, among AIDS patients, Volberding saw the truth of what he long had believed: The viruses that bring disease also bring out the best in people. This certainly was true with AIDS. Dramas of courage and reconciliation played daily in the clinic rooms and hospital deathbeds. On the streets, there was talk of lovers abandoning their AIDS-stricken partners, but the most commonly enacted stories were of unparalleled fidelity. Some families abandoned their "leper" children, but most often mothers and fathers, sisters and brothers, crowded around the sick men's bed, often returning to offer a last measure of devotion after years of estrangement. For many families, news of a Kaposi's sarcoma or *Pneumocystis* diagnosis rendered a dual diagnosis, informing the parent both of the child's disease and sexual orientation. Still, it mattered little, Volberding saw. Reconciliation was a far more common scenario for AIDS patients and their families than abandonment.

There was also the bravery of these men facing an early death. Routinely, they allowed Volberding or the other AIDS Clinic doctors to poke, prod, and puncture them in a vain attempt to find something that might offer a clue to the disease's cause. Although it was clear that any medical discoveries would come too late to help these patients, few failed to voice the hope that maybe that last blood sample, painfully drawn from a near-collapsed vein, would save others from suffering. Maybe it would save others from dying.

On July 26, the day the Medical Special Care Unit for AIDS opened in Ward 5B, all but two of its dozen beds were filled. Within days, however, an AIDS patient occupied every bed in the ward, and there would be no vacancies from then on.

○

After he saw the death notice of someone with whom he had gone to bed a couple of years back, Gary Walsh had stopped scanning the obituaries in the *Bay Area Reporter* for signs of the person who might have infected him. Lesions were coating Gary's stomach, making it difficult for him to eat. He had occasional dizzy spells, and his doctors were testing him for cryptococcus. Walking was painful because of severe athlete's foot that had appeared from nowhere one day. God only knew why his joints ached so much. But he still thought he might make it. The press was full of talk about promising breakthroughs. Maybe he still had a future.

In the meantime, everybody in the gay community was at everybody else's throat. Gary's friend Joe Brewer had written a series of articles in the *Bay Area Reporter,* urging gay men to modify their sexual life-styles. For this, Joe was denounced as a "sexual fascist." Gary had developed his own plan for AIDS prevention in San Francisco. "They should put one of us at the end of every gay bar in town," he told Lu Chaikin. "Then they would know what AIDS is really all about."

○

The University of California AIDS researchers had broken ranks with the university to get funds directly from the legislature. By late July, it was clear they were going to pay for that aggressive move.

The state government of California moved with amazing speed to fund the AIDS research grants assembled by Marc Conant in April. Without any serious opposition, the legislature passed the $2.9 million; by late July, the governor had approved the funds. Although the legislature cannot allocate funds for specific university projects, Assembly Speaker Willie Brown's staff thought they had an agreement with university officials that the funds would be released immediately for AIDS doctors. Unfortunately, the appearance of a windfall in research money stirred a hornet's nest of jealousy among other researchers. Suddenly, doctors who had demonstrated no interest in the epidemic before began calling UC administrators with ideas for AIDS research, and university officials announced they would not release any funds directly to AIDS researchers. Instead, doctors would submit grant proposals, which would undergo the same languorous reviews that any funding applications faced in the UC system. With the sluggishness that characterized the academic response to the epidemic, funding requests were shifted from committee to committee within the university system. Finally, the university announced a deadline for applicants in October and slated the first meeting of the university review committee for October 15. With luck, the university could start releasing funds in December.

Marc Conant couldn't believe it. The reason the funds had been sought in the first place was because of similar delays at the National Institutes of Health. The university made some deference to AIDS doctors' pressure by releasing $819,000 in small grants to researchers. These grants were so small that some researchers refused them, saying the amounts were not enough even to buy equipment, much less begin any serious research. The university also set aside $740,000 for clinical research centers to be headed by Paul Volberding in San Francisco and Michael Gottlieb in Los Angeles. But most of the money that had been assigned for scientific, nonclinical research was untouchable.

Word quickly spread through the UC system that administrators were exacting academic retribution on researchers who had dared defy university hierarchy to get funding directly from the legislature. As pressure mounted on university officials, however, they only dug in their heels. It soon became clear that doctors who complained about delays also would pay.

$\bigcirc$

Larry Kramer had been in Europe for a month. In late July, in Munich, Germany, he was killing time; he had no idea what to do with himself. It was three years since that summer on Fire Island when he had talked to Enno Poersch about the mysterious disease haunting Enno's lover Nick. It was barely two years since he had held the first AIDS fund-raiser in his apartment and organized the Gay Men's Health Crisis. Christ, it seemed like a lifetime ago, he thought. It was his life Before.

In Munich, Larry saw a sign that said "Dachau." He took the subway to a streetcar, which took him to a bus that made its way through the suburbs to the famous death camp.

"Dachau was opened in 1933," Larry read in the museum.

He stood there stunned. He had had no idea the camp had opened so early, just months after Adolf Hitler assumed power in Germany. World War II started for the United States in 1941, Larry thought.

"Where the fuck was everybody for eight years?" he wanted to shout. "They were killing Jews, Catholics, and gays for eight years and nobody did a thing."

In an instant, his fury turned to ice. He knew exactly how the Nazis could kill for eight years without anyone doing anything. Nobody cared. That was what was happening with AIDS. People were dying, and nobody cared.

As the anger rose again in Larry, he knew what he would do. That night, he jumped a plane to Boston. He quickly made his way to Cape Cod and spent his first night in the States at the Hyannisport Holiday Inn. Within a few days, everything fell into place. He found a cottage on the water and sat down to write a play that would force people to care.

35 POLITICS

Monday, August 1, 1983
ROOM 2154,
RAYBURN HOUSE OFFICE BUILDING,
WASHINGTON, D.C.

The problems that had dogged Representative Ted Weiss's attempts to get investigators into the Centers for Disease Control were resolved quickly on the eve of his oversight subcommittee's hearings on AIDS. Clearly, the administration did not want the story of obstruction and delays to get a messy public airing on Capitol Hill. Still, the administration's stall had been successful in impeding the House of Representatives, dominated by Democrats, from ascertaining the real needs of agencies in time for a concerted AIDS budget plan for fiscal year 1984, which would begin in just eight weeks. The president's budget called for a $300,000 cut in AIDS funding at the Centers for Disease Control for the next year. Total federal spending for AIDS was slated to increase only about 20 percent, from $14.5 million to $17.6 million. There still were no federally funded AIDS-prevention campaigns, and there was nothing resembling a coordinated plan of attack on the disease. The first day of hearing testimony, largely from scientists working on AIDS, became a litany of what was not being done.

"The failure to respond to this epidemic now borders on a national scandal," said Dr. Marcus Conant, who led scientific testimony. "Congress, and indeed the American people, have been misled about the response. We have been led to believe that the response has been timely and that the response has been appropriate, and I would suggest to you that that is not correct."

Conant recited the "unconscionable" funding delays at the National Institutes of Health, maintaining that the institutional sloth "has resulted in loss of lives." He called for a blue-ribbon commission to establish AIDS priorities and set funding parameters independent of the heavy hand of the Office of Management and Budget. "We are in the beginning, not the midst—we are in the beginning of a national and indeed worldwide epidemic that is going to threaten the lives of hundreds of thousands of individuals," Conant concluded. "It would seem clear that the mandate of this government is to respond and to respond immediately."

Dr. Mathilde Krim from Sloan-Kettering in New York suggested a federal program of $200 million and also called for a special AIDS commission, noting that no coordinated plan for AIDS epidemiology, treatment, or basic research yet existed. She also wondered aloud at the federal government's claim that it was spending $25 million directly on AIDS research. "These figures of $25 million spent in 1983 puzzle me," she said, politely. "I don't see any evidence for them among my colleagues. I know of a few hundred thousand dollars that have been spent." Other witnesses suggested that the National Academy of Sciences be enlisted to conduct an independent study of funding needs, even though that august body, like most scientific groups, had shown little interest in the epidemic.

Stan Matek, immediate past president of the American Public Health Association, said that the Reagan administration's policy on AIDS was to order health officials, "Don't ask for any money. Make us look as good as you can with what you've got."

Dr. Mervyn Silverman, San Francisco Public Health director, noted that $100 million was being spent nationally just in the hospital bills of AIDS patients already. He made a pitch for a government AIDS education program and cited the 300-year-old advice from Thomas Adams: "Prevention is so much better than healing because it saves the labor of being sick."

Throughout the day, the increasingly partisan lines on which AIDS funding would be debated became clear. Republican representatives, apparently briefed by the administration, chided witnesses for wanting to "throw money" at the AIDS problem. "We should be careful to avoid the inevitable push for more money as if dollars are a magic potion," said Representative Robert Walker, a Republican from Pennsylvania.

It was the people with AIDS who lent the first day of hearings the most poignant and sometimes humorous moments. This was appropriate, given the fact that although they were only bit players in this political drama, they were the least devoted to any script. They played their roles for their lives' sakes. AIDS sufferer Anthony Ferrara of Washington, D.C., described the depression that followed his Kaposi's sarcoma diagnosis in March with the comment: "I came home that night and my significant other held me in his arms, and I said to him, 'Why do I feel like Ali MacGraw?'" *Pneumocystis* victim Roger Lyon from San Francisco pleaded, "I came here today with the hope that this administration would do everything possible, make every resource available—there is no reason this disease cannot be conquered. We do not need infighting. This is not a political issue. This is a health issue. This is not a gay issue. This is a human issue. And I do not intend to be defeated by it. I came here today in the hope that my epitaph would not read that I died of red tape."

The next day, Dr. Edward Brandt told the subcommittee that the administration had provided the NIH and CDC with all the AIDS funds they could use.

"I am not sure, quite frankly, what further activities we could undertake at the present time in a reasonably meaningful way," said Brandt, who, in truth, had made a list of precisely such further activities only a few days before in his unanswered request for $35 million. Brandt explained that the administration was spending $166 million on studies "relevant to this particular problem."

⊂⊃

The Weiss hearings also gave the blood industry the opportunity to again enact its ritual of denial on the problem of AIDS in the blood supply. At the hearings, Dr. Joseph Bove, chair of both the transfusion advisory committee to the FDA and the similar committee for the American Association of Blood Banks, blamed the concern about transfusion AIDS on an "overreacting press."

"Even if—and it is still a big if—a small number of AIDS cases turn out to be transfusion related, I do not believe that this can be interpreted to mean that our blood supply is contaminated," said Bove. Saying that 10 million people had been transfused with blood since 1980, Bove maintained, "If—and there is no evidence yet that this is so—but if all twenty cases under investigation by CDC finally turn out to be transfusion related, the incidence will be less than one in a million." Bove brought charts and tables that purported to show that the average American had twice the chance of dying in a flood than of transfusion AIDS. A typical Californian was twice as likely to die in an earthquake, he said, as from transfusion AIDS. A hernia operation or appendectomy, he claimed, offered twenty times the chances of death.

August 3
Irwin Memorial Blood Bank,
San Francisco

The day after Dr. Joseph Bove's graphic example of the odds against transfusion AIDS, a male blood donor walked into the Irwin Memorial Blood Bank. The nurse didn't pay much attention to his deferral card and didn't notice that he never answered the question about whether he had had hepatitis. The man did say he was not a member of a high-risk group for AIDS. His pint of blood was properly refrigerated with other units of blood, awaiting the calls from hospitals.

The Next Day
Dublin Street, San Francisco

Frances Borchelt and Bob, her husband of forty-one years, had talked for days before they went to see the doctor about the possibility of an operation. The doctor took X-rays and noted that Frances Borchelt's right hip was degenerating. The hip replacement operation would probably ease the grandmother's chronic pain, the doctor agreed. Frances and Bob decided they needed a few days to think it over. Four days later, the elderly couple returned to the doctor's office resolved. Frances wanted the operation. When Frances made up her mind to do something, she moved. One of her sons was to be married in October. Frances wanted to be fit enough to dance at his wedding reception. The doctor scheduled the surgery for a week later.

During all the explanations and consultation, nobody ever mentioned anything about a blood transfusion.

August 13
CASTRO STREET

Gary Walsh had been too sick to celebrate his thirty-ninth birthday a few days before, so Matt Krieger was overjoyed when Gary felt well enough again to enjoy a night out on Castro Street. A week before, a huge feature article on Gary had appeared in the *San Francisco Chronicle* with pictures of Gary at home, Gary at the doctor's office, and Gary with Matt.

As one of the first AIDS patients to go public, Gary Walsh had opened his life like a book for interviews and televised guest shots. But reporters' questions about how many sexual contacts he'd had in his lifetime, and the gay community's maudlin fawning over AIDS patients rankled him.

Gary told Matt that somebody he didn't know had shouted "I love you" from a car on Castro Street earlier in the day. "If one more person says they love me, I'll punch them in the mouth," he said.

The previous day, Gary's doctor had found eight new lesions. Life wasn't proceeding like a Marcus Welby episode, as far as Gary was concerned. He spent his days getting stuck with needles. Then, he'd have to wait five days to see if the needles had ferreted out some deadly new disease that he had never heard of.

Matt admired Gary's courage through all this. After he dropped Gary off at home, Matt called his sister Susan. He hadn't planned on talking about Gary or AIDS, but his sister asked about vacation plans, and Matt mentioned he and Gary were planning to go to Hawaii for Christmas. He worried whether Gary would make it because of his health.

"What's wrong with his health?" she asked.

Matt had told both his mother and another sister that Gary had AIDS. Apparently, nobody had bothered to tell Susan. He trembled with anger as he recounted Gary's travails.

"He was back in the hospital last week for tests for cryptococcus meningitis, which were negative," said Matt.

"I don't believe it!" said Susan.

"He's going to die," he said.

"I don't believe it!" she said.

"If he lives a year, it will be a miracle."

"I don't believe it!" she said.

"We're very close," Matt continued, wishing his sister would say something else. "We're closer than ever. Not in a sexual romantic way. But we're going through this together. We talk about all of it very openly. I can't believe Mother or Mary didn't tell you."

"Maybe they haven't known for long," offered Susan.

"They've known for months."

"Maybe they didn't think it was serious."

"They know it's serious," he said. "It's another way of invalidating my relationships. If it had been a girlfriend, or even an ex-girlfriend, you would have heard about it."

"You're right," said his sister softly.

"Straight folks don't think enough of my friendships and relationships to talk about them," Matt continued. "That's why I sometimes get angry and keep my distance from straight folks, even if they're my family."

"I'm sorry," Sue said. "I really am sorry. I had no idea."

August 14
PERTH, AUSTRALIA

Cleve Jones's camera bag bulged with snapshots of boyfriends he had courted in Florence and Mykonos, Athens and Bangkok. On the flight from Bali to Perth, Cleve had met a group of Australian gay men. Already, in his sixth week away from San Francisco, Cleve was planning to help them put together their own AIDS help-line, based on the model he had developed in San Francisco. They've got the chance to do it right from the start, he exclaimed to himself. Cleve's heart sank when he stepped into a men's room at the Perth airport and saw the graffiti over the urinal. "GAYS," it read, "Got AIDS Yet Sucker?"

The next day, the Centers for Disease Control released figures showing that the nation's AIDS caseload had exceeded 2,000. As of August 15, 2,094 AIDS cases had been reported to Atlanta; of these, 805 had died.

August 17
CABRINI MEDICAL CENTER,
NEW YORK CITY

To ease AIDS hysteria, Secretary of Health and Human Services Margaret Heckler wanted to be seen taking the hand of an AIDS victim, touching him. For a week, her aides scoured New York City hospitals for the ideal site for this photo opportunity. A dozen hospitals were approached but declined to participate, because they saw the press conference as a cynical attempt to create the illusion of action on the part of an otherwise inactive federal government. With the highest number of AIDS patients of any hospital in the nation, Bellevue would have been ideal. However, hospital administrators insisted that Heckler wear a mask and gown before she step into an AIDS victim's room. Such a picture, Heckler thought, would do more to inflame hysteria than quell it. The appropriate bedside was found at Cabrini.

Heckler used the hospital visit to announce that President Reagan would ask Congress for an extra $22 million for AIDS funding for the upcoming fiscal year, more than doubling the planned allocation of $17 million. Despite Assistant Secretary Ed Brandt's pleas, the money was not in new funds but in appropriations already designated for existing health programs—in this case, mostly pirated from the National Health Service Corps and the Rural Development Fund of the Office of Community Services. Heckler said that the new funding proposal was being submitted because AIDS researchers wanted more money.

"If they feel they need more, I will submit the request to Congress," she said.

◯

In Washington, Congressional aide, Tim Westmoreland watched the televised coverage and gave Heckler points for being an excellent publicist for the administration, even if she was not a distinguished administrator.

Like a handful of other Washington insiders, however, Westmoreland knew the truth about the proposal, which had nothing to do with whether AIDS researchers wanted it. Already, in secret session, a subcommittee of the House Appropriations Committee had approved a $40 million appropriation for AIDS research for the next year. Given the mood in Congress, nobody doubted the money would be passed. Even Republicans were taken aback by the nickel and diming at the Office of Management and Budget over AIDS. The vote was supposed to be kept confidential until the entire budget went before the full appropriations committee. However, Reagan loyalists had leaked the news to the White House, where an inevitable allocation was transformed into a public relations coup for Secretary Heckler. This was how AIDS policy was conducted in the summer of 1983.

What few people outside the Public Health Service knew was that Heckler's request was still $13 million less than Dr. Brandt had requested a few weeks earlier. That proposal had been deep-sixed by the budget people.

That Day
SETON MEDICAL CENTER,
DALY CITY, CALIFORNIA

Frances Borchelt had been born in the Excelsior District in San Francisco with "the caul," meaning that she had the second sight, according to the Slavic traditions of her immigrant family. As a small child, Frances wore around her neck the remnants of the caul that the midwife had carefully sewn together on the day of her birth. It would bring her luck, although Frances always complained that all her luck was bad. Still, she did have uncanny precognition. Bob Borchelt had noticed it not long after he married Frances and the pair moved into a home on Dublin Street, four blocks from the house where she was born. Whenever the phone rang, the Borchelt's children got in the habit of asking Frances who it was before they'd answer. Frances always seemed to know who was calling.

The one trait that overshadowed Frances's sixth sense was her fastidiousness.

She was always cleaning. Every morning she'd dust. It seemed she washed her hands twenty times a day. Frances's younger daughter Cathy joked that they'd bury her with a can of Mop 'n Glow. When pressed, Frances admitted she was just one of those people who didn't like the idea of germs.

At about the same time that Secretary Margaret Heckler was stepping into her limousine to drive away from her press conference at Cabrini Medical Center, a doctor walked into the suburban San Francisco hospital waiting room where Bob Borchelt and his four children waited for news of their mother's hip replacement operation. The doctor declared the surgery a success. The family was relieved. Nobody could remember the last time Frances was ever sick with anything, but she was a seventy-one-year-old woman, they knew, and any surgery, however routine, could be risky.

A few days later, Frances Borchelt was her old feisty self and fell into a fierce argument with a niece. A doctor had wanted to give her a blood transfusion, she complained.

"I told them I don't want one," she said.

Her niece argued that doctors knew what was best, and she should pay attention to them. As usual, Frances was obdurate and could not be budged.

"I won't let them give me a blood transfusion and that's final," she said. "They can give me iron pills if they want my blood better."

At the time, her family figured the obstinance stemmed from a lifetime as a clean freak. She couldn't adjust to the idea of somebody else's blood in her; no telling where it had been, she'd say. Later, however, the family would recall the argument and talk about the caul.

⬭

Frances did not know that loss of blood during her surgery had required the transfusion of two pints of blood. The third unit, doctors said, was transfused as a precaution. It was this last unit that had been donated by the young man two weeks before—the man who did not fill out his donor deferral card properly.

36 SCIENCE

August 25, 1983
CENTERS FOR DISEASE CONTROL,
ATLANTA

Eager to form a top-rate retrovirus lab at the CDC, Dr. Don Francis had recruited a retrovirologist from Robert Gallo's lab at the National Cancer Institute, Dr. V. S. Kalyanaraman. Kaly, as everybody called him, most recently had achieved notice for his discovery of HTLV-II, the second variant of the Human T-cell Leukemia virus, which Gallo had discovered in 1980. Long frustrated in Gallo's large Bethesda laboratory, Kaly looked forward to working on a smaller team, where he would have greater responsibility. He also hoped he would leave Bethesda with the blessing of his mentor, Dr. Gallo, figuring his success at tracking an AIDS virus at the CDC would be only to the greater glory of Bob Gallo.

That, however, was not how Dr. Gallo saw it. When cajoling did not persuade Kaly to stay in Bethesda, Gallo resorted to threats: He would not let his researcher take any reagents to any retrovirus from his NCI lab to the CDC. He'd have to culture his own viruses and antibodies, Gallo said. Meanwhile, Don Francis heard in early August that Gallo had asked top officials at the National Cancer Institute to stop the CDC from hiring the younger researcher. By this morning in late August, Gallo knew these efforts would not succeed, and he phoned Don Francis directly.

AIDS research was "at a crossroads," Gallo said, so there was no need for the CDC to launch its own retrovirus research. It was a "duplication of government expenditures."

When this tact failed, Gallo pushed harder.

"There's no way we will collaborate with you," said Gallo, saying he saw "no evidence of CDC goodwill" toward the National Cancer Institute.

For that reason, he would not release reagents or antibodies to the HTLV virus.

"Kaly will get nothing," he said. "You ain't ever going to have any retroviruses."

The battle with Bob Gallo came as an unwelcome distraction for Don Francis but was no surprise. Gallo already suspected that the CDC was not sending him their best specimens for analysis. He had voiced the fear to a number of close colleagues that the CDC was plotting to find the cause of AIDS themselves and then "run without me," meaning Gallo would get no credit.

Feuding between the National Cancer Institute and the National Institute for Allergy and Infectious Diseases also had assumed legendary proportions. The NCI claimed primacy in AIDS research because it had staked the territory first, back when AIDS most commonly appeared as skin cancer. Although the NIAID only recently had demonstrated much interest in the epidemic, it now had asserted that it should carry the dominant role in AIDS research because the syndrome was an infectious disease.

Bob Gallo had also drawn battle lines with the French retrovirologists at the Pasteur Institute and their virus, LAV. "The European press is full of the French have the cause," Gallo complained to Don Francis. He worried that if they were later disproved, he would look bad because he had reviewed the first LAV paper that was published in *Science,* in May 1983.

Gallo also worried that the French would be proved right, and he would not get the credit for discovering the AIDS agent. Privately, he spread the word that the French isolates were not human viruses at all but contaminants from other viruses kicking around their labs. In various calls, Gallo warned Francis away from working with any other researchers, particularly the French. "Don't form tertiary relationships," Gallo told Francis. "Keep me in a prime relationship with AIDS and cherish the goodwill."

Don Francis had spent the summer trying to grow the virus in anything he could think of, including the fetal cord of newborn infants, bat lung, monkey kidneys, and dog thymus. He had ordered the French-discovered LAV from Paris, but it had not arrived. Gallo still thought that HTLV-I caused AIDS, outlining all the evidence in a long memo to NCI officials in early August, but that didn't make any sense to Francis. The AIDS virus did not cause the multiplication of infected lymphocytes; it heralded their mass destruction. It didn't act like a leukemia virus. Moreover, the HTLV focus was extremely time consuming. Each cell-line infection took about three months to culture, and after each culture the researchers came up empty-handed. Dr. Walter Dowdle, Chief of the Center for Infectious Diseases, worried that the CDC had put too much emphasis on the retroviral hypothesis, leaving the Center barking up the wrong virological tree. Francis counted on Kaly's expertise on retroviruses and HTLV to help make the lab investment pay off.

At the NCI, Kaly was dejected at the bitter turn his seven-year relationship with Gallo had taken. The job at CDC was a marriage, Kaly thought, but Gallo was family.

Kaly had been born to a poor family in India on Victory Europe Day, 1945.

He had come to the United States on a fellowship and enlisted in the war on cancer's push to isolate cancer-related viruses in the 1970s. He had worked in Gallo's lab since 1976. Recently, Kaly had been working with AIDS. Like Gallo, he was frustrated by the inability to propagate the virus. He remained excited about AIDS research and viewed his tenure with Gallo as the tree from which he would branch out. Now, he felt Gallo was treating his staff like flunkies: Once in, they could never leave. Even when it was clear that Kaly intended to depart, despite the doctor's protestations, Bob Gallo pressed on with his strategy of intimidation.

"I will destroy you," he said.

The annual International Congress of Immunology met in Kyoto that August. The CDC's Dr. Dale Lawrence could see the AIDS epidemic had piqued the curiosity of the world's immune experts as had few problems before. Although, the organizers of the Japan conference were reluctant to sponsor a special session on AIDS, Lawrence insisted, and the turnout was so large that the AIDS meeting had to be moved from a modest conference room to the largest auditorium on the site. However, in private discussions, when Lawrence flatly stated that within a few years 20,000 AIDS cases would be diagnosed in the United States alone, he was greeted with blank stares. Few among these leading world experts, he thought, had yet grasped the enormity of what was unfolding.

The same day that Bob Gallo had called Don Francis, pledging to withhold NCI cooperation from CDC AIDS research, the tale of the University of California's withholding funds appeared in the *San Francisco Chronicle*. Dr. Art Ammann, an eminent pediatric immunologist, was one of the handful of doctors with the courage to go public, saying AIDS researchers were being punished for committing a "bureaucratic offense" against the university hierarchy. Dr. Marc Conant infuriated university officials by leaking the memo that described the serious public relations consequences of further university delay. By now, of course, all the AIDS researchers in the UC system suffered from lack of funds. Dr. Jay Levy still could not buy the ultracentrifuge his retrovirus lab needed, stalling his search for an AIDS virus.

For the record, the medical school dean stoutly told reporters that he now saw that the AIDS money needed to be expedited and that he would get the money freed if he had "to walk across the Bay Bridge to Berkeley" and force administrators to do it. Once the reporters' backs were turned, however, the dean told colleagues he had been misquoted. There would be no speedup in the release of funds.

Indeed, the university held on to the money for another three months, and then the funds went largely to the scientists for whom they were originally intended. There was one exception, however. Dr. Art Ammann was cut out of the AIDS money entirely. Ammann was the doctor who had first alerted the nation to the threat of AIDS in the blood supply in December 1982. His actions probably resulted in the saving of many lives, but saving lives was not the criteria upon which university officials based their decisions. Before long, Ammann made plans to leave the university for work in the private sector.

That was how the science of AIDS unfolded in August 1983.

August 27
35 Alpine Terrace, San Francisco

While he washed Gary Walsh's dishes, Matt Krieger talked to Gary about their *Family Portrait* project. It was a book idea promoting the concept of the chosen family, as opposed to the biological family. For many gay people, friends often were closer than brothers and sisters, and Gary wanted to demonstrate this new family theory in a book with pictures of his chosen family, including Matt, Lu Chaikin, and Gary's nephew, Rick Walsh.

"Are you still excited about the project?" asked Matt.

After a long hesitation from the bedroom, Matt heard a weak, "Yeah."

Matt walked into Gary's comfortable bedroom and put his arms around him, holding his frail body close.

"It's just that I know I'll never see it," Gary said. "I won't be here when it's published."

"But you might be," said Matt. "Can't we still hope for miracles?"

"We can hope, but I know I'm dying."

Matt asked whether Gary actually felt death physically, or was just intellectually weighing his chances of survival.

"I can feel it in my body," said Gary. "I can feel the increasing weakness, and it's almost like I can feel the cells dying . . . this morning I felt so horrible, I thought I was dying today."

$\bigcirc$

According to figures released August 29, 1983, by the Centers for Disease Control, 2,224 Americans were stricken with AIDS, of whom 891 had died.

$\bigcirc$

Frances Borchelt was released from Seton Medical Center in the San Francisco suburb of Daly City on August 30. Although the doctors said the surgery was successful, Frances still had not regained her strength from the operation. She was weak, running continuous, unexplained fevers. She was released from the hospital with a temperature of 100 degrees. Once home, she was so fatigued that she was incapable of performing the exercises necessary to regain use of her new hip. The family doctor advised Bob Borchelt to watch his wife for a few days and report her condition.

It was during this anxious time that the bill for Frances's operation arrived from the hospital. Because Medicare did not pay for blood transfusions, the cost of three units of blood from Irwin Memorial Blood Bank was included on the invoice. That was how the Borchelt family learned about their mother's blood transfusion.

○

On September 9, 1983, the first Norwegian to contract AIDS died in Oslo; he was also that country's first AIDS fatality. The thirty-three-year-old man's death followed the death of Sweden's first AIDS victim by three weeks. In Mexico, health authorities were now formally reporting their first AIDS cases. Haitian authorities responded to a year of publicity about the links of AIDS to that impoverished nation by going to the country's only gay bar in Port-au-Prince and jailing everyone.

Although the intense media coverage of the past six months was fading as summer turned to autumn in the United States, Europeans remained jittery about the new disease. In early September, British health authorities distributed leaflets urging people in high-risk groups to stop donating blood. Evidence linking AIDS to blood transfusions continued to mount. Doctors in Montreal had reported an AIDS case in an infant whose only risk was the bad luck of having a transfusion at birth. The CDC now linked twenty-one U.S. AIDS cases to transfusions. In only one case, however, had a victim's blood donor actually come down with AIDS, leading CDC officials to agitate for tighter screening of donors, because it was clear that blood donors with no AIDS symptoms could give a lethal dose of AIDS. Blood banks, however, maintained that donor-deferral guidelines were adequate and said any future transfusion-AIDS cases would stem from transfusions given before the guidelines went into effect. Dr. Edward Brandt also assured gay groups that he would not require more stringent donor screening. He met with gay leaders after word leaked out that White House aides had met with leaders of Jerry Falwell's Moral Majority to discuss legislation banning gays from donating blood. Brandt was said to be furious that the White House would meet not with health officials about such an important health issue but with the Moral Majority.

On September 15, the House Appropriations Committee voted to approve a $41 million AIDS budget for the next fiscal year. The committee issued a report saying it would review the progress of AIDS programs in the coming months and push for supplemental appropriations as necessary. In a pointed directive, the committee noted the absence of any programs of public education and AIDS prevention, and ordered Secretary Margaret Heckler "to mobilize available Public Health Service resources to assist the CDC in implementing a timely and effective public education effort."

The same day the House committee passed its AIDS appropriations, seven U.S. senators issued a joint statement asking Lowell Weicker, the chair of the appropriations subcommittee that handles HHS funding, for monies to support a Public Health Emergency Fund. The senators had learned that the CDC and NIH had actually requested more than $50 million in funds for AIDS research, about $10 million more than Heckler had announced on the day she said she would give AIDS researchers whatever they felt was necessary to stop the epidemic. Although the Public Health Emergency Fund was authorized by a unanimous vote of Congress in July, no money had been set aside for it. "Without availability of these contingency monies and the coordinated effort the Fund would provide, HHS's only way to react to public health emergencies is the same way it is proposing to react to the AIDS crisis—by siphoning resources out of other programs to which the same immediacy may not attach, but which are equally important to protecting the health of our Nation's citizens," the senators wrote. "Moreover, when these other resources cannot be found and diverted quickly, we experience dangerous delays in our efforts to stop the spread of diseases that can cause widespread suffering and death."

The statement carried intriguing political significance, coming on the eve of the 1984 presidential election year. It was not lost on pundits that AIDS might play a role in the election, given the fact that the signers included presidential aspirants Alan Cranston, John Glenn, and Edward Kennedy.

September 17
PASTEUR INSTITUTE,
PARIS

Dr. Luc Montagnier was exasperated when he returned from the conference of AIDS researchers at the federal research facility at Cold Spring Harbor, Long Island. He had been cautious in his presentation but had delivered the full hand of what nine months of intensive research on the French AIDS virus had unearthed. By now, the French were conducting blood tests on AIDS patients from both Claude-Bernard and Pitie-Salpetriere hospitals, and they were getting results. Although they did not find LAV antibodies in every AIDS patient, they did show higher levels of LAV antibodies than Robert Gallo had reported with HTLV-I. Moreover, Gallo's results, they felt, were suspicious because he included HTLV antibodies found in the blood of Haitian AIDS patients. HTLV was endemic to the Caribbean and could reasonably be expected among such people even if they did not have AIDS.

A week before the Cold Spring Harbor conference, the Pasteur researchers had passed their first independently administered test. Don Francis from the CDC had sent the group four blood samples drawn from San Francisco gay men who had participated in the hepatitis B study. Two of the samples had been drawn early in the study, probably before the men were exposed to the AIDS virus; the other two samples were drawn from the same two men after they presented AIDS symptoms. Francis asked the French to determine which samples came from which time. In both cases, the Pasteur doctors accurately found no LAV antibodies from the serum that was coded earlier and LAV antibodies in the more recently drawn blood. Francis was clearly impressed, and Montagnier hoped the other Americans would be convinced as well.

Instead, the Cold Spring Harbor conference had become "a festival of HTLV," Montagnier reported. The scientists could not stop talking about the possibility that Dr. Gallo's leukemia virus might cause AIDS. Montagnier's presentation was shunted to the end of the proceedings. Some scientists chuckled aloud when Montagnier insisted LAV bore no relation to HTLV and instead resembled the equine anemia virus. A horse virus, indeed, they thought.

Gallo himself led a grueling interrogation of Montagnier, mocking the supposed link to the equine lentivirus. Behind the scenes, talk spread that the French isolates were contaminated. Any real breakthroughs, the scuttlebutt went, would come from Gallo's lab.

The news dispirited the other researchers gathered for the regular Saturday meeting in Montagnier's paneled office at the Pasteur campus. Virtually all the prestigious scientific journals were American, and few seemed interested in publishing French research. Most often, the comment upon rejection was: "We'll wait and see what Bob Gallo comes up with." Even in Paris, scientists were split on the significance of the Pasteur studies. Jacques Leibowitch, still hurting over his rejection as a Pasteur job applicant, had become a partisan of Gallo, deprecating the Pasteur doctors as amateurs.

But the Parisian "amateurs" had made dramatic progress in recent months. They now had a blood test, and immunological work by Dr. David Klatzmann defined how the virus attacked the T-helper lymphocytes. Moreover, Willy Rozenbaum's tests with the antiviral drug HPA-23 showed some results in the pioneering area of AIDS treatments. The delay in accepting French research was not merely another episode of international rivalry, they felt, but a development that would cost science its most crucial weapon in fighting the epidemic: time. And they needed time to start testing anti-viral drugs for treating AIDS, to develop a widely available antibody test, to begin blood testing and serious control measures. With the virus spreading around the world, scientists did not have the luxury of engaging in parochial disputes. The French understood that Gallo and the National Cancer Institute carried more weight in the United States than the Pasteur Institute. They assumed, however, that an entire nation of scientists would not be wed to one notion of such an important disease, particularly when it was as unconvincing as HTLV-I.

Willy Rozenbaum dismissed the problem as "scientific imperialism" from Americans, but Montagnier knew that the rivalry between the NCI and the Pasteur Institute would not easily be resolved. The handful of French researchers, working with a fraction of the budget available to the Americans, would have to push on without much financial support or recognition.

"We are in the tunnel," he said. "We are in the dark."

San Francisco

Bob Borchelt spent late September in a state of sustained anxiety over the deteriorating health of his wife, Frances. On September 10, she was readmitted to the hospital and immediately diagnosed with hepatitis. The doctors reluctantly confided she had contracted the disease from her blood transfusion. But Frances seemed far more afflicted than a typical hepatitis sufferer. She had a violent cough, spitting up white gobs of mucus. Nothing tasted right, so she wouldn't eat. In the course of her seventeen-day hospitalization, she lost twenty pounds. The doctors blamed the weight loss on "anorexia." At one point during that time, the family doctor told Bob Borchelt that he was worried Frances might die, but, somehow, the feisty grandmother pulled through. Later, Bob and the kids would note ruefully that she would have been far better off to die that September than to suffer what lay ahead.

September 22
MATT KRIEGER'S JOURNAL

Despair is what I hear in Gary's voice tonight. . . . He has just reason for despair. He fell down three times today when his legs simply gave out on him. He had an infection in one eye and now the same infection in the other eye.

He went to the dentist for a routine checkup and learned he has an infection and may well need a root canal. And he has a new infection of the prostate for which his doctor told him beating off may alleviate the pressure and pain. Masturbation is a distant memory for him and holds no appeal.

"You may not believe this," I tell him, "but you'll get past this depression. You've been in this spot before and you will beat it. I wish I could do it for you or make it go away."

I wonder how he *can* sustain this relentless series of devastating and painful illnesses. Horribly, I recognize that dark corner in my mind that wishes it were all over and I could talk about Gary and his illnesses in the past tense.

My mind plays that game. Sometimes I think it is all over. Gary is dead. Back in the eighties, I had a best friend and former lover, a wonderful man whom I loved very deeply, and he suffered and he died in that terrible epidemic that hit the gay community nationally, the disease we hardly remember now. It was called AIDS.

37 PUBLIC HEALTH

October 4, 1983
SAN FRANCISCO AIDS FOUNDATION

The ambulance stopped on 10th Street, double-parked, and quickly bundled a young man onto a gurney. The ambulance driver and a second man carried the stretcher to the second floor offices of the AIDS Foundation and set the stretcher on the floor. A nurse walking with them hurriedly put down a few plastic bags containing all the young man's possessions. Then, they turned and walked out, leaving the gaunt man lying on the floor.

Confused staffers at the foundation pieced together his story. Since July, Morgan MacDonald had been treated at Shands Hospital in Gainesville, Florida, for severe cryptosporidiosis, stemming from AIDS. When his state Medicaid benefits ran out, Shands, a private hospital, ordered MacDonald to leave by October 7. However, there was no place for the twenty-seven-year-old to go. No nursing home would accept him; and although Florida had the third-highest AIDS caseload in the nation, the state had no public programs of any type for AIDS patients, beyond those provided by volunteer groups in Miami and Key West.

Shands Hospital doctors called San Francisco General Hospital to see whether that facility would accept MacDonald. The hospital said it did not accept acutely ill transfer patients and suggested he stay in Florida. Then the AIDS Foundation started getting calls from Florida, inquiring how a man with AIDS, who wanted to move to San Francisco, could get on the outpatient treatment program.

Early Tuesday morning, Shands Hospital officials loaded MacDonald in a private Learjet air ambulance with a doctor and nurse. Although the plane cost $14,000 to charter, it was a cheaper alternative to the $100,000 in hospital bills an AIDS patient typically accumulated. The hospital also took $300 from money raised in the gay community to help AIDS patients and put it in the stricken man's pocket for spending money.

Unable to even raise his head, MacDonald was instantly taken from the AIDS Foundation to San Francisco General's AIDS Ward, where his health immediately turned worse. Dr. Mervyn Silverman, San Francisco Public Health Director, was infuriated and accused Shands of "dumping" the patient when he was gravely ill. The hospital responded that it had sent MacDonald to San Francisco "for humanitarian reasons." He was ambulatory when he left the Florida facility, the hospital said, suffering only from anorexia because he hadn't eaten well lately. As for MacDonald's acute illness within hours of his discharge from Shands, a hospital spokesman offered, "AIDS is a disease where your condition changes."

San Francisco Mayor Dianne Feinstein immediately denounced the transfer as "outrageous and inhumane" and demanded that the governor of Florida investigate the dumping. Both San Francisco daily newspapers editorialized on the "unconscionable act." When a state spokesman announced a Florida Health Department investigation into the MacDonald case a few days later, he admitted, "We are having problems in Florida because medical professionals are reluctant to provide care because they know so little about AIDS. We are seeing people take any opportunity within the law to avoid providing care."

SAN FRANCISCO DEPARTMENT OF PUBLIC HEALTH

Dr. Selma Dritz looked weary as she glanced up from her desk in her crowded office in the health department's Civic Center headquarters. In the upper right-hand corner of her blackboard, she had listed the latest number of reported AIDS cases in San Francisco—292—with a breakdown separating the numbers of patients suffering from KS, PCP, and other opportunistic infections. Selma Dritz kept the list of all the AIDS sufferers in the San Francisco Bay Area, marking off their names in red ink, one by one, as they died. An epidemiologist from San Francisco General Hospital's AIDS Clinic recently had used Dritz's methodical tally to calculate the various survival rates by disease group. Of the men stricken by *Pneumocystis carinii* pneumonia and other opportunistic infections, none were alive within twenty-one months of diagnosis. All the patients suffering from both Kaposi's sarcoma and PCP were dead within fifteen months. The best prognosis came for men suffering only from Kaposi's sarcoma, half of whom remained alive twenty-one months after their date of diagnosis.

In her office, Selma Dritz looked back down at her manila folders. The enthusiasm that had marked her early work in the epidemic had waned.

"During the wars with Napoleon, when Admiral Nelson asked for the numbers of men killed and wounded in a week of action, he said, 'Let me have the butcher's bill for the week,'" Dritz sighed to a reporter one day. "As I make out these reports with the new numbers of AIDS cases each week, and as I check them off when they die, I feel like I am writing the butcher's bill of this epidemic."

When mild-mannered Bill Cunningham was pulled from retirement and given the task of heading the San Francisco health department's AIDS Activities Office, he received one piece of advice: "Involve all the different gay groups in your planning or they'll fight whatever you want to do." In the first months of his tenure in the politically sensitive post, the former deputy health director walked delicately through the sensibilities and competing agendas of sundry gay factions. He learned not to offend. To accomplish this, Cunningham observed the central ritual of public health policy on AIDS: He held committee meetings. No action was taken until everyone agreed it was appropriate; this was called consensus. For months, that had meant not taking any action at all since nobody could agree on much. This was appropriate, however, given the fact that the rituals of AIDS, whether enacted in Washington or San Francisco, rarely demanded action, just rhetoric.

Cunningham's problem was that Supervisor Harry Britt, Bill Kraus, and the Harvey Milk Club had been leaning on the health department to issue some kind of coordinated AIDS education plan for San Francisco. Charting such a plan was no easy task. First, Cunningham had to consult the city's AIDS Coordinating Committee, a nebulous group of gay activists composed of anybody who showed up at meetings. That committee next appointed a twenty-five-member subcommittee for AIDS planning, consisting of representatives of every gay political club and all the various organizations petitioning for city funds. Only three members had a professional background in public health education. This subcommittee then broke into more subcommittees and spent three months in meetings.

The result was a lackluster seven-page "plan" that did little more than restate what the city already was doing in AIDS education. Even this plan, issued in late September, was tentative since it would not be adopted until after a month-long "feedback" period. Cunningham himself admitted the plan didn't present much in the way of innovation, but he maintained that the city needed to follow "the process" so it would not anger gay activists.

After Supervisor Britt read the health department's long-awaited plan, he fired off a letter to Dr. Mervyn Silverman. "How will the Department assure that those people it contracts with to conduct any further educational activities have the skills and experience necessary to do the job? It appears that a great deal of leadership is still required on your part to see that the education program is carried out as thoroughly and quickly as demanded by this emergency. I do not believe the city can put up with any further delays without an outcry from the community and without assuming responsibility for the lives of thousands of San Franciscans."

In response to a reporter investigating what the city had to show for its hundreds of thousands spent on AIDS education, Britt bluntly said: "The public health department is treating this like an outbreak of psoriasis, not an epidemic that is killing people."

Without a concerted educational effort by the city, the gay community's approach to AIDS was transformed. To be sure, tens of thousands of gay men were, quite literally, dying to know more about the epidemic. They crowded lectures on safe sex and burgeoning therapy groups on "AIDS anxiety" for the "worried well." They educated themselves on all things relating to the immune system, often placing themselves in the unfamiliar position of lecturing less informed physicians on the intricacies of T-cells, B-cells, and macrophages.

This collective concern fueled the most dramatic shift in behavior since the contemporary gay movement was forged in the Stonewall riots of 1969. Non-sexual social alternatives thrived. A half-block off Castro Street, the Castro Country Club flourished, offering gay men a relaxed, alcohol-free environment in which they could play "Trivial Pursuit" and canasta away from the heavy cruise scenes in gay bars. Gay Alcoholics Anonymous groups proliferated in church basements of gay neighborhoods throughout the city. Weekly bingo at the Most Holy Redeemer Church, two blocks off Castro Street, found an un-tapped market among gay men, who started crowding the church basement every Wednesday night. Some private sex clubs found popularity sponsoring J-O nights, in which partners were encouraged to recall the nostalgic, teenage masturbation of "Boy Scout sex." With the national popularization of videocas-sette recorders, gay men realized they need never go home alone again, even if they didn't pick someone up in the local meat rack. Dating and matchmaker services enjoyed a comeback.

At the bars, the gay men who were still cruising rarely admitted to being single. Instead, it seemed, everybody in every gay bar had a lover who was out of town. Telephone sex services also prospered. Rates of anal gonorrhea, an indicator of the prevalence of passive anal intercourse, plummeted that year. This new toned-down gay life-style had started as a vogue in early 1983; by the end of that year, it was a trend; in the year that followed, it would turn into a full-scale sociological phenomenon.

The gay community, however, remained at crosscurrents with itself. Even as behavior shifted for significant numbers of gay men, others managed to party on, like the revelers in Edgar Allan Poe's "Mask of the Red Death," oblivious to the plague around them. When the summer's intensive media blitz eased, bathhouse attendance picked up and lines formed around the sex emporiums every weekend.

The odious biological realities of a deadly epidemic encouraged paradox. At a dinner party one night, Cliff Morrison, the nursing coordinator for the AIDS Ward at San Francisco General Hospital, was introduced to a man who later scolded his host, "You should have told me who he was. I never would have shaken his hand if I knew where he worked." After dinner, the anxious guest left the party for an evening at the baths. In line at the Club Baths at Eighth and Howard streets, patrons jokingly called the facility "AIDS and Howard," even while they fished membership cards and locker fees from their wallets.

In a local gay newspaper, writer Paul Reed summarized the various styles of gay response to the epidemic. There were the "What Crisis?" types, who denied there was an epidemic at all, as opposed to the "Nervous Nellies," who were paralyzed with dread. The "Ozzie and Harriets" had settled into monogamous relationships, while the "Superman" types tricked on, convinced they were somehow immune to AIDS. The "Doris Day" types invoked fatalism to ratio-nalize their continued cruising, singing, "Que sera, sera." Reed counted himself in the last category: "The Utterly Confused."

Psychologists studying the gay community compared the contradictory trends to the reactions men typically have when facing their mid-life crisis. Psychologically, the mid-life crisis marks the period of individual redefinition. Friends begin to die, sparking the sudden realization of mortality. There is a sense of loss: Is my life really half over? Some men run off with their younger secretaries in an attempt to recapture their lost youth; others find that adversity engenders a new maturity and a more meaningful posture in every aspect of their lives. The gay community's confused response marked the start of its own collective redefinition, a process that, for all its early silliness, would become one of the more profound effects of the AIDS epidemic in the coming years.

More gay newspapers circulated in San Francisco than in any other city in the United States, but often these publications did more to cloud than to define the challenges facing gay men. *Bay Area Reporter* columnist Konstantin Berlandt had recently begun a new attack on the Harvey Milk Club, branding club officers as "our own worst enemies" for their "anti-sex" brochure on safe sex called "Can We Talk?". Berlandt wrote, "Advice on safe sex, while perhaps well meaning, is actually collaboration with the death regime that delights in blaming ourselves and would pin the blame on us. The myth of 'safe sex' fosters the finger pointing when anyone of us does come down with a disease: 'You see, we told you so. We brought it on ourselves.' "

A week later, Berlandt followed this essay with a treatise that announced, "I love to rim. To some people, a tongue up the asshole can be relaxing, mesmerizing, even spiritually uplifting." Berlandt maintained it was society's responsibility to find the medical technology to prevent all sexually transmitted diseases, rather than the gay community's responsibility to keep sexuality in line with what medical technology could cure. As for safe sex, he wrote, "I don't mean we can't make such changes if absolutely necessary, but why must we?"

In the area of medical coverage, the *Bay Area Reporter* devoted the most space to a San Mateo doctor who claimed he could cure the syndrome through megadoses of vitamin C. A gay psychologist also wrote a series of articles on the "psychoincubation" of AIDS, maintaining that AIDS victims all had suffered an "emotional emergency" as children that made them feel abandoned. The abandonment now was being played out with AIDS, he said, meaning that a change in psychological posture toward the world could be the best prevention against the disease.

The contribution of the *Sentinel,* the second largest gay paper in San Francisco, was a huge series of articles blasting Marc Conant's fledgling National KS/AIDS Foundation. The stated reason for the merciless attacks was that staffers at the foundation had given AIDS patients free tickets to the Debbie Reynolds fund-raiser in June. The real reason for the assault was less savory. The *Sentinel* was then owned by a man who long had been in heated competition for circulation with *BAR* publisher Bob Ross, who was treasurer of the foundation. The attack on the foundation was little more than an attack on a business competitor.

Nevertheless, the national foundation foundered under the criticism. In late August, a second Debbie Reynolds fund-raiser in Los Angeles flopped when local AIDS groups refused to cooperate. Demoralized by the constant criticism and bickering from other gay leaders, board members began resigning. One attorney bitterly told Marc Conant, "Let them all die if that's what they want to do."

NEW YORK CITY

The Hispanic man arrived at a meeting of the People With AIDS group looking confused. He had just been told he had contracted a deadly disease of which he had never heard. It was called AIDS.

"How come nobody told me there was an epidemic?" he asked the PWA president, Michael Callen.

"Don't you watch TV?" asked Callen.

"No."

"Don't you read the *Native?*"

"No."

For all the problems in San Francisco, at least the West Coast city had a program for AIDS, however torpid. In New York City, an interagency task force met monthly to discuss the epidemic, but meetings were little more than a chance to enumerate all the things that the city was not doing to meet the challenge of AIDS. Official inaction was not a matter of neglect; now it was elevated to the level of policy. Unlike San Francisco, where the health department assumed a direct role as service coordinator, New York City Health Commissioner David Sencer maintained that the proper role of the health department "should provide those services that others have not, will not, should not, or cannot provide." The interagency task force defined its role as "seeking not to direct, but to provide a neutral meeting ground." Essentially, Dr. Sencer said, the health department should fill gaps, not launch any ventures of its own.

This was a fortunate ideology for David Sencer, since he maintained that few gaps existed in New York. He opposed establishing coordinated care facilities like those at San Francisco General Hospital, saying that "attempts at the municipal level to bundle these [preventive, ambulatory, and institutional] services too closely are dangerous." Sencer maintained a similar lack of enthusiasm for education and prevention programs. At the Weiss subcommittee hearings, one Republican congressman suggested that Sencer "ought to be really quite loud about . . . methods of prevention." Commissioner Sencer, however, responded, "I think that there are ways in which this could be accomplished without taking to the soapbox. I certainly believe that the information is going to be better accepted and come from a stronger support if it comes from the affected communities themselves." Sencer said he was working with gay newspapers, adding, "I think that public exhortation has not stopped the spread of venereal disease."

The reliance on gay newspapers was a curious position for a public health education program. New York City had only one gay newspaper, the *New York Native*. Its circulation was about 20,000, in this city with an estimated gay population of 1 million. That meant that 49 out of 50 gay men did not read the publication upon which New York City based its entire AIDS education effort.

By the end of 1983, the entire contribution the government of New York City had made to AIDS services or education was a $24,500 allocation to the Red Cross to provide home attendant care to AIDS patients. Even that program started three months late because nobody bothered to get phones hooked up so prospective clients could call. The Red Cross service was designed to serve 200 AIDS patients. In the fifteen months before the contract was canceled, however, only 80 patients were helped, because of bureaucratic problems in administering the agreement.

Meanwhile, Gay Men's Health Crisis was running its entire operation out of five small rooms in a boarding house. The group had enlisted 300 clinical volunteers and coordinated twenty training sessions a months for doctors and nurses seeking information on treating AIDS. They trained 50 new volunteers every month for new clients. Although the GMHC space was woefully inadequate, few landlords wanted their buildings to become the site of Manhattan's "leper central." Dr. Joseph Sonnabend, one of the city's leading AIDS doctors, filed suit against his co-op association after he was ordered evicted from his offices because of the large number of AIDS patients visiting his West 12th Street address. When GMHC asked the city if it could use an abandoned high school on West 13th Street as an AIDS service center, the city demanded $2 million cash up front. Gays were not about to get charity from the Koch administration.

After meeting with Mayor Koch, Dr. Mathilde Krim sat down with Joseph Sonnabend and GMHC Executive Director Rodger McFarlane to write a proposal for a coordinated city response. Based on the San Francisco program, the group described a plan for diversified care alternatives, including hospice beds, AIDS wards, and clinics. Krim took the idea to public officials but found few interested in the epidemic. Carol Bellamy, the New York City Council president, wouldn't see the researcher. Andrew Stein, the Manhattan Borough president, chatted politely with Krim but declined to take any action. Krim later summed up New York City's official attitude in four words: "Nobody gave a damn."

When Larry Kramer checked his mail on one of his trips back from Cape Cod, he found five letters. Four of them were from doctors worrying that gay men were returning to their old licentiousness now that AIDS was out of the headlines. They also despaired that the gay political leadership had not challenged the mayor or health department to do something, anything, about stemming AIDS. The fifth letter was the announcement of a memorial service for a friend who had just died of AIDS. He was the thirty-second friend of Larry's who had succumbed to the syndrome.

GMHC was having a hard time selling tickets for its latest Madison Square Garden fund-raiser, so a private donor took out a full-page *Village Voice* ad and asked Larry to write a plea for support. In the appeal, "2,339 and Counting," Larry lashed out at the two evils upon which he blamed the sorry state of affairs in New York—Mayor Koch and the newspaper that continued to ignore the local policy aspects of AIDS, *The New York Times*.

After writing the appeal, Larry traveled to Little Washington, Virginia, where he was polishing his play, still not sure of what he should call it. "City of Death," his first idea, was too depressing, he decided. One night, perusing a book of W. H. Auden's poetry, Larry found the perfect title in the classic poem "September, 1939." He'd call his play *The Normal Heart,* he decided, from the verses:

> *What mad Nijinsky wrote*
> *About Diaghilev*
> *Is true of the normal heart;*
> *For the error bred in the bone*
> *Of each woman and each man*
> *Craves what it cannot have,*
> *Not universal love*
> *But to be loved alone . . .*
> *And no one exists alone;*
> *Hunger allows no choice*
> *To the citizen or the police;*
> *We must love one another or die.*

⬭

In the first five years of the AIDS epidemic the brightest moments only served to illuminate how bad things really were. That San Francisco had managed the best response to the AIDS epidemic in the United States was the pride of the city; that San Francisco had managed the best response to the AIDS epidemic in the United States measured the shame of the nation.

By late 1983, San Francisco had put together the only thing resembling an official response to the epidemic thus far mounted in the country. Although New York City had no services beyond what an overstrained gay community provided themselves, patients at least could look forward to reasonably decent care in the city's hospitals. In other parts of the country, public health mechanisms and the medical community were so poorly prepared for the epidemic that patients could not even expect this ration of comfort.

The report submitted to Florida Governor Bob Graham on the Morgan MacDonald incident concluded that hospital officials had "acted in good faith" when they loaded the young man on a plane and dispatched him to San Francisco. The hospital had only wanted to put the patient in a city where support services existed, the state health department decided. The transfer, of course, could have been avoided if Florida had adequate facilities to treat patients who no longer needed acute-care hospital beds, but no such facilities existed outside San Francisco. Partially in response to the furor surrounding the MacDonald case, the American Hospital Association was putting together recommendations requiring all healthy hospital employees to work with AIDS victims. The guidelines followed the logic laid out by the University of California in September that stated, "There is no scientific reason for healthy personnel to be excused from delivering care to patients with AIDS."

Morgan MacDonald died a "quiet death" of cardiac arrest on Ward 5B of San Francisco General Hospital on October 20, 1983. He was the 111th person to die of the disease in San Francisco. Health Director Mervyn Silverman sent the Shands Hospital in Gainesville a bill for the $6,500 it had cost the city to care for the man, and accused the hospital of "hastening" MacDonald's death through its actions. At Morgan MacDonald's passing, Mayor Dianne Feinstein issued a statement. "It is sad," she said, "that a young man had to spend his final days as a medical outcast."

○

The day that Morgan MacDonald died, Gary Walsh was walking across Union Street, his favorite sixties songs running through his head from the soundtrack of the new movie he had just seen, *The Big Chill*. Suddenly, he felt dizzy. He waved his cane for a cab. The next thing he remembered was being put in an ambulance, telling somebody, "I've got AIDS. Take me to Franklin Hospital."

Gary was convinced he was dying. If he wasn't now, he wasn't sure how much longer he wanted to continue his posthumous existence. He had been thinking about it for a week anyway. In little ways, he had begun tying up the loose ends of his life. By the time Lu Chaikin and Matt Krieger visited him that evening, he had talked to a doctor friend about his plans. Reluctantly, the physician told Gary he'd give him whatever he needed.

The next day, Gary called Matt and said he planned to commit suicide if he recovered. Weeks earlier, Matt and Gary had had a bitter confrontation on the issue, because Matt bitterly opposed suicide. Knowing Matt's moral qualms about suicide, Gary was surprised when Matt simply said, "I support and respect your decision."

"Really?" Gary asked.

"You've been enormously brave and courageous for so long," Matt said. "You've been determined. Even your going to the movie alone yesterday was brave. I admire you and love you very much."

They talked about Gary's fears.

"That the Catholics are right," Gary said. "That I'll go to hell for taking my life. And that it won't work."

A few days later, the doctor put Gary on morphine. With his pain at a tolerable level, Gary retreated from his plan for suicide. He told Matt he was glad to have considered the issue and would now hold it open as "an option" if the pain returned.

○

On October 31, 1983, the Centers for Disease Control counted 2,640 AIDS cases in the country, of which 1,092 were dead. Of these, 1,042 were from New York City and 320 were from the San Francisco Bay Area. As the disease began spreading more thoroughly across the country, the geographical focus of the disease began to shift. In October 1982, about three-fourths of the nation's AIDS caseload had lived in one of the four cities hardest hit by the epidemic: New York, San Francisco, Los Angeles, and Miami. By now, however, fewer than two-thirds of the people with AIDS lived in these cities.

Gary Walsh lay awake in his bed when she appeared to him, with long white hair and outstretched arms. Gary recognized the woman as the mother of a good friend; she had died just a few months ago. She was stunningly beautiful and beamed a spectacular smile as she assured him, "Don't worry, honey. I'll help you over that line. And it ain't bad at all here."

38 JOURNALISM

November 4, 1983
SAN FRANCISCO PRESS CLUB

The press club had recruited Bill Kurtis, co-anchor of the "CBS Morning News," to deliver the keynote address for the group's annual awards dinner. As keynote speakers are wont to do, Kurtis opened his talk to the assembly of journalists with a little joke.

"I was in Nebraska yesterday and when I said I was going to San Francisco, people started talking about AIDS," Kurtis said, smiling. "Somebody said, 'What's the hardest part about having AIDS?' "

Kurtis paused for his punch line: "It's trying to convince your wife you're Haitian."

An uncomfortable laugh skimmed the surface of the crowd. Most people did not think it was funny. Several reporters nodded knowingly to each other, as if to say, "This is what you can expect from somebody who lives in New York."

Kurtis clearly had misjudged his audience. Nevertheless, the joke reflected the dormant feeling among national news organizations, all of which were headquartered in Manhattan. AIDS remained something of a dirty little joke. Moreover, it was something you could josh about in crowds of reporters because you could safely assume that the disease had not touched the lives of the people who wrote the news and scripted the nightly newscasts. Homosexual reporters, particularly in New York, tended to know their place and keep their mouths shut, if they wanted to survive in the news business.

Newspapers like *The New York Times* and *Washington Post* solemnly insisted that they did not discriminate against an employee on the basis of sexual orientation. In practice, however, such papers never had hired anyone who would openly say they were gay, and homosexual reporters at such papers privately maintained that their careers would be stalled if not destroyed once their sexuality became known. Gays were tolerated as drama critics and food reviewers, but the hard-news sections of the paper had a difficult time acclimating to women as reporters, much less inverts. Few in the business ever talked about this. American journalism was always better at defining others' foible than its own.

In New York, editors complained that nothing new was happening with the epidemic. Indeed, the more obvious breaking angles—such as the discovery of an accepted cause or a breakthrough in treatment—had not yet happened. Still, the numbers of new cases were rising exponentially, and even a modicum of investigatory journalism revealed a trove of flashy new angles for news stories.

The *San Francisco Chronicle* struck pay dirt in late November when a Freedom of Information Act request unearthed hundreds of pages of internal memoranda revealing the serious funding shortages at the Centers for Disease Control. The duplicity of many of the nation's top health officials was also apparent by comparisons of the newly released memoranda and conflicting congressional testimony offered on virtually the same days. In Washington, administration officials braced for a torrent of journalistic investigations after the front-page *Chronicle* stories, but nothing happened. To other news organizations, AIDS was a science story or a human interest story, but for years to come, AIDS would not be a story to which standard journalistic techniques applied. Thus, the federal government did not have to fret that news hounds would dog their AIDS efforts. It wasn't going to happen.

News coverage and the lack of it left a profound mark on local public policy. When the Institute for Health Policy Studies at the University of California in San Francisco later analyzed the differences between the municipal responses to AIDS in New York City and San Francisco, it concluded that the disparate quality rested in part on the vast difference in news coverage by the two cities' major newspapers. Between June 1982 and June 1985, the *San Francisco Chronicle* printed 442 staff-written AIDS stories, of which 67 made the front page. In the same period, *The New York Times* ran 226 stories, only 7 of which were on page one. From mid-1983 on, the coverage of the *Chronicle* focused on public policy aspects of the epidemic, while the *Times* covered AIDS almost exclusively as a medical event, with little emphasis on social impact or policy. The study concluded, "The extensive nature of coverage by the *Chronicle,* aside from providing a degree of health education not found in New York, helped sustain a level of political pressure on local government and health officials to respond to the AIDS crisis."

Nationally, the problem was not so much in what the press covered as in what they did not print. Indeed, throughout the epidemic, well-intentioned journalists went out of their way to calm hysteria. Particularly since the "routine household contact" fiasco, virtually every news story stressed that AIDS was not casually infectious and that it posed no threat to "the general population." In the soul-searching that came later, journalism reviews criticized news organizations for not discussing the specific sexual practices that spread AIDS, most notably anal intercourse. This was a proper criticism, but it was a minor one. The fact that it was the only major self-criticism by the news business was a measure of the epidemic's continued trivialization, even after AIDS was a major national news story.

It wasn't that the news organizations weren't thinking about AIDS during this time. Everybody talked about it; everybody joked about it. Planning for coverage of the 1984 Democratic National Convention in San Francisco created unusual concerns for sophisticated Manhattanites journeying to what they considered the AIDS capital. NBC News, for example, queried local caterers as to whether homosexuals would be serving food if hired to cater the NBC news staff. NBC wanted assurances that their staff would not be served by gays, it turned out, because they were afraid of getting AIDS.

NATIONAL CANCER INSTITUTE, BETHESDA

The laboratory of Tumor Cell Biology fills the B corridor of the sixth floor of red-brick Building 31 at the National Cancer Institute. The cinder block walls are painted a cheerful yellow; the sound of centrifuges echoes behind gray doors sealed with double air locks to keep the labs' deadly retroviruses from escaping. For six months, B corridor was headquarters for the nation's laboratory war against AIDS, and the man in office 6B03 was Dr. Robert Gallo, its commander.

In September, the Pasteur Institute had sent to Gallo isolates of its LAV to help establish their case that LAV was not a relative of HTLV-I but a distinct virus. The chronology of this virus' arrival in Bethesda would later prove very important.

Shortly after receiving the virus, Dr. Gallo had started forging major breakthroughs in his AIDS research. For more than a year, Gallo's progress had stumbled on one key point. His laboratory staff could not grow whatever virus was causing AIDS. It kept killing his cell lines. Gallo was sure some kind of retrovirus was at work. For months, he had detected reverse transcriptase activity, but that didn't do him much good when he needed to isolate the specific virus, sustain the microbe's growth, and establish that this was the cause of AIDS. Gallo had a nagging fear that the retrovirus he was seeing was simply another opportunistic infection. Without isolates of a specific virus, there was no way to resolve this question.

Gallo also was getting impatient. In the fall, he had confided to an AIDS writer from the gay paper the *Advocate* that if his HTLV studies did not prove fruitful soon, he would shift his research to other diseases and more promising fields. By November, however, his doubts had passed. Although Gallo told few colleagues, he believed he had now isolated the virus that caused AIDS.

Meanwhile, rivalry continually dogged AIDS research at the National Institutes of Health. Robert Gallo's temper had earned him many enemies within the NIH. Some NIH doctors wouldn't allow their lab techs to deliver tissue samples to Gallo, so Dr. Sam Broder, who was working with AIDS patients at the NIH hospital, took to walking specimens from patients to Building 31 himself.

Sniping also continued between the National Cancer Institute and the National Institute for Allergy and Infectious Diseases. The strangest twist came in late October when Dr. Ken Sell and other NIAID researchers announced that they had discovered a fungus they believed might cause the syndrome. The fungus, they said, mimicked the immune suppression caused by drugs used to artificially slow immune response. NCI doctors believed that the announcement by Sell, who had served as AIDS coordinator for NIAID, was made to embarrass Gallo and detract from his retroviral theories. Researchers at the Centers for Disease Control thought the fungal theory bordered on witchcraft. Few suspected that the announcement was anything other than the continuation of the NIAID–NCI feud over which institute should have primacy in AIDS research.

Scientists outside the NIH expressed more open skepticism about the HTLV-I hypothesis. In no study had HTLV been found in more than 25 percent of AIDS patients. These isolates tended to come from Haitians who hailed from a region where the leukemia virus is endemic anyway. Harvard's Dr. Max Essex, the leading proponent of HTLV-I, argued that the HTLV-I antibody tests might not be sensitive enough, but this convinced few scientists. By October, Dr. Paul Black of Boston University School of Medicine warned in the *New England Journal of Medicine* that HTLV-I had been "overplayed to the point where I worry that it will diminish interest in other viruses. . . . I think it's getting an overwhelming emphasis. There's a lot of hype associated with it." In backing his "serious doubts" about HTLV-I, Black noted that HTLV "immortalized" cells, allowing them to propagate madly, while the AIDS virus had the opposite effect and was killing lymphocytes.

Research in other government laboratories continued to bog down because of the lack of resources. Dr. Bill Blattner, division director of the NCI Environmental Epidemiology Branch, where NCI AIDS research began in June 1981, continued to pilfer from other research projects to support his AIDS studies. Although money now existed for AIDS research, a hiring freeze had aborted Blattner's attempts to add scientists to his staff. Even worse, Blattner was unable, because of the freeze, to replace researchers when they left his division. At times, when he heard NIH officials tell Congress that AIDS researchers had all the money they needed, he wondered whom the officials were talking to. They obviously weren't talking much to the researchers.

At the Centers for Disease Control, laboratory work stalled because Dr. Gallo had made good on his threat to deny HTLV reagents to Dr. V. S. Kalyanaraman as punishment for leaving the NCI. Dr. Kaly was left to start his retrovirus lab from scratch and hunt down people who were infected with HTLV-I and HTLV-II so he could culture the retrovirus and antibodies himself. Don Francis opened all his lab reports at every weekly meeting of the CDC AIDS researchers in Atlanta with an enumeration of the problems caused by lack of space, lack of staffing, and lack of money. Money had started to trickle in from the various congressional funding initiatives, but, as was always the case in AIDS studies, it tended to come a day late and a buck short.

When the *San Francisco Chronicle* pressed Dr. James Curran for an assessment of funding needs in the wake of the Freedom of Information Act disclosures, Curran conceded that problems had troubled the early efforts of the AIDS Task Force at CDC but that everything was fine now. "This is cursing the darkness after the candles have been lit," said Curran. "You can't single out the government; everybody was late in picking up on how serious this was. The media wasn't around two years ago and neither were the congressmen who are talking so much now."

At both the NIH and CDC, anxiety grew more profound. In early 1983, virtually everyone had expected that the AIDS virus would have been found by then.

◯

In Paris, over six months before, scientists had published articles on the virus that caused AIDS, but few were paying much attention to them. With characteristic French understatement, Pasteur Institute researchers recalled the fall of 1983 as the time of "the long walk across the desert."

The Pasteur scientists were convinced they had accumulated enough evidence to decisively demonstrate that they had isolated the virus behind the epidemic. They had cultured virus or detected LAV antibodies in all ten lymphadenopathy patients on whom they had performed blood work, and they were working on a standardized test to detect LAV antibodies for use in blood banks. They had sent the virus to both the CDC and the Max-von-Pettenkofer Institute in Munich for inoculation in chimpanzees. Exhaustive immunological work determined that the virus selectively targeted the T-4 lymphocytes, the very cells that disappeared in AIDS victims, setting the stage for the final collapse of the immune system. Trials of the antiviral drug HPA-23 were under way among sixty French AIDS patients to determine the toxicity of the drug.

Despite all their evidence, the Parisian doctors found that the American scientific establishment was reluctant to take their work seriously. Their research papers were subjected to lengthy delays. In rejecting one paper, an American reviewer took a nationalistic tact when he dismissed LAV as "the French virus." Behind the scenes, Robert Gallo at the NCI continued to spread the word that LAV was nothing more than a laboratory contaminant. Repeatedly, Pasteur researchers heard from their American counterparts that, yes, the Pasteur work was interesting, but they would wait to see what Gallo came up with. Willy Rozenbaum, returning to his tropical disease ward after such conversations, continued to see new patients parading by with their grisly array of diseases, and wanted to shout: "People are dying. We are losing time." But there was no one to hear him.

The disheartened doctors often ended their fourteen-hour days commiserating at a Left Bank cabaret, the Paradise Latin, where they pondered what more they could do to make people believe them. The researchers' spouses joked that they would form an anti-SIDA committee to get the researchers' minds off the relentless frustration of having the answer but being ignored.

In November, Francoise Barre, the Pasteur researcher who had discovered LAV the previous January, ran into Bob Gallo at the international airport outside Tokyo. Both were bound for the same scientific conference, so they shared a cab into Tokyo. During the ride, Gallo confided that at last he had discovered the retrovirus that caused AIDS. It might even prove to be similar to LAV, he said.

Back in Paris, the Pasteur researchers had no doubt that whatever AIDS virus Gallo had discovered would indeed prove to be LAV. Perhaps, finally, they would gain their long-denied recognition.

◯

Dr. Jay Levy, researcher at the University of California at San Francisco, had done a sabbatical with Dr. Jean-Claude Chermann at the Pasteur and had maintained his links to the institute over the years. When Levy visited Paris in September, he was impressed by the Pasteur's research, although he turned down an offer to take LAV back to San Francisco with him. He intended to find the AIDS retrovirus himself and did not want skeptics to later charge that his own research was tainted by lab contamination. Within a month of his return, Levy had cultured six isolates of a retrovirus from the blood of local AIDS patients. He decided against speeding the research into publication until he could accumulate more definitive proof that his agent was indeed the cause of AIDS and not an opportunistic infection.

It was November 1983, and science at last was closing in on the viral culprit that bred international death. Unfortunately, the scientific intrigue that would surround the discovery had only begun.

November 7
MATT KRIEGER'S JOURNAL

For the third time in some four weeks, Gary is in the hospital. This time with pneumonia. Not *Pneumocystis* pneumonia, just regular pneumonia.

Pneumonia, Kaposi's sarcoma, severe psoriasis, herpes, an anal fissure, a bad tooth that needs a root canal (but can't be treated because of risk of infection and the fact that he couldn't withstand the procedure). Probably more infections that I can't think of.

He's been extremely weak, especially the last three or four days. Too weak to walk, to eat his food, to shower, even to squeeze a tube of toothpaste or push the button on the shaving cream can.

I stayed with him three of the last four nights. . . . During these times, his conversations go to his inability to withstand the pain. "This is no way to live. I've lost my fighting spirit. I don't know how much longer I can make it." And that's so understandable to me now, even though I can never even vaguely comprehend the severity of his pain.

To my surprise and pleasure and at his suggestion, I slept on his bed two of the three nights. We sleep on far opposite sides of his big platform bed. Still I have sexual feelings for him. Although I haven't felt very sexual in a while. . . .

[This morning] it was the talk with the nurse just before I left that first disturbed me. She told me of Larry, a guy with AIDS on the floor. Larry and Gary never met but exchanged greetings through their doctor. Everyone said Larry was friendly, wonderful, terrific, fun, and caring. Now he's crazy, senile, and psychotic, they say. He thinks he's being raped. Thinks he's dead. Thinks he's at home. Outbursts of anger at people he loves. Doesn't recognize people. He's given up and he's mentally gone. He'll be dead very soon.

What must this do to Gary to hear this? It must be horrible.

Then, after I left Gary's room, I ran into a nurse, Angelina. She confirmed the report about Larry. "And this one in here, with KS," she said to me just outside a patient's open door, "he's going to die in two or three days. He's been here two months. His face, it's horrible. Do you want to see it?"

No thanks.

"I'm afraid for Gary," she said. "Larry had the same terrible headaches just a few weeks ago."

I went into the hospital with hope. I left with a sickness in my stomach.

What lies ahead? Gary will not go through that, I know. . . . When I left the hospital, I stopped by Gary's apartment to pick up clothing and my tape recorder, which I had left there over the weekend. I ran into the man who delivers videotapes to Gary. He was there to pick up some tapes, which I got for him from the apartment.

"How's Gary?" he asked.

"Not so good," I said.

"My best friend died of AIDS in Los Angeles this morning," he told me. "He got a respiratory infection three or four days ago and his whole system just went whammo."

I feel surrounded by inevitable painful death.

⬭

Gary was awake in bed when another image appeared to him. This friend had been a writer and aspiring stand-up comedian before he died of leukemia in September. Gary was excited to see him.

"There is a passageway you have to go through," he told Gary. "I'll help you get through it. You'll like it here."

Gary asked him to come back again, and a few days later he did.

"I'm scared," Gary said.

"I told you not to worry about it," his friend said, seeming impatient at the interruption. "Now stop bothering me. I've got writing to do."

⬭

The off-year municipal elections on November 8 produced a bonanza for a gay political movement that had worked long to broaden its political base nationally. Openly gay men were elected to the city councils of both Boston and Minneapolis, while a gay art dealer became mayor in Key West. Virtually all the major Democratic presidential contenders were now on the record in favor of gay civil rights. Within days of the election, Senators Alan Cranston, John Glenn, and Ernest Hollings, who were all announced presidential hopefuls, included their names among the fifteen solons seeking Senate AIDS hearings in the fall. Mayor Dianne Feinstein rolled up the largest margins in San Francisco history to win her second full term. The city got a collective chuckle from an obscure opponent named Brian Lantz, who was the northern California field organizer for an equally obscure extremist presidential candidate named Lyndon LaRouche. Among Lantz's claims in the race was that the city should abandon pro-gay politics, because he could establish that homosexuality was a temporary condition that could be "cured" with proper treatment.

The disclosure in mid-November that Dr. Selma Dritz had sought a legal opinion on whether she could ban people with AIDS from the city's gay bathhouses resurrected some gay leaders' convictions that a general lock-down of the city's homosexuals was imminent. Dritz had sought the city attorney's opinion about the legality of forcing AIDS sufferers out of the baths after continuing reports that patients were routinely using the sex palaces. The stories came at a time when bathhouse patronage was soaring again. A deputy city attorney ruled that Dritz would be on shaky legal ground because scientists had yet to discover a viral agent behind the epidemic, thereby proving conclusively that AIDS was a communicable disease.

Dritz leaked the story to the *San Francisco Chronicle,* hoping at least to warn gay men of the risk in continued attendance at bathhouses. Meanwhile, at the state health department's infectious disease headquarters in Berkeley, meetings were being organized to determine state policy on what to do about recalcitrant AIDS patients. Ultimately, state health authorities listed an array of options, beginning with community dissuasion of such behavior and ending with possible quarantine of obdurate individuals. Ritualistic denunciations from gay leaders and civil liberties lawyers followed such talk. More imaginative gay leaders insisted that the suggestions were preludes to the internment of the entire gay community. The civil rights of people who might contract the deadly syndrome from these patients was rarely considered in these arguments.

Dritz tried to keep the debate elevated to the level of policy discussion. She never publicly discussed the individual who had inspired her to explore her options in restricting bathhouse patrons.

In Vancouver, Gaetan Dugas's health was beginning to fail. He had already defied all odds by surviving over three years after his June 1980 diagnosis with Kaposi's sarcoma. As his energy faded, he confided to friends that he was growing tired of the fight.

On November 21, 1983, the Centers for Disease Control reported that 2,803 Americans had been diagnosed with Acquired Immune Deficiency Syndrome. Of these, 1,146 had died.

November 22
GENEVA, SWITZERLAND

By the time thirty-eight AIDS experts from around the world gathered at the World Health Organization headquarters in Geneva for the first meeting on the international implications of the AIDS epidemic, the disease had been reported in thirty-three nations on five continents.

Canadian health authorities had logged fifty cases throughout the confederation. Six cases had been reported in Israel in the past year, and four in Australia. On the eve of the conference, Japan had reported its first two AIDS cases, making it the first Asian nation to be touched by the epidemic. The brothels, Turkish baths, and sex parlors in Tokyo's famed Yushiwara District were refusing entry to foreign visitors for fear that they might spread AIDS. Baths posted signs reading: "Japanese Men Only."

At the end of 1982, European health authorities had reported 67 cases of AIDS. By the time conference participants gathered in the aluminum-and-glass WHO headquarters, 267 cases were reported in fifteen western European nations. West German epidemiologists were now uncovering their own sexually related clusters of cases. Although early patients could virtually all be linked to sexual activity in the United States, it was clear by late 1983 that Germany now had its own pool of infected men who were spreading the disease. In Denmark, the national health board already had moved to establish specialized clinics and screening centers for the disease. With 27 cases now reported in Great Britain, doctors were clamoring for research money from a conservative prime minister who did not include the epidemic on her list of health priorities.

France reported the highest AIDS caseload on the continent, with 94 diagnosed patients. As in Belgium, more than half of the cases reported were natives or tourists of five African nations—Zaire, Congo, Mali, Gabon, and Rwanda.

French and Belgian research in these Central African nations, particularly Zaire, had recently led NIH and CDC scientists from the United States to Kinshasa. Shortly before the Geneva meeting, Dr. John McCormick had discussed his findings at a meeting of CDC AIDS researchers in Atlanta. In just two weeks, McCormick had confirmed 37 AIDS cases at two hospitals in Kinshasa. The CDC was stunned that McCormick could find so many cases in just two hospitals in so brief a time. The disease was obviously widespread in Africa, although it had not been noticed because of the lack of sophisticated medical care. Searching through hospital records and death certificates, the epidemiologists made an even more disconcerting finding. The disease had killed nearly as many women as men, leading researchers to believe that in these poor Equatorial nations, AIDS was spreading as a heterosexually transmitted disease. The typical female patient was a young unmarried prostitute, while the male victims tended to be the older single men who used them. Nine cases could be linked in two clusters. The epidemiology suggested that, unlike in the United States, where most heterosexually transmitted cases were spread from men to women, AIDS was spreading bi-directionally in Africa, from men to women and from women to men.

The findings were consistent with research in Haiti that found that one-third of the 202 reported Haitian AIDS cases were among women, again suggesting heterosexual transmission routes. The initial routes of the epidemic's spread became clear by virtue of the link between Haiti and Zaire in the early 1970s, when the African nation imported many better-educated Haitians who, as

French-speaking blacks, could take the role of the Belgian colonial administrators who had been expelled. Given the longer history of AIDS in Africa, it appeared that the Haitians had taken AIDS back to the island of Hispaniola at about the same time that the first cases of AIDS, virtually all of which were linked to Central Africa, appeared in Europe.

The WHO conference room overlooked Lake Geneva and a panorama of the Swiss countryside. Delegates gathered around M-shaped tables. Don Francis sat with Marc Conant, with whom he had found a common concern about what lay ahead. Health officials from the Soviet satellite nations of eastern Europe sat across from them, although Czechoslovakia was the only communist nation to concede that AIDS could spread within socialist borders. Throughout the four-day meeting, representatives of the Union of Soviet Socialist Republics stoically insisted otherwise.

"We will not have any of these cases in the Soviet Union," said a Soviet delegate confidently.

Don Francis couldn't resist saying to Marc Conant in his loudest stage whisper, "And they won't, all right." In a stern Russian accent, Francis continued: "You have AIDS—bang, bang, bang."

The Soviets were not amused.

The more serious discussion centered on the problem of blood, the one area in which officials felt they could slow the scope of the epidemic. Nine European hemophiliacs had contracted AIDS from Factor VIII manufactured in the United States, including three of the first four Spaniards to be stricken with the syndrome. Most suggestions centered on banning the shipment of blood products from the United States, a move that several European nations already had implemented. But in the Netherlands, the Dutch Red Cross backed off on screening plans in the face of rigorous gay opposition. The British health ministry had countered fear of AIDS in blood by echoing the U.S. blood centers' claims that there was "no conclusive proof" that the ailment could be transmitted through transfusions.

$$\bigcirc$$

That night, at a Swiss bistro, Don Francis had dinner with Jim Curran and Ed Brandt.

"What went wrong with AIDS?" Francis asked Brandt bluntly.

"What do you mean?" Brandt asked.

"It seems like we're always behind in funding," Francis said. "We're always piecing things together."

"Bill [Foege, CDC director] and I thought it was poppers," Brandt said. "We thought it would be over by now."

Francis was disbelieving. He played killer racquetball with Foege every week, and he knew that the CDC director had not believed AIDS was caused by poppers since late 1981. That was two years before.

39 PEOPLE

December 1983
WARD 5B,
SAN FRANCISCO GENERAL HOSPITAL

Chanteuse Sharon McKnight tugged her black-and-white feathered boa over the web of clear plastic tubes threaded into various patients as she stood to examine a light blue hospital gown.

"Love it," cooed McKnight, a popular cabaret singer. "It looks designer."

"See the Dior label?" parried the patient, tugging the gown around his neck like a precious mink.

"San Francisco General Hospital," gushed the entertainer, fingering the gown. "Yes, yes. This is the only place where I like not playing to a full house."

Everybody laughed, except for the man with the scars from two holes drilled in his head earlier that week. The doctors had tried to find out what bizarre infection had virtually robbed him of his mind. That patient stared straight into space, fidgeting occasionally when McKnight's boa ran across his leg. The dozen other patients sipped champagne and smiled at the doctors and nurses crowding the AIDS Ward's largest room for McKnight's performance. Everyone at San Francisco General knew that the unconventional AIDS Ward was the most entertaining unit in the hospital. Gay nurses took their breaks there, joking with the patients or, sometimes, just quietly holding their hands. Throughout the holiday season, gay volunteer groups tromped through the hallways giving massages, handing out presents, and dishing out gourmet dinners. The extraordinary charity efforts were an aspect of the gay community that didn't get much press. On this cold drizzly night, Sharon McKnight had rolled her own piano in to sing "Stand By Your Man" to men who would probably never get to a nightclub again, because they all were going to die.

More people died in Ward 5B than in any other ward of the hospital; more diseases raged in a typical 5B patient's body than could be found in an entire ward in any other part of the hospital. And there were more such patients checking into the hospital every day. In just four months, the ward had had over 100 admissions. The unit was filled to capacity now, and another three patients waited in other wards for transfer to 5B.

The AIDS Ward had created an unheard-of situation at the county hospital:

Well-heeled, respectable gay men clamored to get in. To say the least, San Francisco General had suffered more than its share of image problems and was frequently on the brink of losing its accreditation. But the innovations undertaken by AIDS nursing coordinator Cliff Morrison had returned some luster to the hospital's reputation. Other doctors, convinced that Morrison had political pull with the gay community, deferred to him, giving him leeway to continue his unorthodox approach to health care.

The most recent innovation Morrison instituted concerned visiting privileges in a patient's final days. Normally, the ailing man's biological family was given all prerogatives in deciding who saw a patient in the critical care unit. However, an unseemly conflict had arisen recently when one patient's mother marched into her dying son's room and ordered out his longtime lover. "I'm his mother and I don't want any faggots in this room," she announced brusquely. "And I don't want any of those nurses who are faggots. They did this to him."

The patient broke down crying but was unable to speak because he was on a ventilator. A few days later, he died without seeing his lover again.

Morrison announced the new 5B policy: that all patients designate their significant others who would have visiting privileges. As far as Morrison was concerned, the definition of the American family had changed. It should be the right of patients themselves to define their families, not the right of the hospital.

As the months progressed, Ward 5B developed its own rituals. During the days, patients pushed their IV feeders around with them in the hallways and talked to each other about their release dates, like prisoners looking ahead to the day they would be sprung. Conversations sometimes evolved into high camp, eerily punctuated by painfully long coughs that echoed from the rooms of the many PCP patients. At night, amid the humming of the refrigerated blankets that kept the *Pneumocystis*-bred fevers from spiking above 103 degrees, there was only the sound of heavy breathing and, occasionally, the mournful groans of nightmares.

Bruce Schneider was one of the residents of 5B whose recurring nightmare had him fading, dissolving like some phantasm into the air. His friends hovered in the vague distance, asking him: "Bruce, why are you fading away?" He tried to answer, but they didn't hear; he just continued to fade.

The dream came many times in the two months Bruce was in the hospital. Until August, he had been a regular hardworking guy in the Castro, holding down a weekday job with the phone company and pulling in weekend shifts as a brunch cook. Then, he felt steel bands wrap around his chest, and he had a hard time breathing. The doctors told him he had *Pneumocystis*. Now he lay in the bed at the end of the hall, watching television. And much of what he saw wasn't relevant to him now—all the commercials about retirement accounts, pension funds, and IRAs, for instance.

A normal thirty-year-old single male like Bruce could expect to live another 43.2 years, according to insurance actuarial tables. But he now knew that, if typical, he would live only ten more months. He felt as though he were on Death Row.

Three doors down from Bruce was Deotis McMather, tossing in the throes of his nightmare. A native of the hills of southern Virginia, Deotis had lived a seamy life in San Francisco, hustling tricks and shooting drugs in the Tenderloin neighborhood. In April, he noticed bruises all over his body. He had no way of knowing that his body had stopped producing blood cells called platelets, which help blood to clot. Instead of clotting, Deotis's blood began to leak from his capillaries with each bump he suffered. In October, a trick told Deotis that his back was covered with purple spots. When Deotis went to San Francisco General for AIDS tests, his roommate had Deotis's belongings packed and sent off to a friend's house with instructions that Deotis should not return. It didn't matter much because Deotis would never be able to leave the hospital.

A week into his hospital stay, the doctors determined that Deotis had idiopathic thrombocytopenic purpura, which is why he was lacking platelets. Because this condition had left a good portion of his abdominal organs inflamed, doctors cut out Deotis's spleen and part of his liver and stomach. When a newspaper reporter came by to talk, Deotis raised his light blue hospital gown to show him the long, slashing scar, all held together with staples. Deotis was retaining fluids, so the scar looked like a big zipper stretched across his bloating stomach. Deotis smiled as a photographer took a photograph of him holding his gown up. The photo never made it into the paper because an editor thought he'd throw up when he saw it.

Deotis's nightmare started after his operation. He was running, running hard, among the cold concrete towers in downtown San Francisco. Nobody was on the streets. He was alone except for the policemen chasing him down. Deotis stumbled. The police caught him and started kicking him in the stomach. "Can't you see I'm sick?" Deotis asked. "Stop."

But they continued kicking him. He started throwing up. Brown clumps of maggots and crawly worms spewed from his mouth. He was coughing up the maggots when he awakened.

About two weeks after his operation, Deotis's already melancholy disposition turned grim. He started telling nurses that he didn't want to be a drain on people. His condition deteriorated when his lungs started filling with fluid. He was put on a respirator, but after a few days, he asked to be taken off the machine. Within an hour, twenty-seven-year-old Deotis McMather was dead. He was one of three patients on 5B who died that day.

Such stories helped convince the nurses on the AIDS Ward that the will to live was not fantasy but was probably the single most influential factor in determining how long patients survived. People who decided it was time to die, very often did; the young men who fought the disease, often lived longer. Bruce Schneider talked a lot about fighting in December 1983. Maybe he'd get that silver bullet, or that "reprieve from the governor," as he called it. Something was bound to come along soon, he figured. He'd read in the paper that the Reagan administration was calling AIDS its number-one health priority. Maybe soon it would all be over, and he'd get back to those carefree picnics in the Marin countryside and long walks in the Redwoods he liked so much.

December 6
CAPITOL,
WASHINGTON, D.C.

NEWS RELEASE
HOUSE REPORT DOCUMENTS INADEQUATE RESPONSE TO AIDS

The Department of Health and Human Services has failed to adequately fund
Federal efforts to fight the Acquired Immunodeficiency Syndrome (AIDS)
epidemic, according to a report prepared by the Intergovernmental Relations and Human Resources Subcommittee chaired by Representative Ted
Weiss (D-NY).

. . . The subcommittee investigation revealed that despite Administration claims that sufficient funds were being spent on AIDS, important surveillance, epidemiological studies, and laboratory research at CDC and
NIH were undermined because of inadequate resources.

"Tragically, funding levels for AIDS investigations have been dictated
by political considerations rather than by the professional judgments of
scientists and public health officials who are waging the battle against
the epidemic," said Weiss. "The inadequacy of funding, coupled with inex-
cusable delays in research activity, leads me to question the Federal Government's preparedness for national health emergencies, as well as this
Administration's commitment to an urgent resolution to the AIDS crisis.

The subcommittee's thirty-six-page report, "The Federal Response to AIDS,"
accompanied the shorter press release announcing the subcommittee's findings.
It was never clear how many reporters read anything other than the press
release, since few news organizations proved very interested in the story. There
was a *New York Times* story and a shorter wire service piece that included press
release quotes and the administration's ritual denial.

The lack of attention was unfortunate because the report marked the only
comprehensive investigation of federal AIDS policy yet undertaken by anybody. The months of poring through CDC files had produced a highly detailed
summary of every problem the CDC, NIH, and extramural researchers had
faced in their attempts to secure an adequate response to the epidemic. Many
of Don Francis's memos were on the report's pages, as well as other memoranda
written at the ascending levels of the health bureaucracy during the course of
the epidemic.

Probably the most startling revelation was the continued absence of any
coordinated plan for attacking AIDS, even at this time in late 1983. After
months of pressure, the Department of Health and Human Services had submitted a six-page document to the subcommittee in late October. The congressional
report, however, had little praise for this effort.

"The so-called 'operational plan' is, on its face, a document created for the
subcommittee, and serves only to highlight the lack of comprehensive planning
and budgeting by the PHS in response to AIDS," the report said. "It provides
no specific information about future research and surveillance plans. It barely
mentions, if at all, HHS strategy, timetables, contingency plans, and vehicles for

evaluating the Government's activity. Essentially, the plan submitted by HHS is an abbreviated fact sheet about past activities, rather than a program for dealing with the Nation's 'number-one health priority.'"

To prevent similar problems with other health emergencies, the report recommended funding of the Public Health Emergency Fund. The subcommittee also recommended procedures to expedite NIH resources during emergencies. As for the specific problem of AIDS, the subcommittee recommended that the federal government establish an independent commission to both recommend a comprehensive strategy to fight AIDS and suggest resources necessary to carry out the battle.

"The committee believes that PHS researchers and physicians are eminently qualified to plan and conduct the nation's response to health emergencies, including AIDS," the report concluded. "At the same time, these scientists are subjected to severe political and fiscal constraints especially in times of shrinking federal budgets for public health programs. Unfortunately, the lives of countless Americans may be jeopardized when the scope of AIDS research and surveillance is dictated by budget considerations rather than the professional judgments of public health and medical experts."

As was now common in matters of AIDS policy, support and opposition to the unusually hard-hitting report fell along party lines. Ten of the subcommittee's fourteen Republican members added their dissenting opinion to the report, calling it "misleading" and denouncing the idea of an independent panel to review AIDS strategy as "unnecessary." The Republican members wrote, "The PHS already has the responsibility and expertise to develop the proposed plan."

Dr. Edward Brandt accurately noted to reporters that the president had never vetoed congressional efforts to add AIDS funds. "By the time I put a request in and it goes through all the processes, Congress passes the money," he said. "The administration has never taken the position to fight congressional moves for more money. We have spent all the dollars made available to us." As for extramural funding delays, Brandt conceded, "I wouldn't argue that we're perfect and we haven't made some mistakes, but our efforts have been comprehensive and responsible." The criticism of early sluggishness was so much Monday-morning quarterbacking, he said, and was the product of "the 20/20 vision of hindsight."

In San Francisco, Bill Kraus waited for the shoe to drop. Like other gay congressional aides, Bill was convinced the report would spark tough journalistic investigations of the federal AIDS program. Never had so much information on such a hot topic been so neatly tied together and placed in reporters' laps than in this report.

Bill waited, and he waited. By the end of December, it was clear that the report would pass with no impact on the federal government.

During the rounds of Christmas parties that year, Bill couldn't say enough bad things about the television networks and national newsmagazines who were letting the administration off the hook.

"They're not going to do anything," he said. "They're going to let us all die because we're queers."

◯

In Atlanta, little in the report surprised anyone. Despite the infusion of supplemental appropriations, the CDC's AIDS effort remained grossly underfunded. Dr. Walt Dowdle, director of the Center for Infectious Diseases, bluntly told the weekly meeting of AIDS researchers the day after the report's release that "There's more needs than funds."

A week later, Dr. Dowdle asked the new CDC director, Dr. James Mason, for an extra $3 million and, more significantly, forty-six staff positions for AIDS work. By now, Dr. Mason also saw the lack of AIDS resources as a huge problem for the agency. Like Ed Brandt, Mason proved an unusual ally for AIDS researchers. Until recently, he had served as state public health director for Utah. It was his friendship with conservative Utah Senator Orrin Hatch, the chair of the Senate committee in charge of HHS, that had netted him the job as CDC director. Gay leaders at first were suspicious of Mason, noting that he couldn't bring himself to utter the word "gay" when he met with a gay delegation on his first day on the job. Like Brandt, however, Mason had an ingrained American sensibility about fairness and couldn't see the sense in letting a horrible epidemic rage through the nation, even if he personally objected to the sexual proclivities of the people it largely struck.

In his own agency, James Mason thought the constant diversion of staff from other essential CDC activities was undermining morale. Still, Mason was in conflict over how to handle the resource problems. Members of Congress called him frequently to ask about AIDS funding needs, but Mason felt a loyalty to the administration. He sympathized and fundamentally agreed with the president's philosophy of cutting back domestic spending. Weeks after Walt Dowdle's request, Mason decided on a move that he considered both fiscally reasonable and morally responsible, and he established a special committee to start an exhaustive internal review of all CDC AIDS activities. He'd use the report as the basis for his future funding requests.

◯

By the time Dr. Mason's report was written, Bruce Schneider had died at San Francisco General Hospital, hoping until that last day for the reprieve that never came.

NEW YORK CITY

The tragedy of the AIDS-stricken children from Bronx slums was almost numbing now for Dr. Arye Rubinstein and his researchers working at the Albert Einstein College of Medicine. Eighteen months before, he had counted seven AIDS-stricken infants in his practice; a year before, thirteen; by the end of 1983, he was treating twenty-five children. A $27,000 grant from the state allowed him to hire one fellow who became the nucleus for virtually all psychosocial services for AIDS patients in the Bronx slums. Rubinstein could see that soon more children would live in city hospitals, like little Diana, the child who had now spent most of her life in Jacobi Hospital. Her brother, long suffering from AIDS-Related Complex, was near death now from *Pneumocystis,* and still, there was no imminent help from the city on Rubinstein's stalled plan to establish a day-care center for the children.

The strategy of both state and city health officials continued to minimize the severity of the AIDS problem, lending credence to their contention that they were doing enough to fight it. Both the state health commissioner, Dr. David Axelrod, and the city health commissioner, Dr. David Sencer, had cheerfully announced that AIDS diagnoses were decreasing in New York in the last months of 1983. The analyses were based on the fact that rather than doubling, as cases had been for two years, the rate of *increase* had gone down by 30 percent. This did not mean fewer cases; this only meant that instead of doubling in, say six months, the numbers of AIDS cases in New York City would double in nine months. Axelrod attributed the improvement to a "change in life-styles" among gay men. Sencer indicated that the drop-off showed that the health department's low-key approach to education was working. Dr. Herbert Dicker-man of the New York AIDS Institute, a new state-funded group, compared the number of AIDS cases to estimates that between 3 million and 7 million gay men lived in the United States, and he determined that only 1 in 1,000 had AIDS. "I wouldn't consider that an epidemic," he said.

The CDC wasn't impressed with the complacent outlook of health officials, given the fact that it was common knowledge that Manhattan gay doctors weren't reporting many of their cases because of the confidentiality dispute with the CDC. Dr. Richard Selik of the AIDS Activities Office responded to the reports of New York AIDS decreases by ordering an investigation on local reporting practices. In the end, it turned out that the rate of AIDS cases wasn't decreasing in New York but was increasing there as fast as elsewhere in the country. This did not deter the state and city health officials from continuing to announce, at virtually every juncture of the epidemic, that the rate of new AIDS cases was "leveling."

The only education program in New York City was still that of the Gay Men's Health Crisis, which had coordinated $3 million worth of volunteer time and services for AIDS in calendar year 1983 on a budget of only $120,000.

In the same week that New York officialdom was seeing a slowdown in the epidemic, San Francisco Mayor Dianne Feinstein approved spending another $1 million for AIDS services, bringing city spending on AIDS services for calendar 1983 to $4 million.

⬭

In the last weeks of 1983, newspapers were filled with year-in-review pieces. The Associated Press editors released their annual compilation of the year's top ten news stories. The terrorist bombing of the Marine headquarters in Beirut, in which 240 servicemen were killed, was voted the top story, followed by the downing of a South Korean airliner by Soviet jets, and the American invasion of Grenada. The year's top movies were *Silkwood* and *The Big Chill,* and nobody could talk enough about Michael Jackson's Moonwalking and *Thriller,* his huge comeback album. Although AIDS reporting had been the vogue earlier in the year, attention had now fully waned and nobody included the epidemic as a noteworthy benchmark for the year.

Hidden away on back pages, therefore, was the story from Atlanta, reporting that as of December 19, 1983, the CDC reported 3,000 Americans now stricken with Acquired Immune Deficiency Syndrome; of these, 1,283 were dead. Of all cases, 42 percent were reported in New York City, 12 percent in San Francisco, 8 percent in Los Angeles, and 3 percent in Newark. The only states in which no cases had yet been reported were Alaska, Idaho, Maine, Montana, North Dakota, South Dakota, West Virginia, and Wyoming.

By Christmas, Dr. Robert Gallo had told the director of the National Cancer Institute that he had discovered the retrovirus that caused AIDS.

December 26
MATT KRIEGER'S JOURNAL

This morning my anger ganged up inside me with nowhere to go.

Gary woke up after me, weak and in pain. He walked hunched over from pain in his legs. . . . I fixed him tea and loaded my red Mexican shopping bag for what seemed like the thousandth time in the past five days with things shuttled between my house and his apartment. I was running a little late already, and Gary asked me to run to the store to get cigarettes for him. That's when something snapped inside.

Driving to get his cigarettes, I just started screaming aloud: "My whole fucking life runs around Gary. Every goddamn minute. I can't stand it anymore. I want a lover who can do things with me. I want a lover who is healthy!"

It's an irrational anger. And I can't let it out at Gary. He's doing the best that he can. But it just seems like I don't have a life of my own. I don't have a home where I live. I'm in constant flux between his place and mine and constantly at his calling.

I'm scared because I see he's weaker and far less active than a week ago. Has Christmas tired him out? Is he deteriorating again? Was the recent improvement just getting ready for the holidays? . . . I'm scared he'll get sick again. I don't know that I can go through the long, horrible hours of watching him in pain, seeing him suffer and getting ready to die. I don't know how I could live today with death and his impending loss again. It's painful and exhausting for me. . . .

Gary is still very, very sick. He's weak and dependent. His body is still covered with purple lesions. I forget they're there, that they're real, when I hold him at night praying for his health, trying to literally transmit strength from my body to his.

I know I should be thankful for this time, no matter how difficult it is for me. It's much harder for Gary. If I'm scared, Gary must be terrified.

December 30
CENTERS FOR DISEASE CONTROL,
ATLANTA

The question of the length of the AIDS incubation period had troubled Dr. Dale Lawrence ever since July when he had visualized the epidemic as a series of marathons, with thousands racing toward their deaths. The CDC now had documented twenty-one AIDS patients whose disease was linked to blood transfusions, and another ten were under investigation. These cases were unique in that they provided researchers with a specific date on which they could pin the time of infection. In early December, Lawrence took all these dates to a statistician. Although these transfusion cases were among people with shorter incubation periods, Lawrence figured that the time between initial infection and the emergence of disease could be plotted on a mathematical curve.

Thus far, estimates of AIDS incubation represented little more than a hodge-podge of guesses. Most scientists used the two-year figure, although some transfusion cases reached back four years. Lawrence thought that a mathematical curve should be able to offer the first scientific assessments of the shortest and longest incubation periods for the disease. The CDC statistician devised seventeen pages of complicated formulae to plot the survival analysis.

On the last working day of 1983, the statistician gave Lawrence the results. Lawrence was horrified. According to the analysis, the mean incubation period for the disease was 5.5 years. It appeared that some cases would take more than 11 years to incubate, based on the mathematical projections, although some people would come down with AIDS in as little as six months.

Lawrence rushed from his office in the Division of Host Factors to the AIDS offices. He saw Jim Curran in the hall talking to Harold Jaffe and Bill Darrow.

"The incubation period is along the lines of five years," said Lawrence.

He explained the curves. Jim Curran grasped his logic immediately.

"It makes sense," Curran said.

That's what Lawrence was afraid of. He had believed that tens of thousands would die in the AIDS epidemic. This long incubation period, however, meant that the genetic machinations of the still-unknown virus had permitted it to sleep for years before anyone even knew it existed, before anyone knew it was spreading. It just hadn't shown up yet in a dramatic way because of the long incubation. The 3,000 AIDS cases now reported marked the barest beginning of the havoc the epidemic would bring. The future these projections promised was going to be worse, far worse, than anyone had ever imagined.

PART VII

LIGHTS & TUNNELS
1984

Thus, too, they came to know the incorrigible sorrow of all prisoners and exiles, which is to live in the company of a memory that serves no purpose. Even the past, of which they thought incessantly, had a savor only of regret. For they would have wished to add to it all that they regretted having left undone. . . . And thus there was always something missing in their lives. Hostile to the past, impatient of the present, and cheated of the future, we were much like those whose men's justice, or hatred, forces to live behind prison bars.

—ALBERT CAMUS,
The Plague

40 PRISONERS

January 3, 1984
NATIONAL INSTITUTES OF HEALTH,
BETHESDA

Larry Kramer had spent much of the past month visiting the federal agencies involved in AIDS work. His agent was reading the early draft of his play *The Normal Heart,* and having been out of AIDS action for nine months, Larry wanted to review government efforts against the epidemic. In a December trip to Atlanta, he was not surprised to see that the Centers for Disease Control seemed as underfunded and overworked as ever. He was taken aback, however, when one prominent staffer in the AIDS Activities Office bluntly asked him, "Why don't you guys get married?" When Larry started to explain that most states have laws specifically barring same-sex matrimony, the CDC doctor got impatient. "I don't mean marry men," he said. "I mean women. If you guys had been married to women, this never would have happened." The comment, from one of the CDC's top AIDS people, gave Larry insight into why, nearly three years into the epidemic, the CDC still did not include even one openly gay person on their burgeoning staff at the AIDS office.

Interagency rivalry between the CDC and the National Cancer Institute was frequently alluded to during the Atlanta trip. One CDC official candidly admitted, "We don't even talk to them."

In early January, congressional staffer Tim Westmoreland arranged a visit for Larry Kramer to the home of the director of one of the largest and most prestigious institutes among the National Institutes of Health. Like several of the other top NIH directors, this agency chief lived in a baronial mansion on the Bethesda campus, surrounded by antiques and a doting staff.

During the luncheon, Larry excused himself to visit the lavatory. Upstairs, he was attracted to a crowded bookshelf that faced an open bedroom door opposite the stairs. Convinced that you can judge a lot about a person by their books, Larry wandered in. The shelves had an eclectic assortment of volumes: popular fiction, philosophical texts, and scientific volumes, except for one shelf, on which were several expensively framed photos of handsome men in bathing suits, posing with muscles flexed and arms wrapped around each other. In one, a prominent NIH official struck a campy Charles Atlas stance.

Back at the luncheon, the prominent institute director excused himself to return to his office after earnestly impressing on Larry how much his agency had done for AIDS. Larry remained unconvinced, knowing that this particular agency had been extremely slow to respond to AIDS. Much of its current energy, he suspected, was spent squabbling with the National Cancer Institute over which arm of the NIH should be most prominent in the fight against AIDS.

The director's top assistant chatted with Larry as he took the meal's last dishes into the kitchen. Once alone with the author, the assistant confided, "My friend and I loved your novel, *Faggots.* We'd love to have you to dinner the next time you're in town."

Larry could have been knocked over with a feather.

"Is that one of the reasons this institute has been so negligent with AIDS?" he asked. "Because the director is in the closet?"

The assistant looked at Larry with an embarrassed expression and did not answer.

The situation was achingly familiar to Larry. It was a truism to people active in the gay movement that the greatest impediments to homosexuals' progress often were not heterosexual bigots but closeted homosexuals. Among the nation's decision makers, the homophobes largely had been silenced by the prevailing morality that viewed expressions of overt hostility toward gays as unfashionable. In fact, when not burdened by private sexual insecurities, many heterosexuals could be enlisted to support gays on the basis of personal integrity. By definition, the homosexual in the closet had surrendered his integrity. This makes closeted homosexual people very useful to the establishment: Once empowered, such people are guaranteed to support the most subtle nuances of anti-gay prejudice. A closeted homosexual has the keenest understanding of these nuances, having chosen to live under the complete subjugation of prejudice. The closeted homosexual is far less likely to demand fair or just treatment for his kind, because to do so would call attention to himself.

Again and again, this sad sequence of self-hatred and policy paralysis played out in the AIDS epidemic, just as it did in Bethesda.

In Washington, one of the top officials in the Department of Health and Human Services was a closeted homosexual. Dr. Marcus Conant had once hoped that this official, who had an important role in the department's budget process, might prove a valuable ally in securing more AIDS funds. Instead, the man was a haughty defender of administration policy in his meetings with gay leaders and AIDS researchers.

In California, a top health official in conservative Republican Governor George Deukmejian's administration was a covert homosexual. His job, however, required that he appear before legislative committees to argue vociferously against allocating funds for AIDS education programs in the gay community, and he performed his duties with gusto. On the municipal level, the public health director of one of the four American cities hardest hit by the AIDS epidemic was a closeted gay doctor. This man distinguished himself by presiding over a public health department that did even less than New York City's to combat AIDS. Leaders of AIDS groups in that city privately agreed that the official declined to seek money for AIDS education from the county government because he did not want to draw attention to himself and his secret. Among gays, however, the health director was an expert articulator of AID-Speak and talked convincingly of confidentiality and what wonderful places bathhouses were. Grateful gays made him board chairman of the city's major AIDS group.

As Larry Kramer shrugged on his heavy winter coat and stalked out of the agency chief's home in Bethesda, he wondered when the deception would end. Just days before, he had met one of the nation's most influential closet cases at a cocktail party in Washington. Larry immediately recognized Terry Dolan when he arrived at the party. The millions Dolan raised for his National Conservative Political Action Committee had been almost solely responsible for electing the New Right senators who tipped the balance of Senate power to Republicans in 1980. And in the 1980 presidential race, he had raised $10 million for Ronald Reagan. Dolan's brother was now a White House speech writer.

The advertising that the committee sponsored sometimes chastised Democrats for coddling homosexuals. Terry Dolan, however, was fresh from an affair with a staff epidemiologist from the New York City Health Department, Larry knew, and was thoroughly enjoying the gay life his political fund-raising sought to squash. With characteristic reserve, Larry threw a drink in Dolan's face.

"How dare you come here?" Larry screamed. "You take the best from our world and then do all those hateful things against us. You should be ashamed."

January 7
UNION SQUARE, SAN FRANCISCO

Cleve Jones could barely drag himself out of bed that morning, but these were demonstrations that he could not miss. Dan White was being released from Soledad Prison after serving five years, one month, and thirteen days of his prison sentence. Cleve remembered the day when he saw Harvey Milk's corpse being rolled over and stuffed into a black plastic body bag, and knew he had to join in protesting the killer's release.

Speakers told the crowd at the Union Square rally that the Dan White story should inspire them to work at rooting out the deeper social bias that had allowed White to think it was entirely moral to murder a gay man. The crowd, however, wanted no part of such cool analysis, and they booed these speakers down with chants of "Kill Dan White." Some protesters wore lapel buttons announcing themselves as members of the "Dan White Hit Squad."

By the time the marchers had wound their way through the financial district, more than 5,000 had joined the cacophonous procession, many in three-piece business suits. On Castro Street that night, 9,000 held a rally against the release, again chanting their mantra of hate: "Kill Dan White. Kill Dan White." The anger was problematical. It was doubtful that the fury was connected as much to the now five-year-old murder of Harvey Milk and Mayor George Moscone as to the simmering rage at the AIDS epidemic.

Cleve marched and shouted with the throngs, ecstatic that some of the old fighting spirit had returned to the gay community. As the afternoon waned, however, Cleve left the march and returned to his apartment off Castro Street. The exertion had exhausted him completely. In fact, persistent fatigue had dogged him for months. At nights, he sometimes broke into unexplained sweats.

○

Prejudice makes prisoners of both the hated and the hater. That truth would surface less than two years later, when Dan White put his car in his closed garage and turned on the motor, killing himself. Even outside Soledad, he lived as a prisoner and died as one.

January 26

Dr. Marcus Conant avoided memorial services for his patients, but Paul Dague had not merely been a patient. In August 1981, Conant had recruited Paul to counsel newly diagnosed Kaposi's sarcoma patients at Conant's KS Clinic at UCSF. It was Paul who enlisted a floundering Berkeley grief-counseling group, the Shanti Project, to help in the epidemic. In the years since then, Marc Conant and AIDS Clinic doctors Paul Volberding and Don Abrams increasingly had called on Paul Dague to help them as they coped with their daily stress of telling thirty-year-old men that they were about to die.

As Marc Conant listened to the speakers eulogize Paul at the memorial, he remembered how devastated he had been when he told Paul Dague that the purple spots that had appeared on Paul's skin were Kaposi's sarcoma. That was in June 1982, when Paul was the 52nd local man to be diagnosed with AIDS. Now, in January 1984, Paul was the 149th San Franciscan to die of the disease. It was the week that the city's AIDS caseload surpassed 400.

Conant remained unsettled throughout the service. Glancing around the crowded room, he noticed Gary Walsh, sitting with a worried-looking friend. It had been a year since Conant had told Gary that he suffered from KS—one year and one day, to be exact—and Conant noticed that Gary looked as though he didn't have much longer to live.

Gary Walsh also usually avoided AIDS memorial services, but he had known Paul Dague for years and felt obliged to attend this night. Lu Chaikin was there with him. As she fidgeted in her folding metal chair, Lu reflected that out of love she had allowed most of her life the past year to revolve around Gary Walsh. Already, she recognized, she was suffering anticipatory grief for Gary's death. Through all the eulogies, she could only think that soon she would be sitting through a service like this for her closest friend. Always the streetwise tomboy from Flatbush, Lu knew she could endure the grief; always the psychotherapist, she also knew she would learn from it.

The memorial service impressed upon her, however, how much she already had learned about feelings this past year. In her earlier relationship with Gary, he was the sweet one, while she was strong. As Gary's disease progressed, however, Lu noted that Gary had gained an inner strength, confronting fate's cruel prognosis. Lu had learned about vulnerability; she had opened herself completely to Gary, without procrastination, because they had so little time. Even now, as their time together evaporated, Lu saw that during the past year she had learned from Gary much about being a woman, and Gary acknowledged that he had learned from her much about being a man.

Such realizations tended to overwhelm Lu with sadness, because she saw again how much she would miss Gary when he was gone. At the end of the service, Lu felt weak and borrowed Gary's silver-headed cane so she could walk out.

CENTERS FOR DISEASE CONTROL, ATLANTA

On the same day that Marc Conant, Gary Walsh, and Lu Chaikin attended Paul Dague's memorial service, Dr. Max Essex at Harvard told Don Francis that Robert Gallo had twenty different isolates of the retrovirus that caused AIDS. That week, Gallo also told Jim Curran at the CDC that he had isolated the elusive AIDS agent.

Gallo now was trying to culture as many different isolates of the AIDS virus as he could. He wanted the evidence to be overwhelming when it was announced, so there would be no lingering doubt as to what caused AIDS. Gallo decided the new retrovirus was the third variant of the Human T-cell Leukemia virus family he had discovered in 1980, and so he called it HTLV-III.

Four days later, researchers from the Pasteur Institute provided Don Francis with convincing proof that their virus, LAV, caused AIDS. In October, Francis had sent the French scientists thirty blood samples, including ten from the San Francisco hepatitis B cohort of gay men who had developed AIDS, ten from gay men with lymphadenopathy, and ten from heterosexuals not at risk for AIDS. The samples were sent blind, marked only with code numbers. The French researchers reported to Don Francis their results: positive LAV antibody tests in twenty of the samples and negative tests in ten. Francis quickly paged through his notes to compare the code numbers. The French had accurately sorted the blood of AIDS and lymphadenopathy patients from the blood of uninfected people. Francis was elated. With the cause of AIDS found, scientists could now get on with the business of controlling the spread of the epidemic and finding a vaccine.

One building away from Don Francis's office at the CDC that day, the secretaries in the CDC Public Affairs office neatly typed out the new updates on AIDS casualties that were released to the press every week. As of January 30, 3,339 AIDS cases had been reported to the CDC, of whom 1,452 had died. Of these cases, 38 had occurred in people whose only risk for contracting AIDS was that they had received a blood transfusion.

STANFORD UNIVERSITY,
STANFORD, CALIFORNIA

The early February call to Dr. Ed Engleman at the Stanford University Blood Bank confirmed all the blood banker's worst fears about the voluntary donor-deferral guidelines that remained society's only protection against AIDS-infected blood. A blood bank in Davis, California, had called Engleman because a donor had listed Stanford as one of thirteen blood banks at which he had given blood in recent years. The Davis facility had discarded his blood because it showed severe immune abnormalities. Stanford also had thrown out the man's blood in August. None of the other blood banks to whom the donor had given blood, however, had discarded the donation, and eleven people were on record as having been transfused with this man's blood.

Nothing, it seemed, would awaken either the blood industry or the industry's regulators at the Food and Drug Administration to the dangers of transfusion AIDS. Throughout 1983, Engleman had been a lonely voice calling for blood screening in his industry. For this, he had been vilified in local blood banking circles. At the end of 1983, one of the nation's leading blood bankers told the *Wall Street Journal* that Stanford's own testing program was merely a commercial ploy to try to lure patients from other Bay Area hospitals.

By early 1984, however, concern was spreading. Recalls of Factor VIII were now routine news stories. In one instance, 3 percent of the national supply of the clotting factor was taken off the market after an alert blood banker in Austin, Texas, saw a news story on that city's first AIDS case and recognized him as a regular paid donor for a local plasma collection center. In that recall alone, 60,000 vials of Factor VIII were rounded up. So far, sixteen hemophiliacs were suffering from AIDS. In just two years, the disease had emerged as the leading cause of death among hemophiliacs in the United States, even surpassing uncontrolled bleeding.

The blood industry continued to stonewall. A CDC study in the *New England Journal of Medicine* warned again of the problem of transfusion AIDS and was roundly criticized by blood bankers, who picked apart the methodology of the research. Among the most vociferous critics was the spokesman for the American Red Cross, Dr. Gerald Sandler, who maintained that "most of the seven patients in the study were very sick people who required many more units of blood than the average three per patient." Thus, the American Red Cross took the position that only people who needed a lot of blood might be at risk for contracting AIDS from transfusions. The president of the Council of Community Blood Centers told the *Journal of the American Medical Association* that his group believed there might be a blood-borne AIDS virus, but that it probably was not highly infectious. In a January essay in the *New England Journal of Medicine,* industry spokesman Dr. Joseph Bove wrote, "Whether the disease is caused by a transfusion-transmitted infectious agent is still unknown and will continue to be until further data are gathered and the agent isolated. . . . Patients should be reassured that blood banks are taking all possible steps to provide for safe blood transfusions."

By now Dennis Donohue, director of the FDA's blood and blood-products laboratory, was not convinced that all possible steps were being taken. In December, Donohue began pushing the industry to adopt the hepatitis core antibody test that the CDC had first proposed at the disastrous Atlanta blood meeting a year before. In early January, Assistant Secretary for Health Ed Brandt set up a conference call of blood bankers and CDC officials to discuss the AIDS problem. The upshot of all the talk was no new FDA policy; instead, the blood bankers agreed to form a task force to study the issue. The task force moved with the speed that characterized government response to virtually every aspect of the AIDS epidemic: The group decided to hold its first meeting in three months.

DUBLIN STREET, SAN FRANCISCO

In the six months since Frances Borchelt had been given the transfusion of three pints of blood, she had not regained her health. Her spirits dropped. Her fatigue was so relentless that she could no longer bustle through the busy days that had characterized her life. She felt a prisoner of the small home she shared with her husband in San Francisco's Excelsior District.

In early February, however, the nightmare turned darker. It started with a psoriasis rash on Frances Borchelt's arms. Before long, the itchy red rash covered her entire body, from the top of her scalp to the soles of her feet. Bob Borchelt took his wife to every specialist he could think of, from dermatologists to gynecologists. Each offered a different diagnosis, but none could offer a cure. It was during this outbreak that Frances's daughter Cathy began to fear that something was wrong with her mother beyond this or that ailment she had suffered since the August operation. It was just a suspicion at this time, and nothing that Cathy voiced to her apprehensive parents, but she now had started paying close attention to news reports about something that had seemed very removed from her life—the epidemic of Acquired Immune Deficiency Syndrome.

February 2
ALPINE TERRACE, SAN FRANCISCO

Throughout the year since Gary Walsh's AIDS diagnosis, he had busied himself with a major redecoration of his Castro District apartment. The refurbishing had become something of a joke among Gary, Lu Chaikin, and Matt Krieger, because it seemed that Gary always had something to buy for this Sisyphean task. It seemed that he was never going to see his plans completed. Finally, on this Thursday morning, the embellishments were to be completed with the delivery of a new couch.

Gary had spent the night before the sofa's arrival sleeping only fitfully. He was in constant pain. Breathing was difficult. In the morning, his doctor told Gary to check into the hospital, but Gary had insisted on an appointment first. He didn't want to sit for hours in some sterile hospital room unless it was absolutely necessary on this particular day. A quick checkup confirmed what

Gary's doctor had feared—the *Pneumocystis* was returning. Matt rushed to the doctor's office so he could drive Gary to the hospital.

"Are you scared?" Matt asked. He was helping Gary walk up the stairs to his apartment, so Gary could pick up some belongings.

"Yes," Gary confided.

"Well, we'll get you through this one," Matt said. "Good grief, I leave you alone for one night and look at the trouble you get into."

As Gary and Matt stepped out of the apartment building, the delivery truck arrived with the sofa that completed the redecoration.

At Davies Medical Center, the morning seemed like a three-ring circus to Matt. Nurses, phlebotomists, X-ray technicians, and various orderlies streamed in and out of Gary's room, hooking up machines to test for this vital sign or that possible ailment. Amid it all, Gary signed papers renewing his insurance policy so he wouldn't lose the disability payments that had permitted him to live fairly comfortably over the past year. Already, the insurance company had dropped the group policy that covered the other psychotherapists with whom Gary shared a building in the Castro. His own premiums were now up to $300 a month because of his astronomical medical expenses. Given the fact that Gary's health care over the past year had totaled $75,000, the premiums were a bargain.

The lung X-rays proved inconclusive—Gary could have either regular pneumonia or *Pneumocystis,* his doctor reported later. Whatever type it was, the physician felt optimistic that they had caught the bug early enough to stop its progression.

That night, Matt wrote in his journal: "The day left me feeling exhausted. But I don't feel scared for Gary's well-being. Somehow I feel confident that he will be home in a few days. I have an increased confidence that Gary will be well and that he will beat AIDS. I almost feel that the determination on both of our parts will accomplish this. We have many things to do together in the years ahead."

QUEBEC CITY, QUEBEC

From his bed in the Catholic hospital, Gaetan Dugas had never looked so scared, his friend thought. Like Gaetan, the friend was an airline steward, and he had arranged his visit to Gaetan between flights. This third bout with *Pneumocystis* had prompted Gaetan to move back to Quebec, where he could enjoy the care of his devoted family. His family was constantly at his bedside, and Gaetan was in good spirits, but he had wasted away to almost nothing and suffered from a perpetual fever. His old drinking buddy didn't think Gaetan would make it this time.

The winter in eastern Canada was bitter cold, Gaetan complained, even as the first warm days of February were hitting British Columbia. Before long, he started talking about returning to Vancouver, looking for somebody to fly to Quebec and escort him back to British Columbia, because he didn't want to make the flight alone.

"I am trapped in a dungeon where the guards wear white coats," he pleaded. "Please rescue me."

41 BARGAINING

February 1984
UNIVERSITY OF CALIFORNIA,
SAN FRANCISCO

Dr. Marcus Conant completed his examination, marveling again at the strange twists of this most eccentric syndrome. The patient was suffering from idiopathic thrombocytopenic purpura, which meant that his blood had stopped producing the platelet cells necessary for blood clotting. The condition also had all but destroyed his spleen, and he obviously did not have much longer to live. Still, the man had no visible health problems beyond a few dermatological glitches. He remained the picture of Castro Street handsome. As he put his hand on the knob of the examining room door to leave, he told Conant, "Well, I'm off to the baths."

Marc Conant could tell the patient had made the comment to see how he would react.

"Do you have sex?" Conant asked.

"Of course," the patient said.

"When you have sex, do you tell the guy you have AIDS?"

Of course he didn't.

Conant immediately recalled the French-Canadian he had seen almost two years ago, the airline steward who had sparked all the controversy about AIDS patients going to bathhouses. As far as Conant was concerned, however, Gaetan Dugas was a sociopath, driven by self-hatred and inner turmoil. This patient, Conant knew, was an intelligent man with a doctorate in computer sciences and a solid reputation in the community.

"Somebody thinks you're smart—they gave you a Ph.D.," Conant began. "Don't you think it's your responsibility not to spread this disease any further? At the very least, you should warn the people with whom you have contact."

The patient bristled.

"Anybody who goes to the baths is a goddamn fool and deserves anything he gets," he said.

Conant thought of the roller coaster he recently had ridden at the big beach-front amusement park in Santa Cruz. At first he had had trepidations about getting on what seemed a rickety old mechanism, but he had figured that if it was unsafe the government wouldn't let it operate. He thought of the guys who would line up to have sex with this attractive patient and made a quick parallel: They must be thinking that if these bathhouses really were dangerous, some responsible authority would not let them operate. Instead, the bathhouses, all licensed by the city, were prospering.

Rather than condemn the institutions, Public Health Director Mervyn Silverman had adopted the latest neologism of AIDSpeak and had begun praising the bathhouses as wonderful places to conduct educational campaigns. That was where the people who needed education the most congregated, he reasoned. Although, privately, he preferred that they be shut down, Silverman did not want to endanger the relationship his department had with the gay community, a relationship he considered essential to facilitating public health education.

Marc Conant had never been enthusiastic about the continuation of commercialized sex during the epidemic, but like most doctors, he hated entering the local political fray, particularly over an issue that so inflamed gay community passions. A few days after his disconcerting conversation with the AIDS patient, however, Conant was talking over the bathhouse issue with Bill Kraus. As far as Bill was concerned, bathhouses had become dens for publicly licensed murder. He considered Silverman an accomplice to the killings for letting them stay open so long. Urging people to go to bathhouses for AIDS education, Bill Kraus contended, was like telling people to stay in a burning building so they can learn about fire safety. Bill thought it was time to resurrect the issue and was organizing a forum on the bathhouses for the March meeting of the Harvey Milk Gay Democratic Club.

Marc Conant agreed with Bill Kraus. "I'll speak at the forum," Conant said, "but the ideal scenario would be to get the gay community to shut down the bathhouses themselves. Without state action, the closure could be hailed as the work of people taking responsibility for their own lives."

Conant was not prepared to come out and say public officials should shut the baths down. Rather, he'd say the community needed to start discussing whether to close them.

Bill Kraus was not confident that the community would move. Nothing had happened since the last bathhouse controversy nine months before. Everybody seemed hopeful that the whole controversy would go away; instead, it was gay men who were going away.

Bill also was alarmed at data collected by Drs. Leon McKusick, William R. Horstman, and Thomas Coates in their continuing surveys of changing sexual behavior among San Francisco gay men. The psychologists had queried nearly 700 gay men from a sample drawn among men handed questionnaires as they left gay bars and bathhouses. A third group of men in monogamous relationships, recruited through gay newspaper ads, received questionnaires by mail. When broken into three groups—the bar group, bathhouse patrons, and married men—some startling differences in sexual behavior emerged.

While all three sectors had the same awareness of the AIDS problem and how to avoid contracting the disease, men who went to bathhouses were far less likely to be following safe sex guidelines than any other group. Even worse, 68 percent of bathhouse patrons said they used "anonymous sex as a way of relieving tension." This compared with 29 percent of the total survey who acknowledged such behavior. Sixty-two percent of the bathhouse group said, "Sometimes I get so frustrated that I have sex I know I shouldn't be having."

Also revealed in the welter of statistics gathered by the health department was that 8 percent of the men at bathhouses had enlarged lymph nodes. This meant that 1 in 12 patrons probably was already in the early stages of AIDS infection. A bathhouse customer netting three trysts in one visit would have one chance in four of bedding with one of these men. Not surprisingly, the study concluded: "The efforts of the Public Health Department have been ineffective in influencing sexual activity at the bathhouses."

Although many gay men had changed some sexual behavior, the study found, only a minority had entirely eliminated all behavior that would put them at risk for contracting AIDS. Collectively, the gay community was going through the phase in the grief process known as bargaining. On the individual level, this stage follows denial and anger; it is characterized by the desire of the terminally ill patient to try to strike a bargain with the fatal disease, or with God. The classic example is the dying patient who pleads to be just well enough to attend this last wedding or give that last performance. Once the wedding is attended and the performance sung, there often is another marriage to celebrate or another song to sing. The bargaining is an attempt to postpone. So gay men bargained. Safe sex had come to mean eliminating your least favorite sexual activity and hedging on the rest. Maybe if I give up getting fucked, I can still have oral sex, many reasoned.

Politically, gay leaders bargained as well. It was all right to have warning posters, but they didn't want to give up bathhouses just yet—not until an AIDS virus actually was found and the means of transmission was proven. Of course, once the virus was found and the transmission routes were completely established, there would be further demands; this bargaining was not a reasonable process. In this sense, the bathhouse issue for gays continued to play like the blood banking issue for heterosexuals. There was denial and then bargaining. The gay response to the bathhouse problem was not a homosexual reaction; it was a human reaction.

The gay psychologists understood this and pleaded for patience. Bill Kraus figured that by the time the gay community had run through this complicated psychological marathon to acceptance, a good share of them would be dead. Time was a luxury the gay community could not afford. All the psychological pampering wasn't saving lives, Bill decided. Politically, he felt that efforts for closure had to move ahead now, despite the fact that researchers at the San Francisco General Hospital AIDS Clinic had warned him that city leaders would want to sweep the issue under the rug before the Democratic National Convention, which was to convene in five months.

It was time to reach over the heads of the health department and gay community leaders, Bill Kraus decided. On Thursday morning, February 2, he called a reporter at the *San Francisco Chronicle* and casually mentioned the statistics from what had become known as the McKusick study.

The reporter's subsequent visit to Dr. Selma Dritz revealed more concern about the bathhouses. Dritz had just completed a chart of the city's rectal gonorrhea rate. Although the statistics had been plummeting, the number of rectal gonorrhea cases for the final quarter of 1983 showed the first increase of the disease in five years. The rise was not dramatic, but Dritz was stunned that the disease—which could only be contracted through unprotected, passive anal intercourse—should increase at a time when gay men were being told that passive anal intercourse was a ticket to oblivion.

Selma Dritz handed the graph to the reporter. "This says that at the same time we noticed increased activity at the bathhouses, we started seeing another increase in rectal gonorrhea," she said. "This is very strong presumptive evidence of a parallel."

As the reporter was leaving, Dritz glanced at the blackboard with all its circles, arrows, and numbers. "On Monday alone, I logged in eight new cases," she said, her voice sounding tired. "Eight young men and they're probably all going to die."

Dr. James Curran needed little goading when he was contacted by a San Francisco newspaper reporter. As a federal official relying on gay community cooperation for much of his research, Curran wouldn't go so far as to tell Dr. Merv Silverman to close the bathhouses, but he did opine, "I wish the gay community would officially express concern over bathhouses. I'd like to see all bathhouses go out of business. I've told bathhouse owners they should diversify and go into something healthy—like become gymnasiums. Gay men need to know that if they're going to have promiscuous sex, they'll have the life expectancy of people in the developing world."

Gay community leaders became choleric at the resulting bathhouse story in the *Chronicle*. The reporter, they agreed, suffered from internalized homophobia. Anger exploded into fury when the following day's paper carried a long news analysis on the challenges that bathhouses posed to the city's AIDS educational program. The article quoted prominent AIDS researchers who mocked the accentuate-the-positive tack taken by the San Francisco AIDS Foundation. Rather than focus on the harsh realities of AIDS, the city-funded foundation's educational campaign now featured full-color posters graced by the backsides of two nubile men. "You Can Have Fun (and Be Safe, Too)," the cheerful slogan advised. Publicly condemning the health department's don't-panic-gays posture, Supervisor Harry Britt announced that he would meet with doctors and AIDS researchers to start organizing his own educational campaign to inform gay men that "sexual activity in places like baths or sex clubs should no longer be associated with pleasure—it should be associated with death."

Dr. Silverman maintained that he would not take any action on the bathhouses, even to enforce his own much-publicized edict that the businesses should post warnings.

"Any action on this is going to have to come from the gay community, not my office," Silverman said. As for the city's educational program, he insisted, "I think the record shows we've done everything we possibly could do to educate people about this. I've been thinking about this every day and every night for a year—it's not something I take lightly."

By Monday, February 6, behind-the-scenes maneuvering on the bathhouse issue escalated. Bathhouse owners met and issued a statement, condemning the "uncaring and unscrupulous theocrats [who] have stooped to manipulating public fears about AIDS in order to serve their own private, political goals of eliminating first the gay baths, then the gay bars, then all gay businesses and organizations, and possibly the jobs of every gay person." The *Bay Area Reporter* readied its own editorial, blasting the *Chronicle* and anybody who doubted that the bathhouses were terrific places for AIDS education. As usual, the issue was framed in terms of human rights, not human life. "If the baths pulled their own plugs and died a natural death—like some of their patrons—no one would be the richer or the poorer," the *BAR* editorialized. "The issue in this case would be constitutional, not a health issue. A major segment of the body politic would be denied the right to assemble in a place where nothing illegal was taking place."

Meanwhile, the National KS/AIDS Foundation's board of directors met a few blocks away. Bill Kraus wanted the foundation to approve a warning card that all bathhouse owners would be required to give to patrons as they walked in. The warning card would bluntly tell customers that they might die if they participated in unsafe sexual acts. If the bathhouse supporters were going to argue that gays had a right to an informed choice, then there should be assurances that all patrons were indeed informed, Bill Kraus said. Ten of the twelve board members agreed on the warning, but it faced vociferous opposition from foundation treasurer Bob Ross, the publisher of the *Bay Area Reporter,* a publication that reaped hefty advertising revenues from bathhouses. Faced with certain condemnation in the *BAR* if they called for the warning card, the board deferred action. Marc Conant and Bill Kraus left to attend another meeting that Harry Britt had called with Merv Silverman, public health director.

By the time that meeting convened, the battle lines were clear. The only gay political leaders supporting action against the baths were allied with the Milk Club. Of course, longtime public health veterans like Selma Dritz supported closure, as did the increasingly vocal doctors at the AIDS Clinic. But physicians' advice had carried little weight in decision making at any governmental level during the first five years of the AIDS epidemic, and nobody paid much attention to them now. Lined up against closure were most of the city's other gay leaders, the Bay Area Physicians for Human Rights, and the advertising-conscious gay newspapers. Bathhouse owners, some of whom had spent much of the last decade barring racial minorities from their businesses, themselves had become new champions of civil liberties.

Dr. Silverman agreed that his department needed to step up educational activities in the bathhouses, and he praised the bathhouse owners for pledging their cooperation. That should take care of the problem, most of those at the meeting agreed. More pamphlets.

Privately, Silverman felt that if people like Bill Kraus were so goddamned opposed to the bathhouses, they should take picket signs and stand outside the doors, warning people away. That would draw more media coverage of the issue and give him a demonstration of community support that, in turn, could justify his closing the baths. Without such support, Silverman did not feel that closure would serve a constructive end. Gay leaders lauded Silverman for taking the most appropriate action. The foes of the Milk Club could barely restrain a smirk at Bill Kraus. Everybody figured he was behind this burst of attention on the bathhouses, as he had been last year. Once again, he had lost.

⬭

Controversy also swirled around the bathhouses in New York in February. A *New York Native* writer had spent a night at various bathhouses to see if they had indeed turned into campuses for AIDS education. He found that nobody used rubbers, few paid even cursory service to safe-sex guidelines, and that most patrons laughed at the writer's suggestion that sexual activity be restricted to healthy endeavors. Larry Kramer took to pasting AIDS warning stickers on bathhouse doors, a move that only earned him more derision.

The pages of the *Native* were crowded with the obituaries of dancers and architects, priests and poets, university professors and civil engineers who had all died young from AIDS. Still, there remained little pressure for any frontal assault on the disease.

Larry Kramer engaged in a long campaign to regain his seat on the board of directors for Gay Men's Health Crisis, but he was rejected in an overwhelming board vote in early February. As intemperate as ever, Larry fired off a letter to the board, calling them a "bunch of ninnies, incompetents, cowards."

The minutes from Mayor Koch's InterAgency Task Force on AIDS continued to read like a laundry list of the substantial problems that persisted in New York because of the lack of coordinated care facilities or any social support services. One man was literally pushed out onto the cold street in February after he was denied placement in a city housing facility because he had AIDS. At GMHC, people seeking clinical services had increased from 40 a month in early 1983 to between 80 and 100 each week. The group was turning about half of them away now because of lack of resources. Even as problems mounted, the task force voted in February to stop meeting every two weeks and assemble once a month instead.

February 7
PARK CITY, UTAH

Michael Gottlieb had never seen such an electric level of scientific exchange as what had coalesced at the scientific conference he had organized under the auspices of UCLA. The 150 scientists were most of the top people working in AIDS across the country, either as researchers or clinicians. The tremendous strides the field of immunology had made since Gottlieb announced the first four cases of *Pneumocystis* in the *MMWR* just thirty-two months ago was evident. For all the funding problems and rivalries, scientists clearly had responded more swiftly than any others challenged by the AIDS epidemic. After the intervention of Assistant Secretary for Health Ed Brandt, scientific journals recently had agreed to expedite publication of AIDS-related breakthroughs. The release of new federal and state funds had attracted more top minds to the intriguing medical mysteries posed by the epidemic.

On the conference's second day, Gottlieb scheduled the climactic panel on lymphotropic retroviruses that would include Drs. Robert Gallo, his close associate Max Essex of Harvard University, and Jean-Claude Chermann of the Pasteur Institute. Gallo privately belittled the French research, but Gottlieb suspected nothing when Dr. William Haseltine, another Harvard researcher with close links to Gallo, asked to speak for ten minutes before Chermann. Gottlieb granted the time, although the scheduling would be tight. There was good snow for skiing that Tuesday afternoon, and one lure for the five-day conference had been the promise that scientific sessions would end by noon so doctors could hit the slopes.

Dr. Gallo started the session with a talk on "the family of HTLV viruses." Although his talk implied that he had made unspecified research breakthroughs lately, he gave the audience no hint of what other NCI researchers knew—that Gallo was on the verge of announcing his discovery of the cause of AIDS. The crowd already was getting restless when Haseltine rose to speak on arcane matters of gene regulation in the HTLV-I virus. After Haseltine had talked for half an hour, Gottlieb grew worried. He asked a Harvard colleague who was moderating the panel to interrupt Haseltine. The researcher acknowledged the moderator's signal but turned back to the audience and continued to talk.

As Haseltine droned on, Chermann paced nervously on the side of the room. He was self-conscious about his English, and now it appeared that he might not get a chance to speak at all. Gottlieb was dumbfounded. Haseltine was not even an invited speaker and he was taking up all the session's time. What was going on?

Other scientists familiar with the simmering rivalry between the National Cancer Institute and the Pasteur Institute had no doubt about what was going on. Haseltine was trying to block the French from giving their research, they thought. Finally, however, Haseltine finished, and Chermann got the chance to speak to the impatient crowd.

Minutes into his presentation, a hush fell over the conference room as Chermann outlined what the year of French research had uncovered. In halting English, he described the LAV virus, explained its selective taste for T-4 cells, and laid out the impressive evidence from widespread blood testing linking LAV to AIDS. The audience was expecting some interesting findings about LAV, but few were prepared to hear the welcome news implicit in Chermann's message. The mystery disease was no longer a mystery.

Bob Gallo visibly blanched.

"Look, Bob Gallo is speechless," said one New York scientist in a stage whisper. "He's just figured out that the other guy is going to get to go to Sweden to get the Nobel Prize."

In the question-and-answer session, Gallo questioned Chermann aggressively, making it clear to everyone that he disbelieved the work of the French scientist. Couldn't this LAV have been the result of some contaminant? he asked. He also proposed that the French should not call their virus LAV, but

HTLV-III. Chermann held his ground, noting that the virus bore no similarities to the HTLV microbes Gallo had discovered. Gallo's request was indeed impudent, since it is traditional that the researchers who discover an organism have first prerogative in naming it. Despite Gallo's efforts, the elite scientists attending the Park City conference left saying the French had discovered the cause of AIDS.

A year ago.

February 10
DAVIES MEDICAL CENTER,
SAN FRANCISCO

On the day that Jean-Claude Chermann informed America's top AIDS researchers of the cause of Acquired Immune Deficiency Syndrome, a biopsy of tissue from Gary Walsh's lung showed that the *Pneumocystis* protozoa were proliferating. In the days that followed, Gary's temperature routinely peaked at 104 and 105 degrees. All week, he had shown severe reactions to Bactrim, a drug normally used to treat the pneumonia. His doctor put him on pentamidine and now Gary was sleeping between sixteen and twenty hours a day. The longest he could stay awake was forty-five minutes.

On his way to the biopsy, Gary talked to Lu Chaikin and Matt Krieger about his memorial service. On Friday, he reminded his nurse that he did not want code-blue status. Matt overheard the conversation.

"I can't take it anymore," Gary explained when they were alone. "I'm tired of one infection after another. I just don't know if I want to live like this."

Three days later, Gary's doctor informed him that the pentamidine wasn't working. His lungs were still filling up with *Pneumocystis* protozoa. The doctor mentioned a new experimental drug he might want to try.

"And if I chose not to, or if it doesn't work?" Gary asked.

"Then we send you home or keep you here and put you on a morphine drip to make you as comfortable as possible," his doctor said.

Gary decided to try the experimental drug.

February 15
CENTERS FOR DISEASE CONTROL,
ATLANTA

Jean-Claude Chermann was persuaded to speak in the CDC auditorium while he was in Atlanta to give Don Francis samples of LAV. Most of the researchers in the AIDS Activities Office wedged into the chamber. By the end of the afternoon, the agency's headquarters was buzzing with the near-unanimous assessment that the French had indeed discovered the cause of AIDS.

Harold Jaffe, who now was chief of epidemiology for the AIDS branch, also came away from the speech convinced that the French had isolated the AIDS agent. He immediately plotted the work that could now be done. With an antibody test that could detect asymptomatic carriers in the early stages of infection, scientists at last could begin to chart the natural history of the disease, an aspect of AIDS that remained largely unexplored. Was AIDS-Related Complex a different manifestation of infection by the AIDS virus or merely a prodrome to the more deadly opportunistic infections? To what extent had the virus penetrated the population? How serious was the prevalence of AIDS infection in the Third World, particularly the already troubled nations of Central Africa?

WARD 86,
SAN FRANCISCO GENERAL HOSPITAL

By late February, the doctors in the AIDS Clinic had decided to support closure of the bathhouses. Although they preferred not to get involved in political issues, they could no longer pretend to be cool and objective about bathhouses. Day after day, Dr. Don Abrams, clinic assistant director, took the sexual histories of men who appeared at the clinic with their first lesion or that terrifying shortness of breath. Day after day, the young men told him about their bathhouse experiences. Many were not very sexually active, living out of the gay fast track in suburban homes. But, when the itch hit, they'd go to the baths. The baths simply were more convenient than the bars.

AIDS Clinic epidemiologist Andrew Moss frequently said that the only bathhouse warning poster that would offer patrons truly informed consent would be one featuring full-color photos of a person in advanced stages of the disease. In a February 21 letter to Merv Silverman, Moss urged the health director to promote more aggressive public information and to continue public discussions on the future of the bathhouses. "As you know, all evidence points to a resumption of the previous level of sexual activity once the media attention went away," he wrote. "Thus I do not feel it is appropriate simply to wait and see what happens."

As the bathhouse question simmered, Don Abrams and Paul Volberding decided to invite bathhouse owners to the AIDS Clinic to talk about AIDS. Volberding assumed that the bathhouses remained open in large part because their owners did not understand how serious AIDS was. Once they understood, certainly they would move to close the facilities themselves, Volberding reasoned.

The bathhouse owners who attended were hostile. Some had come only because they felt pressured to attend, because San Francisco General Hospital was an arm of the SF Public Health Department. Other proprietors couldn't be bothered and simply sent their attorneys. One bathhouse owner became queasy when he saw the slide projector that Volberding had brought for the talk. He didn't want to see any pictures of AIDS victims, he said. Abrams and Volberding had planned to show just such photos but changed their minds.

After Abrams and Volberding spoke, one of the owners of the largest bathhouses took them aside and tried to reason with them. "We're both in it for the same thing," he said. "Money. We make money at one end when they come to the baths. You make money from them on the other end when they come here."

Paul Volberding was speechless. This guy wasn't talking civil liberties; he was talking greed. Volberding felt hopelessly naive. The bathhouses weren't open because the owners didn't understand they were spreading death. They understood that. The bathhouses were open because they were still making money.

42 THE FEAST OF THE HEARTS, PART II

February 17, 1984
ROOM 213, WARD 2–NORTH,
DAVIES MEDICAL CENTER,
SAN FRANCISCO

"I've decided to stop all therapy," Gary Walsh told Matt Krieger and Lu Chaikin. "My body is too worn out. The side effects of the drugs are too much. I give up."

Matt and Lu understood. The time of anger, denial, bargaining, and depression were long past; now there was only acceptance.

"I understand your decision," Matt said, "and I respect it."

Matt was being utterly sincere. Still, he felt like he was in a play, performing on stage. The words and thoughts were so out of proportion with anything he had confronted in his life before.

February 18
MATT KRIEGER'S JOURNAL

Random notes.

"I wonder if I've made the right decision. The others fought to the very end. I'm taking the easy way out."

"Gary, your decision was very brave and courageous. You're not taking the easy way out. You're living your life now in the beautiful way you always have. You're facing death fully conscious. It's an incredibly brave thing to do. It's not easy."

"Really?

"The morphine takes all the pain away. I feel good. It's hard to stay with my decision when I feel this good. I have to remind myself of the pain without morphine."

Setting up a visiting time with Joe Brewer, he says, "That hour's taken." We all laugh.

He [Gary] tells [his nephew] Rick that Monday night will be too late. I'm dying. Come tomorrow.

He sweats so heavily, it's like someone spilled a gallon of water on his bed. He woke from three naps this way.

He's very much at peace. He's not in pain. He drifts in and out of sleep. Sometimes he's fully awake, alert, funny, wise, childish.

Sometimes, he's delirious, eyes half open, mumbling incoherent thoughts. Good humor, interest in others is remarkably intact.

One of the nurses told Lu, "We don't feel like we're here for Gary. We feel like Gary is here for us."

Another nurse told me, "It is a treat to take care of him. He says the most profound things every time you go in there. You want to touch him and you wonder, 'Is he a saint?' "

I asked him if he wanted me to sleep in the other bed overnight. He said that if he's going to go through this bravely, he has to spend the night alone.

"I'm scared," he said. "I'm scared of death. What if this is all. What if there's a hell. You think of the terrible things you've done in your life now."

"What do you think it's like where you're going?" I asked.

"I don't know. I really don't know. When I was further away from it, I felt like I knew better. But I don't know."

Lu and I were with him all day. It wasn't unpleasant. It was like all our times together. Rich. With laughter. Wit. And love.

I know that I don't really comprehend that he is dying, nor the impact of that. I sleep at his apartment with a feeling like he's just in the hospital again and will be home soon.

There is a dull, throbbing pain in my stomach and my heart.

February 19

Matt Krieger met Rick Walsh and his wife Angie at the hospital elevator. Rick's dad, who was Gary's older brother, had come too. Gary and his brother had not been close in recent years, but as soon as he walked in the room and saw Gary on the bed, he blurted out, "I love you."

"This is it," Gary said. "It's probably the last time we'll ever see each other. It's coming and I wanted to talk to you before I left. I love you and I'm going to miss you."

After the visit, outside Gary's room, Rick fell into Matt's arms and started crying. He saw his father was crying too; he had never seen his dad cry before.

As Angie watched the family reunion, she was struck by how much Rick and Gary resembled each other. They were almost identical. Rick Walsh couldn't get over how much Gary's best friend Lu Chaikin resembled Gary's mother. They were almost identical, he thought.

That Night

Lu Chaikin had always loved Gary, even when he was willful, self-centered, and sometimes defensive, because she saw the essence of Gary Walsh, and she saw that it was good. This essence explained why Gary had devoted his career to helping others accept and integrate themselves, and why his political ideology had never strayed far from the Flower Child credo that the world's problems could be solved if people just cared for each other as much as they cared for themselves. In the year since his AIDS diagnosis, Lu had watched adversity transform her friend. The pretensions of personality had dropped away, layer by layer, until that altruistic essence was all that remained. Gary had forgotten the hurts of his Catholic childhood and the abuses he had suffered as a gay man. He now offered his friends unconditional love. People came away from conversations with Gary like pilgrims leaving a holy shrine. Lu wasn't sure whether Gary knew the effect he was having on others. She wasn't sure whether he understood that, finally, he had become totally himself and that he was very beautiful.

After all the relatives and friends had left, Lu went back into Gary's room and tried to express again what she had tried to tell Gary before. Gary smiled his mischievous grin and interrupted her.

"I got it, I finally got it," he said. "I *am* love and light, and I transform people by just being who I am."

Gary recited the words carefully, like a schoolchild who had struggled hard to master a difficult lesson. Lu broke down and started weeping.

Gary reached to the table near his bed and handed Lu a small brass figure of a magician, holding a crystal ball in one hand and a book in another. Gary knew that Lu had loved it.

"I want to give you this while I'm still alive," he said. "You should have it."

Lu felt that a flame had been passed. Their relationship, Lu knew, was completed.

The Next Afternoon, February 20

"It used to be us and them," Gary said. "And now I'm one of them."

"Who are they?" Matt asked.

"People with AIDS," Gary said. "People dying of AIDS. I'm dying of AIDS. I used to see a corpse or something. That's bullshit. What's going on?"

Gary was delirious. Matt could see that pain racked his body, even though he was being dosed with 50 milligrams of morphine per hour, up from 30 the previous morning. Every breath was labored and achingly brief.

"I'm leaving my body," Gary told Matt between breaths.

"Maybe you are," Matt said. "And I want you to know that as much as I want you here with me, I want you safe and peaceful. And it's okay if you go."

Gary slept into the afternoon, awaking briefly to talk to Lu and Matt.

"Dying consciously and naturally is very hard, harder than I thought, the hardest thing I've ever done," he said. "Death is right around the corner. I know it is. I couldn't do it without the two of you. I'd give up. The things they say about death, they sound trite. But they're all true. I see the stairs."

At dusk, he awoke again.

"I want to leave," he said. "I want to go."

Gary struggled to get up from the bed. His face and voice were expressionless now. There was only supplication for escape. Lu and Matt tried to dissuade him, because he obviously did not have the strength to rise. But he insisted. The two friends and three nurses pulled him upright, so he could sit on the edge of his bed. After they held him there for a moment, Gary stopped pleading and allowed himself to be lain back down.

Three hours later, he awoke again and once more begged that he be allowed to leave his bed. Lu, Matt, and a nurse helped Gary up. He was so weak he could not lift his head. Somehow, he managed three steps with his arms wrapped around Matt's neck. He fell into a deep sleep as soon as his head was again settled onto his pillow.

Gary's lungs filled with fluids all night. Matt took the chore of putting a tube down his throat to drain them. Gary lapsed into a coma. His breaths were short but no longer labored. Lu recalled an old hypnosis trick and took hold of Gary's hand.

"If you can hear me, lift your index finger," she said.

Gary did nothing.

Lu repeated the command, and Gary's finger moved.

Late into the night, Matt and Lu whispered phrases of love into their friend's ears. Long after midnight, Lu again asked Gary to move his finger but got no response.

The Next Morning, February 21

A cool white fog had enveloped the Castro District by the time Matt and Lu awoke early the next morning. Matt felt Gary's forehead and noted that his skin was cold to the touch and no longer pliable. As the morning progressed, Gary's inhalations became less regular. There were longer breaks between breaths. At about 8:40 A.M., Gary let out a series of brief gasps, and then his breathing stopped.

Lu and Matt sat with Gary's body for five minutes and talked to him one last time. Lu told him again how much she loved him and would miss him and what an enormous void his passing would create in her life.

The color had drained completely from Gary's face when Matt returned with the nurse. Matt gathered up Gary's belongings in a shopping bag. Lu told the nurse she was Gary's aunt and gave instructions for the disposition of his remains.

The sun had broken through the fog by the time Lu and Matt left the hospital. Lu was numb with fatigue when she let herself back into her home. Something very important had happened in her life, she knew, and so it automatically occurred to her that she should call Gary and tell him about it. She always called Gary when something important happened. Then she remembered that she could never call Gary again and the emptiness opened up for her and she wept.

⬭

As soon as the phone rang in Rick Walsh's ranch house, he knew it was Matt. Rick was shattered at the news, and Angie sat down to explain to their four-year-old daughter what had happened.

"Gary was one of your dad's favorite people," she said. "But he has gone far away now. He is dead."

"Why?" the little girl asked.

"I don't know," Angie Walsh said. "I don't know."

The little girl looked toward her father, and for the first time, she saw him cry.

After he composed himself, Rick called his grandparents in Sioux City to tell them that Gary, their youngest son, had died. Gary's parents had anxiously awaited the call, but once told, they didn't talk with Rick long; it wasn't their way.

Rick had told only his closest friends that his uncle had AIDS. The next day, he felt estranged from the people in his everyday life. He didn't feel he could share his sadness without going into a complicated explanation. You couldn't go around telling people that your uncle had just died of that gay disease.

$\bigcirc$

Gary Francis Walsh died 997 days after the first *MMWR* report on the mysterious cases of *Pneumocystis carinii* pneumonia among Los Angeles gay men. About an hour after Gary's death, the Centers for Disease Control released its weekly update on the number of people stricken by AIDS since that first report. As of February 21, 1984, some 3,515 Americans had been diagnosed with Acquired Immune Deficiency Syndrome, of whom 1,506 had died. The thirty-nine-year-old psychotherapist was the 164th San Franciscan to die in the epidemic.

$\bigcirc$

A year before, Gary Walsh had been among the thirty-five AIDS sufferers to sign a letter asking that *Bay Area Reporter* editor Paul Lorch be fired. Lorch pulled out the letter when he heard that Gary had died and drew a line through Gary's name.

February 24

Gary had wanted Beatles' songs for his memorial service, so the 300 mourners who went to the chapel at the community center where the Shanti Project held its services were treated to the strains of "Let It Be" as they entered. By now, AIDS funerals had taken on the cast of social events for many in the gay community. Among those who gathered for the service were aspiring gay political personages who may not have known Gary but understood that this was a correct event to attend. However, most in the crowd were people whose lives Gary had touched—his old boyfriends and psychotherapy clients, friends, and the other AIDS sufferers to whom he had lent so much support.

Given the times, AIDS services had taken a high-tech twist, and so Gary was able to appear in full-color at his own funeral in a videotape of an interview he had given three months before. People were warmed by Gary's talk of visions of people who promised to help him to "the other side." It was a strange paradox to see people smiling at the mystic visions of a man who had achieved acclaim for putting one over on Jerry Falwell.

Rick and Angie Walsh weren't sure what to make of the practiced rituals of AIDS death. Still, Rick wept openly when Lu Chaikin concluded the service with her eulogy.

"How do you describe a star whose too-brief journey lit up so many lives?" Lu asked. "And now I say to my sweet, dearest friend—go well and be at peace. And as we had so often promised, we will always be with each other, with love."

Everybody sang "Amazing Grace," and as the people left, Matt played Gary's favorite song, "All You Need Is Love."

43 SQUEEZE PLAY

February 26, 1984
CENTERS FOR DISEASE CONTROL,
ATLANTA

The vial with two ounces of LAV arrived at the Atlanta airport shortly after midnight. Given the fact that the last batch of LAV, packed in dry ice in Paris and shipped to Atlanta through the mail, had been dead on arrival, Dr. Cy Cabradilla from the CDC molecular virology lab took no chances this time, clearing the virus's passage through New York quarantine authorities himself and personally waiting for the plane from JFK airport to arrive. As soon as he got the virus back to his CDC lab, Cabradilla started tests to make sure it had survived. By the next morning, he had isolated the virus and begun growing it in lymphocytes extracted from the umbilical cords of newborn infants. With this virus, the CDC could make its own antibody tests, which would allow researchers to trace LAV in the blood and tissue samples they had been collecting in the two and a half years of AIDS work.

By the end of the week, excitement had spread through the cluster of brick buildings on Clifton Road. The virus was growing rapidly. Soon, lab staffers were to test stored specimens. One after another, the blood revealed the presence of LAV antibodies. The positive antibody tests came from all the AIDS risk groups, including gay men, Haitians, drug abusers, hemophiliacs, addicts' female sexual partners and their babies. Fresh blood samples from AIDS patients were flown in from Los Angeles and San Francisco, and the results were the same. These people were infected with LAV. The French had discovered the cause of AIDS.

March
WASHINGTON, D.C.

"We know we have the cause of AIDS for sure," said Bob Gallo.

Jim Curran had flown to Washington from Atlanta with the codes on 200 blood samples of AIDS cases and controls that the Centers for Disease Control had sent Gallo in January. Sitting with Gallo in a French restaurant, Curran compared the code numbers for the various samples to the HTLV-III antibody tests Gallo had performed on the blood. Gallo's lab work was right on target; Curran could see that Gallo had isolated the long-sought AIDS virus. Curran also figured that the retrovirus was the same microbe isolated by the French a year earlier. Curran was relieved both research groups had discovered the same virus separately, convinced that the dual studies would hasten the acceptance of the discovery in the scientific world. Gallo was evasive when Curran asked him when the National Cancer Institute would release its conclusions.

Gallo was reticent to provide much information, both because of the tensions between the CDC and the NCI, and because the question of how to announce the HTLV-III discovery had become so entwined with election-year politicking that it was out of Gallo's hands. The NCI director, Dr. Vincent Devita, had wanted to go public with the information, but was overruled by Assistant Secretary for Health Edward Brandt, who had been informed of the discovery in February. Rather than be heralded as an accomplishment of the National Cancer Institute or the National Institutes of Health, credit for the break-through was to go to the Reagan administration. The announcement would counter liberal criticism that the government had dragged its feet on AIDS research. With Democratic presidential hopefuls becoming more critical of federal AIDS funding, the administration was eager to eliminate AIDS as a possible issue in the November presidential election. Brandt ordered that any announcement would be made by Health and Human Services Secretary Margaret Heckler when she determined it was wisest to proceed.

That time was rapidly approaching. Gallo had submitted six papers to the medical journal *Science,* all nailing down HTLV-III as the cause of AIDS. Already, the researcher had isolated the virus in forty-eight patients, many more independent isolates than the French had cultured for their LAV. By the time Gallo met with Curran, Heckler had also been briefed on HTLV-III. Now, it was up to her to make the discovery public.

Bob Gallo had politics of his own to consider. Like a number of NCI research-ers, he was worried that this concrete evidence of the AIDS infectious agent would put the syndrome firmly under the aegis of the National Institute for Allergy and Infectious Diseases, and the NCI would lose its central role in AIDS research. Gallo also continued to be obsessed with whether the Pasteur Institute would get credit for the discovery of the AIDS virus. He was suspicious of Curran, aware that the CDC had embarked on cooperative studies with the French after Jean-Claude Chermann had addressed the CDC in February. To keep his advantage, therefore, Gallo told the CDC as little as possible about NCI studies. When discussing the virus with Curran, he made no reference to the six *Science* papers or the forty-eight isolates.

SAN FRANCISCO CLUB BATHS

Larry Littlejohn pulled a towel around his waist and began his informal inspec-tion of the city's largest gay bathhouse. Although he had once enjoyed weekly bathhouse romps, he hadn't stepped into the tubs for a year. The sprawling sex palaces reminded Littlejohn of how far the city's sex industry had come since he had moved to San Francisco in 1962. His first home in San Francisco had been the Embarcadero YMCA, a precursor to the modern bathhouse. After Littlejohn helped organize the city's pioneering gay group, the Society of Individual Rights, in 1964, he had opened one of the city's first private sex clubs. He took some credit as one of the businessmen who introduced a whole generation of gay San Franciscans to the joys of orgy sex.

In the years since then, Larry Littlejohn had served two terms as president of the Society of Individual Rights and was widely recognized as one of the city's first gay activists. He had at one time or another walked into every sex club and bathhouse in San Francisco, developing a personal preference for the more leather-oriented establishments. AIDS was a distant concern until he read Larry Kramer's "1,112 and Counting." A cursory examination of the evidence led him to believe that AIDS was a sexually transmitted disease, which drew him to one quick conclusion: The bathhouses couldn't go on as they were without killing thousands of gay San Franciscans.

Through 1983, Larry Littlejohn wrote various letters to San Francisco Public Health Director Mervyn Silverman, the board of supervisors, and the AIDS organizations, pointing out what he considered to be a rather logical argument for stopping bathhouse sex. He assumed somebody would act. After all, lives were at stake. A city health department that would yank a restaurant license for cockroach infestation certainly would pull a bathhouse license for fostering a far more lethal activity. Yet, by the first months of 1984, it was clear that nobody would do anything. Most recently, Dr. Silverman had written Littlejohn that bathhouses were valuable sites for AIDS education. That was what had brought Littlejohn to the city's largest bathhouse in early March. He wanted to see what kind of education patrons got.

Littlejohn walked out of the locker room and down the hall; he saw none of the safe-sex posters Silverman had ordered posted nine months before. At the dimly lit end of another hall, he did find a poster—in the least conspicuous place possible. The active orgy rooms and the squealing behind the closed doors of private cubicles at the Club Baths that night also implied to Littlejohn that patrons were not perusing safe-sex guidelines before exchanging bodily fluids.

Silverman obviously did not want to take responsibility for protecting the public health, Littlejohn thought. And gay politicos were still talking about whether it was permissible to talk about bathhouse closure. The day after his bathhouse inspection, therefore, Littlejohn called a friend who had been instrumental in placing initiatives on the San Francisco ballot. Littlejohn knew what Mayor Dianne Feinstein had learned a year ago. In San Francisco, you can put just about anything on the city ballot. In his apartment just one block from the Club Baths, Littlejohn drew up an initiative that would ban sexual activity from the city's bathhouses. He knew that such an initiative would force every politician in the city of San Francisco to take a stand on bathhouse sex. And it would force Silverman to explain to the city's electorate exactly why bathhouses were such wonderful sites for AIDS education, if such an explanation could be seriously made. The debate had gone on long enough, Littlejohn decided: It was time to call the question.

◯

That same week, another question was being called at the Irwin Memorial Blood Bank in San Francisco. The woman who had inadvertently raised the issue was Mary Richards Johnstone, a wealthy matron from the affluent suburb of Belvedere.

During heart surgery in December 1982, Mary Johnstone had received twenty units of Irwin blood. Eight days after the operation, she was struck by a mysterious lung virus. She barely survived that ordeal, but in the succeeding months she was plagued continuously with exhausting fevers and strange ailments like oral candidiasis. The doctors couldn't explain what was wrong with her.

Only in February 1984, while leafing through her medical files, did Mary Johnstone see the October 19, 1983, letter from one physician to another at the University of California Medical Center, where she had her surgery. "We have discovered that one of her blood donors is an AIDS patient," the letter said. The doctors had concealed this from Mary Johnstone, however, and if she had not happened across the correspondence, there is no indication she would ever have been informed. Later, the fifty-five-year-old housewife kept her sense of humor when her doctor concluded that she was suffering from the syndrome. "Here I've got AIDS," she said, "and I didn't even have any fun getting it."

In Los Angeles, meanwhile, a thirty-eight-year-old nurse who had received a blood transfusion during a hysterectomy was ailing from *Pneumocystis.* Her condition had been watched anxiously by Los Angeles health officials ever since one of the donors for her November 1982 transfusion answered affirmatively to Question 44 of the questionnaire given to all local AIDS patients: "Have you been a blood or plasma donor in the last five years?"

Within two weeks of the transfusion, the nurse was suffering from lymphadenopathy. Blood tests showed that her T-4 lymphocytes were beginning to disappear.

The two cases marked the first time two adults were proven to have AIDS after being transfused with the blood of diagnosed AIDS patients. In all the other suspected transfusion AIDS cases tracked by the Centers for Disease Control, the donors had fit into the high-risk groups for AIDS but had not actually been diagnosed with CDC-defined AIDS. The first transfusion AIDS case, detected at the University of California at San Francisco in December 1982, was an infant, raising questions about congenital immune deficiency.

The blood industry had discounted all previous transfusion AIDS cases in evaluating the extent of the transfusion AIDS problem. With these two adult cases and the San Francisco baby, however, there were now three cases featuring both a donor and recipient who suffered from the syndrome. Altogether, the CDC counted seventy-three transfusion AIDS cases by March 12, including the twenty-four hemophiliacs. Of these, twenty-two already had died. When the stories of Mary Johnstone and the Los Angeles nurse came out in March, however, faithful medical writers almost unanimously followed the blood bankers' rhetoric that they were the first two adults diagnosed with transfusion AIDS in the United States.

Despite the unstinting support of the news media, Brian McDonough, president of the Irwin Memorial Blood Bank, faced a dilemma with Mary Johnstone's diagnosis. Two of the three AIDS cases to which the blood industry did admit had come from Irwin blood. Another fourteen diagnosed AIDS patients were among Irwin donors in recent years, McDonough also knew. Mary Johnstone was only one of twenty-two recipients whom the blood bank was tracking for signs of AIDS. Already, eleven of these people were having problems with their immune systems. Most significantly, at least one of the donors had given blood after the deferral screening had begun last year. When asked by the blood bank why he had donated, he explained that he never considered himself at high risk for the disease, even though he was a sexually active gay man. It wasn't like he was some fist-fucker who hung out in leather bars.

With Mary Johnstone's husband making noises about a lawsuit, McDonough decided his blood bank could no longer take the wait-and-see attitude that characterized his industry's response to the AIDS problem. He knew he would face the wrath of the blood industry for breaking ranks, but he made his decision nonetheless. Even before disclosing the Johnstone case, the Irwin Memorial Blood Bank announced that, as of May 1, the blood bank would begin testing for antibodies to the core of the hepatitis B virus, the test that the Centers for Disease Control had urged blood bankers to start in January 1983.

"Self-exclusion has not worked well enough in the San Francisco area," McDonough said, "and some individuals are giving blood who should not." In announcing that the testing would begin in May, Dr. Herbert Perkins, the Irwin medical director, tried to reassure a jittery public about the safety of the blood supply. The risk of getting AIDS is extremely low, he said, and was less than 1 chance in 500,000.

Other Bay Area blood banks quickly announced that they would follow Irwin's example and begin core hepatitis testing, albeit reluctantly. When the San Jose Red Cross announced that it would start testing, it did not cite safety concerns as its impetus but "competitive pressure from other blood banks in the area." In other words, the Red Cross was worried that it would lose customers to Irwin if it did not start the hepatitis screening.

Brian McDonough came under immediate attack by his colleagues in the blood industry after the announcement. Industry spokesman Dr. Joseph Bove told the *Wall Street Journal* that "more people are killed by bee stings" than by transfusion AIDS.

The newsletter of the American Association of Blood Banks gave the most telling report on industry response to McDonough's announcement: "Aaron Kellner, M.D., of the New York Blood Center, stated that his facility was 'not about to make a decision in favor of anti-core testing,' not because it would cost $10 million and defer six percent of donors, but because they don't believe it would do anything to improve transfusions safety. 'We're not convinced that AIDS is transmitted by blood transfusion. . . . the evidence is very shaky,' said

Kellner. None of the [blood industry] panel spoke out in favor of anti-core testing for AIDS."

It was against this backdrop that Dr. Dennis Donohue, director for the blood and blood-products laboratory of the Food and Drug Administration, met with the AIDS task force of the FDA Blood Products Advisory Committee. The task force had been established to study Donohue's four-month-old suggestion that hepatitis core antibody testing be instituted for the entire nation's blood supply. While commercial blood companies, sensitive to the demands of hemophiliacs, supported testing, nonprofit blood banks, most notably the American Red Cross, continued to oppose it. As usual, the blood bankers argued cost, saying that testing would add $12 to the cost of a unit of blood and that they would have to recruit new donors to replace the 6 percent of donors whose blood would be rejected because of the testing.

Donohue later said that, given the task force membership, all efforts at initiating testing were doomed. Members were either in the blood industry or allied with blood interests. There were no members whose role was to protect the interest of the customers of these business executives. And, ultimately, that is how the eminent doctors who ran the nation's blood banks behaved—like business executives. Both the task force and the blood advisory committee were clubbish groups devoted to little more than protecting the interests of blood banks. Both voted in March to take no action on Donohue's recommendation for hepatitis testing. That largely marked the end of the Food and Drug Administration's meager effort to protect the nation's blood supply from AIDS. When pressed later about why this agency forswore its mandated duty to guard the integrity of America's blood, FDA spokesmen declined comment.

CENTERS FOR DISEASE CONTROL, ATLANTA

James Mason, the CDC director, had a blunt directive for Don Francis on March 21.

"Get it done," he instructed.

In his scientific notebook, Don Francis wrote PRESSURE and underlined the word twice. The heat was on to resolve the AIDS mystery, and Francis didn't have any doubts that the proximity of the presidential election motivated the unusual administration concern. Nevertheless, Francis was pleased that scientific evidence was accumulating rapidly for the French virus. All the CDC experiments were conducted with LAV, because Robert Gallo at the National Cancer Institute, still angry at the defection of Dr. Kalyanaraman, continued to refuse to provide samples of his HTLV-III virus for experiments. By late March, Francis had detected LAV among asymptomatic people who were in AIDS risk groups. The CDC's own LAV antibody tests proved even more sensitive than comparable tests used at either the Pasteur Institute or the National Cancer Institute. At the CDC, 75 percent of AIDS patients tested positive for LAV antibodies. In a complicated process of viral isolation, LAV itself was recovered in seven of eight AIDS patients tested.

Don Francis felt confident enough to take the costly step of inoculating two unfortunate chimpanzees named Manvel and Chesley with the French virus. By now, Francis knew that his efforts to infect marmosets with AIDS were a failure that had cost the CDC much time. He had used marmosets instead of chimpanzees in order to preserve scarce funds, but the smaller monkeys obviously were not susceptible to AIDS. He could only hope now that the costlier chimpanzees were.

The most significant breakthrough for CDC AIDS research came a few weeks later when Dr. Kaly independently isolated LAV from the blood of the Los Angeles nurse who had contracted AIDS through a blood transfusion. The discovery of LAV, in blood drawn before the nurse came down with AIDS, marked the first time scientists could begin to meet the demands of Koch's postulates, and became the single most important step in proving that LAV was the cause of the syndrome. The presence of the virus in the nurse's blood showed that infection with LAV preceded the onset of AIDS, eliminating suspicion that LAV was merely an opportunistic infection taking advantage of the AIDS patient's compromised immune system. The subsequent isolation of LAV in the blood of the transfusion donor showed direct evidence of transmission of the virus in a natural setting, another prerequisite to nailing down a certain microbe as the cause of a disease.

The scientific politicking surrounding the announcement of HTLV-III began to take increasing portions of Don Francis's attention. On March 27, Francis talked to Bob Gallo in an effort to reach some agreement for a joint announcement from the CDC, NCI, and Pasteur. Gallo wanted to delay any statement. "If we make an announcement, AIDS research will be taken over by NIAID," he said. "We need to keep it quiet."

But Gallo was also concerned that, if the Americans waited too long, the French would preempt them and take the credit for the virus's discovery. "They better have what I have or there will be a major battle," he told Francis, noting that Pasteur researcher Francoise Barre, who first detected LAV, had trained in Gallo's lab. "I think I gave a lot to the French," he said.

Bob Gallo continued to be angry that the European press was giving the French credit for discovering the cause of AIDS. "Montagnier is in the papers every day," he said. Don Francis knew this was a sore spot with Gallo. In February, Gallo had called the Pasteur scientists "whores" for so aggressively courting the media.

By the end of that day's conversation, however, Gallo agreed he would share credit for the HTLV-III discovery and acknowledge the CDC for performing the epidemiology on the isolates he had cultured from AIDS patients. He also would give the French their credit as first discoverers if he was convinced that LAV was the same as HTLV-III.

Francis believed that agreement among the American and French scientists was essential to achieving the acceptance of the scientific data and getting on to the subsequent business of finding AIDS treatments, a vaccine, and some way to control the disease. Francis began to work furiously to set up a meeting with the NCI, CDC, and Pasteur Institute to reach an agreement for a joint announcement.

March 28

The morning paper carried a front-page story about Larry Littlejohn's initiative to ban sexual activity in gay baths. The political reality that gays now confronted became instantly clear.

Littlejohn had five months in which to collect a mere 7,332 signatures to qualify his ballot proposition. Nobody doubted that the signatures could be collected easily. Once placed on the ballot, few doubted that it would pass overwhelmingly. No politician could afford to put his or her reputation on the line for bathhouses. Even worse, the controversy would flare through the summer, while the international spotlight shone on San Francisco during the 1984 Democratic National Convention. Although Mayor Feinstein made no on-the-record comment about the bathhouses, off-the-record sources confirmed that she had spent much of the past two weeks in private meetings with gays, trying to persuade them to close the facilities themselves. And she told the newspapers now, "I am watching the situation as closely as I can."

At first, Bill Kraus was furious with Littlejohn. Such a volatile issue in a citywide election could only bring disaster for the gay community, he said.

"But do you agree that what's going on in the baths is killing people?" Littlejohn asked.

Bill Kraus didn't answer.

"I'm only doing what needs to be done," Littlejohn said. "It can't go on the way it is."

Still, he offered a compromise. If the public health director, Merv Silverman, instituted the regulations that Littlejohn proposed through the use of Silverman's quarantine powers, Littlejohn would withdraw the initiative petitions.

Bill Kraus's anger dissolved in the light of the opportunity Littlejohn's petition availed. Nobody, he reasoned, would want the measure to go on the ballot—not the liberal public officials who would be caught in a no-win choice between alienating gays by opposing bathhouses or offending straights by supporting them. Obviously, the bathhouses now were doomed. The question was only who would kill them, heterosexual voters or the gay community itself. As far as Kraus was concerned, the only obstacle was Dr. Silverman, who would not close the baths without community support.

Kraus conceived his squeeze play. Silverman would be told that gay leaders were now willing to support bathhouse closure. In the meantime, gay leaders would be told that Silverman planned to close the bathhouses whether they supported him or not. They had the choice of claiming victory when Silverman shut the facilities, seemingly at their request, or being cast as losers if he closed the baths without their assent. Kraus explained the strategy to Marcus Conant, who subscribed to its wisdom.

Of course, bathhouse closure was not a fait accompli. The acquiescence of gay leaders and Dr. Silverman to closure came only because each side felt compelled to action by the other. Kraus was not stricken by pangs of guilt at his chicanery.

As far as he was concerned, the continued operation of bathhouses amounted to little more than officially condoned homicide. The ruse was a necessary, if unfortunate, way to get Silverman to finally do what he should have done a year ago, Kraus thought.

The newspaper report on the Littlejohn initiative set off a stampede of public officials and gay leaders, all of whom were suddenly urging Silverman to close the bathhouses. Mayor Feinstein again deferred public comment, even while a spokesman confided that she believed they should be closed. Longtime gay ally Supervisor Richard Hongisto said most eloquently: "I have too many beloved friends in the gay community who have died or who are dying of this. I'm going to too many funerals. It's time the bathhouses be closed."

Pressure from gay leaders also mounted, and the *Chronicle's* story included a not-for-attribution comment from Bill Kraus: "Silverman can defuse this issue, make it go away, by just closing the bathhouses now. When the Democratic Convention comes to town with 10,000 reporters, we don't want the big local issue to center on gays' right to commit suicide in bathhouses."

Marc Conant called Merv Silverman.

"I've got what you've said you needed," he said, explaining that gay leaders were ready to support Silverman in closing the baths.

That night, Conant left a retirement dinner for Selma Dritz and joined Bill Kraus and his friend Dick Pabich. Together, the three men went to the home of Dr. David Kessler, where a number of doctors from the Bay Area Physicians for Human Rights were working on a long-planned statement asking gay men voluntarily to stop going to bathhouses.

Conant told them that Silverman was about to close the bathhouses. Pabich suggested that gay community leaders should endorse the move to make the decision appear as a community victory. The doctors were reluctant, but after much discussion, ten of the twelve people in attendance agreed to support Silverman and drafted a statement: "This is an extremely painful and difficult decision which we make reluctantly after serious soul-searching and consultation with many members of our community. Bathhouses have long been important for gay people, but clearly now, saving lives is of greater importance. . . . Therefore in the interest of saving lives, we call on the director of public health to temporarily close such establishments for the duration of this public health emergency."

David Kessler was one of the two doctors who was anxious about how the community would react to such a statement and decided against putting his name on it. As the meeting concluded, Kessler's young lover, Steve Del Re, stomped into the room and started shouting at Marc Conant.

"You're doing a dreadful thing—you'll rot in hell," he screamed, his face turning red with anger. "Blood will be flowing in the streets. You have all made a serious mistake."

◯

The next morning, Bill Kraus called Cleve Jones, asking him to attend a press conference with the health director to support "Merv's decision" to close the baths. Cleve had not been gung ho about closing the facilities, but he certainly did not want the issue on the ballot, and he never considered bathhouses worth fighting for.

"Let's close them and get it over with," he agreed.

Like Bill Kraus and Dick Pabich, Cleve Jones had worked the phones all day, enlisting support. Within a few hours, he had lined up all eleven members of the board of supervisors for closure. Since he had the best rapport with gay street radicals, Cleve also got assurances from many leftist gays that they would not actively oppose closure, even if they did not support it. Later that day, Cleve received a call from Merv Silverman.

"I'm sorry it's come to this," Silverman said.

Cleve didn't know what he was talking about.

"I think it's a sad day for your community," Silverman said.

"If you feel it needs to be done," Cleve said, "I'll go along with you."

Then the light began to dawn. Cleve called Marc Conant and demanded, "Are we acquiescing or are we initiating?"

Later, Cleve heard that pro-bathhouse staffers at the San Francisco AIDS Foundation had called a community meeting for that night, with Silverman and all the bathhouse owners scheduled to attend. He wondered how well Bill Kraus's strategy would hold together.

Bill had no such trepidations. By the end of the day, he had fifty leaders from a broad spectrum of community, political, and professional groups who would endorse Silverman's closure. Lawyers in the city attorney's office spent the day drawing up quarantine orders for the city's fourteen bathhouses and sex clubs.

By early afternoon, Silverman announced he would hold a press conference the next morning.

Toward the end of the afternoon, Selma Dritz received an anonymous phone call in her office. "Silverman will be killed tomorrow if he closes the baths," the caller said.

$\bigcirc$

In Atlanta, Don Francis had by now made the final phone calls to finesse the meeting between the NCI, CDC, and Pasteur Institute. The next week, he and Bob Gallo would fly to Paris to work out all the details for a joint announcement on the discovery of the AIDS virus.

QUEBEC CITY

The morning newspapers on Monday, March 26, carried stories of a study about to be published in the *Journal of American Medicine*. News of this formal publication of the cluster study, two years after the CDC's Bill Darrow had pieced the tale together, was accompanied by complicated diagrams, with all the arrows and circles centered on one person—the now-famous Patient Zero. The study and the news stories, of course, did not name Gaetan Dugas, although they did allude to the fact that researchers believed he was still alive.

Gaetan had survived his fourth bout with *Pneumocystis* and appeared to be on his way to recovery. He spent much of late March on the telephone with friends in Vancouver, talking about how much he hated cold and dreary Quebec City and how he wanted to return to Vancouver. As always, Gaetan had managed to nurture a torrid love affair in his last months in Vancouver, with a handsome male model. By the end of March, he persuaded the model to fly to Quebec and accompany him back to British Columbia.

The model was on the plane east when Gaetan died in Quebec City. It was March 30, a month past Gaetan's thirty-first birthday, and it had been nearly four years since he first had gone to see the doctor in Toronto about the purple spot near his ear. In the end, it wasn't an AIDS disease that killed Gaetan—his kidneys, strained by the years of infection, simply gave out.

Whether Gaetan Dugas actually was the person who brought AIDS to North America remains a question of debate and is ultimately unanswerable. The fact that the first cases in both New York City and Los Angeles could be linked to Gaetan, who himself was one of the first half-dozen or so patients on the continent, gives weight to that theory. Gaetan traveled frequently to France, the western nation where the disease was most widespread before 1980. In any event, there's no doubt that Gaetan played a key role in spreading the new virus from one end of the United States to the other. The bathhouse controversy, peaking so dramatically in San Francisco on the morning of his death, was also linked directly to Gaetan's own exploits in those sex palaces and his recalcitrance in changing his ways. At one time, Gaetan had been what every man wanted from gay life; by the time he died, he had become what every man feared.

44 TRAITORS

March 30, 1984
SAN FRANCISCO

Marc Conant got the first indication that the plans to close the bathhouses were unraveling when a frazzled Merv Silverman called him at home at about midnight. Silverman had just returned from the community meeting organized by opponents of bathhouse closure. He had spent hours being pulled over the coals for his decision to close the facilities. Earlier, Conant had said he would attend the meeting, but over dinner he had changed his mind. It was clear that the forum, a congregation of closure opponents, would present all the old arguments that had stalled action for over a year.

"You let me down," said Silverman. "Where were you?"

"Merv, there are just some meetings it's better not to attend," said Conant.

Conant was surprised that Silverman had only now discovered that opposition to bathhouse closure persisted in the community. Was Silverman going to wait until *every* gay leader backed him?

Two leaders of the Bay Area Physicians for Human Rights who had enclosed Bill Kraus's letter of support for closure had told the health director that they were withdrawing their names. At one point in the forum, Silverman looked forward to some support when a gay leader sought recognition to speak. This leader had gone to Silverman's office two weeks before, after visiting a friend who was near death from AIDS, and begged Silverman to close the baths. Tonight, however, this same leader denounced the plan for closure. It was just what Silverman wanted to avoid—a confrontation that pitted gays against the health department. He wanted them all on the same side, fighting this damned disease, not in opposition, fighting each other.

Meanwhile, dozens of the gay leaders who had signed on as supporters of closure were calling Dick Pabich, begging that their names be taken off the list. It wasn't that they harbored any newfound affection for bathhouses, of course. They had heard that Silverman had wavered in the public forum earlier in the evening. They thought they had put their names on the line to support a decision Silverman earnestly wanted to make. Instead, they were the ones coming out as the heavies, and they could only imagine what the gay press would do to them for calling for the closure of the gay community's biggest advertisers. Most had political careers to think about, and nobody wanted to end up being branded a sexual fascist like Bill Kraus.

One of the last to call Dick Pabich was Cleve Jones. The ugliness that had emerged in the community made Cleve want to sit down and have a drink. He hadn't been feeling well for some time. He was coming down with staph infections and bizarre skin rashes on his legs. He felt so tired all the time that he slipped out of the office every afternoon and went home for a nap. His lymph nodes had been swollen for months. He couldn't stand all the screaming and hatred; he wanted out of the whole controversy. When Cleve called Pabich, he said that his boss, Assemblyman Art Agnos, had demanded that he not add his name to the list.

Neither Dick Pabich nor Bill Kraus believed this. Bill swore he would never forgive Cleve for deserting him at this most crucial juncture. But Cleve couldn't focus on that. Two years of gay fratricide over AIDS had thoroughly exhausted him. As he slumped into his bed after calling Pabich, Cleve just wished it would all be over.

$$\bigcirc$$

The next morning, Merv Silverman, Marc Conant, and City Attorney George Agnost were huddling in Mayor Feinstein's office before the scheduled news conference when Silverman dropped his bombshell. After the city attorney had assured the health director that he had the power to close the bathhouses, Silverman turned to the mayor.

"I'm going to say that I'm not going to say anything," he said.

Feinstein looked like she was about to fall off her chair.

"We don't have compelling medical evidence," he said.

"Of course you do," she said.

"Are you ordering me to close them?" Silverman demanded. Silverman felt the mayor wanted the baths closed for the Democratic Convention. He would consider closing the bathhouses for public health, but he would never close them as part of a campaign to clean up the city. That, Silverman thought, would be a perversion of his public health powers.

Feinstein retreated from Silverman's challenge. She knew that the value of closure as a public health decision would be destroyed if word got out that she ordered Silverman to close the bathhouses. Her order would make closure a political decision.

In any event, she also knew that under the city charter, she couldn't order Silverman to do anything. He was accountable only to the man who acted as city manager.

As the police chief helped Silverman into a bulletproof vest, Feinstein took Marc Conant into the small parlor adjoining her large office. Conant felt chills when he recognized the room as the place where Mayor George Moscone had been assassinated.

"Please watch Merv," Feinstein told Conant. "I'm worried about him."

Conant was worried too. He believed that the Mafia, who maintained strong links to bathhouses in other cities, was behind the quick change in the health director's thinking.

Silverman was filled with doubts, engendered anew by the previous night's stormy confrontation with the gay community. Would the cause of public health be served if bathhouses became the central issue instead of the more fundamental concern about AIDS transmission? Moreover, given the fact that he could not point to a specific virus as the cause of AIDS, would closure stand up in court? Silverman wanted more time to ponder all these things. He did not want to be rushed.

Silverman and Conant left City Hall to attend a meeting of gay community leaders preceding the news conference. On the way to the meeting, Conant could see that an only-in-San Francisco morning was taking shape. Protesters on the steps of the health building had stripped down and were wearing only towels. They held signs: "Today the Tubs, Tomorrow Your Bedroom," "Out of the Tubs and Into the Shrubs," "Out of the Baths, Into the Ovens."

Scores of television crews, reporters, and wire-service correspondents were assembling for the press conference. Every news organization in the United States—including all three television networks and every major daily—had dispatched reporters to cover the first decisive public health move against the AIDS epidemic, coming, of course, in exotic San Francisco, "the nation's AIDS capital."

Marc Conant took Bill Kraus aside as the meeting was about to begin and told Kraus that Silverman was backing away from closure.

"He just doesn't have the courage," Kraus said.

Kraus's face turned red when Silverman said he had to delay making a decision on the bathhouses, that he needed more time to think.

"When?" Kraus shouted. "We've been hearing this crap for years. When will you do something?"

The normally taciturn Dick Pabich was dumbfounded.

"I think it's the stupidest thing I've ever heard," Pabich shouted at Silverman. "You're derelict in your duty. You've embarrassed everyone who has supported you. You've set the stage for a political disaster."

Dick Pabich and David Kessler, one of the gay doctors who had come to oppose closure, started a fierce argument on the issue. With the meeting disintegrating, Silverman raised his voice over the din.

"Let's put it to a vote," he said. "Everybody in favor of closing the bathhouses, raise their hands."

Kraus was stunned that Silverman was putting a crucial public health decision up to a show of hands. The room was split evenly between opponents and supporters. Silverman said he would tell the reporters he was delaying a decision.

The health department's auditorium was crowded with journalists, cameras, and the towel-clad demonstrators when Silverman arrived, nearly an hour late and escorted by plainclothes police officers.

"I am not discussing the opening or closing of the bathhouses at this point," Silverman said. He would delay that decision, he said, until he studied other "facets of this issue, some of which had basically nothing to do with medicine and some of which do.

"There are many, many complex issues. I was unaware of a number of facets," he said. "I apologize for moving so hastily. I want to make it clear this action—leaving the bathhouses open—is mine and not based on any pressure from any groups."

Silverman said he would announce his decision within a week.

○

Perhaps the most telling sign of gay community sentiment occurred the next night when bathhouse supporters announced a Castro Street protest to demonstrate support for sex clubs. Only twenty-two people showed up, and they were outnumbered by reporters. Nevertheless, the political momentum within the gay community shifted away from bathhouse closure in the days that followed.

"It's obvious to me it's not a medical decision being made; it's a blatant political decision," said Gerry Parker, president of the Stonewall Gay Democratic Club, one of the groups on record as opposing closure. "What makes a medical decision turn upside down within minutes?"

The mood of gay leaders in other cities was summed up by the national gay newspaper, the *Advocate,* which editorialized that people who wanted to close baths were "like Chicken Little." The paper did concede, however, that "at a time when the community in general is winning enormous sympathy from non-gay people because of its considerable suffering, gay leaders are reluctant to defend the rights of gay men to, say, be urinated on."

Nathan Fain, the writer who had so vehemently denounced Larry Kramer in New York, wrote in the *Advocate* that "there is no proof that even one of the 3,775 cases of AIDS tallied by the Centers for Disease Control had involved sexual transmission." The gay-backed move to close baths in San Francisco, he wrote, showed that gay leaders were prepared "to make criminals of their own people."

The Northern California Bathhouse Owners Association announced they were seeking $100,000 from sex club owners nationally to mount a legal challenge against any actions that Silverman might later propose.

Meanwhile, the city attorney backed off his original blanket endorsement of closure and advised Silverman that he would have a stronger case if he merely banned the sexual activities that were shown to spread AIDS.

As the situation became more complicated, Mayor Feinstein made her first on-the-record statement about the baths. To the end, the mayor was not forthcoming on the issue, giving her views only when she was cornered in her limousine by the *San Francisco Chronicle* political editor who had followed her on an official visit to New York City. "My own opinion is that if this was a heterosexual problem, they would have been closed already," she said. "The bottom-line question here is death. AIDS means only one thing, and that is that you die. And therefore, if you want to avoid it, the message has to go out. Not in a namby-pamby way."

April 3
CENTERS FOR DISEASE CONTROL, ATLANTA

The AIDS Review Group that Dr. James Mason, CDC director, had appointed in December turned in its report on the adequacy of AIDS resources. The review group found that the diversion of resources was taking a toll on other CDC activities. Some 70 percent of the CDC's AIDS staffers were people diverted from other programs and not funded by federal AIDS appropriations.

"Opportunities have been lost and the overall CDC work has been impaired by this depletion in resources needed for the AIDS effort," the report stated. The review group termed the CDC AIDS lab "not adequate" and suggested an "immediate and intense exploration of the possibility of accelerating the construction of a more suitable facility." The group recommended that Mason seek $20 to $25 million more in AIDS funding for the CDC.

April 4
PARIS

Negotiations among Robert Gallo from the National Cancer Institute, Don Francis from the Centers for Disease Control, and Jean-Claude Chermann from the Pasteur Institute quickly acquired the mood of delicate arms negotiations among parties who shared only mutual distrust.

Gallo flatly refused to discuss the details of his upcoming publications on HTLV-III in front of Francis, so a game of musical chairs enveloped the meetings. Francis frequently had to leave the room while Gallo and Chermann conferred privately. The Pasteur scientists were astonished that one branch of the U.S. government should hold another in such low regard.

Don Francis had brought to Europe electron micrographs that laid to rest any dispute about whether LAV and HTLV-III were different viruses. They were both extremely unusual human retroviruses; they were the same. Moreover, Dr. Kaly had run his comparisons of HTLV-III to HTLV-I and HTLV-II and found that the AIDS virus bore few similarities to the two previously discovered HTLV retroviruses; they were not related.

Francis felt this was a prima facie case for the French naming the virus. At the end of the negotiations, however, the taxonomy issue remained unresolved. The three researchers ultimately were able to work out an agreement for a joint announcement by the CDC, NCI, and Pasteur. They agreed they would share preprints of articles they were about to publish on LAV and HTLV-III and orchestrate their first public declaration of the breakthrough.

That night, they went to the bawdy Paradise Latin in the Latin Quarter and watched barebreasted women descend from the ceiling on swings. Both Gallo, with his roguish charm, and Chermann, with his movie-star good looks, were in their element in such informal settings. As Chermann and Gallo stood side by side in the pissoir, Gallo had a proposition.

"We can do this together—just the Pasteur Institute and the NCI," he said. "We don't need the CDC."

Chermann dismissed the idea.

The next morning, over croissants and tea with Don Francis, Gallo confided that he would probably get the lion's share of the glory in the announcement because he had a lot of HTLV-III isolates. Gallo then put a different spin on the proposal he had made the night before to Chermann.

"We don't need the Pasteur Institute," he suggested. "The CDC and the NCI can announce this ourselves."

◯

In the first week of April, the number of AIDS cases in the United States surpassed 4,000. The first AIDS death in New Zealand was reported from New Plymouth on April 4. A few weeks earlier, British health authorities reported the first AIDS death in Scotland. The epidemic had spread to thirty-three countries worldwide.

April 4
SAN FRANCISCO

At about the same time Don Francis was boarding his plane back to Atlanta, the new edition of the *Bay Area Reporter* with an editorial by Paul Lorch called "Killing the Movement" was being delivered to Castro Street gay bars.

"The gay liberation movement in San Francisco almost died last Friday morning at 11 A.M. No, that's not quite it. The Gay Liberation Movement here and then everywhere else was almost killed off by 16 gay men and lesbians last Friday morning. This group, whose number changed by the hour as people got on and off what they hoped would be a roller coaster, signed a request or gave their names to give the green light to the annihilation of gay life."

These "collaborators," Lorch wrote, were the people who supported bath-house closure.

"These 16 people would have killed the movement, glibly handing it over to the forces that have beaten us down since time immemorial. . . . The gay community should remember these names well, if not etch them into their anger and regret."

The "traitor's list," as it became known, quickly followed. In many ways, it was an honor roll of veterans of local gay politics. Number one was Supervisor Harry Britt. Number three was gay campaign strategist Dick Pabich, the aide who had discovered Harvey Milk's body five years earlier. Number six was Dr. Marcus Conant, who first conceived the idea of San Francisco's coordinated care model for AIDS patients. Science fiction author Frank Robinson, number nine, had written Harvey Milk's campaign speeches, the speeches that gave the gay liberation movement its most idealistic articulation; Robinson made the traitor's list because he was heard to speak for bathhouse closure in one public meeting. Milk Club vice-president Ron Huberman was traitor number eleven. Bill Kraus was number twelve. Larry Littlejohn, who had founded the pioneering group that had made all the later gay politicking possible, was listed as "traitor extraordinaire."

Hearing that he was going to be put on this list, Cleve Jones had gone to the gay paper and begged that his name not be included. Instead, he was listed merely as someone who "waffled" while others were killing the gay movement.

Bill Kraus was devastated by the criticism. He had spent the past decade doing little else than promoting gay rights. Now he was chastised as a "traitor" for his efforts to ensure the biological survival of gay men. He felt that a homosexual McCarthyism had descended on the gay community. You could be homosexual and be homophobic, by the logic of this McCarthyism, just as McCarthy had denounced American citizens as "un-American." McCarthy felt he could proscribe all the political views a true American should have; the *Bay Area Reporter* and its like-minded gay leaders now felt they could order all homosexuals to think exactly as they did or be branded unhomosexual traitors. With such logic, the heroes had become the bathhouse owners, who had assured doctors at the AIDS Clinic that bathhouses were fine because "we both make money off" the people who were killing themselves there.

What disturbed Bill Kraus more than the charges themselves was the fact that there was no one in the gay community who would censure this verbal terrorism. Not one gay politico, writer, or thinker would step forward and say, simply, "This is madness." Insanity triumphed because sane people were silent. Bill felt abandoned and isolated. Publicly, of course, Bill put the best face on his reaction and feigned to be honored at making a list of such esteemed personages. Privately, he complained to his friend Catherine Cusic: "Those bastards. If I get it, it's because of them."

On the morning of April 9, Dr. Silverman announced a decision that further complicated the bathhouse issue. Flanked by twenty-two gay physicians and community leaders, the health director announced that rather than close the baths, he would propose regulations to ban high-risk sexual activity.

"What we are doing today is taking steps, with the support of many community members, to eliminate bathhouses, bookstores, and sex clubs as places of sexual encounters between individuals, places where multiple sex takes place," he said. "We want these places to continue to operate, to be places for social gatherings, for exercise, for a number of things. They just won't serve the purpose that they have served in the past. What we're trying to do is not have sex between individuals."

Silverman's move had the effect of satisfying no one. Bathhouse supporters were angry that anything was being done to impede bathhouse sex, so Silverman was denounced in the gay community as a homophobe. People who wanted the facilities shut down were dissatisfied by the fact they would remain open, and months of political dilly-dallying clearly lay ahead. Mayor Feinstein was said to be livid at the decision. With this announcement, however, the political heat was off the issue, because Larry Littlejohn said he would not pursue his ballot measure, which had in effect asked for the same restrictions that Silverman had announced.

Nationally, gay leaders turned rabid on the issue. On the afternoon Silverman announced the restrictions, *New York Native* publisher Charles Ortleb left a message with Jim Curran's secretary, asking, "Now that you've succeeded in closing down the baths, are you preparing the boxcars for relocation?"

The *Native*'s next cover story, "I Left My Towel in San Francisco," obscured a story Ortleb had unearthed in an interview with James Mason, CDC director. Buried in the *Native* was the first report anywhere from a government official stating flatly that the cause of AIDS had been discovered. The virus, Mason said, was called LAV and had been discovered by the French.

NATIONAL CANCER INSTITUTE, BETHESDA

The same day Dr. Silverman announced his bathhouse sex ban, a doctor from the National Cancer Institute went to Building 31 on the NIH campus and picked up a bottle that had been carefully packed in a double-sealed plastic bag. He drove the bottle to the "P3 containment facility" at the Frederick Cancer Research Facility in suburban Maryland. The bottle contained 100 million particles of HTLV-III. The center, which once housed the nation's biological warfare research, was beginning to gear up to produce the 750 gallons of virus that would be needed each month for blood assays to test every unit of blood used in transfusions. Although one branch of the U.S. Public Health Service, the Food and Drug Administration, continued to maintain that the threat of transfusion AIDS was so minimal that it did not need regulatory action, another PHS branch, the NCI, had made the blood test its top AIDS priority.

Evidence supporting HTLV-III as the cause of AIDS mounted. Since 1981, Drs. Bob Biggar and James Goedert from the NCI's Environmental Epidemiology Branch had been collecting blood from gay men in Washington and New York as part of a prospective study on AIDS in this high-risk population. As various theories for different AIDS agents emerged in the following years, the blood was tested for a host of agents, including African Swine Fever virus, parvo viruses, and even interferon levels. By the time HTLV-III tests were available to Biggar in April, there was only enough blood from each study subject to conduct this one last blood test. Fortunately, his tests showed that HTLV-III was not another bum lead.

In San Francisco, an AIDS researcher inadvertently speeded the timetable for the HTLV-III announcement with an offhand remark to a radio interviewer. Like just about everyone in AIDS research, Dr. Donald Abrams, AIDS Clinic assistant director, knew of the breakthrough. He alluded to the discovery of "the AIDS agent" during a radio interview with the local CBS affiliate on Sunday afternoon, April 15.

"Is that a scoop?" the reporter asked.

Abrams immediately regretted mentioning it. It broke all rules of scientific courtesy to announce somebody else's discovery. The reporter, however, seemed innocuous enough in her Snoopy sweatshirt. She probably didn't understand the significance of what he had said, Abrams thought.

"This is just for the local audience," she assured him, for airing in "the next week or so."

"What's an agent?" she asked casually. "Is that a virus?"

"An agent is anything that causes a disease," Abrams said. "But in fact, this is a virus."

Abrams didn't think much more of the interview until he got a phone call from a cousin in New Jersey the next morning.

"Mazel tov," he said. "Everybody heard you on the radio this morning when you announced the discovery of the AIDS virus."

When more newspapers and networks started calling, Abrams declined to comment. CBS upped the ante, however, when a reporter demanded that he either retract his statements or reveal the researchers.

That afternoon, Don Francis got a call from the CBS News bureau in Paris. "What is this?" the reporter asked. "Gallo says *he* has the cause of AIDS."

The *San Francisco Chronicle* was going with its own story on HTLV-III the next morning, and a number of other newspapers were calling to demand a press conference on the "new virus."

In England, also, the news was about to break because a few weeks earlier a BBC correspondent had persuaded Bob Gallo's secretary to give him copies of Gallo's *Science* articles, promising not to air the information until July. He then released the reports to *New Scientist,* which quickly ran with the HTLV-III news. When the journal contacted Jean-Claude Chermann for a comment, the Pasteur Institute researcher called Don Francis in a rage.

"If Gallo violates our agreement, I'll kill him," Chermann said.

The National Cancer Institute scheduled a press conference to make the announcement, but Secretary Heckler was on the West Coast and could not attend. The press conference was ordered delayed until Monday, April 23.

Days before the announcement, Don Berreth, CDC public affairs chief, got a draft of the NCI's press release. Their announcement made no mention of LAV or the Pasteur Institute. Although Assistant Secretary for Health Edward Brandt now had preprints of the papers to be published in *Science,* neither he nor the NCI had shared them with the CDC. James Mason, Jim Curran, and Don Francis put through a conference call to Brandt, pleading with him to delay the announcement until it could be orchestrated with the French. Francis explained that HTLV-III and LAV were the same virus, that this was not an American discovery.

By coincidence, *The New York Times* science writer, Lawrence Altman, had been at the CDC in Atlanta a week earlier. Mason had told Altman then that the Pasteur Institute's work with LAV was "highly significant" and that it looked "like they have the AIDS virus." Late in the afternoon on Friday, April 20, Altman called Mason. He had heard of the hubbub surrounding the impending HTLV-III announcement and wanted to put Mason's earlier comments in the Sunday *Times.* Mason knew that it would look as though he were upstaging Heckler's announcement and asked Altman not to print the story.

"Anything you say I say will get me in trouble," Mason said.

April 20
SAN FRANCISCO DEPARTMENT OF PUBLIC HEALTH

By that Friday afternoon, Dr. Selma Dritz had heard of the imminent HTLV-III press conference. The news brought a natural end to the phase of the epidemic that had involved people like herself, Dritz thought. It seemed appropriate that this was her last day of work. With the cause of the disease found and the routes of transmission established, the focus of the next phase of AIDS research would shift to the lab, where scientists could develop the vaccine and treatments. Selma Dritz's legacy was written into the notebooks she had carefully kept since the first day she had heard of the mysterious case of Kaposi's sarcoma in Ken Horne. Dritz felt a serenity with her retirement. She had done her share of the world's work, she felt, and she had done a good job.

At her retirement dinner, somebody recalled a talk he had heard Dritz give in 1980 at UCSF about venereal diseases in gay men. In the talk, Dritz had warned that "too much was being transmitted" and there would be "hell to pay" if any new infectious agent made it into this population. The statement showed uncanny prescience, the colleague noted. Selma Dritz didn't remember.

45 POLITICAL SCIENCE

April 23, 1984
HUBERT H. HUMPHREY BUILDING,
U.S. DEPARTMENT OF HEALTH AND HUMAN SERVICES,
WASHINGTON, D.C.

Bob Gallo was weary and nervous when he arrived in the office of Health and Human Services Secretary Margaret Heckler. He had come straight from the airport, having flown all night from Italy, where he had delivered the closing remarks at a human retrovirus conference. Only yesterday had he learned that his presence was required this morning at a press conference in which Heckler would announce the discovery of HTLV-III. Gallo was stunned to hear that the previous day's *New York Times* carried a page-one story in which Dr. James Mason from the Centers for Disease Control gave credit to the Pasteur Institute for isolating the AIDS agent. Knowing that the *Times* writer who broke the story, Dr. Lawrence Altman, was a former CDC staffer, Gallo figured the leak was a salvo meant to upstage his research at the NCI. And Gallo had no doubt that Don Francis, who was collaborating with the Pasteur, was the man behind the *Times* story.

Indeed, James Mason, who had flown to Washington for the press conference, was made aware in no uncertain terms by HHS officials that his comments in the New York daily were not appreciated. Before the press conference, a shouting match had broken out between Bob Gallo and one of Heckler's top aides when the HHS staffer had the temerity to scold Gallo, NCI Director Vincent Devita, and NIH Director James Wyngaarden about the leak. After the hollering subsided, the scientists briefed Heckler and walked down to the massive auditorium in the Hubert H. Humphrey Building.

Gallo had never seen so many reporters, lights, and cameras. He quickly realized that the announcement would be a major international news story and that the French scientists would be furious with him. Heckler opened the press conference with a six-page statement that had both a nationalistic and political tenor.

"Today we add another miracle to the long honor roll of American medicine and science," she declared. "Today's discovery represents the triumph of science over a dreaded disease. Those who have disparaged this *scientific* search— those who have said we weren't doing enough—have not understood how sound, solid, significant medical research proceeds. From the first day that AIDS was identified in 1981, HHS scientists and their medical allies have never stopped searching for the answers to the AIDS mystery. Without a day of procrastination, the resources of the Public Health Service have been effectively mobilized."

The doctors who accompanied Heckler to the podium blanched visibly when she proclaimed that a blood test would be available within six months and a vaccine would be ready for testing within two years. None of the doctors with Heckler on the stage believed this claim, and nobody could determine where she had conceived such deadlines, which they knew would never be met.

Because of the CDC's prodding, Heckler had added a nod to the efforts of the Pasteur Institute. Heckler went out of her way, however, to enumerate why the NCI research was particularly "crucial." She noted, accurately, that Gallo alone had figured out how to reproduce the virus in large quantities, a discovery that continued to elude the French. Only this ability made the mass production of a blood test possible. Somehow, however, Heckler also managed to deduce that the Pasteur Institute's research "has in part been working in collaboration with the National Cancer Institute." With further studies, Heckler added, scientists expected that LAV and HTLV-III "will prove to be the same."

After the years of frustration, the announcement of the HTLV-III discovery deserved elation, Don Francis thought as he watched the live Cable News Network coverage of the Heckler press conference in the CDC's television studio with other members of the AIDS Activities Office. Instead, he felt burdened by the conflicts he saw ahead. The French were being cheated of their recognition and the U.S. government had taken a sleazy path, claiming credit for something that had been done by others a year before. Francis was embarrassed by a government more concerned with election-year politics than with honesty. Moreover, he could see that suspicion would play a greater, not a lesser role in the coming AIDS research. Competition often made for good science, Francis knew, lending an edge of excitement to research. Dishonesty, however, muddied the field, taking the fun out of science and retarding future cooperation.

The New York Times echoed the concern in an editorial shortly after the announcement. "What's going on?" the piece asked. "Since even certain discovery of the guilty virus will not produce a vaccine for at least two years, and even better blood screening cannot occur for months, what you are hearing is not yet a public benefit but a private competition—for fame, prizes, new research funds. . . . Some kind of progress is surely being made. The commotion indicates a fierce—and premature—fight for credit between scientists and bureaucratic sponsors of research. Certainly no one deserves the Nobel Peace Prize."

In Paris, the Pasteur scientists were aghast at the short shrift their work was given. Willy Rozenbaum considered Heckler's performance no more than a political stump speech. "Elect us and we give you antibody test in six months," he mimicked bitterly. "Elect us and we give you vaccine in two years."

Three days later, Luc Montagnier revealed his own suspicions when he told

United Press International, "I don't say Gallo took our virus. He worked independently."

Officials at the National Cancer Institute had no reluctance about taking center stage in the discovery of the AIDS agent. As far as they were concerned, the Pasteur and NCI did not deserve equal credit because the NCI clearly had done more extensive and definitive work on the virus. Beyond perfecting the means for its mass production, Gallo had cultured many more isolates and perfected a more sensitive blood test. Complaints from the Pasteur and the CDC were sour grapes, they thought.

○

How timely was the discovery of the long-sought AIDS virus? Partisans of the scientific establishment and the Reagan administration pointed out that the mystery of the AIDS epidemic was solved much faster than for any comparable disease. This is an accurate observation. Such analysis, however, ignores the fact that AIDS did not emerge in the days of Antonie van Leeuwenhoek or Louis Pasteur. The outbreak occurred in an era marked by exponential growth of medical knowledge and technology. Rather than compare the research on AIDS to disease research in earlier eras, it is more to the point to look at the chronology of the actual AIDS research.

As it turned out, the AIDS virus was not a particularly difficult microbe to find. The French took all of three weeks to discover LAV and had published their first paper on it within four months. This early publication lacked the certainty of a definitive discovery, but the French had enough evidence to assert they had found the cause of AIDS by the summer of 1983, seven or eight months into the research process.

Nor was the NCI research marked by great longevity. Gallo's announcement of forty-eight isolates of HTLV-III came just twelve days past the first anniversary of the April 11, 1983, NCI meeting in which the researcher swore he would "nail down" the cause of AIDS. Meanwhile, at the University of California in San Francisco, it took Dr. Jay Levy about eight months to gather twenty isolates of a microorganism he called AIDS-associated retrovirus, or ARV, which he too believed to be identical to LAV. Levy's research was hampered by lack of resources and did not begin in earnest until after the arrival of his long-sought flow hood and the release of impounded UC research funds the previous autumn. On the date of the HTLV-III press conference, Levy also was on the verge of announcing his discovery.

Therefore, by April 1984, isolates of the AIDS virus had been made at the Pasteur, NCI, CDC, and UCSF, all of which were discovered after substantially less than a year of research.

What delayed the NCI, therefore, was not the difficulty in finding the virus but their reluctance to even look. Most CDC researchers privately believed that if the NCI had begun serious laboratory efforts in 1981, the virus could have been detected by 1982, before it had made its vast penetration into American life. Although all the scientists who made the viral isolations certainly deserved applause, the discovery of the AIDS agent ultimately was not a contest for accolades but a race against time. Once again, time, the true adversary, had won.

$\bigcirc$

As of April 23, 1984, there were 4,177 cases of Acquired Immune Deficiency Syndrome in the United States, the CDC announced that afternoon. Of these, 1,101 had been reported in 1984. The disease had spread to forty-five states. About 20 new cases were reported on every working day. Thus far, 1,807 AIDS deaths had been counted nationally. New York City reported nearly 1,657 cases. That week, the numbers of AIDS cases in San Francisco surpassed 500.

May 4
UNIVERSITY OF CALIFORNIA,
SAN FRANCISCO

Within days of the HTLV-III announcement, Marc Conant had issued invitations to a high-powered group of health educators, AIDS specialists, and media professionals for a symposium to develop an "AIDS Prevention Media Project." Supervisor Britt would try to secure city funding for the project.

The gay press, still angry at Conant's involvement with bathhouse closure in March, counterattacked with a savage character assassination, rehashing Conant's efforts against the bathhouses. The headline in the *Bay Area Reporter* announced: "MD's Plot 'Behavior Modification' for Tricking Gays," and characterized the campaign as an Orwellian conspiracy for thought control. Sensitive to anything that might upset gay voters in an election year, the board of supervisors began wavering on the program.

The prevention program was not the only controversy snaring the mayor in May. The bathhouse issue was stalled, as was the city's AIDS prevention campaign. Silverman subsequently said he was disappointed with the AIDS education campaign mounted by his department and the San Francisco AIDS Foundation, although he never expressed his reservations in public. He felt he had no choice but to include all the various gay factions in his considerations, aware that any one of the groups would move to sabotage prevention efforts if they felt excluded. As he said later, it was better to have all the Indians inside the tent pissing out than to have them on the outside pissing in.

It was about this time that Steve Del Re, the young man who had so bitterly chastised Conant for wanting to close the baths, appeared in Conant's office. By now, Conant had heard the rumors about the twenty-seven-year-old's liaison with Rock Hudson, but Steve hadn't come to gossip.

"I have this purple spot," he said.

$\bigcirc$

Gay leaders in other cities had by now moved to head off action against their bathhouses by public health authorities. A spokesman for New York State

Health Commissioner David Axelrod termed actions against the bathhouses "ridiculous," citing the sex fiend argument that gays would be screwing in the bushes if they didn't have the baths. Both New York Governor Cuomo and Axelrod referred discussion of closure to the advisory council of the AIDS Institute, which was dominated by gay leaders opposed to such a move. When Dr. Roger Enlow of the New York City Health Department announced the city's opposition to bathhouse regulation, he noted with obvious satisfaction that Robert Bolan had lost his BAPHR post in supporting closure. "At times like these, we are tempted to turn to authority figures, as we did when we were children, to ask them to protect us, to take the responsibility from our shoulders, to tell us that they can save us from ourselves," Enlow wrote.

The speed with which New York officials jumped to the defense of civil liberties was not matched by an enthusiasm to spend money to prevent the disease. Even as Governor Cuomo assured gay leaders he would never move against the bathhouses, he opposed—for the second year in a row—allocating state funds to fight AIDS. After Cuomo neglected to put any money into his state budget for AIDS, the legislature voted to spend $1.2 million for AIDS research and $400,000 more for education.

In Los Angeles, public health moves against bathhouses were also dismissed out of hand. UCLA researcher Michael Gottlieb was growing more convinced that gay community should act against the facilities, but gay leaders continued to talk convincingly of their strategy to "engineer out" the riskiest playrooms of the baths, such as orgy chambers and glory holes. Privately, gay leaders sometimes confided that the cat was already out of the bag in the AIDS epidemic and that closing the bathhouses would no longer do much good to slow the tide of infection. Gottlieb considered this unusual logic from leaders who publicly maintained that bathhouses did not contribute to the spread of AIDS. He also wondered whether public health officials were saying that the epidemic was out of control long before it actually was.

Gottlieb had already fallen into conflict with public health authorities on the issue of contact tracing. Gottlieb thought that health officials should track down sexual contacts of AIDS patients much as they did the contacts of syphilis patients. Health officials argued that authorities had no magic bullet to offer people exposed to AIDS, like that offered to syphilis patients. Contact tracing would only scare people, they said. There were also civil rights concerns of privacy to consider. The issue of people who might unknowingly be spreading AIDS to others—and the rights of this next generation of victims—was not considered.

Southern California also was running its scant education programs on a shoestring. The city's major AIDS service group, AIDS Project–Los Angeles, continued to be funded exclusively by private contributions. Only eight paid staffers coordinated services to the city with the nation's third highest AIDS caseload. Since the county board of supervisors was dominated by conservative Republicans, there was no hope of county funds. Los Angeles education efforts, therefore, depended on state money.

As in New York, state funding requests met with gubernatorial opposition. Although California's Republican governor George Deukmejian was ready to approve $2.9 million for AIDS research, he opposed the legislature's plan for $1 million in AIDS education monies. At a legislative hearing, Peter Rank, the head of the state Department of Health Services, said the funding was unnecessary, because, "We spent $500,000 on education last year."

Legislative efforts to plan California's AIDS program also were stymied by the governor, who opposed long-term planning for the epidemic. The previous year, the legislature had established an advisory committee made up of both legislative and gubernatorial appointees to make budget recommendations for AIDS. By early 1984, all the legislative slots on the committee were filled, but Governor Deukmejian had resisted nominating a single member for the group. Despite the Deukmejian administration's rhetoric about AIDS being the state's "number-one health priority," Democrats in Sacramento recognized the governor's strategy as similar to that of the conservative president in Washington. Long-term planning for the epidemic would require a long-term commitment of resources, and that was something that both the Deukmejian and the Reagan administration wanted to avoid.

U.S. Department of Health and Human Services, Hubert H. Humphrey Building, Washington, D.C.

By late May, this truth was dawning on Assistant Secretary for Health Edward Brandt. With the announcement of HTLV-III, Brandt quickly identified the four paths on which research should proceed. Top priority was the development of a blood test. Federal researchers also had to start seeking an AIDS vaccine and effective AIDS treatments while nailing down HTLV-III as the cause of AIDS. Brandt by now knew the conclusions of the CDC director's review committee on that agency's research needs. He also felt that now that the AIDS virus was discovered, the NIH should receive enough money to explore every avenue for fighting the disease. Brandt put a $55 million price tag on the new initiatives with $20 million to be immediately infused into AIDS research for the remaining four months of the current fiscal year. He made the requests in a May 25 memo to Secretary Heckler.

"These exciting discoveries bring us much closer to the detection, prevention and treatment of AIDS," Brandt wrote. "There is much left to do. . . . In order to seize the opportunities which the recent breakthroughs have provided us, we will need additional funds both for the remainder of this fiscal year and for FY 1985. Although I realize that general policy would discourage supplemental and amendment requests at this time, I believe that the unique situation with respect to AIDS justifies our forwarding the requests at this time."

Brandt attached twenty-one pages of detailed breakdowns of how the money would be spent. Once again, he began what would be a long process of waiting. And more waiting.

AIDS may have been the number-one priority of the Department of Health and Human Services, he later observed, but it certainly was not a priority for the Office of Management and Budget.

Other controversies continued to distract Brandt. Earlier in May, he had agreed to attend the annual awards dinner of the Fund for Human Dignity, the fund-raising arm of the National Gay Task Force, to present an award to the Blood Sister Project of San Diego. The group had enlisted hundreds of lesbians to donate blood, which was virtually pristine because of the noted dearth of social disease among lesbians. The blood then could be used to help San Diego County AIDS patients. Brandt considered the project a worthy example of the kind of community program called for in President Reagan's cry for more volunteerism. When a number of conservative "pro-family" groups heard of Brandt's appearance, however, they inundated the White House with telegrams demanding that Brandt be fired if he went to the dinner.

"We are utterly outraged and appalled at this presentation by Dr. Brandt, who has himself identified AIDS as the number-one priority for the U.S. Public Health Service," said Gary Curran of the American Life Lobby. "This is an outrageous legitimization of a life-style repugnant to the vast majority of Americans." Other fundamentalist groups quickly joined in the chorus. The organizations had long been suspicious of Secretary Heckler, whom they considered far too liberal for their tastes. When Brandt met with Heckler to discuss the fracas, she was worried about the political fallout.

"This is going to blow up into a mess," Heckler said.

"I can smell it already," Brandt said.

That afternoon, an HHS spokesman announced that Brandt had a meeting to attend the night of the awards dinner. Although "disappointed," he would not be able to present the award.

$$\bigcirc$$

On May 31, 1984, the number of Americans killed in the AIDS epidemic surpassed 2,000. But the deaths of the 2,000, and the diagnosis of 2,615 others who now awaited death, had not moved society toward mobilizing its resources against the new epidemic. Even the pleading of the Assistant Secretary for Health would not make much of a difference. What did make a difference began on June 5, 1984, when a man went to his doctor's office to learn the results of a biopsy. The biopsy had been performed on a pesky purple spot on the fifty-eight-year-old's neck. The doctor suspected what the spot signified as soon as he saw it. Nevertheless, he waited until the biopsy confirmed the diagnosis before he told Rock Hudson that he was suffering from Kaposi's sarcoma.

46 DOWNBOUND TRAIN

June 1984
CENTERS FOR DISEASE CONTROL,
ATLANTA

The brightest moments in the first five years of the AIDS epidemic tended to do little more than illuminate how truly dark the future would be. Never was this truth more conspicuous than in the first months after the acceptance of the LAV and HTLV-III viruses as the cause of AIDS. Antibody testing gave researchers their first glimpse into the number of Americans infected with the virus. Past epidemiology could only chart the course of the epidemic through full-blown AIDS cases, which meant in effect that researchers were following routes the virus had traveled several years before. With AIDS antibody testing, scientists learned where the virus was traveling now. This understanding produced a welter of bad news in the summer of 1984.

At the CDC, Don Francis supervised this bleak work at his virology lab. Of 215 men whose blood was drawn recently at the San Francisco venereal disease clinic, 65 percent, or 140, had antibodies to LAV. Moreover, an unsettling proportion of these test subjects already had symptoms of immune problems, most commonly swollen lymph nodes. When local health officials tested blood from 126 subjects who had shown no early signs of either AIDS or ARC, they found that 55 percent were infected with the virus. Although their presence at a VD clinic meant they were more sexually active than the typical San Francisco gay man, that extraordinarily high infection rate meant the virus was already pandemic in the San Francisco gay community and probably other major metropolitan areas as well. Testing of East Coast gay men by Bob Gallo's lab found that 35 percent had HTLV-III antibodies, while comparable screening in Paris found an 18 percent infection rate.

Testing among people exposed to the virus through blood contact—either through the use of illicit drugs or by transfusion—produced even more depressing results. Of eighty-six intravenous drug users tested from one New York City drug clinic, seventy-five, or 87 percent, were infected with LAV. Tests on twenty-five hemophiliacs with no AIDS symptoms revealed that 72 percent, or eighteen of them, had LAV antibodies. Severe hemophiliacs who used Factor VIII more than once a month demonstrated an even higher infection rate, 90 percent. CDC studies on recipients of blood transfusions from high-risk donors found a similarly high rate of infection. This indicated an exponential increase in future transfusion cases as late-arriving runners from these AIDS marathons approached the finish lines.

The testing also laid to rest lingering doubts about the relationship of AIDS to the unexplained immune abnormalities that were appearing with greater frequency among children of drug abusers. Strict CDC guidelines had long kept many such infants out of official AIDS tallies. Arye Rubinstein was treating 128 patients from the impoverished Bronx for what he considered to be AIDS. The CDC would count only between 10 and 15 percent of these cases as meeting the agency's requirements for such classification. When Rubinstein ran HTLV-III antibody tests, however, he found that all were infected with the AIDS agent. Such results sparked early calls for the CDC to expand its definition of AIDS. After all, many were dying in New York and San Francisco as an effect of LAV/HTLV-III infection, even though they were never counted as AIDS patients. The CDC, however, resisted.

Antibody testing lent scientists their first insights into the progression of AIDS infection. The gay men studied in the San Francisco hepatitis vaccine research during the 1970s again proved a singularly valuable tool in this research. In June, Don Francis put on his long johns and ski parka to pull the tubes of blood he had collected from the 6,800 men for vaccine research. He selected 110 blood samples drawn in 1978 and about 50 taken in 1980. Only 1 person in the 1978 study had LAV antibodies, while 25 percent of the group studied two years later were infected. Since then, the infection rate had more than doubled. The retrospective testing bolstered the hypothesis that a new viral agent had appeared among San Francisco gay men in 1976 or 1977 and spread rapidly through the city well before Ken Horne first saw the purple lesions on his chest in 1980. Since then, the virus had proliferated even more wildly.

When Dr. Bob Biggar from the NCI returned to Denmark in June to test the gay men he had recruited for his prospective AIDS study in 1981, he was jolted to discover that 9 percent of them already had HTLV-III antibodies. Biggar was particularly distressed because this was not a group of big-city Copenhagen gay men but people from Aarhus, the more remote city north of the great fjord—the city where Grethe Rask once attended medical school. Biggar started advising colleagues that such an infection rate had "horrifying" implications. Although few in his Danish study group had AIDS yet, the San Francisco study confirmed that impressive numbers of cases could lag years behind the first infection with the virus. Other scientists told Biggar that he needed to study larger groups of gay men before he started trumpeting such alarmist declarations.

Biggar's studies also pointed toward the emerging infection routes. In Denmark, for example, infected gay men tended to be the very men who had visited New York City. In a similar vein, Biggar also found that Danish hemophiliacs who used Factor VIII made in Europe did not have HTLV-III antibodies; the hemophiliacs who were infected with HTLV-III got their Factor VIII from the United States.

Antibody testing in Africa by the Pasteur Institute defined the earliest paths of AIDS transmission. From their testing, the Pasteur researchers estimated that the incidence of AIDS in Zaire was probably on the order of 250 cases per million. This compared to 16 per million people in the United States, the nation with the highest officially reported AIDS cases. Biggar tested blood he drew in the remote Zairian bush country north of Kinshasa and found that 12 percent of local people were infected with HTLV-III. Such statistics led researchers to conclude that AIDS had come from somewhere in Equatorial Africa. Certainly, no one proposed that American gay men had visited that neck of the savannah recently. Such theorizing on AIDS origins, however, made African governments uneasy. As a condition for entering Zaire, authorities demanded that American and European research teams pledge not to release AIDS data.

With no direct links to African governments, Dr. Max Essex was at liberty to hypothesize openly about how AIDS started. His own studies on outbreaks of an AIDS-like disease among research monkeys in both Massachusetts and California had led him into research on Simian AIDS, or SAIDS, and the discovery of STLV-III, or Simian T-lymphotrophic virus. The similarities in proteins between STLV-III and HTLV-III led Essex to believe that AIDS may have been lying dormant in some primate population for thousands of years before being transferred to humans.

Given the abrupt sociological dislocation in equatorial Africa in recent years, the rest of the story was fairly easy to piece together. A remote tribe may have harbored the virus. With the rapid urbanization of this region after colonization, the virus may have only recently reached the major cities, such as Kinshasa. From Africa, the virus jumped to Europe, where AIDS cases were appearing regularly by the late 1970s, and to Haiti, through administrators imported from that island to work in Zaire throughout the 1970s. From Europe and Haiti, the virus quickly made its debut in the United States, returning to Europe in the early 1980s through gay tourists.

For all the insight the antibody testing offered, substantial mysteries remained in mid-1984. The most important question concerned exactly what the presence of HTLV-III antibodies meant. The large number of people infected with the AIDS virus might mean that it was less lethal than scientists had imagined, some researchers hoped. The early prospective studies of people with lymphadenopathy, for example, found that relatively few were developing AIDS. Perhaps, some thought, this meant that ARC was a mild form of AIDS infection, and the worst thing that ARC patients might contract was a hard lymph node and a few dermatological problems. Maybe some of the antibodies could be protective and neutralize the effect of the AIDS virus, other scientists hoped. Although the presence of AIDS antibodies in so many patients indicated that this was not always the case, there was not enough known about the antibodies to draw any definitive conclusions yet.

Substantial debate continued as to whether the AIDS virus—whether LAV or HTLV-III—acted alone or in tandem with another infection to produce AIDS. Again, this could explain why some people infected with the AIDS virus came down with the full-blown disease while others got ARC and many more had no symptoms of malaise. Cytomegalovirus and the Epstein-Barr virus were the most-nominated candidates for AIDS co-factor. Others voted for gastrointestinal parasites.

Against all this uncertainty, Dale Lawrence's research into AIDS incubation gained a more pressing import. With an average incubation period of 5.5 years, there didn't have to be many cases in 1984 to substantiate the fatality of the AIDS virus. According to his calculations, because the virus had not invaded the bodies of very many Americans until 1980, the huge number of AIDS cases would not start appearing until late 1985. Still, throughout 1984, the CDC made no effort to reveal Lawrence's disquieting research.

Lawrence discerned a pattern in this. All along, the agency had routinely delayed making public its new discoveries for at least six months. Other staffers' work on intravenous drug users and their female sexual partners had encountered such delays. Leading CDC researchers assured journalists that there was "no evidence" that AIDS was an infectious disease even as they prepared the tale of Patient Zero and his clusters for official publication. Warnings about possible heterosexual transmission of AIDS were also stalled, in part because Assistant Secretary for Health Brandt did not believe AIDS could become a heterosexual problem.

Lawrence understood the wisdom of such caution. The agency's credibility could be undermined if it had a reputation of shooting from the hip on issues of key national health policy. Still, Lawrence was concerned that health officials across the country were relying on estimates of a two-year incubation period to support optimistic analyses that AIDS would reach a plateau soon because of recent changes in gay behavior. Those were not the statistics on which to base intelligent planning, he knew. However, from the day in December 1983 that Lawrence first advised Jim Curran of his research, it was sixteen months before scientists learned this bitter truth about the AIDS virus.

Don Francis knew enough about the vagaries of retroviral incubation to quickly draw some depressing conclusions from the various studies on the prevalence of AIDS virus among the various high-risk groups. Gay men in major urban areas, he could see, stood to be devastated by the epidemic. Hemophiliacs faced decimation. Intravenous drug users would be wiped out in astounding numbers, taking with them their sexual partners and infant children. Equatorial Africans faced death on the scale of the Holocaust. The light at the end of the tunnel was an oncoming train.

Grim prognostications were nothing new to the AIDS epidemic. The new wrinkle for Francis was the scientific rancor between Robert Gallo and the Pasteur Institute over credit for the AIDS virus discovery. Rather than settling the dispute, the HTLV-III announcement had enlarged it, and the fallout was profoundly frustrating Francis's work at the CDC. Because Gallo remained angry with the CDC for leaking news about LAV on the eve of the Heckler press conference, he was reluctant to provide the CDC with substantial amounts of HTLV-III. A thimbleful of virus had arrived from the NCI in May, but the CDC lab had difficulties culturing it, so Jim Curran requested more.

The CDC knew that plenty of this virus existed. In May, the NCI had sent out 25 liters to the five private pharmaceutical companies who were chosen to manufacture the blood screening test. However, the NCI refused to give the CDC anything but token amounts of HTLV-III. Gallo was convinced that the CDC was not sharing its best specimens with his lab, and he would not cooperate with the CDC as long as he suspected the CDC was not cooperating with him. Not until the end of the year did the NCI relent and finally enter into a purchase agreement with the CDC for 100 liters of HTLV-III.

Gallo was also adamant that the CDC not perform genetic comparisons between HTLV-III and the French LAV. Gallo promised to do his own comparison between HTLV-III and LAV, but the results weren't forthcoming. Francis knew the comparison could settle whether the two viruses were identical; if identical, it also would settle the question of who discovered the AIDS virus first. Gallo did not want this settled, Francis thought, because it would show he had lost the great viral competition of the twentieth century. Francis anticipated that Gallo would spend a year publishing reams of scientific papers on HTLV-III. Later, when he was internationally recognized as the virus' discoverer, he would allow that HTLV-III and LAV were the same. Gallo viewed this as part of normal scientific competition; Francis thought it smarmy.

At the Pasteur Institute, French researchers were miffed at being treated as pretenders to the throne, awaiting Bob Gallo's confirmation that their claim to the coveted discovery was rightful. Internationally, scientists working on AIDS were forced to choose sides between the French and the Americans. Within a week of the announcement, Francis got into a bitter public argument at a scientific conference in France with Dr. William Haseltine, a Harvard researcher aligned with Gallo.

"How can you share specimens with the French and not with Bob Gallo?" Haseltine shouted at Francis.

Around them, other scientists fell silent. Don Francis was stunned. The comment revealed that Gallo had shown Haseltine the private memos he had been circulating in the NIH complaining about the CDC.

"Don't get involved with things you don't know anything about," Francis shouted back. "Keep your nose out of it."

Because the Reagan administration had relied on Gallo to take the political heat off the AIDS epidemic, the top officials at HHS and the Public Health Service supported the NCI. At one point, they ordered the CDC to stop referring to the virus as LAV in their research papers and instead defer to Gallo's taxonomy of HTLV-III. The request was ludicrous: All CDC research was on the French-supplied LAV, if for no other reason than they couldn't get HTLV-III from Gallo. Ultimately, the CDC persuaded higher administration officials to accept the compromise moniker of LAV/HTLV-III.

There were also problems publishing studies. During an argument over hiring Dr. Kaly, Gallo had sworn to Don Francis that "you'll never get anything published." Francis dismissed the pledge as an empty threat.

As the imbroglio grew more bitter, Francis noticed that good virologists were shying away from AIDS research, reluctant to become stuck in what had become a quagmire of scientific politicking. AIDS research had become "wretched, rank with politics," Francis wrote in his journal that summer. "It's lost all the fun and excitement of science."

The intrigue played against the usual backdrop of funding shortages. By the summer of 1984, of course, Francis's lab technicians were working with large quantities of the deadly LAV as well as large amounts of tissue from AIDS patients. His antiquated laboratories, however, did not have an autoclave to sterilize pans and instruments. Instead, technicians carried their contaminated trays and instruments down a hallway to another lab for cleaning. Doing this required the workers to precariously balance their materials in one hand while they turned the doorknob with their contaminated lab gloves. In the summer of 1984, Francis's problems with doorknobs came to summarize his despair over adequate resources.

Fearing a viral spill or the spread of the pure AIDS virus from the contaminated doorknobs, Don Francis asked the building engineers for swinging doors so his employees could back out of the lab. Such doors were too expensive; it would take months to get approval for them. Francis then asked for the doorknobs to be replaced with the European-style hooks that hospitals routinely use instead of knobs. Thus, the techs could open a door with an arm while keeping both hands on AIDS-infected materials.

Francis wrote out his request, but nothing happened. He wrote more memos and discussed his safety concerns at every staff meeting, but nothing happened. Altogether, Francis agitated for four months before he was able to negotiate two $2.75 hooks for his lab doors.

Francis figured the funding problems dominated nearly 90 percent of his time. For example, he had conducted a nationwide search for another virologist to ease his staff's load. Once employed, the scientist had to wait two months before he could get to work, because there wasn't enough lab space for him. Francis gave up his office so it could be converted into a lab, but conversion took three months because the CDC didn't have enough building engineers to do the construction.

Francis and his scientists were forced to do their paperwork on desks in hallways four floors above the sub-basement where their labs were located. The constant problems were taking a toll on his lab crew. Everybody worked until 2 A.M. every day. By that summer, one researcher in the virology lab was hospitalized with an ulcer; another developed severe hypertension.

As far as Don Francis was concerned, the reward for government work rested in impact. You didn't get a hefty salary, a fancy office, or elaborate perks as a government scientist, but you could make a difference. Francis had beaten every virus he had fought; that was impact. He had helped wiped out smallpox and the dreadful Ebola Fever virus. But he couldn't beat the system when it conspired to help the viral enemies of humankind. By the summer of 1984, Francis was beginning to feel thoroughly beaten down.

◯

Resource problems frustrated every aspect of AIDS research. Until the end of 1984, only two scientists had received grants to conduct research on retroviruses and AIDS—Drs. Bob Gallo at NCI and Max Essex at Harvard. Despite his achievements, Gallo was given no new personnel for the stepped-up AIDS work his lab was expected to perform. When Gallo frequently mentioned his problems to other scientists, they laughed. Nobody believed him.

Most striking, however, was the deficiency in funds for research into treatments for AIDS. The LAV/HTLV-III discoveries opened the way for testing of experimental anti-viral drugs. One CDC doctor wanted to test ribavirin, a drug that had had some success against flu viruses. To test the drug's efficacy, however, the doctor needed viral cultures on the blood of his subjects. Only with this capability could he determine whether the drug was reducing the level of virus in his test subjects' blood. Don Francis had to reject his request because the CDC lab could make only fifteen viral cultures a week, and this capacity was required for more pressing work.

At the National Cancer Institute, Dr. Sam Broder was in charge of treatment strategies, and he too found little interest in developing anti-AIDS drugs. After all, the "miracle drug" advances of the past decades had come in treatments for bacterial organisms, which are independent life forms. Viruses and retroviruses, however, are not independent life forms but are pieces of genetic material that actually become part of the infected cell. Killing the virus means killing the cell. Science had yet to develop any successful treatments for viral diseases. Vaccines could create antibodies to protect people from infection, but they were not cures. Given the lack of success in fighting viruses in the past, some scientists believed that no treatment for AIDS would ever be found. Broder argued bitterly for at least exploring possibilities. "If you declare the patient terminal and don't do anything to treat him, he'll always die," Broder said.

Meanwhile, Ed Brandt was aware of the discontent at all levels of the Public Health Service over AIDS funding, but he could do nothing. His May 25 request for expanded AIDS research continued to sit on Secretary Heckler's desk, unanswered.

SAN FRANCISCO

The shingles had started on the back of his neck and spread over the right side of his scalp to cover his forehead and right eye. Another outbreak had gone down his shoulder and over his chest. Just the movement of wind through his hair caused extraordinary pain. Cleve Jones was frantic by the time he got to the doctor's office.

"Do you know what this means?" the physician asked.

"What?"

"All the young men who I've seen get this are developing AIDS."

Cleve dragged himself to the nearest gay bar for a drink. A few days before, he had been on the assembly floor in Sacramento when he heard a familiar name being read as the day's session was adjourned. It was Frank, the lawyer from

Long Beach with whom Cleve had had his brief affair in 1982. The assembly was being adjourned in Frank's honor that day because he had just died of AIDS. Another boyfriend had died a few weeks before. Cleve's romantic interest from the summer of 1980, civil rights lawyer Felix Velarde-Munoz, had suffered a bout of *Pneumocystis.*

Together, Felix, Frank, and Cleve had helped chart a new world for gay people, and now one was dead and another was doomed. Cleve wondered when this nightmare would consume him too. He gulped another vodka tonic; he knew he would have to get drunk this afternoon. He felt adrift. There was no way out.

Cleve's own aimlessness reflected the gay community's confusion over the epidemic. The bathhouse controversy had defied resolution, turning into an only-in-San Francisco political controversy full of unexpected twists. In early June, it was revealed that Mayor Feinstein had dispatched police investigators into the bathhouses to don towels and write a report on the activities within. She had commissioned the research in March, in the wake of the Littlejohn initiative, presumably to get data that would strengthen her hand with the wavering public health director. The disclosure of the investigation three months later, however, angered the mayor's friends and foes alike, because it conjured memories of the days when police officers raided bars and bathhouses to enforce their Irish Catholic morality.

Feinstein countered her critics by forthrightly demanding that Silverman "have the guts" to shut the bathhouses before the imminent Gay Freedom Day Parade. "You go to the AIDS Ward and you see young people dying and you feel a strain," she said. "Dr. Silverman should take his medical information, make a decision and go with it—not count hands to see what is popular."

The proposed ordinance to transfer bathhouse licensing authority from the police to the health department continued to be stalled in the board of supervisors. After hearing testimony from such noted public health experts as the Bay Area Lawyers for Individual Freedom and the American Association for Personal Privacy, a supervisors' committee decided that they would postpone making any decision. The supervisor proposing the seven-week delay was Supervisor Richard Hongisto, who had said in March the baths should be closed because he was spending too much time at funerals of gay friends. Hongisto was thinking of running for mayor in 1987.

Even while gay political leaders were making bathhouses their top issue, support for the facilities steadily dropped within the community itself. With patronage plummeting, member clubs of the Northern California Bathhouse Owners Association joined to take out full-page ads in gay newspapers offering half-price coupons that carried a full reprint of the group's "Resolution Regarding an Objective Response to AIDS" on its reverse side. The business decline, however, proved lethal for many bathhouses and private sex clubs. The Hothouse, Cornholes, and Liberty Baths were gone. The cells at the Bulldog Baths were locked for the last time. The Cauldron announced "The Last J-O Party" and threw in the sling.

The most festive closing came at the Sutro Baths, the city's only "bisexual bathhouse," which catered to males and females of all sexual orientations. Over 500 went to its three-day Farewell Orgy in early June to nostalgically recall the Sutro's carefree early days. The festivities climaxed when five people who were losing their jobs because of the bath closure lined up on the stage and stood over a barbecue, burning AIDS brochures.

"If we can't pass them out, we might as well burn them," reasoned Sutro's owner. The logic was abstruse for most people, however, and the sight of the bathhouse employees publicly burning AIDS-prevention guidelines became one of the most enduring images of the AIDS-stricken gay community in San Francisco that summer.

◯

With the advent of summer, general interest in the epidemic fell precipitously. Between July and September 1984, the nation's major print news organizations published only 266 articles on AIDS, the lowest level of reportage on the epidemic since the first quarter of 1983. This amounted to about one-third the number of stories written by the same publications during the height of the media blitz in the summer of 1983.

What did increase was the number of people dead or dying. In the last week of June 1984, AIDS cases in the United States surpassed 5,000. The epidemic had spread to forty-six states, and nearly 2,300 had died.

47 REPUBLICANS AND DEMOCRATS

July 1984
RAYBURN HOUSE OFFICE BUILDING,
WASHINGTON, D.C.

In virtually every subsequent interview on the AIDS epidemic, Assistant Secretary for Health Ed Brandt denied leaking a photocopy of his May 25 memorandum to Secretary Heckler seeking $55 million in new AIDS funds. Even so, Brandt frequently joked that he was reading copies of his memorandum in the *San Francisco Chronicle* before his secretary got them out of her typewriter. Tim Westmoreland, counsel to the House Subcommittee on Health and the Environment, suspected Brandt; but when a copy of the memo arrived in a plain brown envelope in his office mail, Westmoreland was less concerned about the identity of his mystery correspondent than jubilant over the memo's appearance. At last, Westmoreland had his smoking gun.

Certainly, the surfacing of Dr. Brandt's twenty-two-page memo proved the watershed event in the AIDS budget battle of 1984. Its delivery could not have come at a more fortuitous moment. Congress was about to begin deliberations on the next fiscal year's budget, and the administration still maintained that AIDS funding was entirely adequate.

Even after the HTLV-III announcement, Reagan officials had not requested any additional AIDS funds for the next year's budget. The official administration request for the fiscal year due to start on October 1 stood at $51 million, a mere 6 percent increase over the previous year's AIDS spending. Although mounting AIDS caseloads indicated the need for drastically increased funding, liberals had no persuasive documentation. Brandt's memo lifted the camouflage off administration claims that doctors had all the resources they needed. Here was the Reagan-appointed health secretary himself making the case for more money.

Within days, Westmoreland had distributed additional copies of the memo to sympathetic legislators on Capitol Hill. Various members of Congress privately relayed their dismay to Secretary Heckler and hoped that the administration would boost its AIDS request. Their entreaties, however, found no response. Westmoreland leaked a copy of the story to the *Washington Blade,* a gay paper distinguished by its investigatory articles on AIDS funding. He hoped some major East Coast paper would pick it up and run with it. The *Blade* ran the story on page one, but the eastern newspapers weren't printing stories on AIDS, so it was ignored.

July 13
UNION SQUARE, SAN FRANCISCO

Six men, dressed as nuns, gathered ritualistically around a table where a woman was being held down.

"We are here to exorcise lies and prejudice," shouted Sister Boom Boom to the crowd of 2,000.

The pinioned woman was playing the part of Phyllis Schlafly, the anti-feminist leader who had spearheaded opposition to the Equal Rights Amendment. Schlafly was appearing a few blocks away at an anti-gay "Family Forum" hosted by the leader of the Moral Majority, Rev. Jerry Falwell.

"Phyllis Schlafly's heart is corrupted with fear and greed," shouted Boom Boom. "We shall remove her heart of lies and fear, and replace it with a heart of purity and love."

From the folds of the woman's dress, Boom Boom pulled a rubber snake and tossed it in the air.

Moments later, a man walked out dressed as Falwell, and the assembled Sisters of Perpetual Indulgence ripped off his pants, exposing fishnet stockings and a black corset.

"Cast off the demons of shame and repentance," Boom Boom intoned.

The Democratic National Convention had arrived in San Francisco.

More than 2,000 reporters had gathered for the meeting, due to start in a few days, and they were being treated to much local color in an unusual array of demonstrations and political protests. Delegates from the Second International Hookers' Convention marched for Prostitutes Rights; advocates of marijuana legalization held a "smoke-in." At the site of the Family Forum, earnest members of the Revolutionary Communist Party and the Spartacist League were fighting with police officers. At City Hall, an environmentalist named Ponderosa Pine, who frequently dressed up as a tree, was leading an "All Species Rally" of fellow ecologists who had donned plant, bird, and fish costumes to call attention to the "fate of other species."

Unable to resist, Jerry Falwell also came to the city and took out newspaper advertisements, asking Democrats to "return to moral sanity" and not provide homosexuals with "special recognition and privileges under the law." The fact that both the Catholic archdiocese and the San Francisco Council of Churches had officially asked Falwell to avoid San Francisco did not deter him and thus came the predictable protests from gay men dressed up as nuns.

Republican leaders were privately ecstatic that Democrats had chosen the gay mecca as their convention site. This allowed the Sisters of Perpetual Indulgence to stroll into America's living rooms on the evening news as an unofficial welcoming committee for the loyal opposition. Fundamentalist ministers across the nation asserted that the Democrats had become the party of the "three A's"—acid, abortion, and AIDS. Mainstream Republicans were more circumspect, although campaign rhetoric routinely included references to the "San Francisco Democratic Party."

The fear of just such a label had created some reluctance among Democratic leaders to include overt references to gay rights and AIDS in the party platform, setting the stage for Bill Kraus's last political battle. Once again, Kraus served as a member of the party's platform committee. The committee chair, Representative Geraldine Ferraro, was eager for the platform to contain only generic language opposing discrimination against all minorities. With sixty-five lesbian and gay delegates from a score of states, Kraus threatened a floor fight over gay rights. You don't beat the redneck Republicans by becoming one of them, he maintained. Privately, he also alluded to the fact that he wouldn't predict what those unruly street radicals might do if the platform didn't include explicit support for gay rights. In the end, Kraus finagled the most sweeping endorsement that any major party had adopted for gays, including a pledge to end the exclusion of gays from the military and as immigrants. The platform put the party on record as promising to end violence against gays and to bolster spending to "learn the cause and cure of AIDS."

The priority that Bill Kraus and San Francisco gay leaders put on AIDS irked gay activists from other parts of the country. As they gathered in San Francisco for the convention, they gossiped that California leaders were obsessed with the disease. The National Gay Task Force had not even wanted to address AIDS as a separate issue, arguing that it should be included as a subcategory in an overall statement about "health concerns." For their part, gay Republican groups heartily endorsed President Reagan's reelection, determined to show that they were not "single-issue" political activists. Meanwhile, the American Association of Physicians for Human Rights largely avoided any stand on the federal role in the AIDS epidemic, channeling its energies into such issues as criticizing medical journals for using such "judgmental" terms as "promiscuous" in articles about AIDS risk factors.

Two days before the convention opened, bathhouse owners quickly let their priorities be known in a meeting of the National Coalition of Gay and Lesbian Democratic Clubs. For the preceding two years, Gwenn Craig, former Milk Club president, had served as co-chair of the group. However, bathhouse owners controlled gay Democratic clubs in Miami and Chicago. Even before arriving in San Francisco, they were campaigning against Craig, frequently referring to her support for bathhouse closure. As a first order of business at the coalition's San Francisco meeting, Craig was ousted from her post, although she continued to serve as chair of the convention's gay caucus.

◯

The next day, 100,000 lesbians and gay men gathered on Castro Street to march to the convention site. Their numbers filled the neighborhood. Demonstration leaders were busily reassuring the press that the march was not a protest but a show of support for Democrats, and, as he had on the sunny June day four years before, Bill Kraus walked at the front of the throng with other delegates and party officials. As the group strode toward downtown, Kraus thought back to the Gay Freedom Day Parade on that sunny afternoon in 1980.

How different the goals and the future of the gay movement seemed now, Kraus thought, and the nagging question returned to him: How many of these people will be alive for the next presidential election?

July 25
NEW YORK CITY HEALTH DEPARTMENT

The city-sponsored conference on the implications of the HTLV-III antibody test marked a novel development for AIDS policy in the United States. For the first time, officials were planning for a problem before it happened. The unprecedented foray into intelligent AIDS policy planning was indeed timely. No issue would prove as complicated and potentially volatile as AIDS testing, and the battle lines drawn at the New York City conference would mark debates that accompanied use of the AIDS test for years to come.

Within days of the Heckler HTLV-III press conference in April, scientists and AIDS organizers knew that the advent of the blood test would create a public policy problem. Federal health officials saw the test as a rare opportunity to define the extent to which the AIDS virus had penetrated the United States. At last, they would be able to see the part of the iceberg of AIDS infection that lay below the visible tip of full-blown, CDC-defined AIDS cases. Traditionally, efforts to control any disease began with authorities determining who was infected and who wasn't, and then keeping the infected people from giving it to the uninfected. Obviously, the antibody test, once licensed for widespread use, would be an essential tool in making such a determination.

Don Francis, for one, was itching to implement widespread voluntary testing for gay men. Jim Curran also viewed testing as essential to any long-term strategy in fighting AIDS. That's what Curran told the 200 health officials and AIDS workers who had assembled for the New York conference.

Paul Popham, president of Gay Men's Health Crisis, moved uncomfortably in his chair when he heard the enthusiastic support for antibody testing. The antibody assay, he knew, could be used in effect as a blood test for sexual orientation. He thought about the new estimates that the typical AIDS patient needed $100,000 in medical care, and wondered what insurers might do once they got this test. "If the insurance industry can find relief from these enormous expenditures, it will," Popham said, voicing concern that no gay man would be able to get an insurance policy once the test became available.

Other gay leaders cited concerns with employment and confidentiality. If test results were easily accessible, people with antibodies could be subject to a wide array of discriminatory moves. Already, the *New York Native* had written a story predicting that people with positive antibody tests might at some point be ordered to report to quarantine camps.

Either the Food and Drug Administration or the National Institutes of Health could have allayed such fears had they simply announced that test results were subject to federal confidentiality guidelines, such as those used routinely in other federal health projects that involve such sensitive personal matters as alcoholism and drug abuse. The mechanism for granting confidentiality was already in place; it could be enacted with the stroke of a pen.

Federal health officials were reluctant to take this act, fearing it would be viewed as coddling homosexuals at a time when the election-minded administration was taking a more forthright anti-gay stance. For public consumption at the New York meeting, however, the agencies maintained that such a federal move would be "too restrictive," and that gays should lobby each institution administering the test to issue such assurances. The suggestion brought loud guffaws from the audience.

"Why burden the community with that?" asked Rodger McFarlane, GMHC executive director. "The feds should require uniform statements of confidentiality." Without such guidelines, McFarlane added, he would suggest that gay men not participate in AIDS research involving the antibody test.

Cooperation remained the trump card that gay community leaders held in negotiations with the federal government. For the past three years, the gay community had provided some of the most helpful study subjects in the history of medical science. Virtually everything the federal researchers understood about AIDS epidemiology stemmed from this unprecedented cooperation. The gay community's good faith, however, was running short, given the lack of reciprocation on the part of the federal health establishment.

Already there was difficulty enlisting volunteers for a NIAID study of San Francisco gay men by University of California researchers because it involved antibody testing. The threat of noncooperation was the only leverage gays had in the debate. Federal officials were sufficiently uneasy at the end of the New York City meeting that they pledged to listen to more "community input" on the issue before making any final policy determination.

━━━━━━

Although the meeting was short on definitive policy recommendations, it left Paul Popham troubled. The growing rift between AIDS groups and the federal government troubled the Republican streak in Popham's personality. At one point, he would have considered rhetoric about quarantine camps to be so much paranoia from fringe radicals, but his old-fashioned trust in the government had been profoundly shaken by the AIDS epidemic.

By now, it was clear to him that the government would do as little as possible to research AIDS as long as only homosexuals were dying. This thought bothered him. Before AIDS, Paul had never believed that gays really were all that oppressed; now he was worrying about wholesale employment discrimination and quarantine camps. Paul had spent a lifetime believing in his nation, and he had fought in Vietnam to protect it. One of his greatest disappointments in the AIDS epidemic was that he felt robbed of his faith in the United States.

Paul had another reason for concern with the antibody test. In 1982, he had enrolled in one of the first prospective studies of gay men. Blood drawn for the past three years had been ferreted away in the freezers of St. Luke's–Roosevelt Hospital in Manhattan. A few weeks before, Dr. Michael Lange had sat down with Paul to tell him that he had been infected with this new virus since the study began, probably longer. In fact, 50 percent of the sixty men participating in the study were antibody positive, and they were now the first gay men in the United States to be given the disquieting news that they were carrying the AIDS virus.

The news didn't surprise Paul. After all, his old boyfriend, Jack Nau, was one of the first dozen AIDS cases diagnosed in New York City. It also explained why his lymph nodes had been swollen for so long.

The confidentiality issue dominated AIDS concerns in the summer of 1984. The particulars often demonstrated the complexity of the question, even as it defined the shape of things to come in the AIDS epidemic.

In late July, Jim Curran caused an uproar when he sent a memo to all state and territorial epidemiologists asking whether authorities should start keeping a registry of everyone whose blood donations proved to be infected with HTLV-III once the blood test was available. Already, authorities throughout the nation kept a similar registry of people infected with hepatitis B and syphilis. Adding HTLV-III to the list would help avoid situations like that of the California man who had donated blood to eleven different centers even though he suffered from immune problems stemming from his AIDS infection. Gays worried that such a list would amount to little more than a registry of homosexual men and pointed out that the list could be put to nefarious use in the twenty-five states where gay sexual acts remained illegal.

In San Francisco, where health officials anxiously kept track of gay concerns, confidentiality-obsessed health department staffers saw a unique opportunity to advance their privacy agenda with the departure of Selma Dritz. Like a good soldier, Dritz had left the department her plump notebooks jammed with observations on the first years of the AIDS epidemic. The information was amassed on health department time, Dritz figured, so it belonged to the department. And in the summer of 1984, the San Francisco Department of Public Health took the politically correct action of feeding the notebooks into a paper shredder.

The same day that the antibody test conference convened in New York City, the *San Francisco Chronicle* published the contents of the May 25 Brandt memo that had asked $50 million more for the war on AIDS. When questioned, a spokesman for the Office of Management and Budget said the budget agency had never heard of the request. Brandt's plea, it turned out, had never moved off Secretary Heckler's desk in two months.

The next day, Representative Ed Roybal of Los Angeles walked into an executive session of the subcommittee in charge of appropriations to the U.S. Department of Health and Human Services and threw the Brandt memo on the table. The committee immediately approved $8.3 million in additional AIDS research money to be spent in the remaining two months of fiscal year 1984. Senator Alan Cranston put together a Senate bill seeking the full amount of Brandt's request. And the wide circulation of Brandt's memo on Capitol Hill ensured that Republicans would not toe the administration line that government doctors had all the funds they needed to fight AIDS.

On August 8, Secretary Heckler responded to Dr. Brandt's memo and rebuffed his request for new funds for AIDS research. Instead, she gave him authorization to redirect the funds from other projects within the NIH and CDC.

Between the time that Brandt wrote his memo and the date that Heckler answered it, 600 Americans died of Acquired Immune Deficiency Syndrome and another 1,200 were diagnosed with the disease.

It was during these difficult weeks that Brandt decided he would retire from government service at the end of the year. He had been offered the post of chancellor at the University of Maryland in Baltimore, a respected medical school. Gay leaders, sympathetic to Brandt's position as a sincere public servant, spread the word that the doctor was quitting in frustration over his inability to secure a commitment to AIDS research from the administration. But Brandt later said that the problems with AIDS funding had the opposite effect. "I couldn't help but worry about what would happen if I weren't there to fight for the money," he said.

August 1984 was a month of death in San Francisco, as the mounting number of AIDS casualties included increasingly well-known people. Jon Sims, the former Kansas music teacher who organized the San Francisco Gay Freedom Day Marching Band, died of brain infections, having spent the last weeks of his life blind and suffering from dementia. The city's most prominent AIDS sufferer, Bobbi Campbell, died on August 15 of cryptosporidiosis. He was the "AIDS Poster Boy" who went public with his plight in 1981 and ended up on the cover of *Newsweek* two years later. By an eerie coincidence, in the last months of his life, Bobbi Campbell had made his home on 1040 Ashbury Street, in the same apartment that was left vacant nearly three years before by the death of the city's first diagnosed AIDS patient, Ken Horne.

Several weeks earlier, philosopher Michel Foucault also died from AIDS in Paris. To the end, however, Foucault hid his diagnosis from everyone, including his devoted lover. Even though the *New York Native* chastised *The New York Times* for not listing AIDS as a cause of death in its obituaries, the *Native* itself reported that Foucault died of an "infection that attacked his central nervous system."

The reluctance of prominent people to publicly acknowledge their AIDS diagnoses left obituary columns strangely empty of actual flesh-and-blood people who were dying of the syndrome. Only the most knowledgeable of obituary readers could detect the presence of this epidemic in the death notices. A thirty-eight-year-old fashion designer dying of "cancer and pneumonia," for example, was a sure giveaway, as was the man in his thirties who left no surviving widow after succumbing to a "lingering" or "lengthy" illness. How lingering can an illness be for somebody who is only thirty-two years old? Sometimes newspapers concealed AIDS as the cause of death because the news writers found it embarrassing; more frequently, because the family did. In fact, the lack of people dying of AIDS in obituary columns led gay journalist Larry Bush to wonder aloud: "What if they gave an epidemic and nobody died?"

August 18
DALLAS, TEXAS

Larry Bush was wading through a crowd of gay Republicans who had sponsored a party for the eve of the Republican National Convention when he recognized Terry Dolan across the room. Dolan was the New Right fund-raising genius whose National Conservative Political Action Committee had raised over $10 million for Ronald Reagan's reelection campaign.

Publicly, Dolan distanced himself from the gay rights movement. Privately, Bush knew, Dolan took advantage of the more comfortable gay life-style that the movement had created. Dolan regularly appeared in Washington gay bars, and he vacationed at the gay Russian River resort area north of San Francisco. Bush couldn't resist goading Dolan about the Reagan administration's miserable response to the AIDS epidemic.

"We've been able to stop a lot of negative things," Dolan answered. "It's a real horror show, some of the things that have been suggested."

"Are we talking quarantine?" Bush asked, alluding to the rumors that the administration might seek to intern everyone harboring AIDS antibodies.

Dolan got nervous.

"I'm not at liberty to discuss any of the details," he said.

"Are we talking tattoos?"

"I can't talk about it," Dolan said and then excused himself.

A few minutes later, Bush encountered the son of a prominent anti-feminist leader, a woman who had earned a national reputation for spearheading opposition to the Equal Rights Amendment. One of the recent additions to the woman's anti-ERA arguments was that equal rights for women would promote homosexual rights and therefore cause the spread of AIDS. Bush asked the anti-feminist leader's son if his mother knew where he was at that moment.

"No."

"Does she know you're gay?" Bush asked.

"I'd never do anything to embarrass Mother," he said.

"What about your mother's publication linking the ERA to AIDS?" Bush asked. "That embarrasses us, doesn't it?"

"Mother feels very strongly about the ERA," he answered, uncomfortably.

"How do you feel about AIDS? About people dying of a disease while your mother makes political capital off it?" Bush asked.

The young man abruptly excused himself and left the party.

AIDS was a topic of much discussion at the Republican Convention, although all of it was off the convention floor. At a party barbecue held at the estate of a millionaire Republican businessman, a fundamentalist minister delivered an invocation that included a reference to the fact that God was using AIDS to mete punishment to the immoral. At a breakfast for Republican business executives a day later, the president of American Airlines opened his talk by telling guests that the word "gay" stood for "got AIDS yet?" To highlight the link between the party of Lincoln and growing fundamentalist political clout, Republican leaders recruited Jerry Falwell to deliver the benediction for the session in which President Reagan was renominated.

For all the behind-the-scenes talk, however, AIDS remained a largely unspoken subtext in the election. When the issue was considered at all, it was generally in the context of what each political party thought was wrong with the other. For the Democrats, AIDS was another example of the woes that would be cast upon the world by aggressive reductions in domestic spending. For Republicans, the epidemic was a just desert, the result of permissiveness bred by the secular humanism of liberals, being visited on people they largely did not care for. Thus an epidemic that had wholly unfolded within a Republican administration had a distinctly Democratic cast for Republicans; for Democrats, AIDS was a Republican epidemic.

Of course, nobody spoke the A-word aloud from the podium of either convention. The entire subject continued to be embarrassing for most people in the mainstream of society; this uneasiness was something that Republicans and Democrats shared.

STANFORD UNIVERSITY

For AIDS clinicians, the most frustrating aspect of their work was the absence of any effective treatment. When Michael Gottlieb from UCLA read about the Pasteur Institute's work with an anti-viral drug called HPA-23, he was jubilant. Hearing that Pasteur's Jean-Claude Chermann was lecturing at Stanford, Gottlieb eagerly made his way to the university.

Chermann showed Gottlieb a photocopy of HPA-23 research results under consideration for publication in a medical journal. According to the Pasteur research, HPA-23 successfully inhibited the reproduction of LAV in patients. The centerpiece of the French research was an AIDS-stricken hemophiliac whose health had rebounded dramatically after taking HPA-23.

"You mustn't show this to anybody," Chermann said, worried the data would never be published if it were released in the mainstream press.

Gottlieb persuaded Chermann to at least let him be the first American to get HPA-23 for use in the United States. Of course, Gottlieb added, HPA-23 would have to meet the FDA standards.

Chermann said he had never heard of the FDA. He figured he could send some boxes of the drug to the United States and it would immediately start being injected into AIDS victims. Gottlieb's heart sank when he realized the legal barriers that would block testing of this promising drug, but he remained enthusiastic about Chermann's assessment of what was necessary for successful AIDS treatment.

Because the AIDS agent was a retrovirus, Chermann reasoned, it needed to perform an extra chemical feat before reproducing in a cell, releasing the chemical reverse transcriptase that enabled its RNA base to pick up the cell's DNA for replication. HPA-23 interfered with reverse transcriptase, Chermann said, blocking the virus from replicating itself. In this sense, HPA-23 was not a cure. It merely kept the virus from running wild and destroying the immune system.

The logic made sense to Gottlieb, who started pitching American pharmaceutical companies to develop reverse transcriptase inhibitors. Like Sam Broder at the NCI, however, Gottlieb found that most drug companies were not eager to get involved in AIDS work. The potential market seemed small. A drug for a few thousand AIDS cases would never offer the opportunity for profits that a successful potion to help the hundreds of thousands who suffered, say, from hypertension would. Moreover, the chances of success appeared remote.

Drug companies wouldn't invest funds to create new drugs, but Gottlieb found they were game to use on AIDS patients whatever treatments they already had on the shelves. Gottlieb returned to UCLA and started a search of medical literature for retroviral drugs that already had gained FDA approval. He was willing to try anything that offered a reasonable chance of success. Already, a trickle of southern California AIDS patients were trekking to Mexico, where a number of drugs not available in the United States could be easily purchased at the corner *farmacia*.

News about the promising French drug HPA-23 was also spreading on the gay medical grapevine. One of the people who heard the optimistic rumors was Rock Hudson. Gottlieb had been seeing the film star since Hudson was first diagnosed in June. The actor was showing signs of weight loss when he ambled into Gottlieb's office in late August. A friend in San Francisco, Steve Del Re, had told Hudson about HPA-23. He was planning to go to the film festival in Deauville anyway; he wondered whether Gottlieb knew anybody involved with the Pasteur Institute.

Gottlieb called Chermann, who referred him to Dr. Dominique Dormant, an army doctor who had been experimenting with HPA-23 for a number of years. When Hudson arrived in Paris in September, Dormant called Gottlieb to talk over some details concerning the actor's condition. It turned out that Dormant had no idea who Hudson was until the actor stepped into his office. The Frenchman then recognized the actor from his films.

At that time, the Pasteur had two regimens for treating AIDS patients, one in which the patient was given large doses of HPA-23 for several weeks and another in which the patient was given lower doses of the drug daily for a more extended period. Hudson was committed to return to the United States to appear in the television series "Dynasty," so he opted for the short-term regimen. At the conclusion of his treatments, Dormant told Gottlieb that the AIDS virus was no longer detectable in Hudson's blood.

Later, it would be clear that the short treatments were flawed. Although HPA-23 might halt the replication of the virus, as soon as the patient was off the drug, viral reproduction began anew, ravaging the patient's immune system. This would not be clear for several months, however, so Hudson left Paris convinced he was cured of AIDS.

Back in the United States, Hudson, a life-long Republican, attended a state dinner at the White House. Noting that the actor had lost weight, an old friend from Hollywood expressed concern about his health.

"I caught some flu bug when I was filming in Israel," Hudson assured his friend, Nancy Reagan. "I'm feeling fine now."

48 EMBARRASSED

September 1984
DUBLIN STREET, SAN FRANCISCO

More than a year after her hip replacement surgery, Frances Borchelt still had not recovered her health. The painful psoriasis persisted; she never regained the twenty pounds lost during her bout with hepatitis. In August, a case of the sniffles turned into a severe cold that would not go away. Frances either trembled from chills or sweated profusely from fevers that peaked daily at 103 degrees. As usual, the doctors were baffled.

Sometimes Frances asked her husband Bob to hold her. Even as he became drenched in her sweat, Bob stared down on his suffering wife, feeling pity and compassion and sorrow, wishing desperately that he could do something to ease her agony.

The nightsweats started about the same time Frances complained that she was having a hard time catching her breath. Her appetite declined. Bob and the couple's daughter, Cathy, forced her to eat.

Cathy's suspicions continued to grow. Maybe it was the story in the paper about the wealthy Belvedere matron, Mary Richards Johnstone, who had recently died from a blood transfusion supplied by the Irwin Memorial Blood Bank. Cathy insisted that Bob ask the family doctor whether any of Frances's problems resembled what might happen to somebody who got AIDS.

The doctor assured Bob there were no indications of the syndrome, but Cathy was less convinced. Her boss's wife was a registered nurse who had recently attended an AIDS seminar. She gave Cathy some brochures about AIDS and Cathy was immediately struck by how closely her mother's symptoms resembled those listed in the brochure.

Nobody debated whether blood transfusions could spread AIDS anymore. By early September, the Centers for Disease Control counted 80 cases of transfusion AIDS, a quadrupling of confirmed cases in just eight months. A report released several weeks later announced that 52 hemophiliacs in twenty-two states suffered from CDC-defined AIDS, while another 188 had contracted

ARC. The first cases of AIDS in both the wife and infant child of a hemophiliac had just been reported. Even more frightening were new studies indicating that as many as 89 percent of the most severe hemophiliacs were infected with HTLV-III, predicting thousands of potential AIDS cases in future years. The National Hemophilia Foundation reported a 20 to 30 percent drop in the use of Factor VIII among members, indicating that some hemophiliacs would rather hazard the potentially fatal consequences of uncontrolled bleeding than inject Factor VIII and risk AIDS.

Dr. Joseph Bove, who had led opposition to blood screening for surrogate AIDS markers, was so shaken by the unfolding statistics that he shifted views and was arguing for FDA regulations to require hepatitis B core antibody screening. When the FDA advisory panel on blood products considered the issue again during the summer, however, other blood industry spokespeople prevailed and Bove's arguments were rejected.

Irwin Memorial Blood Bank and other Bay Area blood banks had been testing for the hepatitis antibody since May; Irwin was also storing vials of blood taken from every donated unit so they could test donations once the HTLV-III antibody test was available. For taking these precautions, Irwin continued to be chided by other blood bankers. Los Angeles Red Cross spokeswoman Gerri Sohle said in late August that "political pressure" had forced Bay Area blood banks to start the CDC-suggested testing. "I think they've been politically pressured into doing the tests, probably by people worried about the gay community," she said. The executive director of the Council of Community Blood Centers argued that such testing would create "unnecessary anxiety" among donors whose blood might be rejected.

Thus, efforts to protect the nation's blood supply continued to be frustrated for the rest of 1984 by the factors that always seemed to interfere with intelligent AIDS policy—denial and delay, sophistry and self-interest.

NATIONAL CANCER INSTITUTE, <u>BETHESDA</u>

A summer of investigation of HTLV-III by Dr. Robert Gallo had not produced reassuring information. When he began studying HTLV-III, he figured that perhaps 1 in 100 people infected with the virus would develop AIDS. A few months later, he adjusted his estimate to 1 in 25. By the end of the summer, he confided that he thought 1 in 7 people infected with the virus would develop AIDS, and maybe more.

"It's unfortunately as efficient a virus as I've ever seen," Gallo told the *New York Native*.

An even more sobering discovery followed when Gallo began picking up clues that HTLV-III infected brain cells as well as T-4 lymphocytes. The insight solved a key puzzle that had baffled clinicians throughout the epidemic. AIDS patients frequently suffered neurological problems that could not be linked to any particular brain infection. Often, the early symptoms were mild, marked by depression, loss of memory, or a mental disorder that resembled senility. Doctors initially blamed psychological factors such as stress. As problems with the central nervous system became more pronounced and increasingly common, however, this diagnosis began to ring hollow. Some patients were dying from their brain dysfunctions. The observation that the problems might stem from an HTLV-III infection of the brain solved the puzzle but added serious obstacles to the search for a cure.

To infect the brain, the retrovirus had to cross the blood-brain barrier, a metabolic filter that normally keeps microbes away from the body's most crucial organ. Any medication that sought to successfully treat AIDS, therefore, also had to cross this blood-brain barrier. Otherwise, the virus could lurk in brain cells and reinfect the blood. Few medications, however, could do this, setting up still another hurdle that a treatment must leap in order to be effective.

Gallo's genetic sequencing of HTLV-III also revealed variations in the virus as it appeared in different people. Such mutations raised fears that science might not be able to make a vaccine, since a vaccine that worked for one strain of HTLV-III might not work for another.

At the National Institute for Allergy and Infectious Diseases, the news was another piece of gray sky on an already bleak horizon. As it was, the vaccine development field had suffered in recent years for lack of interest. In the 110 years since Pasteur accomplished the first vaccination, science had created only eleven vaccines. In 1980, Dr. Richard Krause, the NIAID director, had proposed a program to develop ten new vaccines over the next ten years, but few pharmaceutical companies were eager to participate. The hepatitis vaccine, for example, had cost tens of millions to produce, but the anticipated market for the product had never materialized. Between hepatitis B and the swine flu fiasco, many pharmaceutical companies had become convinced that vaccine development promised not profits but large research expenses and huge liability lawsuits. Meanwhile, funds to entice scientists into AIDS vaccine development were on the list of Dr. Brandt's AIDS projects ignored by Secretary Heckler.

Despite the hindrances, the HTLV-III/LAV discoveries continued to propel a quantum leap in the understanding of the AIDS epidemic, nailing down aspects of the disease that had lived only in the realm of the hypothetical for the past three years.

By August, Manvel and Chesley, the two chimpanzees that Don Francis had infected with LAV five months earlier, developed swollen lymph nodes and LAV antibodies in their blood. This proof of AIDS infection strengthened the case that LAV caused AIDS and at last provided scientists with an animal model for the disease. Finding an animal susceptible to the disease was a crucial step for vaccine development; a vaccine's effectiveness could be tested on laboratory animals.

Now that scientists knew what they were looking for, researchers were able to study various body fluids and confirm the presence of the AIDS agent. HTLV-III was recovered in the semen of both an AIDS-stricken man and a healthy gay man with HTLV-III antibodies, proving definitively that healthy carriers could spread AIDS. Virus also was recovered in vaginal fluids of an infected woman, explaining the bidirectional heterosexual transmission that clearly was spreading the disease in Africa. The retrieval of virus from the saliva of eight ARC patients was more problematical. Not one of the nation's nearly 6,000 AIDS cases had contracted the disease from saliva. Given the low levels of virus in saliva, Dr. Jay Levy frequently argued that the only way you could get AIDS from spit was to inject a gallon of saliva intravenously. Still, sensing the potential for hysteria, Dr. Edward Brandt held a press conference as soon as the saliva studies were released to assure the public they would not get AIDS from a sneezing homosexual.

By early October, NCI scientists also found a drug they hoped might prove effective in fighting AIDS. Suranim had been used for sixty years to treat African sleeping sickness. In test tubes, the drug interfered with the reverse transcriptase enzyme, disabling HTLV-III's reproduction mechanism. Dr. Paul Volberding made plans to test the drug at San Francisco General Hospital's AIDS Clinic in the early months of 1985.

Antibody testing continued to offer reassurances that the AIDS epidemic hadn't broken out of the afflicted communities to threaten the entire society. The virus simply was not spreading outside the previously defined routes of transmission. NCI tests on the families of hemophiliacs found that no family members were infected with HTLV-III, despite daily contact with HTLV-afflicted hemophiliacs. In labs throughout the country, doctors and technicians who had been working with AIDS for years eagerly tested themselves. Between needle sticks and constant exposure to infected blood, most considered it likely that they harbored HTLV-III in their blood. In test after test, however, their fears proved unfounded. A substantial dose of the virus fed directly into the bloodstream, either through sex or transfusion, was required to get AIDS.

The fact that science was making swift strides in understanding AIDS did not mean that the disease had acquired a new respectability in medical circles. The syndrome still lacked star quality, and most scientists who labored on it did so without much institutional support. Assistant professors who were among the international experts in AIDS research were denied promotions, while associate professorships went to doctors studying more conventional diseases. At the University of California in San Francisco, administrators mentioned to one of the nation's foremost researchers that they wanted less publicity about AIDS. UC officials worried that top interns were choosing to go to other medical centers because the UCSF teaching hospital was San Francisco General, the nation's premier AIDS facility. The best medical school graduates, they feared, would not want to perform internships at a hospital if all they would see was one kind of patient.

Researchers, however, thought the reluctance to embrace AIDS as a legitimate topic for scientific study reflected more than just concern over the quality of interns a university might attract. Put simply, AIDS continued to embarrass people. From the start, it had made people uncomfortable, whether they were in government or media, in public health or prominent universities. AIDS was about homosexuals and anal intercourse, and all kinds of things that were just plain embarrassing. And when UCSF opened its own AIDS clinic in the summer, it did not call it a clinic for Acquired Immune Deficiency Syndrome, but a center for Adult Immune Deficiency.

SAN FRANCISCO

Men carried surgical tubing down the hall of Animals, a popular gay bathhouse, as casually as business executives carried briefcases in the financial district. Once upstairs, one man wrapped the tubing around another patron's biceps, pausing until the vein bulged. A long sigh signaled that the needle had accurately delivered the methadrine to the patron's central nervous system. When the man with the needle noticed somebody watching him, he cheerfully offered the observer a hit of crystal. Across the hall, another man's arm disappeared between the legs of his partner, and throughout the bathhouse, scores of men participated in sexual acts that did not fall under the heading of "safe" in the risk-reduction guidelines passed out by the Bay Area Physicians for Human Rights.

By late September, patrons at the city's remaining bathhouses and private sex clubs included private detectives who had been hired by the San Francisco Department of Public Health to document whether the facilities encouraged sexual activity that spread AIDS. The report was to be used when Merv Silverman went to court in a few weeks to close down the bathhouses.

Silverman had hoped the issue would not come to such a confrontation, but he had no doubt as to what course of action he would take when he read the investigators' reports.

Even Silverman, who was not naive about what went on in gay bathhouses, was shocked by what investigators found. The X-rated, eighty-five-page report certainly documented the fact that condoms and safe-sex brochures were available in almost every bathhouse. Most patrons, however, ignored them. Just about every type of unsafe sex imaginable, and many variations that were unimaginable, were being practiced with carefree abandonment at the facilities. That, after all, was what bathhouses were for.

Of even more concern was new data on gay sexual behavior generated by the first professionally designed random survey of San Francisco homosexuals. The study, undertaken by Research & Decisions, a prestigious marketing firm, found that 12 percent of local gay men had gone to a private sex club at some point during the month of August. During the same period, 1 in 10 gay men had gone to a bathhouse. The fact that so many gay men continued attending the facilities, despite the unprecedented publicity about their dangers, argued against the notion that baths would close for lack of business if gays were educated about AIDS.

Pressure mounted on Silverman not only from political quarters but from medical authorities alarmed at the steep increase of local AIDS cases. At one hospital, sixty doctors signed an open letter to Mayor Feinstein in the *Chronicle,* demanding closure and saying that "there is a strong need for aggressive public policy measures that do not capitulate to any political pressure." On September 14, Silverman met with Mayor Feinstein, hospital administrators, and Jim Curran from the CDC to privately announce that he would close the baths as soon as the private investigators' reports were complete.

○

During the third week of September 1984, America's AIDS caseload surpassed 6,000. Treatment costs for these first patients, the CDC estimated that week, would run at about $1 billion.

ATLANTA

The car swerved, jolting Don Francis awake. Francis regained control of his Volvo and continued home. The night before, he had arrived home at 6 P.M. and was in bed by 8:30 P.M., as usual, so he could slip into the CDC headquarters on Clifton Road by 5 A.M. to get a few hours of work done before the meetings began and the phone started ringing. When he had a paper to write, Francis went to work at 2 A.M., sometimes running into Jim Curran, who would only then be on his way out of the office. Francis had learned such rigorous schedules when he was fighting smallpox in India. It was you against the disease, his ethos went, and the disease might win if you let up for one day. In India, however, Francis had felt he had a chance to win.

By the time he was nodding asleep at the wheel of his car on the way home from a sixteen-hour day at the CDC, he no longer had that confidence in regard to AIDS. More than three years into the epidemic, the CDC still did not have the staff or resources to tackle the syndrome. Francis's proposals were still being killed by budget officials. Meanwhile, scientific politicking continued to taint the field. Bob Gallo had taken an increasingly strong role in AIDS science, exacerbating the divisions among researchers over the NCI-Pasteur feud.

On his rare evenings home, Francis wondered what he was doing with his life. His sons, four and six years old, barely knew their father: He had spent most of their lives waging his Sisyphean struggle against a strange acronym they did not comprehend. All the boys knew was that the neighbors did not want their kids to play with the children of a scientist involved in AIDS research; it might be catching.

Don Francis's wife, Karen, had given up her job with the Epidemiological Intelligence Service to move to Atlanta. She was a highly esteemed epidemiologist in her own right, having discovered the link between aspirin use and Reye's syndrome. Now she was without a job, without her familiar home, and for all practical purposes, without her husband.

Increasingly, Don Francis fell into conflicts with Jim Curran. Francis's orientation was toward control: Find the uninfected people and get them vaccinated. Curran's, however, was oriented in epidemiology, charting the course of diseases through a population. He did not have the background in control. He was also a realist. He favored control programs, but he knew that the money didn't exist for such projects even if he designed them. Other AIDS staffers were not surprised at the clashes between Francis and Curran, only that they had taken so long to surface. Curran was a take-charge administrator who kept firm control over his department. This put him in an awkward position with Francis. On the one hand, Curran was respectful of Francis's international reputation; on the other, he wasn't about to surrender control of the AIDS Activities Office. Increasingly, Francis was on the losing end of policy decisions at CDC.

On September 21, Don Francis met with Walt Dowdle, Director of the Center for Infectious Diseases, and outlined his frustration at the lack of a crash vaccine development project and infection control programs. He wanted out. Dowdle warned Francis against a hasty move and suggested he chart where he'd like his career to move in future years. Francis agreed, although he had resolved by then that whatever his future included, it would not mean working in Atlanta. He had never known defeat before, and he would not stay at the CDC headquarters and endure its daily reminders.

September 23
GAY COMMUNITY SERVICES CENTER,
NEW YORK CITY

The 200 gay physicians munched on *dolmades* and shoved broccoli into vegetable dips. Jim Curran fiddled with his slide projector. Curran was always cautious when he talked to newspaper reporters, fearful that his observations on the future of the AIDS epidemic might be fashioned into the stuff of sensational headlines, but he felt no such inhibition with the gay community. Instead, he felt his mission was to constantly stress the gravity of the unfolding epidemic. With each new epidemiological study revealing a more disheartening future, Curran came loaded with bad news to the general membership meeting of the New York Physicians for Human Rights.

"AIDS will certainly be the major cause of death during the lifetime of everyone here, and probably through the 21st century," Curran said. "In spite of good intentions and continuing efforts of the gay community and scientific sector, we should not expect scientific technology to rescue us from AIDS in the next few years, although eventually technology may help conquer the disease."

An unmarried man over the age of fifteen in New York City now stood a higher chance of dying of AIDS than of heart disease, which is traditionally the greatest killer of men, Curran said. In San Francisco, a single man was five times more likely to die of AIDS than of a heart attack. It was now clear that the CDC had vastly underestimated the scope of the epidemic, he added. Curran recited the statistics garnered from the San Francisco hepatitis cohort and more recent studies among hemophiliacs and IV drug users. Between 200,000 and 300,000 were infected with HTLV-III/LAV—and possibly many more. At least 10 percent would get AIDS, Curran estimated, and perhaps as many as 20 percent. Within five years, he added, the nation could expect 25,000 AIDS cases.

Given the sheer prevalence of AIDS infection, reductions in sexual contacts were not enough to avoid infection, Curran noted. A man who was having one-third the number of sexual partners of a year ago had done nothing to reduce his overall risk of AIDS if three times as many people were infected with the virus. In fact, with increases in prevalence outpacing changes in behavior, it appeared that the typical gay man who participated in any risky sexual behavior stood a greater chance of contracting the AIDS virus.

Curran bluntly addressed the political concerns that these AIDS statistics generated. The question was not if there would be a backlash against gays, but when. It might come soon. "You should get ready for it," he said. And, of course, there would be the loss of lives.

"When I spoke before you two years ago, on a kitchen chair in a living room, I looked out at the audience and felt these guys are the same age as I am. We're the same age as the men who are dying of AIDS. That was two years ago. The average age of men dying of AIDS is now younger than ours. It is time to start thinking about how to save the younger generations of gay men as they move out into sexual activity in a world full of AIDS."

The *New York Native* subsequently chastised Curran for his assessment, saying the federal government had no intention of finding an AIDS cure if it was warning gays that AIDS would be around until the next century. Ironically, Curran's projections that night vastly *underestimated* the scope of the AIDS epidemic. There would be 25,000 AIDS cases within two years, not five, and by then, the estimates of infected Americans would increase fivefold.

Even the milder prognosis, however, stunned most of the earnest physicians at the NYPHR meeting, particularly because it came at a time when the already lamentable state of affairs regarding AIDS in New York City was getting worse.

In August, Dr. Roger Enlow resigned as head of the Office of Gay and Lesbian Health Concerns. Although Enlow declined to give interviews about his experiences, he did offer one comment about his eighteen months working on AIDS in the Koch administration: "I spent a lot of time talking."

Meetings of the Interagency Task Force on AIDS turned into gripe sessions with members fuming about the lack of any substantive action to solve the festering problems. Task force member Arthur Felson came to the September meeting with a detailed review of what the group had accomplished in its two years of existence. By Felson's count, the task force had discussed the problem of housing for AIDS patients sixteen times, the lack of any active surveillance in the city fourteen times, and the need for home health care eight times, all without any resulting moves by the city government. Health Commissioner David Sencer acknowledged that the task force was "better at raising issues than solving them" and announced he would form yet another task force. This one, he said, would be geared at action rather than talk.

The sorry state of affairs led Larry Kramer to try again to be reinstated on the board of directors for Gay Men's Health Crisis. He had four producers making offers on *The Normal Heart;* the play most certainly would go into production in early 1985, but he certainly had time to work on AIDS now. The absence of any official moves against AIDS had only vindicated his anger, Kramer told the board when they met in mid-September. Kramer was devastated when the board voted down his request to be reinstated. Paul Popham said, "He'll join the board over my dead body."

October 1
MUSCLE SYSTEM,
SAN FRANCISCO

Bill Kraus had completed a set of Nautilus exercises and fell back on a bench for a rest. He bent his head down to catch his breath and spotted a purple spot on his right thigh. He told himself it was a blood blister. That night, Bill had two friends over for dinner; they laughed, drank, and argued about movies, and Bill didn't mention anything about the spot on his right thigh. He waited two days before he went to see Marc Conant.

Conant's assistant Mark Illeman saw Bill first.

"I can't tell you for sure that it's not KS," said Illeman.

He could tell Bill already knew it was; he was hoping against hope that he was wrong.

Marc Conant and Bill Kraus had grown so close in the past years of behind-the-scenes maneuvering on AIDS that Conant felt a numbness fall over him when he walked into the examination room. He felt Bill's neck and noted that virtually overnight, Bill's lymph nodes had burst forth with the swelling characteristic of AIDS patients. He could tell right away that the five-millimeter lesion was not a blood blister, but he couldn't offer Bill any definitive diagnosis until he performed a biopsy. Normally, KS biopsies took ten days to perform, but Conant assured Bill he'd have the results right away.

As Bill started dressing, Conant walked into the hall and told Illeman to record a diagnosis of Kaposi's sarcoma on Bill Kraus's chart.

"He's got it," Conant said somberly.

49 DEPRESSION

October 1984
<u>SAN FRANCISCO</u>

So many people had AIDS now that the old Public Health Service Hospital was converted into an AIDS hospital. Bill Nelson was surprised to see that all the old hands from San Francisco General Hospital's AIDS ward were there, serving as administrators. They were together again, like the old days on Ward 5B, back when you could have an AIDS ward that only had twelve beds.

Then Bill noticed that Allyson Moed, who had been the head nurse at 5B, was having a hard time breathing; she had *Pneumocystis*. Another nurse, it turned out, had toxoplasmosis, while nursing unit coordinator Cliff Morrison had tuberculosis.

Bill looked at himself while passing a mirror. Kaposi's sarcoma lesions covered his face.

"I can't go outside with all these KS lesions on my face," Bill said. "I can't be seen in public."

Bill bolted upright in bed, his face covered with a film of cold sweat. Earlier in the day, he had read a story in the paper in which Marc Conant predicted that, by 1988, there would be so many AIDS cases in San Francisco that the city might need an AIDS hospital and that the city should think about converting the shut-down Public Health Service Hospital into an AIDS facility. Everybody was talking about how crazy Conant was. That was where Bill Nelson's dream had come from.

Bill eased back into his bed. In the morning, he would return to his job as a nurse in the AIDS Ward and the nightmare would begin again.

October 4

Bill Kraus took the wheel of the convertible and sped along the back roads of the hill country north of San Francisco, past the geysers and vineyards of Napa County, and the redwoods and lighthouses of Sonoma County. Beatles, Supremes, and Jefferson Airplane songs blared from the car stereo.

"I look in the mirror and it's like looking twenty years in the past," Bill said.

The music and the general aimlessness of the day reminded Bill's friend

Dennis Seely of the past as well, when he met Bill in 1974 and they both were unemployed hippies hanging out on Castro Street. Dennis had known Bill before he had become involved in gay politics; in fact, it was Dennis who had introduced Bill to Harvey Milk. Now, when Bill needed a friend who predated his life as a gay political celebrity, he turned to Dennis Seely. They were wasting time before Bill called Marc Conant for the results of his biopsy.

"I don't know what's going to happen when they tell me," Bill said.

Dennis didn't believe that Bill really had AIDS. After all, Bill had scaled back his life-style before anyone he knew. For most of 1984, Bill had calculated that he would be home free once December came, because that marked two years of completely safe sex. The second anniversary was only six weeks away. It would be a cruel cosmic joke for Bill to get AIDS now, Dennis thought.

"How could you have it?" Dennis said. "You hardly ever got fucked—unless there's something you haven't told me."

"I only have six weeks left to go," said Bill. "It's so unfair. I'm the one who stopped having sex and got called all that shit for being 'anti-sexual.' I was the sexual fascist, and now I'm the one getting it."

Back at Dennis's apartment, Bill didn't want to phone Conant. Dennis cajoled him into making the call. Conant would tell Bill he was fine, and then Bill would leave and Dennis could take a nap. But Conant's nurse told Bill he had to come in, because Conant wanted to check his bandages. Bill started to cry.

"They don't need to check my bandages. It was only a small biopsy," Bill said. "I've got it."

"Stop being melodramatic," said Dennis.

When they got to Conant's waiting room, Bill took a Valium. A nurse asked Bill if he wanted a cup of coffee.

"Did you see the way she looked at me?" Bill asked, crying again.

"She looked at you like you wanted a cup of coffee," Dennis said.

"I've got it," Bill said. "I know it."

They went into Conant's office together. Inside, Conant put his hand on Bill's shoulder.

"I asked them to check it again, because I didn't want to believe it," he said. "You've got Kaposi's."

Dennis started to cry. Bill froze, one tear forming in the corner of his eye.

"I guess you and Kico will get my house," Bill said to Dennis.

"I'm not sharing the house with Kico," Dennis said, trying to joke even as he wept. "He's so irresponsible, he'll never pay his share of the expenses."

"You'll have to share it with him," Bill persisted, "because I'm going to leave it to both of you . . ."

"Wait a minute," Conant interjected. "You don't have to talk about who's getting the house yet. There are things you can do, Bill. With the position you're in, working for Sala, you can pressure for more funding. You can make your position an activist one. The bad news is that this is a life-threatening disease. But there are people who have lived three years. There are a lot of things that can happen."

Bill wasn't paying attention.

"Then I am to die," he said.

Conant paused.

"We're all going to die," he said finally, his voice turning grim. "If something doesn't break, we're all doomed."

◯

William James Kraus was the 728th San Franciscan diagnosed with Acquired Immune Deficiency Syndrome.

◯

By the time Bill Kraus got home, his closest friends had assembled at the two-flat Victorian he recently had purchased with Ron Huberman, Milk Club vice-president. His old friend Gwenn Craig was there. Bill's friends immediately laid plans to tap their lists of campaign contributors and raise enough money so Bill would not be wanting for anything during his ordeal. They stayed up late into the night, drinking and reminiscing around Bill's kitchen table.

"I wish I didn't have to get sick before I saw how many people really like me," Bill observed.

Kico Govantes came late and felt as though he had walked in on a funeral. Except, of course, that the person everyone was mourning was right there.

Bill wept and Kico held him, realizing their roles were now reversed. In years past, he had always needed Bill; now Bill needed him.

◯

The next morning, Bill woke up enveloped in dread. Every physical movement required tremendous exertion. He had not felt this way since his father died.

Was it true? he wondered briefly. Had yesterday really happened?

He realized that it had happened and that he would spend this day, and all the days he lived, knowing that he might die at any time. A microscopic junta had seized control of his body; he was under its command.

◯

"You don't have to die."

Bill Kraus's old friend Sharon Johnson saw Bill becoming more and more morose in the days after his diagnosis. Long ago, Sharon had sensed that Bill had a martyr complex. Like Bill, Sharon had been raised a devout Catholic, and she knew one thing about martyrs: They died. He'd kill himself with his grief, Sharon thought, so she took Bill to a psychic healer she knew, Jocelynn Nielsen.

Bill Kraus was cynical, but he was also desperate. He had been with Nielsen only a few minutes when she began talking about his father's death and the death of someone else very close, someone like a father, about fifteen months earlier. It had been Nielsen's experience that people diagnosed with a terminal disease usually had undergone some kind of trauma fifteen months before the onset of symptoms.

Bill was stunned. Obviously, she had no way of knowing about his father's death a quarter-century earlier, and she had perfectly described his emotional reaction to the death of Phil Burton. Bill poured out his heart to Nielsen. He told her about how for months, he had imagined seeing his own memorial service. Everybody had gathered in an auditorium to talk about him, and he wasn't there. The vision scared him.

Nielsen asked Bill to meditate and tell her what pictures he saw. Bill went into a trance but was quickly fidgeting with fright.

"I see snakes," he said. "They are out to attack me. They want to kill me."

"You can be afraid of them or you can master them," Nielsen said. "Make friends with the snakes. Don't be afraid of them."

And then Nielsen told Bill, quite simply, "You don't have to die."

He had created his own illness, she said. He could heal himself.

Bill was ecstatic at the idea, and he religiously adopted the regimen of diet and meditation she outlined. He gave away all his black and gray clothes to Dennis Seely after Nielsen said he would be healthier if he wore only earth tones. Bill threw himself into the effort to save his own life with a gusto he normally reserved for a political campaign. He ordered all his friends to visualize him well. Nobody was ever to talk about death around him again.

"I created this," Bill told Kico Govantes. "And I can beat it."

October 9
SAN FRANCISCO DEPARTMENT OF PUBLIC HEALTH

Reporters jockeyed for position when Merv Silverman strode into the auditorium and sat before the scores of microphones. Six months before, he had walked into the same room before the same reporters for his now-famous "no comment" press conference on the baths; today, he spoke with unaccustomed decisiveness, comparing the baths to "Russian roulette parlors." It might be legal to play Russian roulette at home, he said, but you can't open a business and charge people $5 a head to come in and play Russian roulette for profit.

"Today I have ordered the closure of fourteen commercial establishments that promote and profit from the spread of AIDS—a sexually transmitted fatal disease," Silverman said. "These businesses have been inspected on a number of occasions and demonstrate a blatant disregard for the health of their patrons and of the community. When activities are proven to be dangerous to the public and continue to take place in commercial settings, the health department has a duty to intercede and halt the operation of such businesses. Make no mistake about it: These fourteen establishments are not fostering gay liberation. They are fostering disease and death."

Within an hour, health inspector Thomas Petty was taping public health notices on the door of The Slot bathhouse on Folsom Street: "The continued operation of the above designated business constitutes a hazard and menace to the public health," the order read. When Petty found the manager, he explained, "I've been directed by the director of public health to order you to cease operations as of noon today." A few blocks away at the San Francisco Club

Baths, an announcement over the public address system told patrons to turn in their towels.

Indignant gay organizations held press conferences throughout the city that afternoon to protest the action. The San Francisco AIDS Foundation called bathhouses "leaders in AIDS education." The gay Golden Gate Business Association said the closure was an intrusion on private enterprise. The Bay Area Lawyers for Individual Freedom, a gay lawyers group with several prominent members on retainer to bathhouse owners, said gays across the country would lose their civil rights because of Silverman's move. The Bay Area Physicians for Human Rights maintained that closure would lead to more cases of AIDS, not fewer. In the end, the only gay group to support Silverman was the Harvey Milk Gay Democratic Club.

Later that afternoon, the owners of six of the bathhouses defied Silverman's order and reopened their doors. Their attorneys hoped that the courts would let them remain open until a full hearing could be held on the merits of closure. The lawyers, however, overestimated the tolerance of the judicial system when it came to violating a public health order. The courts quickly issued a temporary restraining order shutting down the baths, although judges deferred to the First Amendment and reopened a handful of closed pornographic theaters as long as the businesses shut down their orgy rooms and glory holes.

Ironically, in the weeks after bathhouse closure in San Francisco, there was little evidence that very many gays cared much about it. Three weeks of planning for a Castro Street rally protesting the closure brought out only 300 demonstrators. The expected gay outcry that had so paralyzed the health department and intimidated politicians never happened.

◯

The closure of bathhouses in San Francisco engendered a flurry of activity in other cities. In Los Angeles, Mayor Tom Bradley and County Supervisor Ed Edelman convened a task force on the subject of bathhouse closure. Both politicians were largely beholden to the gay community for political support, so neither endeavored to create a committee that was much more than window dressing. The group's chair was Dr. Neil Schram, a former president of the American Association of Physicians for Human Rights. For two years, Schram had championed the cause of bathhouses. Few were surprised when his task force ultimately concluded that the bathhouses should stay open.

When articulating her county's stance, Dr. Shirley Fanin, deputy director of Los Angeles County's Bureau of Communicable Disease Control, used an argument that was increasingly popular among health officials in both New York and Los Angeles. "The die is probably already cast," said Fanin. "It's likely that most of the people who can be exposed through bathhouses have already been exposed." New York State AIDS Institute Director Mel Rosen said closing the baths was like "closing the barn door after the horses are already out."

◯

In the end, the final act of the San Francisco bathhouse drama was anticlimactic, like the denouement of almost every subplot in the AIDS epidemic. Much legal wrangling followed Dr. Silverman's order in the months ahead, but the truly significant act of the controversy had been completed when Silverman held his press conference that October morning. At last, a local public health official had said that AIDS was an extraordinary situation requiring extraordinary action. Political rhetoric bowed to biological reality; saving lives was more important than saving face.

Supporters of the bathhouses said the closure order was politically motivated. This was true, if only because bathhouses had been allowed to stay open solely for political reasons. It was historically inevitable that the authorities would ultimately move to shut them down in all the cities hardest hit by the AIDS epidemic. Within a year of Silverman's orders, baths also were closed in both New York and Los Angeles under pressures that were far more brazenly political than anything seen in San Francisco.

What made the San Francisco closure so anticlimactic, however, was that it came so late. Most of the people still frequenting San Francisco bathhouses in late 1984 were already infected with the AIDS virus. The saved lives were most likely those of a few thousand uninformed gay tourists. In fact, by the time the baths were closed and a truly comprehensive education program was started in San Francisco, about two-thirds of the local gay men destined to be infected with LAV/HTLV-III already carried the virus. Any victories wrung from AIDS education or bathhouse closure would be Pyrrhic indeed.

The health officials who made this point while defending their inaction in New York and Los Angeles were telling the truth—and also confessing their worst sin. They were acknowledging that, in truth, they could have closed the barn door before the horses galloped out. Instead they did nothing, letting infection run loose and defending further inaction by saying it was too late to do anything, because infection was already loose in the land.

Later, everybody agreed the baths should have been closed sooner; they agreed health education should have been more direct and more timely. And everybody also agreed blood banks should have tested blood sooner, and that a search for the AIDS virus should have been started sooner, and that scientists should have laid aside their petty intrigues. Everybody subsequently agreed that the news media should have offered better coverage of the epidemic much earlier, and that the federal government should have done much, much more. By the time everyone agreed to all this, however, it was too late.

Instead, people died. Tens of thousands of them.

$$\bigcirc$$

In no place in the Western world was this despondent future more palpable than on Castro Street in late 1984. As word of Bill Kraus's illness spread, people thought less about what it meant to Bill than what it meant for everyone. Bill had changed his life-style before virtually anyone in the gay community. If Bill Kraus was vulnerable, then so was everyone. When told the news, many echoed the private fears of Marc Conant, who said, "We're all going to die."

By claiming Bill Kraus, the epidemic also delivered early notice to gay San Franciscans of the truth that would panic millions worldwide in later years. Even those who reacted quickly to the epidemic might have moved too late. There was no denying or arguing or bargaining with this virus, gay people could see now. As the winter of 1984 approached and the full weight of the tragedy fell over the neighborhood, a depression settled among the cheerfully painted Victorian houses of gay San Francisco.

Already, at least one in fifty of the gay men in the Castro District was diagnosed with AIDS; within a year, that figure was going to double, researchers warned. A door-to-door NIH survey of gay men in the area produced even more disquieting figures. Nearly 40 percent of gay men in the neighborhood were infected with HTLV-III. One in seven gay men already suffered from lymphadenopathy or ARC symptoms. The dire predictions of yesteryear were becoming the morose realities of today.

For most gay men, the depression was made more frantic by the fact that there was nothing they could do to counter impending doom. By October, a survey of 500 gay men found that two-thirds had changed their sexual habits enough to effectively remove any risk of contracting the syndrome. Ironically, the men who were least likely to have changed their behaviors were better educated, upscale professionals in their thirties. With a certainty that would make John Calvin proud, this group appeared to link their success to a sense of immunity to AIDS. Moreover, their sexual patterns were entrenched during the candy shop era of gay sexuality in the Castro. Younger men, unfamiliar with lustier times, found little difficulty changing.

With life-style changes already made, there was nothing else people could do to improve their future and few positive directions in which to channel the growing anxiety. Many turned to mysticism. Local health food stores did a booming business in tapes by such healers as Louise Hay, who guided listeners on meditations geared to visualizing good health. Thousands more allayed their anxieties by enlisting as volunteers in AIDS groups. But all this did not dispel the aura of gloom descending on the Castro, the sense that there was to be no escape. There was only the hope that the government's huge scientific establishment could create some miracle and the dying would end.

October 11
THE CAPITOL,
WASHINGTON, D.C.

With Congress eager to return home for a last month of campaigning, House and Senate conferees did not need lengthy negotiations on a final spending bill for AIDS research. On the eve of the congressional recess, House leaders agreed to increase their appropriations for AIDS to $93 million to coincide with the funds the Senate allocated after the leak of Dr. Brandt's memo. As it turned out, the Department of Health and Human Services had never forwarded any of Brandt's requests to Capitol Hill for consideration, prompting Representative Henry Waxman to hold a hearing that was little more than an opportunity to rake HHS officials over the coals.

"Every day there are deaths that are a monument to your irresponsibility," Waxman berated the HHS budget chief.

The final allocation passed within hours of the conference negotiations and represented a 60 percent increase over what President Reagan had requested for AIDS funds. It marked the fourth fiscal year in which Congress had constructed its own AIDS budget over the objections of the administration. The budget included $58 million for the National Institutes of Health and $23 million for the Centers for Disease Control.

The day after Congress appropriated these funds, Dr. Edward Brandt announced he was leaving the administration at the end of the year.

Days after adjournment, however, another dispute erupted between Congress and the administration. Included in the last-minute appropriations was an extra $8.35 million for the Food and Drug Administration to rush the development of an HTLV-III antibody test. The administration, however, decided it would only use $475,000 of the funds for the blood test, allowing the rest of the money to revert back to the treasury. Already, the administration was behind on its April promise to have a blood test available in blood banks within six months. The reluctance to spend money to speed the test stupefied both Republican and Democratic senators. The ensuing outcry, however, created little interest within the news media and brought no response from the administration.

October 25
CASTRO THEATER,
SAN FRANCISCO

The premiere of a documentary film on Harvey Milk moved Bill Kraus briefly back to the glory days of the gay movement in San Francisco, when the enemy was Anita Bryant, not some virus, and the dream seemed so clear. After the lights rose and the applause faded, everybody congratulated Bill on how articulate he had been in the movie when he described what it was like marching with candles toward City Hall.

From across the theater, Cleve Jones saw Bill surrounded by admirers. Cleve had heard that Bill had been diagnosed, but Bill's friends had also made it a point to tell Cleve he would not be a welcome guest at Bill's doorstep. Bill's friends had not forgiven Cleve for withdrawing his support for bathhouse closure six months before. Bill's diagnosis came as the latest blow to Cleve, who walked daily in a cloud of constant personal despair. Of four roommates he had had in 1980, two were dead from AIDS and a third was suffering from ARC. Cleve's excruciating shingles infection had cleared, but his lymph nodes remained swollen. And now Bill.

As he made his way out of the theater, Cleve wondered if Bill recalled everything about that night when Harvey Milk and George Moscone were killed. Cleve and Bill had made love that night, after the candlelight march.

Characteristically, Bill tended to be less sentimental about the episode and dismissed it as an aberration in his tastes. Cleve had had a crush on Bill ever since that night, however, and it had never died. Now Bill hated him. The epidemic had barged into all their lives like some rampaging bull and left only destruction. Cleve wandered to the Elephant Walk bar for a drink.

As Bill left the theater, he ran into an old acquaintance, who also had been diagnosed with AIDS. Steve Del Re told Bill about this experimental drug the French were using, HPA-23. He was going to Paris to try the drug. Bill might think about it too.

On Halloween, Bill had dinner with Marc Conant and a journalist friend who had traveled to Paris recently to interview Pasteur Institute researchers. The reporter played a tape of an interview with Dr. Willy Rozenbaum discussing the immune studies of an AIDS-stricken hemophiliac.

"He has the immune system of a normal person," said Rozenbaum. "This drug works."

Bill Kraus was euphoric. All his denial and bargaining had one name now: HPA-23. He was going to survive.

50 THE WAR

November 1984

On November 6, Ronald Wilson Reagan was reelected president with the biggest electoral-vote landslide in nearly fifty years. Democratic candidate Walter Mondale carried his home state of Minnesota and the District of Columbia; Reagan won the rest. Throughout the campaign, the burgeoning AIDS epidemic never became an issue of import. Neither candidate made any public pronouncement on the administration's "number-one health priority," and no reporter thought the issue significant enough to raise. In fact, President Reagan had never publicly spoken the word AIDS or ever alluded to the fact that he was aware that an epidemic existed.

When claiming victory on election night, President Reagan told a cheering crowd, "America's best days lie ahead." It was during the month of Reagan's reelection that the nation's AIDS caseload surpassed 7,000.

PASTEUR INSTITUTE, PARIS

The emergence of the harsh nationalism that marked the French-American rivalry among AIDS researchers was an unusual phenomenon in the scientific world, but the problem continued to fester. Most scientists on NCI grants or collaborating with Dr. Robert Gallo sided with the National Cancer Institute. Since the lines of scientific collaboration tended to follow the routes of the Eastern Airlines shuttle on the Atlantic coast, researchers at such West Coast centers as Stanford, UCSF, and UCLA collaborated more with the French scientists and sympathized with their side of the rift.

Dr. Michael Gottlieb from UCLA, who first reported the epidemic, decided he should be a senior statesman of AIDS research. He also was feeling left out of the virologic action, now that the focus of AIDS research had shifted to East Coast laboratories. The French, constantly overshadowed by the publicity that Gallo and the NCI garnered, were ecstatic at any glimmer of recognition for their research, and they welcomed Gottlieb when he came for a visit in November.

Gottlieb was impressed at the Pasteur team's enthusiasm, as well as with what they had been able to accomplish on extremely limited resources. Like most European governments, the French had not invested in AIDS research, figuring the vast American scientific establishment would make key AIDS discoveries from which the rest of the world could benefit. The entire AIDS budget for the Pasteur Institute was a few million dollars. With this, the Pasteur was coordinating extensive blood testing on serums from Africa, where French and Belgian researchers were tracing the heterosexual spread of the disease. In the Paris labs, the French also were exploring the genetic properties of the AIDS virus in hopes that a successful treatment might be found if they could discover a weak link in the retrovirus's RNA.

Because both the NIH and the scientific establishment in the United States largely continued to ignore research on AIDS treatments, the Pasteur Institute had become the world's most important center for treatment research. The French were eagerly testing all sorts of drugs on AIDS patients, all of whom were more than willing subjects since they knew the alternative to treatment was death. Drs. Willy Rozenbaum and Dominique Dormant were thrilled with the success of HPA-23, the drug with which Dormant had treated Gottlieb's patient, Rock Hudson.

The French focus impressed Gottlieb, because nothing frustrated him more than the inability to offer any hope of treatments to his eager patients. The U.S. government had taken a business-as-usual approach to AIDS treatment. For example, when the FDA had recently approved isoprinosine for experimentation, it allowed for testing on only 200 patients throughout the country. Under standard scientific procedures, the tests would be both controlled and double-blinded. Half the subjects would be given isoprinosine and the other half a placebo. To ensure that no one's expectations biased the results, neither doctor nor patient were allowed to know who was getting which. The protocol made scientific sense. The limitations on study participants ensured that untested drugs that might have serious harmful side effects were not distributed willy-nilly to the population. Moreover, only through such controlled experiments could science really determine whether a drug actually did hold promise as an AIDS treatment.

These scientific principles, however, were difficult to explain to patients facing a death sentence. Gottlieb knew of scores of Los Angeles patients who were driving to Mexico for isoprinosine and ribavirin, another drug reputed to have curative power for AIDS even though it was not licensed in the United States. Every week, more Americans arrived in Paris pleading for HPA-23 treatments as informal word of its potential spread on the AIDS grapevine.

The Pasteur doctors considered Americans barbarous for not aggressively pursuing every possible means of treatment. Double-blind studies were cruel and inhumane, they thought; the patient who receives a placebo might die from lack of treatment. Every patient who wanted it should get some kind of treatment, the French said. "You Americans let people die without any hope," Rozenbaum told a California reporter that autumn. "What do these people have to lose?"

For all their enthusiasm, Gottlieb saw that the French were poor scientific games players. One reason they had found difficulty in getting their research published and accepted in the United States was because they were inexperienced at writing papers for American scientific journals. They did not present their data as well as American scientists. The Pasteur's primary spokesman, Dr. Luc Montagnier, lacked the charisma and forcefulness of Gallo.

In Paris, the Pasteur researchers asked Gottlieb to help frame their article on the early success of HPA-23. One reason the French were eager to publish was because they were afraid they would be upstaged again by Gallo's work on suranim treatments.

The Pasteur team remained dispirited by their inability to gain recognition for their achievements. As they plodded from conference to conference, they continued to see their work slighted and the viral discovery they had made attributed to others. By the end of the year, Montagnier sighed, "I have learned more of politics than of science during all this. I never thought I would have to be a good salesman in order to be heard."

⬭

"The war," as Rozenbaum called it, simmered on the American front as well. Gallo was conducting a memo battle with the Centers for Disease Control because the CDC continued to refer to the AIDS virus as LAV/HTLV-III. Medical journals were returning to Dr. Jay Levy at UCSF his papers on the virus, which he called ARV, saying he should refer to it as HTLV-III. The reviewers who wanted the name change, Levy noted, were usually scientists on NCI grants. At one point, Gallo himself suggested that everybody should "throw out the name AIDS" and instead call the syndrome "HTLV-III disease." This would remove the stigma that the word AIDS now conveyed, he suggested.

UNIVERSITY OF CALIFORNIA, SAN FRANCISCO

When Marc Conant was in college and told his staunchly Catholic mother that he no longer believed in God, she scolded him. "Some day you'll be dying and you'll need it," she had said. "You'll return to the church."

The comment always bothered Conant. The idea that Catholic mysticism might rise again to overwhelm his good judgment ran against the grain of his scientific rationalism. At Duke University, he even minored in theology, hoping that by understanding religious totems, he would not succumb to their superstitions. Conant's lingering fear that he might one day surrender to mysticism is what made Bill Kraus's decision to go to Paris all the more upsetting.

In Bill Kraus, Marc Conant saw a younger mirror of himself. Like Conant, Bill was cerebral and articulate, and he had long ago shed the denial about AIDS. Now Bill was seeing a mystic healer and chasing the rainbow of some untested drug in an exotic, faraway land. It was denial and bargaining, Conant thought. It most certainly was not intelligent.

Bill was equally adamant about the trip to Paris. He had made his decision after the second lesion appeared in November. Walking along the windswept cliffs at Land's End, above the pounding surf of the Pacific, he had told Catherine Cusic that he was frightened of the depression that had settled on the San Francisco gay community. He didn't know what else he could do. Bill bolted at the suggestion that he talk to the grief counselors at the Shanti Project, a group that he frequently called "the Angels of Death." Bill told Catherine, "They tell people how to die—I want to live. I want to go to Paris."

Catherine had to agree that a morbid fascination with death pervaded the Castro neighborhood. And in the growing number of obituaries in the gay papers, people didn't just die of AIDS anymore. Instead they left this plane, departed this incarnation, or went to the other side. Bill chortled when one of his friends confided that, if he got AIDS, he wanted his obituary to read that he kicked the bucket. Nevertheless, Bill had surrendered to his own mysticism as well, spending his hours in visualization of good health or in daydreams about the promise of HPA-23.

Although many of Bill's friends looked askance at his increasingly metaphysical leanings, everyone noticed how his mood lifted when he decided to leave. They made plans to help finance the trip and began scheduling visits to Paris so Bill would never have to live there alone. The pieces fell quickly into place. Through his political connections, Bill would have the best treatment. Research would continue in the United States because of money he had helped to obtain. He would have the support of a community he had helped organize.

Ironically, it was with Kico Govantes, whose superstition had once been the butt of so much of Bill's teasing, that Bill could most freely discuss his changing attitude toward spirituality. For all his Catholic upbringing, Bill was awed at the realization that he did have a soul, that there was a pure spirit within him that he could tap for strength. And Kico had to laugh when he saw a copy of the *Bhagavad Gita* at Bill's bedside one night.

Bill was defensive. "It's a good book," he said. Then Kico reminded Bill of how he had ribbed Kico four years ago when Bill had seen the same book by Kico's bed. That was the night they had met, Kico reminded Bill.

"Four years ago," mused Bill, his voice echoing with wonder at all that had been lost and all that was being found. "Just four years ago."

November 28
SAN FRANCISCO

Before a hushed courtroom, San Francisco Superior Court Judge Roy Wonder issued a ruling aimed at balancing public health and private rights. Wonder said the bathhouses could reopen, but only if they hired monitors who would survey the premises every ten minutes and expel any men engaging in unsafe sexual practices. Moreover, the bathhouses had to remove all doors and private places where such acts might occur unobserved. Any violations of his order could result in closure.

The ruling put into effect the anti-sex regulations that Dr. Mervyn Silverman had proposed in mid-April. Gay attorneys declared the ruling a partial victory, although bathhouse owners were dubious. In the two months since they were shut down by Silverman's order, several had gone out of business. For all the talk of bathhouses as places where gays exercised their First Amendment rights to freedom of association, bathhouse owners understood more than anyone that gay men only went to their establishments to screw. Most of the bathhouses never bothered to reopen in the weeks after Judge Wonder's order. Some did, but business fell dramatically. One by one, bathhouses and sex clubs started shutting down, and the issue largely faded from the city's consciousness.

With the bathhouse issue out of the way, the San Francisco Department of Public Health finally put into place an aggressive education program that minced no words in exhorting gays to change their sexual behavior. Billboards, dramatic ads in gay newspapers, and public service television announcements became part of a hard-hitting program that quickly became a national model. It didn't escape notice among Bill Kraus's friends that the campaign finally instituted in late 1984 was virtually identical to one that Bill Kraus had drawn up over a weekend in mid-1983, sixteen months earlier.

AUSTRALIA

Even as the last news analyses on the U.S. presidential election were being written, AIDS suddenly exploded as a potent issue in an otherwise dull federal election campaign Down Under. The controversy started a week after Reagan's reelection, when the health minister of Queensland Province announced that four babies had contracted AIDS from blood donated by a Brisbane man. Three of the babies to receive the blood, which had been donated in February, were already dead; a fourth was dying. The twenty-seven-year-old gay donor had no AIDS symptoms, although subsequent testing showed he harbored HTLV-III antibodies. To date, the continent had been home to only twenty-six AIDS cases, of whom nine had died. These first deaths outside the gay community, however, proved a lightning rod for critics of the ruling Labor government of Prime Minister Bob Hawke. Within a day, the Queensland legislature passed a law imposing a stiff fine and a two-year prison sentence on any member of a high-risk group who donated blood.

Conservative opponents immediately blamed Labor's support of repeal of the nation's old sodomy laws. "If it wasn't for the promotion of homosexuality as a norm by Labour, I am quite confident that the deaths of these three poor babies would not have occurred," said Ian Sinclair, leader of the right-wing National Party. One National Party parliamentary candidate advocated manslaughter trials for any gay men found to be donating blood; others said they should be indicted for murder.

Leading fundamentalists said this never would have happened if the nation had heeded their 1983 call for a quarantine on all gay men traveling to the United States. Gay rights groups reported numerous gang attacks on gay men, apparently inspired by the AIDS panic.

With clamor rising across the country, Prime Minister Hawke interrupted a campaign tour and called an emergency meeting of AIDS experts and state health ministers in Melbourne. The atmosphere was acrimonious. According to one report, the Queensland health minister refused to so much as walk into the room where an openly gay man was present. A number of committees and task forces were established, and the health ministers agreed to impose national guidelines to deal severely with people who misled blood bankers when filling out questionnaires about their status as possible members of high-risk groups. Hawke issued a national call for female donors.

Although Australia was the hotspot for AIDS hysteria in 1984, concern grew elsewhere as well. The World Health Organization reported a threefold increase of AIDS cases in western Europe during 1984, with 762 cases diagnosed in fourteen nations. About one-third of the cases were in France. The two nations with gay populations most prone to travel, Denmark and Switzerland, reported the highest per capita rates of AIDS on the continent.

Blood testing continued to show the penetration the AIDS virus was making into countries that had yet to report a high incidence of the disease. Finland, for example, reported only five cases, all of which were diagnosed in the last six months of 1984. Testing of 175 Finnish gay men, however, revealed that 10 percent were infected with HTLV-III. Of these, one-third already had developed ARC.

In the Federal Republic of Germany, the second hardest-hit nation in Europe, testing found that two-thirds of hemophiliacs, 20 percent of intravenous drug users, and one-third of gay men carried HTLV-III antibodies. West German authorities predicted 10,000 AIDS cases in that country by 1990. The projections led to the first proposals to place AIDS patients under the same restrictions that apply to people with syphilis or gonorrhea. Under these venereal disease laws, which were in force in virtually every northern European country, it was a crime for a person infected with a sexually transmitted disease to have sex.

The spread of AIDS in Africa most likely outpaced the spread in any other region in the world, although determining this with any degree of accuracy remained problematical. African governments continued to be reluctant to acknowledge that the epidemic even existed within their borders. Therefore, the extent of the problem was most obvious in Europe, where one in six AIDS patients was African. These cases could be traced to eighteen sub-Saharan African nations. Two-thirds of the African-linked AIDS cases in Europe, however, came from one country, Zaire, and 11 percent came from the nearby Congo. Belgian scientists reported only one major risk factor in these nations: heterosexual promiscuity.

In December, a new wave of concern over AIDS flared in England when health authorities reported that fifty-five Britons had been treated with blood products contaminated with AIDS. Within days, the first British transfusion-AIDS case was announced. The victim was a baby whose mother had received an infected unit of blood during pregnancy. Doctors were anxiously watching the mother for signs of the disease.

In the United States, the CDC reported ninety cases of transfusion AIDS by the end of 1984. Another forty-nine hemophiliacs had contracted the disease from infected Factor VIII.

December 10
SETON MEDICAL CENTER,
DALY CITY, CALIFORNIA

One doctor suggested Frances Borchelt was suffering from psitacosis when they admitted her to the hospital this time. Maybe she had picked up the disease from the family parakeet, he said. Frances's daughter Cathy had studied her AIDS brochures and believed her mother had AIDS, but the doctors were adamant that she did not have any of the symptoms.

They cultured Frances Borchelt's blood, tested her bone marrow, and used every gadget of nuclear medicine to see what was wrong. Meanwhile, the grandmother grew weaker with each passing day. Breathing was becoming excruciatingly difficult.

On December 23, Frances went into respiratory failure and was rushed into the intensive care unit. On a respirator, Frances managed to communicate with her worried husband and children by scribbling on a piece of paper. It was the first anniversary of the death of her older daughter and one day away from the anniversary of her father's death, she noted. As orderlies prepared Frances for emergency surgery, the fiercely superstitious woman said, "This time it's my turn."

Christmas Eve

Bill Kraus's mother Mary had looked forward to her Christmas visit with her two boys in San Francisco. She had been devastated since Bill's diagnosis and felt isolated because there was no one with whom she could discuss Bill's plight. She didn't feel comfortable talking to her friends about AIDS. For years, she often avoided saying even that her two sons lived in San Francisco for fear that it would explain why they were still unmarried.

On Christmas Eve, Bill was in bed, suffering from a cold. He was moody and seemed troubled when he talked to his mother.

"I've had this recurring dream that there's a wall of ice in front of me," Bill said.

"Visualize the wall melting," Mary suggested. "Make it go away."

Bill hesitated for a moment, and then confessed, "It scares me."

Christmas Day

Lying on the respirator, with tubes coursing through her, Frances Borchelt was her usual commanding self, writing notes to Cathy about how to cook the roast beef and prepare the mashed potatoes. Normally, Christmas was a major production at the Borchelt household, with Frances ruling the kitchen and doting over the grandchildren. The family tried to be cheerful on this Christmas, even as nurses insisted they don gowns and gloves before seeing Frances. The matriarch's two granddaughters stayed behind in the waiting room; nobody wanted the children to see Frances weak and wasted on the breathing machine.

Three days later, the family doctor told Bob Borchelt that the lung biopsy showed that Frances had contracted *Pneumocystis carinii* pneumonia. He mentioned that it was a pneumonia that people with AIDS sometimes got, but went no further into this troublesome side of the diagnosis. When Bob told Cathy, she wanted to scream.

"Dad, that's AIDS," she said. "Mom has AIDS."

$$\bigcirc$$

In Washington, meanwhile, the Reagan administration had yet to decide whether to release the $8.4 million that Congress had appropriated more than two months before to speed the HTLV-III antibody test to blood banks. The matter was "still under discussion," a White House spokesperson said.

Attempts at the year's end to prod other national institutions toward paying attention to the implications of the epidemic proved unsuccessful. Defense Secretary Casper Weinberger declined to meet with outgoing health chief Edward Brandt, who felt the military needed to face up to the problems that undoubtedly would arise from AIDS infection of U.S. servicemen. In private discussions with insurance lobbyists, meanwhile, congressional aide Tim Westmoreland warned that they should use their substantial political muscle to pressure for more AIDS funding. He predicted billions of dollars of medical expenses in future years that would cripple the corporations. However, like most large corporations, insurance companies supported conservative leaders who were for less government spending, not more. They weren't about to start dallying with a gay issue like AIDS, so Westmoreland found few willing listeners.

Nineteen eighty-four was the year of the films *Amadeus* and *Purple Rain*. Tina Turner made a dramatic comeback, inspiring New Year's Eve costumes for drag queens across the country. And it seemed that every year-in-review piece on the television newscasts featured huge American flags waving at the U.S. Olympics in Los Angeles and at the Republican National Convention, scored to the music of the year's top-selling record, *Born in the U.S.A.* This Bruce Springsteen album was a collection of songs about the ignored Americans who were left out of the American dream, stranded in despairing lives of unfulfilled aspirations. A more powerful message of discontent had not been written in twenty years, and yet, somehow, *Born in the U.S.A.* was seen as part of the flag-waving patriotism that had thoroughly seized the nation that year.

It was easy to ignore anomalies in 1984. President Reagan, who had presided over the greatest deficit spending of any government in human history, won reelection on a platform promising to make deficit spending unconstitutional. And everybody agreed the future of the United States was bright again. On December 31, the Centers for Disease Control reported that 7,699 Americans were dead or dying of a disease that had never been heard of when President Reagan was sworn in during his first term, and nobody paid much attention to the CDC's warnings that tens of thousands more would be dead by the time he was done with his second.

SAN FRANCISCO

In San Francisco, the endgame of AIDS public health politics also came in December when Dr. Mervyn Silverman called a press conference to make an announcement that surprised nobody. After seven years as the city's health director, he needed "to do something else." He was resigning.

The handwriting urging Silverman's departure had been on the municipal wall for several weeks. In November, voters passed a proposition shifting control of the health department from the city manager to a new health commission to be appointed by the mayor. Three days after the election, Mayor Feinstein announced the formation of a high-level task force to chart the transfer of the department; pointedly, she did not appoint Silverman.

Silverman had little support anywhere in the city now. Doctors and politicians who supported a vigorous response to the AIDS epidemic felt Silverman had moved too slowly. Meanwhile, many gays felt Silverman had done too much. The health department's new education program was nothing more than a revamping of the "behavior modification" plan forwarded by Dr. Marcus Conant earlier in the year, they noted bitterly. For months, the gay papers had been crammed with vitriolic editorials and nasty letters condemning Silverman as "homophobic." The criticism was ironic, of course, because so many of Silverman's problems were a direct result of his unwillingness to do anything that might be perceived as even remotely anti-gay.

In any event, Silverman was weary at the end of the year and looking forward to the rest. He was not resigning in disgrace. After all, he was handing his successor an AIDS program that was now internationally esteemed as the model against which all future efforts in other cities would be judged. To be sure, the education and prevention projects had taken years to forge in the highly charged atmosphere of public health politics in San Francisco, but they were now complete. Silverman felt proud of what he had accomplished, and if he had it to do over again, he did not feel he would do it very differently.

During Silverman's press conference, a reporter asked Silverman how he felt to be leaving his job "in the middle of an epidemic."

"I'm afraid we're not in the middle of an epidemic," Silverman answered. "This is the beginning."

PART VIII

THE BUTCHER'S BILL 1985

. . . The weariness, the fever and the fret,
    Here, where men sit and hear each other groan;
Where palsy shakes a few, sad, last gray hairs,
    Where youth grows pale, spectre-thin, and dies;
      Where but to think is to be full of sorrow,
      And leaden-ey'd despairs . . .
            —JOHN KEATS
            "Ode to a Nightingale"

51 HETEROSEXUALS

January 1985
<u>NEW YORK CITY</u>

At the emergency room of St. Vincent's Hospital in Greenwich Village, the patient lay on a gurney, wheezing from *Pneumocystis.* He had lain there for twenty-four hours, waiting for a room. Under normal circumstances, his doctor would have called the hospital and had the man admitted. But hospital administrators preferred not to take any more AIDS patients; they already had so many. The man's doctor had told him to circumvent standard procedures and simply show up in the emergency room, where, under New York law, he could not be turned away.

That's what doctors advised patients who needed hospitalization for AIDS in New York City in early 1985. At Memorial Sloan-Kettering Cancer Center, Dr. Mathilde Krim fielded calls daily from doctors desperate to find hospital rooms for their ailing patients. Physicians were afraid to send their patients to a number of the city's hospitals, given the bad treatment AIDS patients had received in the past; institutions with good reputations for dealing with AIDS already were overwhelmed.

Uptown at St. Luke's-Roosevelt Hospital, one of the largest medical centers in the world, half of the hospital's private rooms were filled with dying AIDS victims. In one well-known New York hospital, the vice-president of one of the largest corporations in New York City, who was suffering from Kaposi's sarcoma, was denied a bed and had to check into the hospital through the emergency room. Even there, running a 104-degree fever, the executive had to wait seven hours for a room. There was talk among AIDS clinicians that one AIDS sufferer had already died while waiting for a room at one of Manhattan's most prestigious university hospitals. Throughout the city, AIDS clinicians could not imagine what they would do in coming months when burgeoning numbers of patients overwhelmed the hospitals' finite resources.

"We're not talking about a nightmare that is going to happen," said St. Luke's-Roosevelt AIDS expert, Dr. Michael Lange. "It already is a nightmare."

At Jacobi Hospital in the Bronx, three-year-old Diana waved wanly at Dr.

Arye Rubinstein, one of the only familiar faces she had known in her life. She had lived in the hospital since 1983, not because she needed hospitalization but because New York City had no place else to put its AIDS patients. There were at least twenty-five children like her in the hospitals of New York and New Jersey, and every month, as the parents of such children died or abandoned them, there were more. Everybody had known this would happen, of course, but nobody had really planned what to do when it did.

The crisis in New York AIDS treatment characterized the new phase the AIDS epidemic was entering. The unheeded warnings of 1983 and the lost opportunities of 1984 were materializing into the tragic stories of 1985. The future shock of the AIDS epidemic was arriving; the butcher's bill had come due.

January 3
THE TENDERLOIN, SAN FRANCISCO

Street lights and blinking neon signs cast shadows across the young woman's face. She pouted histrionically when the undercover police asked for her identification. The other women quickly hustled themselves off the dingy block of Ellis Street in the heart of San Francisco's sleazy hooker district. In this part of town, of course, such arrests were not rare occasions.

Silvana Strangis ignored the stares of passing motorists while the arresting officer waited for the radio to tell him whether the thirty-four-year-old brunette had an arrest record. Her record, it turned out, was unusually impressive, even for this part of town. In the past five years, she had been busted thirty-two times and charged with thirteen felonies and thirty-nine misdemeanors, from robbery and grand theft to tonight's offense, "obstructing a sidewalk."

When Silvana brushed her long straight hair out of her eyes, the arresting officer could see the dark brown puncture marks on her arm where she injected her heroin. He knew her story; it wasn't that different from the other prostitutes who worked the Tenderloin.

Silvana was handcuffed and put in the back of the squad car. Right away, she noticed that the vice cops seemed inordinately chatty. Instead of reading her Miranda rights, they wanted to talk about Silvana's boyfriend and pimp, Tony Ford. They'd heard on the street that Tony had AIDS. Was it true?

Years of heroin addiction had undone whatever Silvana Strangis had learned of discretion, and she admitted that Tony had just been discharged from the AIDS Ward. She was worried that she had AIDS too, she added.

It was then that Silvana noticed that instead of turning toward the Hall of Justice, the patrol car was heading through the Mission District. A little past midnight, the police officers brought the handcuffed prisoner into the emergency room at San Francisco General Hospital.

"We want her to have the AIDS test," one of the officers said.

The hospital personnel were astonished at the request. They carefully explained that so far no AIDS test, per se, existed. The HTLV-III antibody test had yet to be licensed, and that was not an AIDS test. Moreover, they could not force a handcuffed prisoner to take any test so that the results could be turned over to police officers. Maybe the woman should come back when the AIDS Clinic was open and when she could decide for herself what she wanted to do.

The disappointed officers put Silvana back in the cruiser, wrote out a citation for obstructing a sidewalk, and drove back to the Tenderloin. Silvana should go back to the AIDS Clinic, they instructed, and get whatever tests she could. And she should get the results in writing. They'd be back to check up on what the doctors had to say.

Silvana was shaken when she stepped out of the car. She searched out her dealer, scored some heroin, and took it back to her seedy room, where Tony Ford was waiting. They shot the heroin, sharing the needle, just as they always had. Soon, the pair passed out.

The next morning, a *Chronicle* reporter, tipped off by an emergency room attendant, knocked on Silvana's door.

"Tell him to get the hell out of here," Tony grumbled.

"I need a ride to the clinic," Silvana said, pulling a beat-up poncho over her blue jeans.

At the AIDS Clinic, the head nurse, Gayling Gee, cleared her schedule to talk to Silvana Strangis, although the hooker was too embarrassed about her predicament to say much. Instead, she asked the reporter to tell Gee about her profession and the vice cops and her urgent need for AIDS screening. Gee and the other clinic staffers who heard the tale were dumbfounded. They wondered about issues like confidentiality and civil rights.

Silvana didn't want to hear about this. All she wanted was a piece of paper that said she didn't have AIDS. She could show it to the vice cops and get on with the business of turning tricks and buying heroin. Gee gave her an appointment for the next week.

"How did you end up like this?" the reporter asked, as he drove Silvana back to her Jones Street hotel room.

Silvana turned up the Moody Blues tape on the car stereo, sighed, and said she had grown up in a nice Italian family in a San Francisco suburb. When she had graduated from a Catholic high school in 1968, she was full of optimism about a world that seemed on the brink of a New Age. The idealism faded in the years that followed, and she started taking drugs, and then she met Tony and bore his child. It was easy to make money by turning tricks, and life now went from trick to trick, from fix to fix.

By the time the couple heard about AIDS and the threat posed by sharing needles and sexual relations, it was too late. Tony already had the first symptoms of immune disorder, and the threat of some distant health problem paled in comparison to the urgency of getting that soothing rush of heroin. Nobody cared much about this disease in the Tenderloin, she added. When Tony lay in the AIDS Ward a few weeks ago, some of the other players from the neighborhood brought Tony's fixes to his bedside. They'd close the door, make jokes about the gay male nurses, and all shoot up together, sharing the same needle.

There was, of course, no question of what Silvana would do tonight. Tony couldn't work. He certainly didn't want her to stop working either; that would mean the end of his heroin.

"It's the drugs," she concluded. "It's like what they say on TV. You get in and you can't get out."

That was why Silvana was going back to the streets that night. Yes, she was worried about spreading AIDS. In fact, her lymph nodes were swollen, her sleep was disturbed by chronic nightsweats, and she felt dog-tired all the time. But she had to work. She didn't know any other way to make money.

○

The next morning's front-page story about a prostitute raised all the profound public policy questions implicit in the case of a working hooker who almost certainly was an AIDS carrier. Dr. Paul Volberding talked about how the prostitute posed a "monster of a public health issue," with its classical conflict between public health and individual rights. Other news coverage of Silvana Strangis, however, was less delicate.

"A human time bomb is walking the streets of San Francisco," announced the grim anchor at the top of the local evening news that night. Another newscast likened her to "Typhoid Mary."

All weekend, television crews trolled the Tenderloin in their Instant Eye vans, trying to interview anxious streetwalkers. Frightened callers to talk shows almost unanimously opined that the police should lock the woman up and quickly discard the key.

Silvana became such an instant persona non grata in her neighborhood that she was literally chased off the streets and into her residential hotel lobby by four angry prostitutes who threatened to have her stabbed to death if she left her hotel again. The news stories, it turned out, hadn't done much for business. It seemed every john looking for action that weekend started negotiations by asking, "Are you the one with AIDS?"

The uproar illuminated the profoundly heterosexual male bias that dominates the news business. After all, thousands of gay men had been infecting each other for years, but attempts to interest news organizations to pressure the city for an aggressive AIDS education campaign had yielded minimal interest. A single female heterosexual prostitute, however, was a different matter. She might infect a heterosexual man. That was someone who mattered; that was news.

Although evidence of heterosexual AIDS transmission could be dated back to the first epidemiological studies by the Centers for Disease Control in the summer of 1981, it was not until early 1985 that the straight links of the disease garnered much attention. The most disconcerting stories came from Central Africa, where AIDS was simply called "the horror sex disease." Although image-conscious African governments swore to silence the researchers working within their borders, leaks confirmed that thousands of immune-suppressed people were dying in black Africa, usually from gastrointestinal parasites, the most common opportunistic infections of that region. Unaware of foreign acronyms, Ugandans had dubbed AIDS "slim disease" because of the wasting away that marked the virulent parasitic diseases.

In scientific forums, European researchers working closely with teams in Central Africa were the most outspoken about the heterosexual dimension of the epidemic. These doctors, largely in Belgium and France, had always considered the preoccupation with the gay angle of AIDS to be a strange American idiosyncrasy. Given the experiences of such nations as Zaire and Rwanda, these doctors warned that the Western world should not be complacent about the threat that this new sexually transmitted disease posed to all people.

In the United States, the most aggressive research on heterosexual AIDS transmission came from a most unlikely source, the U.S. Army. From his work at the Walter Reed Army Institute in Washington, D.C., Dr. Robert Redfield had documented the ease of male-to-female sexual transmission of AIDS. Of seven married male sufferers of AIDS and ARC, for example, Redfield found that five had wives who were infected with HTLV-III. Of these five wives, three were already showing clinical symptoms of ARC. The fact that one-third of military AIDS and ARC cases claimed that prostitute contact was their only risk behavior also made Redfield a passionate proponent of the threat posed by female-to-male AIDS transmission. His case, however, was problematical because the military was by now routinely dismissing gay servicemen suffering from the syndrome. That provided powerful motivation for military personnel to blame prostitutes rather than homosexual contacts for their infection.

The question of female-to-male AIDS transmission had exploded in San Francisco not long before, when Dr. Paul Volberding at the AIDS Clinic held a press conference to announce the first two local AIDS cases among heterosexual men who claimed no other high-risk activity than sexual relations with intravenous drug-using prostitutes. In San Francisco, the new cases were something of a revelation because AIDS had remained an almost purely gay phenomenon in that city. More than 98 percent of the city's caseload were gay or bisexual men; the transfusion AIDS cases and five drug addicts were the exception proving the rule that, in San Francisco, AIDS was a gay disease.

"We don't usually call a press conference to announce every new AIDS case," Volberding admitted when he announced that two straight men had contracted the disease from women. "But we shouldn't lose track that this might be our last chance to halt an epidemic among heterosexuals."

Days later, Volberding's concern was underscored with the diagnosis of the first local woman to contract AIDS through a heterosexual liaison. Within days, she was in Ward 5B, the first woman on the AIDS Ward, staring at the stark landscape outside her window and wondering how a tryst with a bisexual man several years before had brought her here.

Dr. Mervyn Silverman, in his last weeks as health director, announced that the health department would start updating brochures to include risks to heterosexuals. A new task force was organized to start laying groundwork for more elaborate educational plans in the future. Volberding took things a step further when he suggested that city epidemiologists begin sexual contact tracing on every heterosexual AIDS case. Dr. Dean Echenberg, who had replaced Selma Dritz in the Bureau of Communicable Disease Control, took what became the standard public health argument against such tracing, saying that even if the tracing turned up infected people, there was no medical treatment to offer them.

"You might cause a tremendous amount of damage without doing any good," Echenberg said. Volberding countered that the people who might later get infected from such contacts, however, would not see it that way.

This medical point of view did not prevail. AIDSpeak still dominated public health decision making, and those rules decreed that, even in a deadly epidemic, you weren't supposed to do anything that might hurt somebody's feelings.

For all the concern about heterosexual transmission—and the role prostitutes might play in spreading the disease—there was probably no aspect of the epidemic in which the facts were more arguable. At this point, only 50 AIDS cases nationally were linked to heterosexual transmission. Of these, 45 were women and only 5 were men who appeared to have no other risk except sexual contact with infected women. Five out of nearly 8,000 AIDS cases reported nationally did not constitute an epidemic. And there could be no certainty that those 5 men, 2 of whom lived in San Francisco, were not gay men who were too ashamed to admit it.

The mechanics of female-to-male transmission also were problematical. Which female body fluids are as invasive to men as semen is during vaginal or anal intercourse? In Africa, transmission appeared possible when vaginal fluids connected with blood through open sores stemming from untreated venereal disease. In the United States, venereal disease was almost always treated, and female-to-male transmission was rare. To be sure it did exist, and numbers would probably increase as more women became infected with the virus. However, heterosexuals had no amplification system comparable to the gay bathhouses to speed the virus throughtout the country. In the future, heterosexual AIDS would remain a problem for the people it had already struck; sexual partners of intravenous drug users, concentrated largely among poor and minorities in eastern urban cities. It seemed unlikely that the epidemic would suddenly become a heterosexual blight in the way it had swept the gay community.

Perhaps no single aspect of the epidemic was as instructive in this point than the AIDS-carrying prostitutes. Even while the Silvana Strangis story raged on the front pages, UCSF researchers were completing their journal article on the first person in the United States known to have been infected with the AIDS virus. The first documented carrier was not a gay man, they said, but a San Francisco prostitute. This woman, like Strangis, had a long rap sheet of Tenderloin arrests related to prostitution and intravenous drugs. In 1977, the woman, who was then twenty-five years old, gave birth to a baby girl who began showing signs of immune deficiency eleven months later. While the infant's condition deteriorated, the mother gave birth to a second girl in 1979. This child also showed signs of immune abnormalities, including chronic diarrhea and swollen lymph glands. A third daughter was born in April 1982. Within two months, she had candidiasis in both her mouth and vagina. Three months later, doctors blamed her breathing problems on *Pneumocystis.* By 1984, two of the three children were dead. Any mystery about the source of their immune problems was resolved when UCSF researchers tested their stored blood samples for HTLV-III antibodies. All three children were infected. The mother, who suffered from swollen lymph nodes in 1982, clearly was infected with the virus as early as 1977 and possibly 1976, shortly after the virus arrived in the United States.

During all these years of infection, the woman had been an active prostitute in the Tenderloin, as she would continue to be until her death in May 1987. If she was easily spreading the virus to her clients, there had been plenty of time for the stricken men to surface. Yet, San Francisco counted only two male heterosexual cases. Similarly, New York City was not teeming with straight men blaming prostitutes, even though that city's legion of drug-shooting hookers dwarfed the number of such women on the West Coast. Taken together, it appeared there was more smoke than fire in the prostitution-AIDS debate.

Nevertheless, the outpouring of official attention to the handful of heterosexual AIDS cases in early 1985 proved a crucial event in determining the direction of AIDS debate in the next two years. It instructed health officials and AIDS researchers, who had had such a difficult time seizing government and media interest in the epidemic, that nothing captured the attention of editors and news directors like the talk of widespread heterosexual transmission of AIDS. Such talk could be guaranteed air time and news space, which, in the AIDS business, quickly translated into funds and resources. Thus, even though epidemiological support for fears of a pandemic spread of AIDS among heterosexuals was scant, few researchers would say so aloud. There was no gain in taking such a position, even if it did ultimately prove to be honest and truthful. Five years of bitter experience had schooled just about everyone involved in this epidemic that truth did not count for much in AIDS policy.

January 10

Cathy Borchelt was at work in the San Francisco Police Department's record room when a co-worker handed her the morning *Chronicle* and asked about the story on page eight. It was an announcement by the Irwin Memorial Blood Bank that an ailing, unnamed woman at Seton Medical Center had contracted AIDS through blood provided by Irwin in August 1983.

"Is that your mom?"

It was the first time anybody in the Borchelt family was informed that Frances was indeed suffering from transfusion AIDS.

"I've been suspecting this because the doctors said she had *Pneumocystis*," Cathy said as she scanned the story.

"There's a lot of *Pneumocystis* going around," her colleague agreed.

Cathy knew her mother was an intensely private woman and would not want to see anything about herself in the newspaper, even if it did not carry her name. She called the hospital to make sure nobody put a copy of the *Chronicle* in her room.

That evening at the hospital, Cathy was watching television with Frances when the newscaster began talking about the new transfusion case in Seton Medical Center. Frances Borchelt shook her head sadly at the news.

"That poor lady," she said. "If it were me, I'd sue."

Cathy was shocked. Obviously, nobody had told her mother yet that she had AIDS. That night, Bob Borchelt insisted that the doctors tell Frances what had happened.

The next day, Frances didn't say anything about the conversation she had had with her doctor, although the family noted that she seemed depressed.

$$\bigcirc$$

The woman in Seton Medical Center was the 100th American known to have contracted AIDS through a blood transfusion, Irwin president Brian McDonough said the next day. As part of a new policy of openness, Irwin was now publicly announcing each new case of transfusion AIDS. The intent was to allay any suspicion that the blood bank was whitewashing the transfusion-AIDS problem. In revealing Frances's diagnosis, McDonough added that thirty-two AIDS patients had donated blood to Irwin in recent years and that at least seventy-two local people had received blood products from these donors. The blood bank expected another two dozen AIDS cases from recipients of its products in the next year.

The Irwin policy of candor infuriated other blood bankers who were still clinging to their one-in-a-million rhetoric, if not declining comment on the problem of transfusion AIDS altogether. Blood bankers were anxious to get the entire AIDS problem behind them. That would happen with the release of the HTLV-III antibody test, when at last they could pronounce the blood supply safe from AIDS.

The Food and Drug Administration had announced a February 15 release date for the screening test. Local public health officials and gay organizations, however, continued to be concerned about its vast policy implications. In few issues had social, political, psychological, and medical variables converged to create such a policy morass.

Surveys of gay men indicated that as many as 75 percent planned to take the antibody test once it was available. Concern soared that, once blood banks started screening, the men would go to a blood bank and donate blood in an effort to learn their antibody status.

Meanwhile, scientists were uncertain as to the accuracy of the test. Dr. Robert Gallo said in early January that the test might not detect between 5 and 30 percent of AIDS virus carriers. The problem stemmed both from the test's accuracy and the fact that it did not appear that people developed detectable HTLV-III antibodies until six weeks after infection. Thus, somebody recently infected with the AIDS virus would not test positive on the antibody test. This left health officials worried that if gay men donated blood to learn their antibody status, some infected blood might slip through the AIDS screening, further contaminating the blood supply.

Added to these fears was the growing anxiety about the civil liberties implications of blood testing among gay men. With as many as one-half of gay men testing positive for HTLV-III in some studies, it appeared that the test could well become a de facto test for sexual orientation. Access to test results could possibly result in widespread discrimination against gays by employers, insurers, or a government that might turn repressive toward gays in future years.

All this could happen even while the medical value of the test remained in some doubt. Official estimates still put the number of antibody-positive people who would develop AIDS at between 5 and 10 percent, although it was still not possible to predict which group that might be. Because the test had little predictive value, therefore, the newest axiom of AIDSpeak became "the test doesn't mean anything."

Translating all these concerns to policy became the task of Dr. Mervyn Silverman, who was president of the U.S. Conference of Local Health Officers. Silverman put together a proposal that seemed to meet everyone's needs, seeking money for alternative test sites in which gay men and other concerned people could be tested outside the blood banks. Silverman also wanted the government to issue regulations assuring the confidentiality of blood bank test results, so employers or government agencies could not subpoena them for purposes unrelated to protecting the blood supply.

The proposals were greeted with enthusiasm at the Centers for Disease Control, which had long grappled with the complexities of AIDS policy. In meetings with federal officials, however, Silverman ran into a brick wall of resistance. The alternative test sites would cost money, he was told, and the federal government had no plans to expend more money on AIDS. As it was, the Reagan administration still had not released the more than $8 million that Congress had appropriated the October before to speed the antibody test to blood banks. Moreover, the government would do nothing to assure confidentiality for blood bank test results. That should be handled on the local level, officials said.

In a January 15 meeting with representatives from the Food and Drug Administration, Silverman got tough. If the government did not release funds for the alternative test sites, he would publicly announce that federal officials were fashioning a new threat to the blood supply. He gave the FDA a two-week deadline. Angry at being handed ultimatums, administration officials told Silverman he was just looking for a way to line the pockets of his health department. The charge amused Silverman, coming as it did on his last day as public health director of San Francisco.

⬭

The efficient social services department at the San Francisco AIDS Foundation easily found Silvana Strangis a slot in a methadone program and quickly obtained food stamps and general assistance funds, so she would not have to turn tricks to pay rent. Silvana seemed repentant and ready for a new life. "Nobody should have to see the kind of life I've lived in the Tenderloin," she said tearfully. "At least now I'm beginning to see an end to all this."

The end of Silvana's story, however, was no new life and was emblematic of the complicated problems that intravenous drug users presented in the AIDS epidemic. These people weren't optimistic gay men who would spend their last days doing white-light meditations with their Shanti Project volunteer; they were addicts.

With a terminal diagnosis, Tony Ford had little incentive to quit drugs, and he provided little encouragement to Silvana. Within weeks, Silvana disappeared from her drug rehabilitation program. Two months later, she was arrested for petty theft, the first of five more arrests for prostitution and drug-related charges in the next year.

Tony Ford survived four bouts with *Pneumocystis* before he died of kidney failure on June 20, 1985.

Silvana Strangis died on January 24, 1986, during the eleventh day of her first bout with cryptococcosis. Her remains were interred in the middle-class San Francisco suburb where her story had started, back when she was the beloved daughter of an Italian family and a New Age was dawning.

52 EXILES

January 20, 1985
CASTRO STREET, SAN FRANCSICO

The crowd surged up and down Castro Street, blowing horns, waving banners, and chanting the ubiquitous mantra: "We're number one. We're number one."

All day, the bars of Castro Street, like bars across the United States, were packed with fans awaiting the last touchdown. In Washington, President Reagan delayed his public inauguration by a day so he could watch the Super Bowl face-off between the San Francisco 49ers and the Miami Dolphins. Castro Street was vaguely comforted by the connection it briefly shared with the rest of the world; it was an increasingly rare feeling, now that gay people were suffering the full weight of a situation about which most heterosexuals were oblivious.

When the final pass was thrown and the 49ers had won their second Super Bowl in three years, San Francisco was engulfed in the wildest celebration since the day World War II ended. In no neighborhood was this abandon more pronounced than in the Castro, where people were grateful for any cause to celebrate. Police quickly closed Castro Street to traffic, surrendering the thoroughfare to the swelling throng, waving their red and gold banners. They climbed streetlights and even formed a cancan line atop a trolley car that was trapped amid the crowd.

From the doorway of Bear Hollow, Cleve Jones cheered the crowd on. He didn't care a whit about football, but large crowds gathered for any reason excited him. Cleve also was thrilled that twenty-one-year-old Todd Coleman had taken an inordinate interest in him. Todd had fine brown hair, beautiful eyes, and delicate features that Cleve found alluring. He also was a bona-fide fan who seemed to know everything about Cleve's life, a quality that Cleve found downright irresistible.

Cleve had met Todd in the Bear Hollow during Super Bowl halftime. Cleve pressed the young man for his phone number, but Todd was evasive, so Cleve stuck with him. When Todd and a group of friends left for a night of carousing, Cleve tagged along. Within a few hours, the pair retreated to Cleve's apartment a block off Castro Street, where they spent the night.

A few days later, Cleve was back in Bear Hollow sipping vodka tonics when he saw Todd come into the bar with a group of friends.

"See that cutie over there," Cleve said to an acquaintance, adding with a note of triumph: "I went out with him."

"Yeah, he's got AIDS," Cleve's friend said.

"What?"

Cleve's friend said Todd was living at the Shanti Project residence for homeless AIDS patients.

Suddenly, the pieces fit together. Cleve understood why Coleman was evasive about his phone number and why he seemed to know everything about Cleve's work in organizing the AIDS Foundation.

Cleve was stunned, and he later confronted Todd. The young man admitted he had AIDS. He explained that he had always admired Cleve and had followed his career for years, reading everything he could find on the young activist. As soon as he saw Cleve on Super Bowl Sunday, he'd known what he wanted to do. Cleve hadn't seduced him; he had seduced Cleve.

"Why are you behaving this way?" Cleve demanded. "You have a responsibility to your partners to let them know that you have AIDS. Even more important, you have a responsibility to protect yourself."

"They say at the Shanti Project that it's important for me to have sex," Todd said.

Cleve felt the tide of despair begin to shift again in his stomach. Everybody, it seemed, was going crazy.

For months, Cleve's spirits had been sinking. Hardly a day went by that some crony or boyfriend was not diagnosed. His own health had teetered on the brink of AIDS for a year now. He had contemplated an escape to Hawaii for months. The incident with Todd Coleman cemented his determination to leave San Francisco. Everybody was either dying or going crazy, and he'd die or go crazy too if he stayed.

Cleve periodically called his mother in Arizona to empty his heart; he called her during January, too, to tell her about the death of his old boyfriend, Felix Velarde-Munoz. Gently, Marion Jones began talking about the young men with whom she had graduated from high school over forty years before, during the darkest hours of World War II. "All the boys I knew went off to war and most of them didn't come back," she said. "The ones who did survive were damaged. That must be what it's like for you."

Cleve agreed. That was what it was like.

$$\bigcirc$$

Other thinkers in the gay community believed the homosexual plight was less like being in a war than like living with terrorism. At any time, without any coherent reason, the virus could emerge from its victims' blood and violently seize their lives. There was a terrifying amorality to the epidemic that went far beyond the articulated ideologies that clashed in war.

Gay men who had lived with terrorism in countries like Israel argued that AIDS was an even more insidious enemy. They said that people living in a country stricken by terrorism have a camaraderie, a sense that they need to stick together to survive.

But the stricken in America's gay community were exiles. Most heterosexuals cared about the epidemic only when it appeared that it might affect them. Rather than bring the nation more together, the epidemic had driven Americans further apart. To gays, who emigrated to mainstream society daily to work, the heterosexual life-style seemed surreal. Here people wondered whether they could afford a second color television set or if they should have a child. Gay life now consisted of more prosaic concerns, like whether your lover was going to die next week or if one day you would wake up and find a purple spot that foretold your own death.

Moreover, for homosexuals caught in this cruel new reality, there was no one to say, "Hang in there." Instead, there was a prevailing sentiment that was sympathetic and at times compassionate but still detached and ultimately uncaring, as if to imply that, somehow, this whole mess is your own fault.

January 23

Bill Kraus's older brother Mike had rented a limousine stocked with champagne and Edith Piaf tapes to drive Bill and his friends to San Francisco International Airport. With his new superstitious bent, Bill at first did not want to be sent off in a black car, fearing it looked like a hearse and was a bad omen. Nevertheless, he was coaxed into the backseat, and as he sipped champagne, he joked that if he were to be in exile, it might as well be Paris.

Bill's friends knew he was cloaking his fears. He had no idea whether he would be accepted into the HPA-23 trials. Even more pressing, he still didn't know whether the medication would work.

The Next Day
PARIS

Paris was in the grips of the coldest winter in a half-century when Bill and his friend Sharon Johnson arrived. The pair spent their first day finding an apartment. On the second day, they went to the World War I American military hospital on the outskirts of Paris to see Dr. Dominique Dormant about HPA-23.

Dormant already had heard about Bill Kraus's case. It struck Sharon that the Frenchman thought Bill was much more important than he actually was, an illusion Bill was not going to shatter. Dormant described the comparative benefits of AIDS drugs on trial, such as isoprinosine, interferon, ribavirin, and HPA-23.

"This is not a cure," he warned. It would only impede the virus, and Bill would probably have to stay on the drug indefinitely. The virus appeared to come back as soon as patients went off the medication, and that, most likely, would bring the demise of the patient.

"I want to try it," Bill said. "I want to live."

Dormant said Bill could take his first shot the next week.

In the United States, no issue frustrated AIDS clinicians and researchers in the early months of 1985 more than the lack of experimental treatments to offer AIDS patients. In no area of AIDS research was the paucity of funds having a more devastating impact.

Dr. Donna Mildvan at Beth Israel Medical Center in New York was receiving five calls a day, from lovers, friends, and relatives of AIDS patients, pleading for a treatment, any treatment, that might work. A day rarely went by without some mother sobbing, "Please, doctor, save my son."

Officials at the National Cancer Institute assured everyone that they were screening every possible drug for experimental trials in AIDS patients. What they didn't reveal was that this federal screening program consisted of Dr. Sam Broder and two technicians; a federal hiring freeze prevented the NCI from augmenting this program.

The lack of trained retrovirologists and money for retrovirology labs also proved an impenetrable barrier to drug testing. To determine whether an anti-viral drug was any good at halting viral replication, scientists needed to perform viral isolations on every patient. The cost of one such isolation was $700. Even the NCI, which had the largest budget of any medical research institution in the world, found the cost of extensive drug testing and viral isolations to be prohibitive. Even if the money did exist, there were few facilities capable of performing the isolations and few retrovirologists to do the work. In New York City, for example, there was only one laboratory capable of performing the LAV viral isolations.

The lack of such laboratories was a legacy of the cutbacks of the first years of the Reagan administration. In the early 1980s, when retrovirology grants dried up, scientists simply stopped learning how to be retrovirologists. There wasn't any future in it. Now, research institutions across the nation were desperate for retrovirologists, but there were few to hire. It would take years to train scientists and establish laboratories, once funds were made available.

When the NIH held a meeting in Bethesda to discuss drug studies, Don Francis complained, "We don't need more meetings. We need labs, and we need money."

Neither, however, were forthcoming.

DUBLIN STREET, SAN FRANCISCO

"I feel like a leper," Frances Borchelt told her husband and children when she returned from the hospital. "None of the family will come to see me. I don't want to go out of the house."

"Don't be depressed, Mom," Cathy Borchelt answered. "Get angry. We're going to fight this."

Frances didn't feel angry. She felt tired and ill and alone. Although her psoriasis had receded while she was undergoing antibiotic treatment for *Pneumocystis,* it returned virulently when Frances got home. When Cathy helped her mother into her first shower after leaving the hospital, she was staggered at her mother's appearance. Frances had shrunk to ninety-eight pounds. Her tailbone protruded from her baggy skin. Cathy thought she looked like the pictures of concentration camp victims she had seen in World War II books.

The family soon fell into the same confusion that gay men had faced about their own vulnerability to the syndrome. The doctors told them to take precautions, not to use the same dishes as Frances and to wear gloves when they washed her dishes and laundry. For all they knew, they might already have been infected with the virus. There was no testing yet to calm their fears.

Cathy started researching transfusion AIDS. Dr. Marcus Conant told her about the T-cell tests at Stanford University and the controversy about hepatitis core antibody testing. Conant also told her the family should hire a lawyer.

"Why didn't anybody do anything?" Cathy asked friends.

By coincidence, a series of dramatic transfusion-AIDS stories seized public attention in San Francisco during the early months of 1985. One was a Roman Catholic nun, Sister Romana Marie Ryan, who had broken her hip while sliding into home base during a softball game. During a hip replacement operation in July 1983, the sixty-six-year-old sister was transfused with infected blood. When announcing the death, her priest said Ryan had spent her final days in "excruciating pain," praying for the person who donated the blood to her and for all people who were suffering from AIDS.

Such stories raised the stakes in the drama unfolding around the release of the HTLV-III antibody test. On January 31, Dr. Mervyn Silverman made good on his promise to announce the objections of the American Public Health Association and the U.S. Conference of Local Health Officers. The groups wanted funding for the alternative test sites for AIDS blood tests, Silverman announced, and the federal government's refusal to provide them could result in the contamination of the blood supply.

The officials at Secretary Heckler's office and the FDA had avoided making any decision on funds for the alternative test sites during the months of negotiations, but they were on the phone to Silverman within an hour of the first reports of his press statements, assuring him they would make $12 million available for the program. Then they delayed release of the test for two weeks so the program could be put in place.

Although this settled the public health questions surrounding the test's licensure, it did not resolve the civil rights questions that troubled gay leaders. The federal government had made no provisions about confidentiality of blood test results. As battle lines hardened, the conflict became a classic confrontation of public health and civil liberties. The Lambda Legal Defense Fund, a New York–based gay legal group, threatened to block release of the test in court. How could the government release a test that could have such devastating impact on so many American lives, without any safeguards? they asked. At the CDC, doctors who had worked on transfusion-AIDS research were dumbfounded. How could these people threaten to halt a test that could clearly save lives? By mid-February, the two sides had reached a standoff.

University of California, San Francisco

For the past year, the cooperation that had marked the relationship between Marc Conant's AIDS Clinical Research Center at UCSF and San Francisco General Hospital had been dissipating. With the hospital's growing international reputation and prestige, its researchers had developed leverage for their own government grants. They also were mindful that the focus of local AIDS work had shifted to the county hospital in large part because UCSF officials were uncomfortable with the UC Medical Center becoming a focus for AIDS studies.

Marc Conant continued to argue that the medical center should carry more of the city's AIDS burden, if for no other reason than because of its geographic location on the edge of the largest concentration of gay men in the Western world. Conant's own influence, however, was waning. Ever since he had gone directly to the legislature for state research funding, over the heads of UC administrators, he was something of a marked man at the university. And so he was not surprised to be told at a meeting, on a cold January day, that it would be best for the university if he resigned as director of the Clinical Research Center. The university, of course, presented reasonable arguments as to why Conant should step down. He was a clinical professor, and the center would have more eminence if the title of director was conferred on a full professor with broader scientific credentials, they said.

Virtually everyone close to AIDS research, however, knew the other reasons for the shift. University officials continued to worry that they were losing top applicants for residencies because of San Francisco's reputation as the center of the AIDS epidemic. Four years of Conant's dire predictions had succeeded in convincing university officials of the skyrocketing number of AIDS cases that would come from the nearby Castro neighborhood, so the future did not look more promising to anxious UCSF administrators. Other UCSF scientists were being told to tone down their AIDS pronouncements, and enthusiasm for AIDS research dropped among university officials. Removing Conant would rid the university of a troublesome maverick whose priorities did not lie within academic politics.

The university no longer had to worry about the political ramifications in the gay community of Conant's departure. Conant's role in opposing bathhouses and pushing for an aggressive education campaign had made him persona non grata among most gay political leaders as well as among the gay doctors in the Bay Area Physicians for Human Rights. Hardly an issue of the *Bay Area Reporter* came out without some personal attack on Conant.

The dean who accepted Conant's resignation assured Conant that it was what was best. Conant recalled, however, that this was the dean who also once observed, "At least with AIDS, a lot of undesirable people will be eliminated."

UNIVERSITY OF CALIFORNIA,
<u>LOS ANGELES</u>

Dr. Michael Gottlieb had spent the past two years pleading for an AIDS clinic, but UCLA administrators wanted no part of it. When they finally gave him an office in which to see his patients, Gottlieb could scarcely believe the site—in the corner of the old Veterans Administration Hospital that had been largely abandoned when the newer hospital was built next door. A trip to Gottlieb's office took patients through a dusty and deserted lobby and down dank hallways past gutted rooms. At the sound of footsteps, huge cockroaches scurried out of the walls, many of which were torn apart. This clearly was a place for patients the university was not enthralled about treating. Gottlieb had to remind himself that the University of California system was not one of the worst places for AIDS research; it was among the best.

January 29
<u>SAN FRANCISCO DEPARTMENT OF PUBLIC HEALTH</u>

As the newly formed San Francisco Health Commission began its first meeting, member Jim Foster looked wearily toward the succession of civil liberties lawyers and gay activists who had come to argue against the ban on "high-risk sex" at the city's bathhouses. The debate was rapidly growing moot, Foster knew. Only three of the city's eleven bathhouses were still in business; the owners, who were funding the new Committee to Preserve Our Sexual and Civil Liberties, were here to argue against the sex regulations.

Jim Foster certainly understood the group's rhetoric. As a father of San Francisco gay politics, founder of both the pioneering Society for Individual Rights and the Toklas Democratic Club, Foster had fashioned much of the sexual liberation ideology that bathhouse owners were now championing.

But the words rang hollow to Foster today, and he wondered how gay men at this time and in this place could ask public commissions to campaign for their right to unlimited sex.

Thirty hours before this commission meeting convened, Jim Foster had been in his comfortable Victorian home on Eddy Street, holding the hand of Larry Ludwig, his lover of twelve years. After suffering the ravages of Kaposi's sarcoma for seventeen months, Larry had slipped into a coma. At midnight, Larry took four deep labored breaths and then breathed no more.

It was a horrible moment, and it was a beautiful moment, Jim Foster thought. He certainly had not helped build a gay community so that his generation would spend its middle age in death vigils. Yet, through the ordeal, Foster had seen the incredible courage of people like Larry, and he had experienced the compassion with which gay men were helping each other through this collective trauma. Foster sensed that there was a new community emerging from the AIDS tragedy. It was not the community of politicians or radicals talking about bathhouses, but of people who had learned to take responsibility for themselves and for each other.

This is what a community really is, Foster thought. And ultimately that was what he had been fighting for in all those years of gay politicking: the opportunity for gay people to enjoy their own community. Now, against this backdrop of tragedy, that community was being forged.

After presentation to the health commission, the leaders of the Committee to Preserve Our Sexual and Civil Liberties were shocked when this elder statesman of San Francisco gay politics dismissed them with the comment that their concerns were "trivial."

January 31
CENTERS FOR DISEASE CONTROL,
ATLANTA

Don Francis had finally completed his nine-page program: "Operation AIDS Control." Warning that between 20,000 and 50,000 deaths could be expected from AIDS within "the next few years," Francis had designed a plan that employed the only two weapons with which health authorities could fight the epidemic—blood testing and education. Francis wanted to begin a six-month program to test blood collected at drug treatment centers and venereal disease clinics. The imminent licensure of the HTLV-III test meant that, finally, the CDC could get an accurate grasp on how far the virus had penetrated American society. They could also start warning infected people that they carried the virus and, most significantly, that they were capable of transmitting it to others.

Francis also recommended education programs to reduce sexual transmission that were tailored for the various risk groups—gay men, drug users, and promiscuous heterosexuals. To slow down the soaring births of AIDS babies, the government must begin advising female intravenous drug users on how to avoid pregnancy. Gay men should be encouraged to know their antibody status, Francis wrote, and be tested through confidential programs outside of blood banks. Not until authorities could determine who was infected, and who was not, could they begin to reduce the number of newly infected people through education.

Francis knew that his proposal was fraught with political problems. Gay groups would object to his call for widespread testing of gay men. Conservatives would object to AIDS education programs. Already, he had noted that the federal government had all but refused to start any AIDS education programs for fear that conservatives would object to government instructions on how to have safe gay sex. The only education the government had thus far paid for was a small amount channeled through the U.S. Conference of Mayors.

Even the release of the CDC's data on the possible uses of nonoxynol-9 became mired in controversy. In late 1984, a researcher in Francis's lab ran tests that showed that nonoxynol-9, the spermicidal ingredient in birth-control foams, successfully killed the AIDS virus in test tubes. Francis was excited about the finding, since it finally presented gays with something constructive they could do to save their lives. Using nonoxynol-9 with a condom could help prevent transmission, Francis thought, and he wanted the findings released immediately. But Jim Curran had stalled publication because a number of scientists listed as senior authors on the paper were unsure of the study's methodology. Curran did not want bad science coming out of the CDC that could later be used to attack the agency. Francis suspected politics. The federal government didn't want to concede the value of nonoxynol-9 because that might be interpreted as condoning anal sex.

To some extent, other CDC staffers noted that the conflicts between Don Francis and Jim Curran reflected the underlying tension between Francis's approach to epidemics and Curran's. Under Curran's leadership, the CDC had done an admirable job of collecting AIDS data. He had guided CDC AIDS research on a course that he felt was the best that could be done in a conservative administration.

Francis remained the idealist oriented toward stopping the epidemic. He felt that the CDC had surrendered its role in controlling AIDS in favor of providing the most up-to-date body counts. He also understood that he was losing his battle. "Operation AIDS Control" was his last-ditch proposal to get the CDC in a control modality. The price tag on the program was $32.8 million. Although this was far more than what the federal government had spent for all CDC AIDS research in the past year, Francis thought the cost was modest compared to the billions of dollars in health care costs and prevention programs that would be needed in years to come if the government did not get serious about AIDS today.

On January 30, the day that Don Francis submitted his proposal, the CDC released figures showing that, in the previous week, the nation's AIDS caseload had surpassed 8,000.

February 4
THE CAPITOL,
WASHINGTON, D.C.

Even the most cynical critics of the Reagan administration were staggered when the Office of Management and Budget released its proposed AIDS budget for the 1986 fiscal year. Not only had the administration *not* increased AIDS funding but the budget called for reducing AIDS spending from the current level of $96 million to $85.5 million in the next fiscal year. The 10 percent reduction would be felt across the board in AIDS research but most heavily at the CDC, where funds would be cut back 20 percent to just $18.7 million. The government's planned appropriation for education aimed specifically at the gay community was $250,000, which, again, was to be channeled through the U.S. Conference of Mayors in an effort to ensure that no federal agency was in the business of telling gays how to perform sodomy safely. Altogether, about 5 percent of the AIDS budget would go to AIDS prevention and education efforts.

The cuts came at an inopportune time. Secretary Margaret Heckler had let it be known to gay leaders that she did not want to use her political capital to fight for AIDS funding in the administration when she knew that Congress was going to allocate more funds anyway. As it was, Heckler's stock in the administration had dropped precipitously. In Virginia, Margaret Heckler's husband of thirty-one years was suing for divorce, claiming, among other things, that Margaret had ceased having marital relations with him twenty-two years ago. Margaret, who was a devout Roman Catholic, had refused to get a divorce, he said, because she felt it would hurt her political career. Gay leaders were aghast at the thought that someone who apparently had had no sex since 1963 was presiding over the government's AIDS fight, and the administration was said to be extremely embarrassed by the publicity. Ironically, Secretary Heckler also was criticized within the administration for doing too much on AIDS. Other conservative administration officials were angry at Heckler for the high profile she had taken on the issue. Rumors abounded that the secretary was on her way out.

The Office of Management and Budget was tired of the repeated HHS requests for budget augmentations. As far as they were concerned, Heckler could do whatever she wished with the $8 billion pot of money the administration allocated to all the nation's health agencies. It wasn't that they didn't want to give her more money to spend on AIDS; they just didn't want to give her more money. Budget officials thought the directors of the NCI, CDC, and NIAID tried to gain new money for AIDS research because they were too cowardly to tell their own scientists that their pet projects needed to be cut in favor of AIDS studies.

In Congress, many of the congressional aides were beginning to balk. It had been their behind-the-scenes maneuvering that had secured added appropriations for AIDS research in previous years, and some of them now confided to the National Gay Task Force co-director, Jeff Levi, that they were tired of making President Reagan look good. It seemed that no matter how much administration officials worked to oppose funding initiatives on Capitol Hill, they were always ready to take credit for the research advances that resulted from funds that were provided.

No congressional spokesperson for AIDS issues had yet emerged in either the Senate or the House of Representatives. Most AIDS legislation was handled by Representatives Henry Waxman of Los Angeles or Ted Weiss of New York City, but both were subcommittee chairmen with other issues to attend to. Neither of San Francisco's two representatives, Barbara Boxer or Sala Burton, had made AIDS their top priority; they focused instead on environmental and defense issues. Without a legislative spokesperson, the work for getting AIDS money would again fall to such gay lobbyists as Jeff Levi and a handful of key congressional aides, such as Tim Westmoreland. AIDS remained something of an orphan issue in Congress. Neither the staggering AIDS caseload nor the increasingly apocalyptic predictions of future deaths made much difference.

◯

On the same day the Reagan administration released its budget, health authorities in Hong Kong announced the diagnosis of the first case of AIDS on the Asian mainland. The forty-six-year-old Chinese seaman had spent a vacation in Miami last year, officials said, and now was near death in a Hong Kong hospital.

The AIDS epidemic had now spread to every populated continent on the planet.

CENTERS FOR DISEASE CONTROL, ATLANTA

The chief assistant to Dr. Walt Dowdle, director of the Center for Infectious Diseases, encountered Don Francis in a hallway at CDC headquarters.

He gave Francis the verdict on his ambitious "Operation AIDS Control." The CDC didn't have the funds to finance the project.

The recommendation to Francis was, "Do as little as possible but look like you're doing a lot."

Francis had decided what he would do if he could not initiate his AIDS-control effort. He couldn't stand spending more time banging his head against the administration's stone wall. As it was, the AIDS efforts at the CDC were being reorganized into a separate branch, and the epidemiology and lab work were being merged. It was a convenient time for him to depart. He had informally lined up a new job as CDC liaison on AIDS to the California Department of Health Services. He was going to leave Atlanta.

$\boxed{53\ \text{RECKONING}}$

February 8, 1985
HARLEY HOTEL,
NEW YORK CITY

Dr. Joseph Sonnabend looked troubled. The panel of journalists, which included most of the nation's leading reporters on the AIDS epidemic, looked confused.

"The implications are terribly important," said Sonnabend cautiously.

Sonnabend, one of New York City's leading AIDS doctors, was trying to explain the significance of an earlier presentation by Dr. Luc Montagnier in the day-long AIDS conference co-sponsored by the AIDS Medical Foundation and the Scientists' Institute for Public Information.

In his patrician, professorial manner, Montagnier had described the genetic sequencing the Pasteur Institute had performed on the prototypes of the three AIDS viruses, LAV, HTLV-III, and Jay Levy's ARV. The gene sequences of the French LAV and ARV varied by about 6 percent, which was normal, the scientists at the conference agreed. The genes of any two different isolates of the same virus are expected to deviate from each other, usually by 6 to 20 percent. Montagnier's lips tightened, however, when he said flatly that the genetic sequence of the HTLV-III prototype isolate had varied from LAV by less than one percent.

Those words started the AIDS researchers present mumbling among themselves, even while the reporters yawned. Journalists had long assumed HTLV-III, LAV, and ARV were all different names for one virus. The reporters, however, were missing the point.

"It would appear that HTLV and LAV are too identical," Sonnabend said, stepping delicately around the fundamental issue. "They are identical to a degree that would not be anticipated with two independent isolates from the same family."

The reporters still didn't get it. The doctors did, but they were afraid to say it aloud.

"Would you be brave enough to voice explicitly the implication of what you're saying here?" one doctor shouted to Sonnabend.

"No, I wouldn't," Sonnabend answered. "I'm not the right person to be saying that."

"Neither am I," the other doctor said.

"What are you talking about here?" asked the Associated Press reporter. "Do you know something that you're not saying?"

"They appear to be the same actual isolate," Sonnabend finally said. "Or some strange coincidence."

"What are you suggesting?" somebody asked.

Dr. Mathilde Krim, who had organized the conference, stepped to the microphone.

"Dr. Montagnier," she said, "felt very appropriately that he was not the person to point this out."

"Nobody's pointed it out quite exactly yet," said one of the exasperated reporters.

"It's perhaps a complicated notion for you to understand," Krim said, "but I think you are coming close."

Veteran science writer Donald Drake of the *Philadelphia Inquirer* was one of the two or three journalists in the room who understood the implications of Sonnabend's remarks.

"Are you suggesting that Gallo swiped his virus from the French?" Drake asked.

"Or Montagnier swiped Gallo's virus, or we are dealing with a very strange coincidence," said Sonnabend diplomatically.

"A light bulb goes off," said the *San Francisco Chronicle* reporter on the panel.

The reporters now understood what the scientists had been discussing in Harley Hotel hallways all day. In the world of virology, it was inconceivable that there could be a genetic variation of less than one percent between two different viral isolates. That would be like finding two identical snowflakes. It simply didn't happen.

What made the similarities more unlikely was that the prototype isolates of LAV and HTLV-III were supposed to have been taken seventeen months apart, from two different men living on two different continents. The only way to account for the identical properties of the two prototypes was if they were the same virus taken from the same person.

Montagnier knew enough about the chronology of Gallo's discovery to be suspicious, although he never publicly made the accusation himself. Even by Gallo's own account, he did not isolate HTLV-III until late 1983—well after September 1983 when the Pasteur Institute sent him LAV samples. To both the French researchers and many of the AIDS doctors at the conference that day, Montagnier's comparisons indicated that the NCI prototype of HTLV-III, announced in April 1984, could have been grown from the same virus the French had cultured in January 1983. If it had, this had the makings of a scientific scandal of immense proportions.

On a number of counts, the AIDS Medical Foundation conference in New York on that bitterly cold Friday in February delivered the first sign of what was to come in the AIDS epidemic. The butcher's bill was so high that long-tolerated transgressions could no longer be ignored. Reckoning was at hand.

Always looking for a new way to interest reporters in the epidemic, Krim had put together this conference in an attempt to get the crème de la crème of AIDS scientists and AIDS journalists into one room. Hidden agendas abounded, and many of the key AIDS players who had first committed themselves to attend the conference suddenly took waivers.

At the last minute, for example, Secretary Heckler canceled her keynote address, pleading the flu. Maybe it was because she had heard that Krim planned to talk about the "fabricated figures" the federal government was using to justify its claims that it was spending enough on AIDS research. And Dr. Robert Gallo had also canceled at the last minute.

Pasteur researcher Jean-Claude Chermann attended the conference to present data on the promise of HPA-23 experiments. Not coincidentally, Krim and other New York clinicians were spending substantial time pleading with a reluctant FDA to speed approvals on experimental treatments for AIDS drugs. Meanwhile, Montagnier's talk on the genetic properties of LAV came as a growing body of evidence was accumulating in support of his contention that LAV was not a leukemia virus related to the HTLV family but a lentivirus, as the French had long maintained. The issue now was of more than academic interest, given the fact that some AIDS researchers were diverting their attention to studies on HTLV-I and HTLV-II in hopes that these allegedly related viruses might yield answers to the mysteries of HTLV-III infection. Clearly, such work was wasted if HTLV-III was wholly unrelated to the other HTLV viruses. There were significant points of prestige in this as well, now that Stockholm Fever had swept the small community of AIDS researchers.

And, of course, the appearance of Chermann and Montagnier at the conference was also an attempt to bridge the simmering rivalry between the Pasteur Institute and the National Cancer Institute. Dr. Gallo's abrupt cancelation infuriated Krim, who opened the conference with the observation, "This rivalry stands in the way of the truth and understanding. Dr. Gallo has slapped all of us in the face and apparently does not have the courage to face this group. We will prevail."

Given her years of efforts in trying to interest New York City government in planning for the epidemic, Krim also wanted a public airing of local health policy issues in a two-person panel featuring New York City Health Commissioner David Sencer and Dr. Mervyn Silverman, who just three weeks before had left his post as San Francisco public health director. With the bathhouse issue resolved, Silverman was increasingly considered something of a sainted figure by AIDS clinicians across the country, particularly in New York. After all, Silverman had actually spent money on AIDS facilities and education programs. His past sins of indecision seemed almost trivial next to Sencer, who was asked to explain why it was good public policy not to spend a dime on AIDS education, patient services, or coordination of treatment facilities. In case the more obvious irony of the Silverman-Sencer pairing was not detected, Larry Kramer was on hand to shout a not-so-dispassionate commentary on Sencer's performance from the back of the room. Silverman was embarrassed for Sencer and uncomfortable himself, feeling he had been an unwitting part of a plan to set up the New York health commissioner. However, the time for Sencer's embarrassment, it turned out, was just beginning.

Public Theater,
Manhattan

Dr. Emma Brookner looked up from her wheelchair. Her voice wavered between weariness and despair, like the voices of many doctors who had spent years tending AIDS patients in this city without a heart.

"Before a vaccine can be discovered, almost every gay man will be exposed," she said. "Ned, your organization is worthless. I went up and down Christopher Street last night, and all I saw was guys going into bars alone and coming out with somebody. And outside the baths, all I saw was lines of guys going in. Why aren't you telling them bluntly? 'Stop!' Every day you don't tell them, more people infect each other."

Ned Weeks understood the frustration.

"Don't lecture me," he said. "I'm on your side. Remember?"

"Don't be on my side," Brookner shot back. "I don't need you on my side. Make your side shape up. I've seen 238 cases—me, one doctor. You make it sound like it's nothing worse going around than the measles."

"They wouldn't print what I wrote," Ned confessed. "Again."

Suddenly, all action stopped and the cast went on a break, and Larry Kramer stared at the empty stage. At times, rehearsals of *The Normal Heart* took on a surreal quality for Kramer. This was his life. He, of course, was Ned Weeks, the protagonist who storms and shouts his way through the first years of the epidemic in New York City. Dr. Emma Brookner, battling both an unresponsive federal government and a lethargic city health establishment, was based on the wheelchair-bound pioneer of AIDS work in New York, Dr. Linda Laubenstein. The play faithfully recalled every obstacle Kramer had faced in his years of AIDS activism, drawing a particularly detailed portrait of the foibles and failings of Gay Men's Health Crisis and its leaders.

Kramer hoped desperately that he might accomplish as a playwright what he had failed to do as an activist—to move New York and its gay community into action against AIDS. The play delivered a devastating indictment of official indifference at City Hall. Mayor Koch's supporters spread word that Joseph Papp was only producing the show to even an old score he held against the mayor. Kramer suspected that the Koch administration might well respond to this latest onslaught the way it had answered every criticism of its AIDS policy in past years, by ignoring it or stonewalling. He also knew that, at last, events were conspiring to force the city to take up arms against the disease.

The changing face of the AIDS epidemic in the city heralded serious consequences if AIDS prevention programs continued to be deferred. More than anywhere else in the country, AIDS in New York City was no longer just a gay problem. The proportion of cases among heterosexual intravenous drug users had increased by one-third in just one year. With the epidemic entrenched in the underclass, the new AIDS stats for January 1985 revealed that for the first time, a majority—54 percent—of New York City's AIDS cases were nonwhite.

The proliferation of AIDS among drug addicts bred a host of related social problems, because drug users were the major vector through which the epidemic could spread into the heterosexual population. Most of the city's AIDS babies were born to drug-using parents, and virtually all the cases of heterosexual transmission were among the female sexual partners of minority drug users. Already, AIDS clinicians working with drug addicts worried that the disease would become endemic to the East Coast poor. Dr. Arye Rubinstein was afraid that the virus would spread from addicts into high schools, where it could proliferate among sexually active teens. He called for aggressive AIDS education in schools, a proposal for which he was dismissed as an "alarmist."

Concern about how the city would logistically handle the mounting AIDS caseload had finally gone beyond AIDS clinicians and into city government. In late January, a seven-member delegation of city health officials traveled to California to investigate San Francisco's network of AIDS patient services and community programs. Like an unofficial fact-finding delegation that Dr. Krim had headed late the year before, the city delegation returned to New York proposing AIDS education and treatment programs based on the San Francisco model. Their fifty-nine-page report, which had been forwarded to Commissioner Sencer, stated bluntly that New York "must" start long-range and short-term planning, warning that AIDS "has the very real potential to be crippling to the city's hospital system."

Meanwhile, the city's bathhouse policy also came under greater scrutiny. The *Village Voice,* which had only recently discovered the epidemic, engendered the bathhouse controversy by doing something that no gay newspaper had dared to do—it printed arguments on both sides of the issue. In a long letter published in the *Voice,* Michael Callen, a man with AIDS who served on the New York State AIDS Advisory Council, recounted how gay political leaders had subverted his attempts to discuss bathhouse closure at the state council. It didn't help matters much when Sencer based his arguments against closure on a study done by a city epidemiologist, Alan Krystal, that said that closing the bathhouses would only reduce the spread of AIDS by one-quarter of one percent. The organization that had financed part of Krystal's research, it turned out, was the Northern California Bathhouse Owners Association.

To his friends, David Sencer was a man whose career seemed cursed by bad timing and a penchant for bumbling. As a former director of the Centers for Disease Control, he had presided over an internal investigation of the infamous Tuskegee experimentation in which a group of poor Southern blacks with syphilis were left untreated so doctors could study the long-term effects of the disease. Even as disclosure of the study threatened a scandal, Sencer opposed ending it. Sencer later presided over the swine flu epidemic and had personally persuaded then President Gerald Ford to launch the ambitious swine flu vaccination campaign. Unfortunately, the flu epidemic never happened and more people died from the vaccinations than the disease itself. For his aggressiveness, Sencer lost his job.

Sencer came to New York City as health commissioner in early 1982, when a handful of AIDS cases heralded the start of a new epidemic. Almost from the start, Mayor Koch had put city AIDS policy under Sencer's sole authority. As late as February 1985, Koch still refused to answer reporters' questions about the handling of AIDS in New York, referring all queries to Sencer. For his part, the commissioner demonstrated throughout the epidemic that he was not about to repeat the mistake that had cost him his job at the CDC. Rather than err on the side of action, Sencer had spent the epidemic erring on the side of inaction, comforting himself with the notion that at least he was not feeding panic. For years, this posture had largely spared Sencer the wrath of the gay community, Larry Kramer notwithstanding, since local gays were more concerned with the politics of AIDS than its medicine. And Sencer rarely fell prey to a critical press because mainstream newspapers weren't writing much about AIDS anyway.

Conditions, however, were deteriorating for Sencer in the early months of 1985. In January, he faced tough questioning at a city council hearing called by council members who were worried that the issue might come up in elections. When pressed to state what the city was spending on AIDS, Sencer said it was "about $1 million a year." He could not say where the money was being spent, however, and maintained that it would be impossible to make that determination.

Sencer's subsequent appearance on a panel with Dr. Silverman also proved a major embarrassment. Within a few days, Sencer's public relations aide was telling reporters that they could not interview Sencer if they were going to try to draw direct comparisons between San Francisco and New York.

On the morning of February 12, Commissioner Sencer agreed to meet with a reporter from the *San Francisco Chronicle* to discuss the public health response of New York City to the AIDS epidemic. On the way into the commissioner's office, the reporter passed Drs. Mathilde Krim, Michael Lange, and Joyce Wallace. In the previous days, the three physicians had talked at length to the reporter about the nightmare unfolding in New York because of the city's slothful response to AIDS. As they left the office, they whispered to the reporter that they had spent the past hour trying to persuade Sencer to do something, without any success. Once in Sencer's office, the reporter laid out the criticisms leveled at the city in words that hardly varied from what Sencer had just heard moments before.

"I'm not aware of these problems," Sencer said flatly. "Nobody has ever brought these matters to my attention."

As for AIDS education, Sencer maintained that the city had done enough. "The people of New York City who need to know already know all they need to know about AIDS," he said.

Sencer dismissed suggestions that AIDS was a "crisis" in the city. Everything was under control, he said.

In that week of February 1985, while the official position of New York City was that the AIDS epidemic was not yet a crisis, the number of the city's AIDS cases surpassed 3,000.

A week later, the first series of newspaper articles investigating New York's response to the AIDS epidemic were published, not in New York, but in the *San Francisco Chronicle.*

◯

By now, AIDS education had emerged as a volatile issue in all the cities hard hit by the epidemic. Although the conservative Los Angeles County Board of Supervisors had still not allocated any funds for AIDS education, state grants had financed an ambitious "L.A. Cares" advertising campaign for AIDS information. Billboards, posters, and gay newspaper advertisements showed a short mother in an apron shaking a wooden spoon at a hunky young son and giving such admonishments as "Play safely" and "Don't forget your rubbers."

By definition, however, such AIDS prevention campaigns frankly discussed a subject about which the mainstream society was skittish—sex. The AIDS Project–Los Angeles spent months in meetings with the Rapid Transit District before they got approval to put the signs on buses. Only one television station would air the APLA public service announcement on AIDS. All other television stations in the Los Angeles area refused, citing considerations of taste. It became something of a joke in AIDS circles that the epidemic would mark the first time that homosexuals died from lack of good taste.

When the San Diego AIDS Project started its "Ban-AIDS" campaign, it found opposition from an even more unusual corner. Johnson & Johnson used a "cease and desist order" to halt the campaign, claiming the "Ban-AIDS" slogan was an infringement on their trademark "Band-Aids."

February 21
RAYBURN HOUSE OFFICE BUILDING,
WASHINGTON, D.C.

AIDS was becoming a big enough story that the television cameras arrived at 9:45 sharp for the start of an unusual joint congressional hearing of the two House subcommittees chaired by Henry Waxman and Ted Weiss. Centers for Disease Control Director James Mason, who had served as Acting Assistant Secretary for Health since Edward Brandt's resignation, sat uncomfortably with other administration officials. He knew that Waxman and Weiss had come armed with more than the usual Democratic accusations of administration indifference; instead, they had a potent report drafted by the Office of Technology Assessment, the highly respected arm of Congress that is mandated to offer legislators nonpartisan analyses of complicated scientific issues. The OTA's 158-page "Review of the Public Health Service's Response to AIDS" completed the most extensive investigation yet undertaken on federal AIDS policy. It also was the reason that Dr. Mason was looking uncomfortable in the hearing room.

"The OTA finds that while the federal government has designated AIDS our country's number-one health priority, increases in funding specifically for AIDS activities have come at the initiative of Congress, and PHS agencies have had difficulties in planning their AIDS-related activities because of uncertainties over budget and personnel allocations," the report concluded.

With scores of footnotes, charts, and graphs, the report recounted in excruciating detail every twist in the sad tale of federal AIDS funding. The study documented the problems the CDC and the NIH faced in securing funds through each year of the epidemic, even while HHS officials solemnly talked of their top priority. The bitter rivalry that had engulfed federal AIDS agencies, particularly the ongoing disputes between the NCI and CDC, also were laid bare. Most striking, however, was the revelation that the government still had not created any serious, long-range plan for how it intended to fight and prevent AIDS in future years. Instead, the epidemic seemed to be handled haphazardly from year to year, with programs set not by health officials but by the budget cutters at the OMB.

"The Reagan administration has pretended that AIDS is only a blip on the charts, a statistic that they hope will go away," said Waxman when he opened the hearing. "Under the best epidemic projections, by the beginning of the next presidential campaign, AIDS will have killed as many people as the war in Vietnam. We cannot stand by and let those Americans die."

Privately, Dr. Mason had long felt torn over AIDS funding. He felt a duty to be loyal to the Reagan administration, but he also knew that an AIDS solution required more resources. The money the administration had budgeted for AIDS in the next year, he knew, was horribly inadequate. At least while Dr. Brandt was Assistant Secretary for Health, Mason could be confident that a proponent for AIDS funding was working in Washington. The administration, however, still had not bothered to find a permanent replacement for Brandt, leaving Mason to catch the flak. Like a good soldier, he did.

"We agree with the OTA report that the number of AIDS cases is increasing rapidly and there is a real possibility that the infection may spread beyond current groups at risk," Mason testified. "We are gearing up for a prolonged battle against AIDS."

Mason pointed to the "spectacular" advances made against the disease. "Never before in the history of medicine has so much been learned about an entirely new disease in so short a time," he said. As for the $10 million reductions that the administration sought for AIDS funding in the next year, Mason was left to weakly argue that funds did not have to increase on a "one-to-one relationship" with AIDS cases.

After nearly four years of work on AIDS issues, Waxman aide Tim Westmoreland felt vindicated to see the truth of the administration's duplicity on AIDS policy revealed as graphically as it was in the OTA report. The reporters would never be able to ignore this now.

Although the real blood and guts of the hearing would come in the cross-examination, thirty minutes into the hearing, the television crews started packing up. They had enough footage for their two-minute stories, and that was all they needed.

As the crews trooped out, Waxman was chiding Mason for the budget reductions. Who decided spending, Waxman asked, doctors in the PHS or accountants at OMB?

Of the AIDS funding figures, Mason said, "We did not write them—they were numbers that were written down."

The reporters, however, weren't around to hear this. Once again, the media response to the OTA report and the hearing on the report was truly underwhelming. The *Washington Post* ignored the report altogether. In *The New York Times,* the report merited six paragraphs on page fourteen, which were not published until four days after the report was released.

⊂⊃

Although the administration did not have to fret about reporters investigating their decision making, the report did make some impact on Washington in the weeks that followed, largely because of OTA's credibility in government. Mason was embarrassed at having to defend the administration against such an overwhelming collection of evidence. After the hearing, the National Gay Task Force co-director, Jeff Levi, overheard Mason mutter, "I'm never going to be put in a situation like this again." No longer satisfied to leave AIDS budget matters to Secretary Heckler, who clearly held little clout in the administration, Mason began showing up at the New Executive Office Building, where the OMB accountants worked with their spread sheets. AIDS was like a snowball going downhill, he warned them. It just kept getting bigger and bigger, and it wasn't going to go away.

⊂⊃

One hundred callers a day flooded the phone lines at the AIDS Medical Foundation offices in the weeks after Jean-Claude Chermann's presentation at the AMF conference about HPA-23. In Paris, Dominique Dormant was awakened in the middle of the night at his home by American AIDS patients desperate for treatments and irritatingly ignorant of European time zones. One American man called from the airport, pleading for treatment. He required an ambulance just to get to the hospital and proved too sick to be put on any experimental drug. He died in Paris ten days later.

French scientists warned that the Pasteur Institute was not a temple where an instant AIDS cure could be found, and some resented the U.S. government for placing such a low priority on AIDS treatments that Americans were embarking on the overseas hegira for HPA-23. "The United States is not a Third World country," said Dr. Philippe Sansonetti of the Pasteur. "I don't like the idea of being, sort of, Lourdes."

Jean-Claude Chermann, Donna Mildvan, and Michael Lange had traveled to Washington to meet with FDA officials about speeding approval for HPA-23 and other drugs, but the federal agency was in no hurry. AIDS scientists across the country were convinced that the FDA would make AIDS treatments follow the same luxuriously paced experimentation it required of all drugs. The slow early trials were designed to weed out substances that might have harmful side effects, they noted. AIDS doctors argued that this was a prudent course of action for diet pills or drugs to treat hypertension in middle-aged women, but it made little sense when it was plain that whatever the long-term side effects of these treatments might be, they were no more deleterious than the long-term side effect of untreated AIDS.

American officials, however, were suspicious of the rush to Paris for AIDS treatments. Dr. Mason felt that the French wanted to introduce HPA-23 into the United States because they knew that the FDA would require the kinds of controlled studies that were impossible to conduct in France. Only such strictly supervised tests would determine whether HPA-23 actually did any good. Some researchers thought that the only reason the French permitted Americans to participate in HPA-23 trials was because they knew it would increase political pressure on U.S. authorities to allow the drug into their country.

Treatment dilemmas sharply divided physicians. Some believed that every AIDS patient should be afforded some kind of treatment, even if its value was unproved. The *New York Native* even called on gays to stop cooperating with federal epidemiological studies if the government did not place higher priorities on treatment research. "It seems like a fair deal," the paper editorialized. "We give them epidemiology and they stop dragging their feet on treatment." However, other doctors hearkened back to the basic tenet of the Oath of Hippocrates: "Primum, non nocare," or, "First, do no harm."

Limited studies of an experimental drug on fifteen patients were, in fact, broad enough to determine whether drugs were effective, these doctors argued. It made more sense to try the drugs on limited numbers than distribute them broadly only to find later that many peoples' lives had been shortened because of previously undetected side effects. There were no easy answers.

LOURDES, FRANCE

Both Bill Kraus and his friend Sharon Johnson, who was nearing the end of her month-long stay with Bill in France, were lapsed Catholics who traveled in circles in which it wasn't cool to gush about such things as miracles and the Holy Mother of Jesus. That made their first hours in Lourdes uncomfortable, because neither wanted to be the first to admit how awed they were to be there. Both had spent their childhoods in Catholic schools, hearing nuns talk about the Gates of Heaven and the miracles to be found in the grotto where Bernadette saw her vision of the Virgin Mary. Of course they were excited.

When Sharon had suggested the train trip to Lourdes, Bill hadn't broken character. "What the hell," he said. "I've got nothing to lose."

Even after he stepped off the train, he still didn't want to admit that he did have something to lose and that he, like so many others, was there hoping for a miracle.

Bill and Sharon walked past the basilica and through the square lined with souvenir shops and their bottles of holy water from the grotto. It was off-season, so the usual crowds were gone. Bill scanned the people approaching the grotto. He saw Portuguese housewives who had saved for twenty years for this pilgrimage, and he saw a nun kneeling devoutly, holding her motorcycle helmet. As

Bill and Sharon approached the grotto, they passed through halls adorned with the crutches of the cripples cured in years past.

"All these crutches look forty years old," Bill said. "Maybe she stopped curing cripples in 1945."

Bill fell silent when they got to the grotto where water dripped from the spring. Sharon excused herself to wander the grounds. Alone, Bill sat on a stone bench, staring at the statue of the Virgin Mary in the grotto. The words "Jesus" and "God" crossed his thoughts, and he automatically began to push them out of his mind, as he had for many years. As Bill watched the other pilgrims and contemplated the statue, he realized that he should not dismiss the thought of Jesus, as if he were some nuisance. The essence of the Christ figure was loving and compassionate, no matter how the message of Jesus may have been corrupted by Christianity.

Bill stared toward the Virgin, and he began to see her as the archetypal mother, not the literal mother of God, but the source of all nourishment and hope. He could speak to that mother, and it would mean something. At last, he could pray, and the words would not be empty.

He realized that the bitterness he had held against the church had alienated him from this elemental source of strength. He had been separated from the font of love and forgiveness that Jesus had to offer, and it was not right. God knew that. It all was very clear to Bill now, and for the first time in many years, he prayed.

Sharon Johnson relished the serenity of this special place and walked the grounds for hours before she returned to the grotto and saw Bill sitting in the same spot she had left him. She had never seen Bill's face so soft. His anxiety had utterly disappeared and in its place was a tranquility she had rarely witnessed.

The pair decided to attend Mass in the nearby basilica. There, however, the spell was broken. The holiness of Lourdes was in the faith of the people, not the rituals of the church.

Night fell as Sharon and Bill left the church and grotto. The winding old streets were dark, and there was nobody to show them the way to their hotel because it was off-season and the shops and restaurants were all closed. It was the enduring image Sharon Johnson kept of that day: the two of them lost, wandering confusing streets in the darkness of Lourdes, trying to find their way home.

54 EXPOSED

March 2, 1985
IRWIN MEMORIAL BLOOD BANK,
SAN FRANCISCO

The future of the AIDS epidemic arrived in a black Chevrolet as night fell in San Francisco. Abbott Laboratories had airfreighted to Irwin Memorial Blood Bank the first AIDS antibody tests to be publicly released anywhere in the United States. The blood bank, after all, had the dubious distinction of dispensing more AIDS-tainted blood than any other blood bank in the country. Ray Price, the Abbott Laboratories district representative, had loaded the six boxes of beige plastic test kits into his Chevrolet Celebrity sedan at the airport for prompt delivery to the blood bank.

Just hours before in Washington, D.C., Secretary Margaret Heckler had announced the licensing of the Abbott test, allowing its distribution to 2,300 blood banks and plasma centers throughout the nation. Four other pharmaceutical companies were vying for licenses for their tests as well, all eager for a share in the $75 million-a-year market created by the need to test all blood and plasma in the United States.

Technically, the test worked like antibody tests already commonly in use for hepatitis and a number of diseases. Little plastic beads were coated with pieces of the AIDS virus. When a drop of blood was added to the small well in which the bead rested, antibodies to the HTLV-III virus would grab onto the pieces of virus. Once washed with various dyes and chemicals, the bead would turn purple if antibodies were present. From now on, the chances of contracting AIDS through a blood transfusion were effectively eliminated or, at last, were truthfully reduced to one in a million. That much was simple, but it was probably the only simple aspect of the enormous implications that the beige plastic test kits held for the future of the AIDS epidemic in general and the gay community in particular.

Although public health groups dropped their objections to the test when it was clear the federal government would pay for alternative test sites, gay groups continued to threaten legal action throughout February. Finally, after delaying the test release, the Food and Drug Administration and the Centers for Disease Control held a joint workshop on February 22. Pharmaceutical companies' data on the accuracy of their various test kits was normally held to be confidential until the actual licensing of the product, but the firms released their test results to quiet fears that the tests would not work. Indeed, the Abbott test was found to be 95 percent sensitive, meaning it would detect 19 in 20 people infected with the virus, and 99 percent specific, meaning it gave false antibody-positive readings in only 1 case in 100. Such statistics gave the test a reliability far beyond comparable assays used for other diseases and converted doubters to the test's medical usefulness.

None of this, however, calmed the fears of gay community leaders that the test could turn into a tool of discrimination. At the CDC-FDA meeting, Dr. Stephen King, a state health officer from Florida, noted that he already had been contacted by school districts eager to weed out gay teachers and by country clubs who wanted to use the test to screen food handlers. There were also questions about how the military would use the test, given the armed service's history of discrimination against gays. The federal government still had not offered any assurance that blood bank screening results could be guaranteed to be confidential.

Just forty-eight hours before Heckler announced the Abbott licensure, the National Gay Task Force and the Lambda Legal Defense and Education Fund filed a petition in federal court to stay the licensing of the antibody test, pending verification of the test's accuracy and a guarantee that the test labeling would not mark the start of massive HTLV-III screening of gay men.

Secretary Heckler, fighting for her political life within the administration, was eager to release the test and reap the public relations benefits in finally claiming a victory in the battle against AIDS. The pressure was on. Within hours of the suit's filing, Lambda lawyers and NGTF leaders met with FDA Commissioner Frank Young, who quickly acceded to the gay demand for government-required labeling of the test. Under the agreement, each test was labeled with the warning, "It is inappropriate to use this test as a screen for AIDS or as a screen for members of groups at increased risk for AIDS in the general population." With the test clearly defined for use in blood banks or laboratories, gays hoped to avert its use as a blood test for homosexuality.

Although that resolved short-term fears, it did not help solve the long-term fallout that gays would face for years. Already, one study of people who had learned their antibody status in the course of research indicated that 14 percent of those who tested positive had contemplated suicide. To test or not to test clearly would become the most important personal decision most gay men would make in their adult lives. To be tested meant learning that you might at any time fall victim to a deadly disease; it was a psychological burden few heterosexuals could imagine. However, not to be tested meant that you might be carrying a lethal virus, which you could give to others; numerous studies indicated that gay men were far less likely to have unsafe sex if they knew they were infected and might infect others. There was also the broader public health question of how you can control a disease if you decline to find out who is infected.

In the months before the test's release, health officials and AIDS researchers had undergone a dramatic turnaround on their opinions about the test. Given the psychological ramifications of a positive result, they had initially advised gay men not to be tested. Now many were swayed by the feeling that the test could be a valuable tool in controlling the spread of AIDS. In San Francisco, the split in opinion led the AIDS Foundation to decide against coming down on either side of the issue. Instead, the foundation launched an aggressive advertising campaign in gay newspapers, listing the pros and cons of the test. Gay men were urged to study the complex issues and make up their own minds.

Gay leaders in most other cities, however, viewed this neutral posture as outright treason, and the question of testing was quickly cast in exclusively political terms. Confidentiality became the preeminent issue. Suspicion that the test might be required as a condition for getting a job or insurance coverage fueled the fears. When push came to shove, however, the most adamant opponents to testing generally promoted a more apocalyptic scenario, namely that at some point, everyone who tested positive for AIDS antibodies would be locked up somewhere in medical concentration camps.

This apprehension was rarely confided to heterosexual audiences, but it continued to animate homosexual nightmares in early 1985. *New York Native* publisher Charles Ortleb made his newspaper an important supporter of Mayor Koch's 1985 reelection campaign despite Koch's sorry record on AIDS, in large part because Ortleb was convinced the feisty mayor would stand up to any federal effort for mass quarantines of AIDS-infected gays. At a San Francisco conference sponsored by the Mobilization Against AIDS in late March, participants passed a resolution calling for armed resistance to any effort to intern antibody-positive gay people.

To most heterosexuals, the rhetoric sounded implausible to the point of absurdity, but most heterosexuals remained uninformed as to the lasting legacy that prejudice imprints on an oppressed people. Humans who have been subjected to a lifetime of irrational bigotry on the part of a mainstream society can be excused for harboring unreasonable fears. The general apathy that the United States had demonstrated toward the AIDS epidemic had only deepened the distrust between gays and heterosexuals. Gays could understandably suspect the intentions of a federal government that had spent the past four years doing as little as possible to thwart the epidemic.

In this poisoned atmosphere, the nuances of long-term consequences for control of the infection fell low on the list of gay concerns. Once again, a key AIDS issue was cast in purely political terms. The politicization of the antibody test issue required new additions to the AIDSpeak lexicon.

To minimize the importance of the medical aspects of the antibody test, it was necessary to diminish the value of the test itself. Thus, the new catchphrase of AIDSpeak became, "The test doesn't really mean anything." This thinking stemmed from the belief that only 5 to 10 percent of antibody-positive men would get AIDS. Many researchers suspected that a still-unidentified cofactor might be necessary to transform HTLV-III infection into full-blown AIDS, and the test, they noted, did not reveal the existence of such a cofactor. The test, therefore, detected whether you had antibodies but not whether you'd be one of the unfortunates to get AIDS.

According to this train of thought, the virus recruited its victims like the U.S. Marines—many were selected but few were chosen. Broad acceptance of this doesn't-mean-anything aphorism reflected the surreality that was part and parcel of AIDSpeak. By most people's standards, a test that indicates somebody has even a 1-in-10 chance of dying within a few years is a test that means something.

Perhaps the most pernicious addition to the AIDSpeak vocabulary, however, was the term "exposed." Having HTLV-III antibodies meant you had been "exposed" to the virus, AIDS groups explained; the term soon became beloved by health officers around the country. Dr. Bruce Voeller, a San Diego research microbiologist who once was executive director of the National Gay Task Force, mercilessly derided the euphemism. "If you've got antibodies to a virus, you've been infected by it—you haven't been merely exposed," said Voeller, who favored widespread, voluntary testing in the gay community. "I've checked the medical books and I've never even seen the word 'exposed' mentioned. When people say 'expose,' I get the feeling that they think the virus floats around the room, like the scent of gardenias, and somehow they get exposed. That's not how it works. If you've got an antibody, that virus has been in your blood. You've been infected."

New York AIDS activists, still appalled at the anti-bathhouse sentiment in San Francisco, were shocked at the more open attitudes toward testing on the West Coast. Confidentiality had never been the bugaboo in California that it had been in New York, in large part because San Franciscans were less obsessed with protecting the rights of closet cases. The public policy enacted in California and New York concerning the antibody test reflected the dramatically different ways the issue was cast on the two coasts.

In San Francisco, Larry Bush, an aide to Assemblyman Art Agnos, had already spent four months drafting legislation to ensure the confidentiality of antibody test results. By the time the test was licensed, the state assembly had passed bills that forbade the release of antibody test results to anyone, even if ordered by a subpoena. Employers and insurers were banned from requiring the test of applicants. Nobody could be given the test without written consent. Any doctor who gave the test without consent, or who released a person's antibody status, would be liable for criminal penalties. To allow people to take the test if they wanted it, the state rushed to make available funds for alternative test sites. A bill setting aside $5 million for testing was introduced in February. Given the psychological damage that could follow the disclosure of a person's antibody status, the law also required follow-up counseling.

To protect the state's blood supply until these centers were established, the state health director invoked his emergency powers on the day after the test's licensure to forbid blood banks from disclosing the antibody test results. This policy, which was quickly announced by the Red Cross as well, was designed to keep gay men from going to blood banks to learn their antibody status.

In New York City, gay leaders remained flatly opposed to gay men taking the test for fear of civil liberties violations. Rather than enact laws protecting civil rights, a much more difficult task in New York than California, the strategy was simply to make it impossible for gay men to be tested. Without any public comment, Health Commissioner David Sencer filed a public order declaring that no laboratory in New York City would be permitted to conduct antibody tests except for scientific research. The order did not apply to blood banks.

While the New York City testing ban eliminated the possibility of abuses, it also denied the test to people who might want to take it for a personal reason. A number of gay doctors were stunned. They had looked forward to the test for its possible use on ailing patients who appeared to have bizarre manifestations of ARC. An antibody test would steer them toward immune dysfunctions, while a negative result might guide them toward other non-AIDS diagnoses. There was also the question of women with a history of drug abuse considering having children. A child born to an infected woman would most likely be infected with the AIDS virus and suffer the fate of those lonely infants who were born to die. The value of the test was incalculable in such cases, but doctors were denied its use for their patients because a handful of gay AIDS activists and political leaders had persuaded the health commissioner to ban the test for political reasons.

It was an ironic policy for a group of people who had based their entire AIDS activism, whether on issues of bathhouses or education, on the idea of "informed choice." Critics noted that gay leaders seemed to favor informed choice when the choices gay people made coincided with what the elite thought proper.

Perhaps the most amazing aspect of Dr. Sencer's order was that it was completely ignored in the local press. Even while papers ran extensive stories on the future implications of the antibody test, they characteristically ignored its significance for local public policy. For the next six months, the only mainstream newspaper in which Sencer's unusual policy was reported was, once again, not in New York but in San Francisco.

California's legislation on antibody testing, meanwhile, soon became the national model. Larry Bush, a gay journalist who was keenly aware of the meaning that testing would have for years to come, circulated the legislation throughout the country in an attempt to get other states to consider similar proposals. In time, Wisconsin and Florida followed suit, but Bush found New York Governor Mario Cuomo uninterested. Ultimately, it was conservative Orrin Hatch, the Mormon senator from Utah, who became the legislation's chief proponent, handing it around to other legislators as an example of what ought to be done everywhere. Hatch saw the wisdom of testing and realized voluntary testing of gay men wouldn't work unless they could be assured that it would not destroy their lives. It was this commonsense approach to the legislation that informed Bush again that attentiveness to the AIDS issue was not determined by whether one was liberal or conservative, but by whether one did or didn't care about the public health.

SAN FRANCISCO CHRONICLE, SAN FRANCISCO

"My wife was at the hairdresser, and her hairdresser said that just a day ago the wife of a big shot at UC Med Center was in getting a tint, and her husband said that he heard that a big movie star was getting treated there."

"For . . . ?"

". . . For AIDS."

The reporter had heard this before. This was the fifth call he had received in the past hour on this very subject.

"And the big star was Burt Reynolds, right?"

"You've already heard?"

In years, no rumor had seized San Francisco like the gossip that Burt Reynolds, the muy macho star of countless B-films, was suffering from AIDS and languishing at either UC Med Center or San Francisco General Hospital. Some gossips went so far as to suggest from whom he had contracted the disease, and everybody had a different version of the ruse he was using to conceal his identity. The most popular was that he wasn't wearing his toupee.

At one point, both San Francisco dailies and three of the four local television news stations were trying to track down the rumors. What made the story so irresistible, many agreed privately, was that Reynolds was so masculine. The notion that he might have AIDS tickled the archetypal view of sex roles that lurked in everybody's subconscious. "This is butch Burt Reynolds, not Liberace," said one television assignment editor at the time, unaware of the irony that history would confer on the appraisal.

AIDS rumors about President Reagan's son, Ron, Jr., also were floating around. And a lot of gay "Dynasty" aficionados noted with raised eyebrows that Rock Hudson certainly had been dropping weight lately. The hearsay about Reynolds, however, got the most circulation in San Francisco, Hollywood, and New York. By early March, Reynolds's press spokesman was issuing heated denials that the star had AIDS. The appearance of Reynolds on the Universal lot in Burbank briefly calmed the gossip, although many in San Francisco's gay community were reluctant to let go of the idea, convinced that the epidemic would not gain the serious attention of the press and the federal government unless it hit somebody famous.

"I don't want to hear that it's not true," confided Allen White, a columnist for a local gay newspaper. White was not alluding to Reynolds's health but to the social dynamics a celebrity AIDS case would create. "If we are to survive, we need it to be true."

By now, the epidemic had slain many prominent people, but to the bitter end, the victims remained so embarrassed about having this homosexual disease that they did not acknowledge their ailment. Doctors cooperated and concealed the truth through the falsification of death certificates.

In an eloquent editorial in *Advertising Age,* editor-at-large James Brady wrote, "I am tired of compiling lists of the dead. They are actors and writers and designers and dancers and editors and retailers and decorators and sometimes when you see their names in the obituary pages of the *[New York] Times* you think, yes, I knew that fellow. . . . The dead are homosexuals who have contracted and will perish from AIDS. Almost everyone who knew them knows this, but there is a gentle, loving conspiracy of silence to deny reality. . . . Men are dying and we in the press cough politely and draw curtains of discretion across the truth. Don't hurt anyone. Protect a name, a family, a reputation. A memory. So we write white lies about the cause of death. . . . Can lies *be* a cause of death?"

UNIVERSITY OF CALIFORNIA, SAN FRANCISCO

Marc Conant felt on the ropes throughout March. The National Kaposi's Sarcoma/AIDS Foundation, which he had once hoped would be an American Cancer Society for AIDS, was defunct now for lack of interest. He was stripped of his title as director of the AIDS Clinical Research Center, and the frequent criticism in gay newspapers had robbed him of whatever influence he could exert in the gay community. His private practice as one of San Francisco's leading AIDS doctors also brought little respite.

In March, Conant's bubbly young receptionist, Jim Sheridan, told Conant he couldn't come to work because he was having a hard time breathing. Jim Sheridan had been a computer wizard a few years back when his lover died of *Pneumocystis*. Jim had dropped his promising career to study medicine and had raced through his first years of medical school, working part-time in Conant's office, where he was an irrepressibly cheerful presence.

And now he had *Pneumocystis* too. He told Conant he would refuse treatment. "I've seen how these people die," he said. "I'm not going to go through what I've seen them go through. If I have this, I want to die quickly."

Marc Conant and Jim's sister finally persuaded the thirty-two-year-old to at least check into UCSF hospital, and his condition seemed to improve. The recuperation cheered Conant significantly, and early one morning Conant bounced into Jim's hospital room on the way to his office to share his good mood.

When Conant opened the door, however, he noticed that the bed was stripped down and all the linens were stuffed into a hamper. Shrouded in a black plastic body bag, Conant could make out the form of young Jim Sheridan.

Conant had spent most of the past four years warning people about the death that would come, but now he realized it had been very intellectual. The reality of death was now starkly sketched out before him, like a Japanese ink drawing. Dawn was breaking over the wooded hillside outside the hospital window, and against this backdrop was the silhouette of another young man in a body bag. Marc Conant was not thinking of the future now; he was feeling the future, and for the first time in years, he wanted to cry.

March 23
DON FRANCIS'S JOURNAL

It's 5:00 A.M. I've been up since 4:00 with my AIDS insomnia which has been so frequent over the past two years. This morning, instead of working on my endless in-box, memos, or manuscripts, I read the *S.F. Chronicle*'s special AIDS issue. It sent me into a flood of tears and sobs with its portrayal of Felix Munoz, a young idealistic lawyer with much in common with me—undergraduate at Berkeley, grad degree from Harvard. Such a good man he must have been— now dead because he was gay. The article outlines in small pieces the incredible personal, local and national tragedy of AIDS. I sympathize and am angered by each. . . .

What have we done to stop this horrible scourge? Much less than we should. We saw it coming. It was in mid-1982 that some of us used to dealing with transmissible diseases saw it coming. Why then has it been so difficult to get a control program out to the local level? It is complex and I can't understand all of it. If I had to blame one thing it would be the hunger for power. Somewhere in our pursuit of understanding AIDS, we have failed to turn the corner, to realize that we did understand it, and do something about it. I blame most the Washington hierarchy who cared more about reading the scientific discoveries as political wares than public health breakthroughs. . . . I also blame the lack of vision on the CDC, but much of this is due to the same Washingtonians who squelch any new proposal to prevent disease. . . . And the Felix Munozes keep on dying.

⬭

Within a week, the number of the nation's AIDS cases surpassed 9,000. Of these, more than 4,300 had died.

PARIS

Like most European health officials, French authorities viewed AIDS as an American problem, one that fundamentally did not affect them. The government devoted little attention to AIDS research, and when the Pasteur Institute devised its own LAV antibody test kits, authorities made no move to require their use in blood banks.

Faced with what he considered to be unconscionable denial, Dr. Jacques Leibowitch started screening a random sampling of Parisians. Tests on 7,500 revealed that 1 in 200 were infected with the AIDS virus. By his estimate, hospitals were infecting about 50 people a week in Paris alone, and the flamboyant scientist gave a press conference saying so. Only then did the government announce that it would require testing of donated blood.

April 1985
SAN FRANCISCO

Cathy Borchelt was watching the television news when she saw the president of Irwin Memorial Blood Bank tell a press conference that the blood bank expected seventy-two local transfusion AIDS cases in coming years.

"What about one in a million?" she asked.

Indeed, the first month of blood testing in San Francisco and across the nation indicated that there was, of course, substantially more than a one-in-a-million chance of getting AIDS from a blood transfusion, even in mid-1985. A dozen of 5,300 units of blood donated at Irwin during March were infected with AIDS, meaning that chances of getting infected from a transfusion in San Francisco were about 1 in 440 at the time testing was instituted.

The American Red Cross similarly reported that, nationally, 1 in 500 donors tested positive for the AIDS virus. This certainly indicated that gay men were not going en masse to donate blood and that self-deferral drives were largely successful, but it also boded poorly for the future. Given the millions of Americans who had been transfused in recent years, it was clear that even a 1-in-500 infection rate would mean thousands of deaths. Later retrospective screening, for example, showed that in just the final weeks before the HTLV-III test went into use, 150 infected donors had given blood that was put into the veins of 200 people. An Irwin press release underscored the tragedy by starkly announcing on April 2 that four new transfusion AIDS cases from Irwin blood were reported in the month of March. Most significantly, none of the cases, Irwin reported, came from transfusions administered after the blood bank started hepatitis B core antibody testing in May 1984.

By now, the Borchelt family's lawyers were preparing a suit against Irwin. Unlike previous lawsuits by aggrieved families of transfusion AIDS victims, the Borchelt suit did not claim product liability, a charge from which blood banks were legally insulated by special legislation. Instead, the lawsuit claimed negligence, saying the blood industry was negligent in not moving to do something about AIDS even after it was aware of the problem. The legal briefs traced the history of public policy on AIDS, back to the January 1983 meeting in Atlanta when Don Francis banged his fist on a table and asked, "How many people are going to have to die before we do something?" Now that it was clear that Frances Borchelt was among those who would die, the family wanted restitution.

Frances Borchelt was embarrassed and angry when she saw her name in the newspaper story about the lawsuit. Cathy, however, pressed on, reading everything she could about the epidemic. In April, watching a PBS "Nova" show on AIDS, she saw somebody talk about the early cases of hemophiliacs in the spring of 1982, and she learned that the nation's first transfusion AIDS case was detected in San Francisco months later. Cathy was outraged.

"They knew you could get AIDS from blood in 1982!" she said to anyone who would listen. "Why didn't they do anything?"

⬭

Sharon Johnson recognized Bill Kraus's voice on the phone right away. He had just awakened from another nightmare.

In the dream, Bill was walking through a graveyard when bony hands started coming up from the earth, latching onto the cuffs of his pants, grasping for his ankles, trying to pull him into the ground. Bill started to run, past the gravestones and toward safety, but ghostly forms arose from the graves and chased him, and the hands continued to pull at him.

"Meditate," Sharon said. "Start thinking of a safe place. I'm here with you."

Slowly, Sharon pulled Bill out of his hysteria.

Bill explained that the doctors were thinking of changing his medication. He didn't know what that would mean, and he was afraid. He was also afraid that when he returned to San Francisco, if he ever returned, his friends would abandon him. Everybody whom he had ever loved had abandoned him, he said. He didn't want to be alone again. He felt so alone in Paris.

55 AWAKENING

April 14, 1985
ROOM 304, WORLD CONGRESS CENTER,
ATLANTA

"Don Francis is a Nazi."

The words passed confidently from one gay leader to another as they nodded in disgust at the CDC virologist who was participating in a panel on whether gay men should take the antibody test. The hallways outside the conference room were filling with 2,000 scientists and health authorities who were registering for the first International Conference on Acquired Immunodeficiency Syndrome. Although the conference was not slated to begin until the next day, gay participants had scheduled their own meeting for this Sunday afternoon to discuss issues geared toward their community. This included a panel on the preeminent issue—the Test.

Gay panel participants entertained the audience with different reasons as to why they should all agree to oppose the antibody test. And then Don Francis spoke, summing up his thinking with two lines and two circles.

The two lines fell across each other like the cross of St. Andrew. The line sloping downward represented the overall reduction in the number of sexual contacts that most gay men had accomplished as part of the dramatic sexual counterrevolution that had seized the gay community over the past two years. That development was hopeful. However, the upward slope of the second line, representing the dramatically increased prevalence of the virus among gay men, showed why this was not good enough to save homosexual men from biological obsolescence. Reducing sexual contacts by one-half, Francis explained, was not enough if the people with whom a gay man had sex were four times as likely to infect him with the AIDS virus. The person would still have twice the chance of getting infected that he had had two years before, Francis said. Gay men were playing the AIDS lottery less often, Francis said, but when they did play, they had a far greater chance of coming across a losing ticket.

Handing out pamphlets that advised gay men to reduce their partners was important, but it was not enough, Francis said. Data from the San Francisco hepatitis study showed that gay men were still out there getting infected with the AIDS virus. The gay community needed to start thinking about control.

Francis drew his two circles. One circle represented men infected with the AIDS virus; the other, men who weren't. The point of AIDS control efforts, he said, should be to make sure that everybody knows into which circle they fit. They should be tested, he said. People who are infected with the AIDS virus should only go to bed with people who are infected; people who aren't infected should only have sex with other people whom they know to be uninfected. He was not recommending mandatory testing, Francis stressed, and he believed civil rights guarantees needed to be in place to encourage people to be tested. Ultimately, however, the tough choice would have to be made. The two circles should be separate, Francis warned, or tens of thousands would die unnecessarily.

"I've seen a lot of viruses in my day, and I've come to develop a profound respect for this one," Francis concluded. "There aren't very many viruses in the history of man that kill one-tenth of the people they infect. We need to start thinking about controlling this one."

Francis's call to action stunned and outraged the gay audience. Nothing proved more unsettling than the word "control." "Control, control, control," muttered the AIDS writer for the *New York Native*. "It's so fascistic, the idea of putting people in circles and talking about control."

To some extent, the semantic aversion to this word reflected the gay community's own ignorance of public health vocabulary, a shortcoming that had remained uncorrected throughout the course of the epidemic. For decades, control had been the operative word in the lexicon of epidemiologists whose job it was to eradicate diseases. It had rarely been invoked during the AIDS epidemic, however, because there were so tragically few tools of control. For Don Francis, the most important tool was being marketed now in beige plastic boxes to blood banks. He did not want it denied to him.

More than almost anyone in government, Francis knew that serious control efforts would not be mounted by federal health authorities in the coming years. Neither the money nor the motivation existed on the federal level. He believed the gay community itself would have to be enlisted if control efforts were to be made.

Gay leaders were instantly suspicious of Francis's rhetoric. Already, they were aggravated at his criticism of bathhouses as "commercialized sex" businesses that had served as "amplification systems," allowing the AIDS virus to spread throughout the gay community. And Don Francis was, after all, part of the federal government that had shown precious little concern over the wholesale demise of a generation of gay men. Why, suddenly, had control become such an important goal?

Moreover, the entire thrust of Francis's proposal was entirely foreign to them. After spending four years listening to polite public health officials chatter in the intransitive lingo of AIDSpeak, AIDS activists were unaccustomed to hearing people suggest that they might actually have to do something. So far, most gay action against the disease had consisted of holding sophisticated AIDS education forums in Manhattan auditoriums and handing out condoms at the San Francisco Gay Freedom Day Parade. Faced with the challenge that this was not enough, most of the gay participants on the panel did to Francis what they had spent the past four years doing to gays with whom they disagreed on AIDS issues. They called him names.

While Jim Curran watched nervously from the back of the room, speaker after speaker denounced Francis as a Nazi and a brownshirt who wanted to put homosexuals into concentration camps. Dr. David Ostrow, panel moderator, disagreed with Francis, but he had known Francis since the hepatitis study in the late 1970s and understood his intentions. He pleaded with people who disagreed to hold off on the personal attacks, but the animus of a people wronged was such that it proved impossible.

Privately, Jim Curran agreed with Don Francis. He had recently heard of three San Francisco gay men in the hepatitis study who, to their amazement, had only recently developed antibodies to HTLV-III. They told doctors that they had been completely monogamous in recent years; it didn't make sense. The three men's lovers, it turned out, were infected. These three monogamous men would have been saved, Curran knew, had they known their lovers' antibody status. That was the answer, he thought, but the sight of the hostile audience unnerved him.

"Don Francis does not speak for the CDC," Curran anxiously told any reporter who asked. "He's only speaking for himself."

Yet, in that room on that Sunday afternoon, there was an awakening among these people. To a large extent, the public health issues of the AIDS epidemic had lain in their hands during the first phase of the scourge. Although the gay AIDS activists were fond of lecturing people that "AIDS is not a gay disease," they had in fact treated the epidemic almost solely as a gay disease, the private property of a community that would base public health policy on its own political terms. Now there were other people with other ideas, and perhaps they might stop treating AIDS as a gay affliction. Jim Curran's skittishness indicated that this moment was not at hand, but the debate over antibody testing clearly informed many people for the first time that the day might come.

For many people, the three-day international AIDS conference, co-sponsored by the U.S. Department of Health and Human Services and the World Health Organization, marked a time of awakening.

That Night

Marc Conant was leaving the Westin Peachtree Plaza Hotel when he ran into the president of the Bay Area Physicians for Human Rights.

"Don Francis says that gay men should take the antibody test and that antibody-negative people should never have sex with antibody-positive people," the doctor said sneeringly. "Can you believe it?"

"I agree with that," said Conant. "Makes sense to me."

At the welcoming reception, gay doctors buzzed about Francis's fascism while CDC staffers talked about his petition to transfer to the Bay Area, reportedly after telling Walt Dowdle that "the Centers for Disease Control has never controlled a disease in its history."

Conant caught up with Francis. He was relieved to find somebody who spoke sensibly about the antibody test. Conant agreed with Francis that the test would inevitably find wide use throughout society. The question was only how much suffering and death was necessary to convince people, homosexual and heterosexual alike, of its exigency. Events, thought Conant, would force the issue.

Francis was upbeat about his personal future.

"If there's any chance of stopping this disease, it will happen in San Francisco," Francis said, his enthusiasm already building for the move.

Conant was excited. At last, he had heard somebody in the federal government talk about stopping this disease. Later, Conant heard that other CDC staffers were calling Francis's transfer an "exile to Siberia."

The Next Day
AUDITORIUM, WORLD CONGRESS CENTER

"AIDS has already arrived in every major city in the developed world," said Jim Curran in the opening presentation of the AIDS conference. Between 500,000 and 1 million Americans, he said, were infected with the AIDS virus. The infection was so endemic to the United States that a vaccine, when available, should become part of the standard inoculations administered to all children before they enter school. He suggested that clinics and physicians providing prenatal and premarital screening of people in high-risk groups should consider routinely screening their patients for HTLV-III antibodies.

Robert Gallo followed Curran's talk with the observation that it was outrageously optimistic to be talking of a time when Americans could be vaccinated. Beyond the problems of a rapidly mutating virus that might defy attempts to create one all-effective vaccine, there was the problem of proving a vaccine was effective once it was developed. "Before you talk about a vaccine being used on the public, you have to have testing and trials—and I haven't heard of anyone close to that point yet," said Gallo.

The normal way to test a vaccine was to administer it to people at high risk of getting a disease, and not administer it to others. If the people who don't get the vaccine get sick, and the vaccinated people don't, you have an effective vaccine. This was a simple enough process with, say, hepatitis, because the people who got sick were likely to recover. Such tests for AIDS, however, created enormous ethical questions. Who would be the ones to die to prove that an AIDS vaccine was effective?

Beyond that, there were huge financial risks. What company would withstand the threat of liability lawsuits in order to develop a vaccine? The hepatitis B vaccine had become a major debacle. Enthusiasm for vaccines had dropped considerably since then.

This was only the beginning of the bad news. The scientific observations that emerged from the 392 presentations in the following days did little to cheer up conferees. The medical insights on AIDS ran the gamut from depressing to dismal.

The virus, scientists said, was the nastiest microbe humanity had encountered in centuries, if not in all of human history. The presence of antibodies presented "presumptive evidence" of continued infection with the virus. Once infected, people carried the virus and were capable of infecting others for the rest of their lives. The virus infected brain cells and the central nervous system, creating a host of neurological disorders beyond the immune deficiency caused by infection of the T-4 lymphocytes. As Bob Gallo told the crowd, "We *do* know what the antibody test means. Antibody positivity means virus infective. I don't think there's going to be a better assay [for AIDS] than the antibody detection."

Any hopes that the virus would select many as carriers but few as AIDS victims were subverted by data from James Goedert, who had been monitoring cohorts of New York and Washington gay men since 1982. Of gay Manhattan men infected with the AIDS virus, 20 percent now had AIDS and another 25 percent had serious immune problems that Goedert called lesser AIDS. Only about one-half were healthy. Of the Washington sample, 12 percent had AIDS and 11 percent had lesser AIDS. Eight percent of the Danish gay men that Bill Biggar had tested now had AIDS. Goedert suspected that the differences in AIDS rates among the cohorts only reflected the differing times at which they were infected. The virus appeared to arrive in New York first, giving the Manhattan men more time to incubate the disease. Infections in Washington followed the New Yorkers', and the spread of the virus in Denmark came later.

Goedert felt strongly that the CDC was understating the risk posed by the virus. He was appalled when he heard people using the term "exposed" instead of "infected." According to his reasoning, the AIDS virus needed only one cofactor to produce the fatal disease—time. The virus plus time, given enough of it, would probably kill far more than the 5 to 20 percent being optimistically projected.

Questions about the role of time in the epidemic were dramatically resolved by the incubation studies presented by the CDC's Dale Lawrence. Although Lawrence had arrived at his conclusions in late 1983, they had only been cleared for public disclosure at this international conference one year and four months later. Pencils dropped and jaws gaped throughout the auditorium as Lawrence calmly laid out his projection that the mean incubation period for the AIDS virus was 5.5 years. Some people, he added, would not get AIDS until 14 years after their infection. These figures meant that the typical person diagnosed with AIDS in April 1985 was infected in October 1979. The huge number of people infected with the virus in 1982, 1983, and 1984, when the virus was far more prevalent, would not show AIDS symptoms until the late 1980s. Some people getting infected at the time of the conference, meanwhile, would not come down with the disease until the turn of the next century.

There was also the question of what would happen to people who were infected with the AIDS virus but did not get one of the opportunistic infections that characterized the CDC definition of the syndrome. Jim Curran noted that people whose immune systems are artificially suppressed for transplant operations later exhibit far higher rates of cancer. Combine this statistic with the fact that the virus fed on the nervous system, and, Curran concluded, "The aging of an infected population means more cancer, neurological disorders and other infections from immune suppression among people infected with HTLV-III."

The AIDS diseases themselves were, in the most overworked metaphor of the AIDS epidemic, only the tip of the catastrophic iceberg that would haunt the United States for decades to come.

The extensive reports on the international epidemiology of AIDS also boded poorly. Harold Jaffe and Andrew Moss presented data from the San Francisco hepatitis B study that found the virus was present in the blood of 4.5 percent of study subjects in 1978, 20 percent in 1980, and 67 percent by late 1984. In other words, they noted, a substantial number of gay men were infected with the virus years before people even knew the problem existed.

Studies on the prevalence of AIDS infection throughout the nation underscored this apprehension. In Pittsburgh, a city with a relatively low incidence of AIDS, 25 percent of gay men in one study were infected with the virus, and an additional 2 percent of local gay men were being infected every month. A Boston study found that 21 percent of a sampling of gay men were HTLV-III positive. To a large extent, all these studies were biased by the fact that subjects were selected from more sexually active men who went to VD clinics. In San Francisco, for example, only about 40 percent of a randomly selected sample of gay men were infected, compared with the 67 percent infected in the hepatitis cohort. All the studies indicated the dramatic inroads the virus had made into other cities, very few of which had mounted any campaign for AIDS education and prevention.

There was disquieting evidence that the virus was spreading among heterosexuals as well, albeit much more slowly. In one Manhattan study of 300 young, sexually active heterosexual men, 3.4 percent were antibody positive. Most significantly, none had engaged in gay sexual activity or in drug abuse, although they were far more likely to have had sexual relations with a female intravenous drug user than study subjects who were antibody negative. (As in virtually all of the heterosexual studies, however, the use of prostitutes apparently did not correlate with whether people were infected.)

Meanwhile, studies of Haitians, who had just been dropped from the CDC roster as an official risk group, had largely solved the mystery of how they were infected. The high rates of infectivity were linked to the sharing of needles and heterosexual promiscuity. In Zaire, the virus was so widespread that scientists had a hard time constructing studies on risk factors. It was difficult to find a control group that was not infected.

The studies of infection prevalence all pointed to the need for better clinical treatment of AIDS patients, if for no other reason than that there would be so many patients in the years ahead. In his address to the conference, Dr. Paul Volberding noted that "the quality of AIDS patient treatment in the nation has not kept pace" with scientific research on AIDS. He challenged other cities "to take AIDS half as seriously as San Francisco has" and start coordinated treatment programs like those at his AIDS Clinic.

As if to give statistical basis to Volberding's entreaty, the CDC reported that AIDS had become the fifth leading cause of death among young, single men in the United States, after accidents, homicide, suicide, and cancer. In Manhattan, however, AIDS was responsible for more years of lost life than these other four causes of death combined. The cost to society was skyrocketing as well. The CDC calculated that hospital bills and lost wages and benefits of the nation's 9,000 AIDS patients had already amounted to $5.6 billion. Within a few years the cost to society would begin to approach the $50-billion-a-year price tag of cancer or the $85 billion in health care cost and lost wages that stem from heart disease.

◯

As if all this bad news were not enough, the conference laid bare the problems that continued to retard AIDS research. On its first morning, both Luc Montagnier and Robert Gallo delivered lectures that were largely extensions of the scientific politicking that consumed AIDS virology. Even though Gallo declared that the nationalistic tenor of scientific infighting was "science debased, science degenerated," he devoted much of his talk to explaining why his AIDS virus was a member of the HTLV family. A few weeks earlier Gallo had tried to explain away the surprising genetic comparison between LAV and HTLV-III by saying that the Parisian gay man from whom LAV was culled had had sexual contacts in New York, implying that he had picked up the same strain of the virus that Gallo would later isolate in Bethesda.

Luc Montagnier followed Gallo's talk with a discourse on why LAV was not a leukemia virus but was a member of the lentivirus family. The lectures on retroviral taxonomy accentuated the intercontinental scientific warfare that subsequent handshakes between Gallo and Montagnier could not belie.

The most discouraging note, however, was not struck by battling researchers or depressing studies but by the Health and Human Services Secretary, Margaret Heckler, who came to deliver the conference's keynote address.

In halting and sometimes confused language, Heckler stumbled through her twelve-page speech, recounting the complicated virological issues that scientists needed to confront with AIDS. Even the phonetic spellings of the technical AIDS terms in her text did not help Heckler pronounce the words right. This problem was less embarrassing than the fact that she bothered to discuss such issues at all.

Scientists hadn't crowded the auditorium so they could hear the administration's cabinet officer for health affairs talk about arcane matters of retroviral replication; they wanted to know what the Reagan administration planned to do about it. What kind of money could Heckler promise to AIDS research? When would the government start financing AIDS education? Heckler only promised that "AIDS will remain our number-one public health priority until it has been conquered."

In her only departure from her prepared text, Heckler added, "We must conquer AIDS before it affects the heterosexual population and the general population.... We have a very strong public interest in stopping AIDS before it spreads outside the risk groups, before it becomes an overwhelming problem."

The statement infuriated organizers from AIDS groups who considered AIDS already an "overwhelming problem" and did not consider it a priority of AIDS research to stop the scourge only "before it affects the heterosexual population." Moreover, many gay leaders wondered who had determined that homosexuals were not part of the "general population" that so concerned the Secretary.

Within minutes of the conclusion of the address, gays were organizing a petition campaign to protest the comments, while the red-faced Secretary confronted an incredulous press corps. When pressed as to who determined AIDS funding levels, Heckler insisted that spending was "determined by scientists' requests." A reporter brought up the difficulties that Edward Brandt had faced in accomplishing this goal, but Heckler countered, "Ultimately, Dr. Brandt did win."

The press conference came as a rude awakening for journalists who had largely believed administration rhetoric about its "number-one health priority." The priority clearly was based on how much AIDS would affect heterosexuals.

April 17

Edward Brandt was given an ovation usually reserved for a returning war hero as he approached the podium for his keynote address at the final plenary session of the AIDS conference. Gay leaders applauded him as one of those rare people who had risen above political perspective and background to truly want to join the AIDS battle. Researchers recognized him as the person who had fought for funding against a recalcitrant administration. Aware of the controversy that had swept the conference in the wake of Secretary Heckler's comments about the "general population," Brandt said, "The fact that the people who are at risk for developing AIDS are human is enough to command the attention of all people."

Brandt endorsed voluntary testing of high-risk groups, saying that the nation "must make progress at a faster rate" against the disease. He added that confidentiality guarantees should be in place as well because "numerous groups would create enormous pressure to report the names of people with the disease."

As for the past, Brandt conceded, "I don't think we were as effective as we should have been in the early stages of this epidemic. There must be a mechanism for emergency procedures to deal with epidemics such as AIDS without sacrificing scientific standards. A continuing examination of our response capabilities is necessary. . . . Throwing money does not solve problems such as AIDS. Starving efforts don't help the situation either."

As for the dark visions of the future, however, Brandt recommended calm, and he closed the session with a citation from his favorite book, the Bible.

"This too shall pass."

April 21
Public Theater,
New York City

A thunderous ovation echoed through the theater. The people rose to their feet, applauding the cast returning to the stage to take their bows. Larry Kramer looked to his eighty-five-year-old mother. She had always wanted him to write for the stage, and Kramer had done that now. True, *The Normal Heart* was not your respectable Neil Simon fare, but a virtually unanimous chorus of reviewers had already proclaimed the play to be a masterpiece of political drama. Even before the previews were over, critics from every major news organization in New York City had scoured their thesauruses for superlatives to describe the play. NBC said it "beats with passion"; *Time* magazine said it was "deeply affecting, tense and touching"; the *New York Daily News* called it "an angry, unremitting and gripping piece of political theater." One critic said *Heart* was to the AIDS epidemic what Arthur Miller's *The Crucible* had been to the McCarthy era. *New York Magazine* critic John Simon, who had recently been overheard saying that he looked forward to when AIDS had killed all the homosexuals in New York theater, conceded in an interview that he left the play weeping.

The formulation of AIDS public policy, whether local or federal, had never been animated by rational forces, and nothing proclaimed this truth like the impact *The Normal Heart* had demonstrated in recent weeks. With his drama, Larry Kramer had succeeded where the reasoned pleas of researchers and experts had failed, bringing the issue at last to the forefront of civic issues.

Just hours before the first preview performance, as photocopied scripts of *The Normal Heart* circulated among the city's news organizations, Mayor Ed Koch hurriedly called a press conference to announce "a comprehensive expansion of city services" for local AIDS patients. Koch shifted responsibility for AIDS from Health Commissioner Sencer to Deputy Mayor Victor Botnick and instituted the plans for coordinated care and long-term facilities that had been proposed years before by AIDS clinicians. Included in the new $6 million program were pledges of expanded home and hospice care, day-care programs for children with AIDS, and funds for ten interdisciplinary patient care teams at hospitals with large AIDS caseloads. The initiatives were a small fraction of what a city with one-third of the nation's AIDS cases needed, but it was a start.

In announcing the programs, Koch, who was up for reelection in six months, was characteristically combative. Rather than admit to any past shortcomings in AIDS funding, the mayor claimed the city was already spending $31 million on AIDS, or about 3,000 percent more than Koch's own health commissioner had dubiously claimed in AIDS spending six weeks before. (It turned out that Koch was including in this expense the cost of every AIDS patient residing in a city hospital, expenses that could only be deferred if the city broke the law and evicted AIDS patients from every room. San Francisco and other cities kept no comparable statistics.) With braggadocio, Koch claimed that his new plan was so good that San Francisco might ultimately imitate New York's response to AIDS. He dismissed suggestions that the city needed to do more to educate people, both straight and gay, about AIDS. "I think we'll find out that the city is well informed," he said.

Koch directly answered the charge in *The Normal Heart* that he, a bachelor, had avoided a high profile in the epidemic for fear that his own life-style might be questioned: "Regrettably in our society, one technique used in order to seek to slander an individual is to simply accuse that individual of homosexuality. These charges are made even more frequently if the person is a single individual over the age of forty and unmarried. It is an outrageous charge because in many cases it is untrue and, even if true, is irrelevant."

Although Larry Kramer aspired for precisely such immediate political impact, audiences leaving the play seemed most struck by the broader themes of prejudice that held the play together. As far as Kramer was concerned, AIDS was not the wrath of God but the wrath of heterosexuals. Heterosexuals had decreed that gays could not legally marry or even live together in any semblance of openness without risking ignominy. The gay movement, in Kramer's view, had colluded with straights by becoming a cause of sexual liberation, rather than human liberation. As Kramer's alter ego in the play, Ned Weeks, said, "Why didn't you guys fight for the right to get married instead of the right to legitimize promiscuity?" The play ended with Weeks marrying his lover in a hospital bed, moments before the lover succumbed to AIDS.

As for GMHC, Kramer decried the group as a bunch of "Florence Nightingales" who had turned away from pressuring the government for their share of research funds and services in favor of the melodrama of deathbed scenes. "I thought I was starting a bunch of Ralph Naders or Green Berets," fumed Weeks in Act II, "and at the first instant they have to take a stand on a political issue and fight, almost in front of my eyes they turn into a bunch of nurse's aides."

Insiders gleefully picked out who was who in the cast, since virtually all the play's characters were based on real people within the GMHC hierarchy. GMHC executive director Rodger McFarlane, Kramer's own lover, became Mickey, an adorable southern queen confronting the daily dramas of suffering that comprised so much of GMHC work. Stolid GMHC president Paul Popham became Bruce Niles in the drama, worrying about whether the word "gay" should be openly displayed on GMHC party invitations.

Paul Popham had heard enough about the play's preview performances to decide against attending the show. He had already heard the rhetoric many times over, and he had other things on his mind now.

In March, the doctor had told Paul that the purple spot on his neck was Kaposi's sarcoma. Paul had taken the news stoically and told only a very few close friends. He had noticed that once people knew you had AIDS, they treated you differently, and he did not want people treating him differently. Friends pleaded with him to take advantage of the support network he had played such a central role in creating at GMHC, but Paul declined. That was for other people, he said, not for him.

Paul Popham had no doubt that he had done the right thing in his stewardship at GMHC, despite all the bad publicity GMHC was getting now. He did not feel he was a murderer for not agreeing with Larry Kramer. Paul had given up four years of his life for the organization and, in the process, lost a lot. He had lost the comfortable confidence he once held in his adopted city, and he felt betrayed by a government for which he had fought and in which he had spent a lifetime believing.

He had gained something, as well, something he never knew had value. Being gay, as such, had never meant much to Paul Popham, and he had never seen the sense of all this gay-movement talk. Now, when he saw a GMHC volunteer returning from the bedside of a dying man, he realized he had gained faith in his embattled gay community. Larry Kramer might call it the work of gray ladies, but Paul viewed the GMHC volunteers as pioneers, imbuing this community with a measure of dignity. The vigils at deathbeds testified to the value of each gay life being snuffed out in this epidemic. The presence of just one witness to the deaths of the lonely sufferers said aloud, "This person was worth something. He was a person."

Larry Kramer was fond of saying, "There are no heroes in the AIDS epidemic," but Paul Popham disagreed. There were heroes in the AIDS epidemic, he thought, lots of them.

Within weeks of Paul Popham's diagnosis, Enno Poersch learned that still another friend from the house on Ocean Walk in the summer of 1980 had AIDS. The late Rick Wellikoff's lover, Bob, was preparing to leave for Paris to receive HPA-23 treatments when *The Normal Heart* premiered. It was a shattering time for Enno, recalling that first rush of tragedy that had accompanied Nick's death four years before. Now Rick was dead, and another Ocean Walk roommate, Wes, was dead, and Paul's boyfriend Jack was dead, and Paul and Bob were dying.

This was the last summer Enno would lease the house on Ocean Walk. There were now several Fire Island homes that had earned the kind of ghostly reputation that had accrued to Enno's summer home. People walked by these houses, and somebody would point, and then they'd all nod and walk a little faster. Enno's new lover was so upset by the number of deaths among the house's former residents that he refused to step inside the building.

It had started five years before, when Nick had come home from work with diarrhea. As far as Enno was concerned, however, it could have been a century ago, so much had happened and so much had changed. With so many of his friends dead from AIDS while he remained as healthy as ever, Enno sometimes felt like he was enjoying a picnic lunch in the eye of a hurricane. The only way out was to become part of the hurricane and perish, and so he stayed in the center, his life wholly encompassed by gales of death.

As New York City belatedly began to grapple with the epidemic, AIDS policy matters were becoming local issues in a number of jurisdictions. In Massachusetts, Democratic Governor Michael Dukakis enraged gay leaders by submitting a $3.3 billion health and human services budget that did not earmark one cent for AIDS. In 1984, when Dukakis had made a similar oversight, the legislature had allocated $1.5 million for education and university research. After substantial pressure, Dukakis added $1.63 million to the 1985–1986 budget.

In New York State, Governor Mario Cuomo, another Democrat with liberal credentials, also was accused of shortchanging AIDS research. For the third year in a row, his budget proposal for state spending was below that suggested by health authorities. When pressed as to why New York State would spend only $3 million for education and direct services, compared with the $9 million being spent in San Francisco, Mel Rosen, the New York AIDS Institute director, adopted the rhetoric of the Reagan administration. "In New York, we don't believe in throwing money at a problem," he said. "I don't know what I'd do with $9 million." Health workers in poor and minority communities, where the state had yet to spend any money to stem the tide of AIDS among intravenous drug users, quickly informed Rosen of plenty of ways to spend such funds.

The objections that Democratic governors had voiced against state AIDS spending were a comfort to conservative California Governor George Deukmejian. In May 1985, Deukmejian was embroiled in his ritualistic fight with Democratic legislators over AIDS funding. After an exhaustive seven hearings on the next year's AIDS budget, the legislature approved $21.5 million in AIDS spending. Deukmejian vetoed $11.6 million of it, part of which was restored. When Democrats criticized the governor, Republicans pointed out that California was spending more on AIDS than every other state in the nation combined, and that the western Republican was approving far more AIDS funds than the eastern Democrats. These were difficult arguments to counter.

Public health issues continued to percolate on the local level, giving health officials a taste of what the future would hold. In Oakland, for example, a gay AIDS patient was making repeated visits to a local venereal disease clinic with sundry sexually transmitted diseases. He admitted that he did not warn his contacts of his health problems and ignored advice that he might cut down on unsafe sex. When Dr. Robert Benjamin, the county communicable disease director, gathered gay leaders to discuss the problem, the gay press branded him an anti-gay bigot out to lock up every homosexual in a concentration camp.

Bathhouse owners nervously waited for the onslaught of national closures that was expected after San Francisco banned sexual behavior in bathhouses. The Association of Independent Gay Health Clubs had announced that it had raised $500,000 in pledges to pay legal fees to fight closure. It was more than the group had ever proposed to spend on AIDS prevention, critics noted. Indeed, there was so much nervousness about AIDS education that the Club Bath Association threatened the Key West Club Baths with expulsion if they proceeded with a plan to sponsor a five-part local television program on the syndrome.

In early May, a number of bath owners were considering withdrawing from the Club Bath Association, because of that group's opposition to any AIDS education in bathhouses. The association's executive director, however, stood firm. "Where do we draw the line?" he asked in a letter to shareholders. "If a person died in a sauna, would we instruct all our members to remove saunas from all our clubs?" Rather than rush into handing out AIDS brochures, the director suggested that businesses adopt a "wait and see" attitude toward the epidemic.

The first controversy over the wisdom of California's antibody test law erupted in San Francisco after a gay man, claiming he had AIDS, bit a police officer. The officer wanted the man tested for the AIDS virus, and the district attorney's office said it might press charges of "assault with the intent to do great bodily harm" if the man was infected.

However, the antibody test law gave all the rights to the man who did the biting. He could not be forced to have the test, a judge ruled, and a doctor would be violating the law if he released antibody test results without the man's permission. As far as the officer was concerned, however, he was the victim. What about his civil rights?

AIDSpeakers had not anticipated this. They operated on the principle that a person with AIDS could do no wrong. Therefore, the policeman was subjected to the kind of vicious personal attacks meted out to those who dared to think dangerous thoughts. The only thing that saved the policeman from being accused of wanting all gays locked up in concentration camps was the fact that he was openly gay himself, having been the first person to join the local police force by invoking the city's gay anti-discrimination law.

It was in response to the policeman's suit, however, that the press liaison for the San Francisco AIDS Foundation fashioned the ultimate expression of AID-Speak, when she said that the officer was suffering from "AIDSphobia."

What was AIDSphobia?

"That's acting like AIDS is the worst thing that could possibly happen to you," she said.

CENTERS FOR DISEASE CONTROL, ATLANTA

AIDS statistics were now tabulated on a Model 277 Display computer in Room 274 of Building 6 at CDC headquarters. Every week, a crew of people, whose job consisted of updating weekly AIDS body counts, categorized the deaths by risk group and geographic region. In the last week of April 1985, exactly four years after drug technician Sandra Ford had written a memo about unusual orders of pentamidine from a New York City gay doctor, the computer said that the number of AIDS cases in the United States had surpassed 10,000.

56 ACCEPTANCE

May 1985
MAUI, HAWAII

If he were fated to die of AIDS, Cleve Jones did not want to undergo the public deterioration that had marked the last months of so many of his other friends. When Cleve left San Francisco, he bought a one-way ticket, thinking he might never return alive. Within a few weeks of his arrival on Maui, however, his health problems cleared. The furrows in his brow smoothed, and he began to think he might stay in Hawaii, not to die, but to enjoy life again.

Cleve spent his days smoking marijuana and wandering through the plush forests; every night he went to Maui's gay bar, Hamburger Mary's, and drank vodka martinis until closing time. It was a good life for the first month, but then his conscience started bothering him. One morning, Cleve woke up and announced to himself: "Today, I start taking care of myself. I'm not going to drink. I'm going to get healthy." That night, however, he found himself back at Hamburger Mary's drinking vodka martinis. Day after day, he awoke with the same resolution, and every night he was back at Hamburger Mary's.

The drinking, he knew now, was completely out of control. It had been out of control for years, but he had not admitted it to himself. He had denied his problem, been angry with it, and even bargained with it, assuring himself that he could drink moderately if only he could drink. But Cleve did not control his drinking; the drinking controlled him. His hangovers were worse than ever, and an emptiness seized his spirit. Remorseful mornings followed drunken nights, and still he could not make himself stop.

Who was Cleve Jones? What had become of the idealist who once led demonstrations to protest injustice? That Cleve was gone. There seemed nothing left of him, except the compulsion to drink. It was when this awareness overwhelmed him that Cleve thumbed through the phone book and called the number he knew he had to dial.

That night, Cleve edged nervously into the Wailuku Community Center and slid into a folding metal chair in the back of the room. He listened to a thirteen-year-old boy and an eighty-year-old man talk about their struggles with alcohol; he recognized the common threads that wove their stories into his, and he began to weep.

In the days that followed, Cleve stayed home and read books about alcoholism. He felt fear growing in his stomach, knowing that if he failed to act now, there would be no hope. If he survived the epidemic, he would not survive his addiction to alcohol. He would either learn to live with the truth or be prepared to die with the lie.

After a week of soul-searching, Cleve edged back into the room where people shared their experience, strength, and hope in their efforts to recover from the addiction. When somebody asked if there were any newcomers at the meeting that night, Cleve inhaled deeply and said the words that he had known for so long but had never admitted to himself.

"My name is Cleve," he said, "and I am an alcoholic."

LUXEMBOURG GARDENS, PARIS

After the bitterly cold winter, Bill Kraus was elated at the coming of spring. He had grown increasingly disenchanted with Paris and fretted constantly about running out of money and returning to California a pauper. In April, Representative Sala Burton had taken Bill off the congressional payroll. Although ailing aides routinely keep their congressional jobs, Burton had been persuaded to fire Bill because he was out of the country. Supervisor Harry Britt and a number of Bill's friends had sent out a fund-raising letter for contributions to a Bill Kraus Trust Fund. However, that effort became controversial when the *Bay Area Reporter,* still angry at the role Bill played in the bathhouse controversy, ran an editorial condemning the fund-raising as elitist.

The only advantage to living in Paris, Bill decided, was that, in France, AIDS was considered to be just another disease, like leukemia. The mere utterance of the word did not elicit the visible reactions it engendered among Americans. Still, Bill was lonely for his friends, and he longed to return to San Francisco.

Bill was also unhappy at the course of his treatment. His doctors were less enthusiastic about HPA-23 and were urging him to start taking isoprinosine, a drug believed to act as an immune system booster. The suggestion upset Bill because he had pinned his entire hope for survival on HPA-23. Even the possibility that it might not be a panacea enraged him, cutting to the core of his denial and bargaining with his AIDS diagnosis. In early May, Bill's spirits sank further; several new lesions appeared on his face.

When his friend and housemate Ron Huberman arrived in France for a month-long visit, Bill was visibly relieved. Together, they wandered through the gay neighborhoods of Paris and dined with other San Franciscans who had come for the HPA-23 treatments.

"Maybe we should sell our house in San Francisco and just move here," Ron suggested as they walked through the Luxembourg Gardens. "I love Paris. You'd be near the Pasteur. We could get jobs here."

"No, I want to return to San Francisco," Bill said. "That's where I want to . . ."

Bill paused.

Ron could fill in the blank himself.

". . . That's where I want to be," Bill continued. "I'm really lonely. I can't bear to not be with my friends."

"When you want to go home, just go," said Ron. "We'll all be there for you."

The pair walked among the statues and hedges until Bill broke the silence. "I don't think I'm going to make it," he said simply.

It was the first time Ron ever heard Bill confide his fears about dying. In fact, ever since his diagnosis, Bill had ordered his friends to not even think about the fact he might die, insisting that their mental images of him in a deathbed would harm his health. Many of Bill's friends considered this idea to be flaky, but fundamentally they wanted to deny Bill's condition as much as Bill did, so they complied. Ron was relieved that Bill seemed to be entering the acceptance stage of his terminal diagnosis. Later that night, however, Bill seemed embarrassed.

"Disregard everything I said earlier," he told Ron. "I'm uptight."

Bill seemed most comfortable angry, and throughout Ron's visit, he railed about the lack of treatment programs in the United States. About 100 Americans were part of the AIDS exile community in Paris, making long daily treks to Percy Hospital on the edge of the city for their shots of HPA-23.

From his apartment on the Quai des Celestines overlooking the Seine, Bill furiously wrote letters to his friends and contacted reporters, urging them to write stories on treatment issues. Less than 10 percent of America's AIDS patients were being offered any kind of experimental drug for AIDS. Only an infinitesimal portion of the 100,000 people estimated to be suffering from ARC were being treated, even though scientists agreed that treatments probably would be vastly more successful on such patients, given the fact that their immune systems had yet to suffer the devastation that precedes an AIDS diagnosis. Patients with AIDS and ARC were told to simply wait until the carefully controlled drug studies were completed before trying the experimental drugs—even though many knew they would be dead before that happened.

The federal government continued to be indifferent to the problem. In early May, the Food and Drug Administration announced that it would permit Newport Pharmaceutical International to supply isoprinosine to doctors under protocols for investigational drugs. In order to meet the FDA requirements, however, the company calculated that it would need to spend about $2,000 in blood tests and other costs for each patient taking the drug. Government funding, of course, was not available for widespread tests. Not surprisingly, Newport announced that it could not permit more than a handful of patients in the United States to use the drug. Meanwhile, James Mason, Acting Assistant Secretary for Health answered congressional inquiries about government AIDS treatment efforts with the assurance that "the Public Health Service continues to give the development of new experimental modalities for the therapy of AIDS the highest possible support."

In San Francisco, desperation fueled a vast underground network to supply AIDS and ARC patients with the two most popular underground drugs, ribavirin and isoprinosine. Both drugs were being used in experimental trials on limited numbers of people in the United States, although they were not licensed for general distribution. They could, however, be purchased at any drugstore in Mexico. A Berkeley group calling themselves the Tooth Fairies had put together a guide on how to conceal the drugs from customs agents at the border. In the hands of less socially conscious profiteers, the cost of these AIDS drugs skyrocketed in a bustling black market. A twenty-tablet box of isoprinosine could be purchased in Mexico for $2.50. In San Francisco, anxious AIDS sufferers paid as much as $1.20 a tablet.

Bill Kraus was angry that the AIDS organizations, which had spent so much time defending bathhouse owners, could not take it upon themselves to fight for wider availability of AIDS treatments. He also implored his friends in political groups to take up the cause. "This is absurd," Bill complained. "People are supposed to go *to* the United States for treatment. We shouldn't have to be leaving."

Throughout his stay in Paris, Bill had largely avoided gay night life. Ron Huberman was more of a party animal, however, so Bill accompanied him to the bars and discos for some rare nights out. At the popular dance palace, Haute Tensione, Bill met a handsome young man who showed some interest in him. When Bill said he was from San Francisco, the conversation immediately shifted to AIDS.

"Is this really a terrible thing, or is it something to moralize against us?" the Frenchman asked Bill.

Bill allowed that the epidemic was very real.

"Is it true they have closed all the bars and the bathhouses?" he asked incredulously.

Bill explained the intricacies of the unsafe sex ban and made it clear he thought it was long overdue. In Paris, similar issues were emerging. A number of Parisian gay bars had dark back rooms with enough sexual activity to match the heyday of any San Francisco bathhouse, orgasm for orgasm. The police were demanding that gay bar owners turn the lights up in the back rooms. The local gay press declared this fascistic.

"I think it's horrible," the Parisian said, "the way they would moralize to us."

Bill was overcome with a sense of déjà vu. He had had this conversation hundreds of times in San Francisco. He wanted to shake the young man and shout: "For God's sake, don't make the same mistakes we did."

⬭

By May 1985, concern about AIDS had swept five continents. European health authorities reported nearly 1,000 AIDS cases. More than 300 were French, 162 were from West Germany, and Britain reported 140. Austrian health authorities reported the diagnosis of *Pneumocystis* in a one-year-old infant. The infant's mother apparently was a prostitute, and her child was the first baby AIDS case in Europe. In Sweden, where 8 were dead and 300 showed ARC symptoms, authorities recommended adding AIDS to the venereal disease laws. Under those laws, the government could impose a two-year prison sentence on any AIDS sufferer who knowingly partook in sexual activity that might spread the disease. In England, the government's chief medical officer declared AIDS the most serious health threat to that nation since World War II. Health Minister Kenneth Clarke announced new regulations to give British magistrates the power to order an AIDS sufferer into hospital isolation if he persisted in engaging in sexual acts likely to spread the disease.

Sensational stories about AIDS in the flamboyant British press inflamed anti-gay prejudice. One prominent gay activist was attacked outside a London subway by a gang of knife-wielding youths who suggested that he should be killed before he could spread "the gay plague" to others. When a London gay switchboard's lines broke down because they were so overwhelmed with AIDS calls, telephone company employees refused to fix them because they were afraid of contracting AIDS from the wiring.

In the strangest twist to English AIDS history, the guide to British aristocracy, *Burke's Peerage,* announced that, in an effort to preserve "the purity of the human race," it would not list any family in which any member was known to have AIDS. "We are worried that AIDS may not be a simple infection, even if conveyed in an unusual way," its publishing director said, "but an indication of a genetic defect."

The death of the first AIDS patient on mainland Asia sparked AIDS panic in Hong Kong. Health authorities discovered, however, that their efforts to trace AIDS were hampered by Hong Kong's draconian laws against homosexuality. Under local law, gays faced life imprisonment. Not surprisingly, when the government set up a hotline to answer AIDS questions, few people would give health workers their names and addresses so they could be mailed risk-reduction guidelines. Doing any sort of epidemiology or contact tracing also was rendered impossible by the severe punishments for homosexual behavior. A gay businessman warned that if the government did not decriminalize homosexuality, "it will be guilty of murder."

Health authorities worldwide braced for growing caseloads, given evidence that the virus already had spread widely, even in nations that had yet to see many AIDS cases. In Montreal, 28 percent of gay men in one study were found to be infected with the AIDS virus. Between 20 and 30 percent of gay men in a Melbourne, Australia, study were infected. In England, an organizer of Britain's major AIDS organization, the Terence Higgins Trust, bluntly advised English gay men to avoid sex with any Londoner after one study found that one-third of the city's gay men were infected with HTLV-III.

The governments that were most intransigent about acknowledging the AIDS problem were those that were widely believed to be hardest hit. Although African health officials claimed only a handful of AIDS cases, one CDC staffer reported in March that there were 11,000 AIDS cases in Zaire alone. The huge number of prostitutes infected with the AIDS virus in such nations as Rwanda and Uganda suggested that the heterosexual spread of "slim disease" continued unabated.

There was a familiar element in the policy questions that rose around AIDS in western Europe. By early 1985, Denmark had the highest per capita rate of AIDS in Europe. One study found that 36 percent of gay men were infected with the AIDS virus, and gay men who went to bathhouses were being infected at a rate of 3 percent a month. Clinicians like Dr. Ib Bygbjerg felt that bathhouses should be closed and the country should include AIDS in its venereal disease laws, as Sweden had. However, health authorities made no move without approval of the well-organized gay community. Still unimpressed by the relative handful of cases in Denmark, homosexual leaders viewed the AIDS threat as homophobic hyperbole and persuaded authorities that bathhouse closure would be an unacceptable infringement on their civil rights.

As case after case came to *Rigshospitalet,* the hospital where Dr. Grethe Rask had died eight years before, Bygbjerg despaired. "Gay radicals are holding public policy hostage to their politics," he complained. "We need to stop this disease, and we're not being allowed to."

In Paris in early 1985, Dr. Willy Rozenbaum had examined a lymphadenopathy patient and had given his opinion that the man should not continue to have sex. The man had been outraged at the suggestion.

"It's my right," he said.

Rozenbaum had argued, but he could see he wasn't getting anywhere.

There was, of course, no question that this man was infected with the AIDS virus. Indeed, his body was home to the progeny of the most famous AIDS virus in the world, because it was from his lymph node that the Pasteur Institute had cultured the first isolate of LAV in early 1983.

May 17
DUBLIN STREET, SAN FRANCISCO

The week-long hospitalization at the University of California Medical Center in San Francisco did not cure Frances Borchelt's brutal psoriasis. Bob Borchelt felt his heart would tear apart, watching his wife return to her bed in the home where they had shared so many happy years. Sometimes, Frances sat in her orange overstuffed chair in the living room, but she'd shoo away anybody who tried to give her a hug.

"You don't want to come near me, guys," she'd say.

Frances was no longer interested in food or drink, so Cathy or Bob thought of all kinds of imaginative ways to feed her. They methodically marked the ounces of water she drank on a jar; every gulp became a small victory.

At times, it seemed the grandmother's mind was going. She had proficiently worked her daily *New York Times* crossword puzzle for years, but suddenly she found it impossible to think of the right words and maintain her concentration. It was hard even to hold a pencil.

Throughout the last weeks of May, it seemed there was no end to the litany of ailments that struck Frances Borchelt. She had severe lymphadenopathy, and the doctors had now diagnosed a blood disease, idiopathic thrombocytopenic purpura, as well. She also had mastitis and oral thrush.

Still, Frances tried to act as if she could live a normal life. Every morning, she made her bed, as she had always done during her four decades of marriage.

Now, however, tidying the sheets sometimes took forty-five minutes; she just didn't have the energy. By the time Frances Borchelt developed a coarse cough in the first few days of June, Bob, Cathy, and the rest of the family had no doubt that the end was near.

On Monday, June 10, the family took Frances Borchelt back to Seton Medical Center to be treated for bronchial pneumonia. Her lungs had filled with fluids, and she sweated continuously from fierce fevers. After the hospital priest administered the last rites, Frances looked up to Cathy and asked, "Who was that?"

As the days passed, she began muttering to herself. Cathy noticed that, at times, the babbling had all the inflections of a conversation. At one point, she turned away from her imaginary interlocutor and asked Cathy, "Why am I sick?" Next, she fell into a coma.

On Saturday, June 15, Frances Borchelt went blind.

Frances had been adamant that she did not want to be buried with her wedding rings. As her body began to fill with fluids and bloat, Cathy decided it was time to remove them. However, her mother's fingers were already so swollen, the hospital had to call custodians to cut the plain bands of white gold from her fingers. After that, Frances's muttering stopped.

Weeks before, the blood bank lawyers had scheduled a June 20 interview with Frances so they could take her deposition for the family's negligence lawsuit against Irwin Memorial Blood Bank. When attorneys heard that the woman was in the hospital, they asked to reschedule the appointment. The request made Cathy Borchelt angry.

"They should be forced to come here and see what actually happens to somebody who gets AIDS," she said. However, she did not prevail.

Bob Borchelt sat with his wife all day on Monday, June 17. She had drifted into a deeper coma, and the nurses, seeing Bob's exhaustion, suggested that he go home and rest. They'd phone if anything happened, and the call came not long after Bob got back to Dublin Street. Frances was dead.

On the day that Frances Borchelt died, the Centers for Disease Control announced that the number of Americans stricken with AIDS had surpassed 11,000. New cases could now be expected at a rate of about 1,000 a month. As of June 17, the CDC said, 11,010 Americans had contracted AIDS and 5,441 had died.

On June 21, AIDS patients at George Washington University Hospital opened their eyes to see a woman in a white linen gown moving among them. She wore no mask or gloves and was not afraid to approach their beds and ask the young men about their illness. Mother Teresa came to visit the AIDS patients directly from the White House, where President Reagan, who had yet to acknowledge the disease, had awarded her the Medal of Freedom.

Although the dramatic events of the next five weeks would overshadow such gestures, it was apparent even in the first days of the summer of 1985 that wider interest in the problem of AIDS was growing. The problem was becoming too vast to ignore.

Religious leaders had played a key role in demanding more attention for AIDS. In San Francisco, Episcopal Bishop William Swing delivered a seminal sermon in which he argued that if Jesus were alive in 1985, he would not be standing with the moralists condemning gays but with the people suffering from AIDS. One of the things that made Christ so compassionate, he said, was the fact that he cast his lot with outcasts.

The new scientific understanding of the virulence of the AIDS virus prompted an unprecedented action at the American Medical Association's mid-June national convention. Although the AMA had a long-standing policy against promoting funding of specific medical research, the House of Delegates voted to put the AMA on record as seeking more funds for AIDS research. The resolution passed overwhelmingly with little debate. As one proponent explained, "We now realize that this is not just another disease, but a major epidemic having a serious impact on public health."

In what was to prove a forerunner for many similar stories that summer, *Life* magazine released a dramatic cover feature story and photo essay that grimly announced on the cover: "Now, No One Is Safe from AIDS." In truth, most Americans were safe from AIDS, and there was more fiction than fact in *Life*'s assertion that heterosexual hemophiliacs, heterosexual transfusion recipients, and heterosexual partners of intravenous drug users were the epidemic's "new victims." None of these risk groups were, in fact, new. What was new was that the media was talking about AIDS in a heterosexual context. This context made AIDS newsworthy, and in the summer months, the most common expression among AIDS organizers became, "AIDS is not a gay disease."

And it was in answer to those words that the United States took its first tentative steps toward the realization that a new epidemic would be indelibly written into the history of the Republic, and nothing would ever be the same again.

June 30
SAN FRANCISCO

Bright sunshine turned the sky porcelain blue and brightened the greens on San Francisco's sloping hills. The sun always shone on the San Francisco Gay Freedom Day Parade, it seemed. A crowd of 250,000 clogged sidewalks and streets for two miles in downtown San Francisco, even before the three-hour procession of floats, marching bands, and other contingents began.

The diversity of the world's preeminent gay community, converging again for its annual celebration, created both the point and counterpoint that demonstrated why the gay community defied singular depiction. Men carried on their shoulders six-year-olds who wore T-shirts proclaiming "I Love My Gay Dad." A block away from this wholesome sight, the float from the Chaps leather bar lumbered along, featuring a troupe of men clad in black leather straps and handcuffed into all kinds of fascinating positions; they loved their daddies too. After the usual appearance of Dykes on Bykes came Ducks in Trucks, a float with scores of rubber ducks floating around little plastic swimming pools. Behind earnest lesbian-feminists protesting Central American policy were the satirical "Ladies Against Women," carrying such signs as "Recriminalize Hanky-Panky" and "Suffering NOT Suffrage."

There was a different mood to this parade, as well as to the community it represented. The depression that had marked the penultimate phase of a community coming to grips with widespread death was beginning to lift. In its place was an acceptance. There might have been a time Before, but it was no longer the moment that people longed for; it was gone, everyone understood now, and it would never come back. Life would forevermore be in this After. It was cruel and it wasn't fair, but that was the way it would be, and at the sixteenth annual Gay Freedom Day Parade it was clear that most gay San Franciscans understood this.

After the years of denial and anger, the bargaining and incapacitating sadness, the San Francisco gay community was mobilized to fight the epidemic, as was no other single group in the United States. The parade was dedicated to the memory of Bobbi Campbell, the one-time "KS poster boy" who had died the previous summer. The floats with naked men got less applause this year than the numerous contingents of AIDS-related organizations that, by now, had persuaded thousands of local gay men to spend their after-work hours staffing information hotlines, raising funds for AIDS services, and performing chores in the homes of the stricken. This was the new gay community that paraded by the hundreds of thousands under the afternoon sun, and everybody applauded. When the San Francisco AIDS Foundation's somber float rolled slowly by, with its huge black faux marble tombstone draped with garlands, people seemed to understand that this was part of the gay community too, and the parade judges awarded the float a special prize.

The parade's largest contingent stretched for two full blocks and marched under the banner of "Living Sober." They were the burgeoning ranks of gay people who had given up drugs and alcohol, largely through Alcoholics Anonymous, and were among the pioneers of the new life-style emerging in the gay community. Other groups handed out thousands of condoms without fear that gay men would simply blow them up like balloons and discard them, as they had in past parades. And nobody joked any more that they didn't know how to use the darn things. One Castro Street boutique now reported selling an average of 4,000 rubbers every weekend and had recently started a rack of "designer condoms." A former porn star had come to the parade to promote his own safe-sex campaign called, "Get Butch with Germs."

At the AIDS Foundation booth, staffers were touting the results of a new survey that found that four in five local gay men had totally eliminated high-risk sexual practices from their repertoire of bedroom activities. Only one in eleven gay men still engaged in unprotected oral sex, and only one in fourteen practiced anal intercourse without a rubber. More than half of gay men were ensconced in relationships. No longer was the foundation giving gays a "safe sex can be fun" message. Instead, new ads bluntly admonished, "There is no longer any excuse for unsafe sex."

The gay community had managed to take this dramatic turnaround in sexual norms with typical good humor. Comedian Doug Holsclaw routinely broke up audiences with his one-liner, "I like to fuck with strangers—call me old-fashioned."

What was particularly noteworthy was that rather than dissipating in the wake of the epidemic, gay political strength continued to increase. Nothing demonstrated this more amply than the presence of Alan Cranston, the first U.S. Senator to ever address a Gay Freedom Day audience, at the rally following the parade. "From our freedom, we produce diversity," Cranston said, "and from our diversity we gain strength to overcome our problem."

The loudest ovations of the day came not for politicians or entertainers, but when the rally's master of ceremonies announced the release of two San Francisco gay men who had been among the twenty-nine Americans held hostage by terrorists in Lebanon. The two men, who had been aboard TWA Flight 847 on an Athens-to-Rome leg of a world tour, had spent most of their captivity living with the terror that their fundamentalist Moslem captors would learn that they were gay and kill them, as they had killed an American serviceman on the flight.

Early in their captivity, San Francisco news organizations learned that hostage Jack McCarty had worked as a chef for the Elephant Walk on 18th and Castro streets, one of the city's most famous gay bars, before embarking on the tour with his lover, postman Victor Amburgy. With unprecedented restraint, local news organizations withheld reporting on this angle of the story, fearing the gay story would result in the two hostages' deaths.

In the long days of captivity, McCarty and Amburgy were kept in dark, rat-infested basements while the terrorists played Russian roulette with the hostages, again and again. When other hostages began to crack, some of the Americans turned to McCarty, who had seemed preternaturally calm. McCarty could not tell them the reason he could handle the prospect of imminent death—that he was a gay man from San Francisco. Instead, he adopted the role of an unofficial counselor for the other hostages. It was a role to which McCarty was accustomed; he had been a Shanti Project volunteer.

Throughout the ordeal, the forty-year-old chef recalled Scott Cleaver, a twenty-seven-year-old whom he had counseled as part of his Shanti work. McCarty had watched Cleaver muster incredible strength and courage to fight his terminal disease, and McCarty promised himself that he would be as brave in the hands of these terrorists. The fortitude was something he shared with the other hostages, and it helped them all survive.

When Amburgy and McCarty stepped off the Air Force plane after their release, while a quarter-million lesbians and gay men celebrated Gay Freedom Day in San Francisco, they walked down the ramp arm-in-arm. They loved each other, and they were proud they loved each other, and they had survived in part because of the strength they had developed as gay men in San Francisco.

On that sunny Gay Freedom Day in San Francisco, it was clear that this entire gay community also had something to share with the larger society. Hopefully, Americans could learn from the gay community's mistakes and not waste valuable time floundering in denial; perhaps Americans could learn from the gay community's new strengths, as well. It was a far different vision of strength than what gays had imagined they would fashion when they marched proudly in the 1980 Gay Freedom Day Parade. The outward push for power continued, but it was largely eclipsed by the inward struggle for grit in the face of some of the cruelest blows that fate had meted out to any American community. As gay people had helped each other find this strength, they had forged a gay community that was truly a community, not just a neighborhood. And by now, there was also a shared sense that they wanted the dream to survive. It had been a painful and difficult five years to reach this point, but it had come this day.

57 ENDGAME

Friday, July 12, 1985
RAYBURN HOUSE OFFICE BUILDING,
WASHINGTON, D.C.

Conflicts again arose between the administration and the House of Representatives as Congress entered the final phase of budget writing for the coming fiscal year. For two months, Representative Henry Waxman had prodded Health and Human Services Secretary Margaret Heckler for documents indicating what the nation's health agency doctors had requested for AIDS research. The administration's claim that the researchers were getting all the funds they wanted meant that doctors had asked for a 10 percent reduction in funds to fight the epidemic. Henry Waxman and aide Tim Westmoreland had no doubt that if they could get their hands on internal memoranda, they would find that, once again, government doctors were pleading for more funds, not fewer. Heckler's office ignored the requests.

Meanwhile, Dr. James Mason, Acting Assistant Secretary for Health, was known to be making trips to the Office of Management and Budget to argue for more money. When an interviewer for the Cable Health Network had asked Dr. Robert Gallo a few weeks before whether he had sufficient funds to study AIDS, the normally effusive researcher would only offer a terse "no comment." Privately, Gallo complained bitterly that over a year after the administration's spotlighting of his HTLV-III discovery, the government had still produced no significant increase in funds for his lab. To a group of French journalists, Gallo openly complained, "The work done right now in therapeutic research is insufficient."

Unrest was growing in Congress as well. California Senator Cranston, looking ahead to a difficult reelection campaign in 1986, had become a leading Senate spokesman for AIDS funding. House Appropriations Committee chair Ed Roybal had become radicalized on the AIDS issue after a gay staffer in his Los Angeles district office succumbed to the syndrome.

Representative Waxman had scheduled hearings on the AIDS budget for Monday, July 22. He wanted documentation for the need of more AIDS funds by then, so on July 12, he threw down the gauntlet in a letter to Secretary Heckler.

"If all documents are not received by that date, I will be forced to consider action to subpoena the information," he wrote. "I am indeed sorry to be so blunt in my request. . . . For six months, however, the Congress has awaited the courtesy of a response, and none has been forthcoming. During those six months, almost 1,800 Americans have died of AIDS and almost 3,300 were confirmed to have this almost certainly terminal condition. Under such circumstances and in light of the Administration's previous years of delay and neglect, I do not believe that we can wait longer."

Once again, Waxman felt, the administration would need to be shamed into allocating appropriate funds for its "number-one health priority."

Monday, July 15
CARMEL, CALIFORNIA

Rock Hudson's friends had pleaded with the actor to cancel the planned taping of a television segment with Doris Day, but the affable matinee idol insisted that he had given his word. He knew that Day, with whom he had starred in *Pillow Talk* and other romantic comedies in the early 1960s, was counting on the publicity from their reunion to promote her new animal show on the Christian Broadcasting Network.

When Hudson arrived, the physical deterioration evident in his haggard face and wasted frame stunned Day and the reporters who attended the press conference near her home in Carmel. Hudson barely had the strength to walk, but he went through his two days of taping bravely and told reporters he had the flu. It was Rock Hudson's last public appearance.

When asked if Hudson was ill, the actor's press spokesman, Dale Olson, said he was "in perfect health" and had dropped some excess weight as part of a diet regimen.

When Rock Hudson returned to Los Angeles, he collapsed from fatigue. His Kaposi's sarcoma had been progressing for a year now. A few weeks earlier, he had been diagnosed with lymphoblastic lymphoma, a cancer seen increasingly among AIDS patients. Hudson told his friends he would return to Paris for his HPA-23 treatments as soon as he could muster the strength.

○

On July 17, Bahamian health authorities shut down a cancer clinic that was treating patients with blood-derived drugs. Batches of the drugs, it turned out, were infected with the AIDS virus. As many as 1,000 patients had been treated at the clinic, and after an initial investigation by the Centers for Disease Control, health officials warned patients that they might be at risk for developing AIDS.

Among the patients was former Georgia Governor Lester Maddox. During the height of the civil rights movement, Maddox had found a permanent place in the history of American racism. He had handed out ax handles to white patrons of the segregated restaurant he owned, after civil rights leaders had targeted the establishment for a sit-in. As taciturn as ever, Maddox reacted poorly to the news that he might have been infected with the AIDS virus. "I'd rather go with straight cancer than AIDS," he said. "There's more dignity with cancer."

Friday, July 19
WASHINGTON, D.C.

The subpoena for administration AIDS records was about to be prepared when a messenger hastily delivered Secretary Heckler's missive to Representative Waxman's office late Friday night.

"There has been agreement within the Administration on the necessity of additional funding," Heckler wrote. The Secretary announced that the administration had just discovered "deficiencies" in the AIDS budget totaling $45.7 million, and Heckler authorized the diversion of the funds from other health programs to the AIDS budget. Heckler's redirection of funds increased AIDS spending for the next fiscal year by 48 percent to a total of $126.4 million. The increase, Heckler said, was evidence of the administration's commitment to AIDS as its "number-one health priority."

Sunday, July 21
PARIS

Shortly after his arrival in Paris, as he walked across the lobby of the Ritz Hotel, Rock Hudson collapsed. A doctor examined Hudson in his room and assumed that the heart condition, for which the actor had undergone cardiac surgery in 1981, was responsible. Hudson was driven to the American Hospital in the suburb of Neuilly. Doctors at the hospital were told only that Hudson had a history of heart disease.

Monday, July 22
WASHINGTON, D.C.

The AIDS hearings of Representative Waxman's Subcommittee on Health and the Environment followed the ritual format for congressional inquiries into the government's handling of the epidemic. Various doctors, including Paul Volberding from San Francisco and Michael Gottlieb from Los Angeles, appeared to chastise the government's low funding levels and, in particular, the lack of even fragmentary research into AIDS treatments. Dr. Martin Hirsch of Massachusetts General Hospital pleaded for a "crash program" of research on the disease and warned, presciently, "Before it is finished, thousands, perhaps hundreds of thousands, more will become victims."

Dr. James Mason defended the administration's record, noting the "tremendous progress in a short period of time" and reminding Congress that the epidemic was the administration's "number-one health priority."

This led to the usual angry cross-examination by Representative Waxman, who, nevertheless, thanked Mason for the increase in research funds. Sardonically, he added, "almost 2,000 Americans died and thousands more were infected" with the AIDS virus while Congress had awaited the additional budget request. "For these people," Waxman said, "even this budget is too little, too late."

Tuesday, July 23

URGENT. ROCK HUDSON FATALLY ILL. URGENT

HOLLYWOOD (UPI)—ACTOR ROCK HUDSON, LAST OF THE TRADITIONAL SQUAREJAWED, ROMANTIC LEADING MEN, KNOWN RECENTLY FOR HIS TV ROLES ON "MCMILLAN & WIFE" AND "DYNASTY" IS SUFFERING FROM INOPERABLE LIVER CANCER POSSIBLY LINKED TO AIDS, IT WAS DISCLOSED TUESDAY.

The bulletin arrived after 1 P.M., in time to make the afternoon headlines. Several news organizations had been tracking rumors that Hudson had AIDS, since his appearance with Doris Day a week earlier. The *Hollywood Reporter* ran an item on the morning of July 23, saying bluntly that Hudson had AIDS. That afternoon, American Hospital sources confirmed that the ailing film star had been in the hospital for two days. Lab tests showed that Hudson, an alcoholic, had liver irregularities, so rumors spread that the actor had liver cancer.

Hudson had told only four friends that he had the syndrome, heatedly denying the AIDS rumors to everyone else. Press spokesman Dale Olson issued the first of many denials about Hudson's AIDS diagnosis minutes after the first United Press International bulletin.

"My official statement is that Rock Hudson is in the American Hospital where his doctors have diagnosed that he has cancer of the liver and that it is not operable," Olson said. Hudson's personal doctors in Los Angeles, however, confirmed that the actor was in Paris to consult with doctors from the Pasteur Institute. Given the Pasteur's reputation for its AIDS research, many reporters began to draw the obvious conclusions.

Later in the afternoon, Dale Olson confirmed that Hudson was being tested "for everything." Reporters asked if that included AIDS. "Everything," Olson repeated.

When Nancy Reagan talked to reporters that evening, she recalled the night that Hudson had joined her and the president for a state dinner in the White House. Hudson had told her he picked up some bug in Israel, she said.

Wednesday, July 24

<u>PARIS</u>

A terse announcement from the American Hospital denied that Hudson had liver cancer and said only that he had been hospitalized for "fatigue and general malaise."

Gossip that Hudson was being treated by Dr. Dominique Dormant, who was treating Bill Kraus and most of the other American AIDS patients, sped through the community of AIDS exiles in Paris. As news organizations suddenly became hungry for stories about the miracle drug Hudson had come to Paris to seek, most of the American patients were hounded by reporters who, at last, were interested in the AIDS issue.

"Sorry we haven't done much on this before now," a *Washington Post* reporter told Bill Kraus as they started an interview. "We just haven't been able to find a handle that would make the story interesting to the general population."

It took all of Bill's self-control to keep from throwing the reporter out his window into the Seine.

That afternoon, Rock Hudson took a call from an old Hollywood friend.

"President Reagan wished him well and let him know that he and Mrs. Reagan were keeping him in their thoughts and prayers," said a White House spokesperson.

Dale Olson denied that the liver cancer story was a ruse to conceal the fact that Hudson had AIDS and said the hospital was being "wishy-washy" in denying the cancer diagnosis.

Just the possibility that Rock Hudson had AIDS, however, electrified the nation. Suddenly, all the newscasts and newspapers were running stories about the disease. In Washington, CBS producers called Representative Waxman to ask him to appear on "Face the Nation" that Sunday with Secretary Heckler to discuss federal AIDS policy. Waxman was delighted with the idea, especially since it marked the first time any major network show would devote significant time to discussing the federal government's role in the epidemic.

"Of course, if it turns out that Rock Hudson doesn't have AIDS," the producer said, "we're going to cancel this show."

In New York, Dr. Mathilde Krim, besieged with interview requests, was privately disgusted that President Reagan was shedding "crocodile tears" over Hudson. Where was his concern for the thousands of others who had been dying all these years? she wondered.

At the Gay Men's Health Crisis, Director Richard Dunne saw the explosion of interest in the epidemic as an opportunity to finally put the squeeze on Mayor Koch's administration. After a few well-placed calls alluding to the sudden interest of the press in all AIDS-related topics, Dunne learned that Koch had abruptly acknowledged the public-health merits in increasing funds for local AIDS projects.

◯

The major problem most news organizations confronted with the Hudson story was in explaining how the actor got AIDS. Of course, virtually everyone in the Hollywood film community had known for decades that Hudson was gay. Homosexuality, however, was an issue about which the media still felt much more comfortable lying than telling the truth. Consequently, the news stories about Hudson's health hedged the issue, alluding only to the CDC's standard list of risk groups.

Gay groups and AIDS organizations largely preferred it this way, eager to prove to the world once and for all that "AIDS is not a gay disease." This desire to conceal the truth sometimes went to absurd lengths. A press spokesperson for the San Francisco AIDS Foundation, for example, said that Hudson was proving to the world that "AIDS is not a gay white male disease," as though Hudson were something other than a gay white male. When pressed on Hudson's risk group status, Bill Meisenheimer, executive director of the AIDS Project–Los Angeles, refused to speculate on the actor's sexuality and instead talked about the transfusions Hudson had undergone during his heart surgery.

The embargo, however, broke late Wednesday night when the bulldog editions of the *San Francisco Chronicle* hit the streets with a story describing Hudson's years of personal conflict about remaining in the closet. With on-the-record quotes from a circle of Hudson's longtime friends in San Francisco, the story discussed the torment of a man who had for years struggled with the question of whether he might do some good by acknowledging his sexuality. In an unusual display of what editors considered good taste, the *Chronicle* had decided to play the story off its front page, on page seven. Other papers, however, demonstrated no such restraint, and by Thursday morning, newspapers and newscasts around the country were reporting the *Chronicle's* disclosure of Hudson's homosexuality.

Thursday, July 25

By now, officials at American Hospital had learned that Hudson had AIDS, and they wanted the actor out of their facility. They did not want the hospital's good name associated with a gay disease, fearing they would lose both prestige and patients. Nurses were anxious about treating Hudson.

Dr. Dominique Dormant pleaded with hospital officials to let him see his patient, but the hospital did not even want the AIDS expert to set foot in their building. When Dormant finally did see the actor, he was amazed at how deteriorated Hudson's condition was. Further HPA-23 treatments, he saw, would do no good.

There was also the question of what to tell the press. The hospital bluntly told Hudson's entourage that if they did not explain the actor's condition, the hospital would. A Parisian publicist, who had been enlisted to handle the local press, met with Hudson and gained his approval for the brief statement. At 2

P.M., Yannou Collart told reporters, "Mr. Hudson has Acquired Immune Deficiency Syndrome."

Collart's explanation, however, tended to complicate the situation further, because she insisted that the actor was "totally cured." When asked how the actor may have contracted the disease, she said, "He doesn't have any idea how he contracted AIDS. Nobody around him has AIDS."

In San Francisco, Marc Conant heard that Hudson had been Michael Gottlieb's patient.

"That's pretty courageous of him to admit that he had AIDS," Conant said to Gottlieb in a phone conversation.

"Courageous, hell," said Gottlieb. "He collapsed in a hotel lobby."

Still, Conant was thrilled with anything that brought the media spotlight to the epidemic. "Now there is a new risk group for AIDS," he told a reporter. "The rich and famous."

Friday, July 26

The revelation that Hudson had felt obliged to leave the United States for AIDS treatment cast the international spotlight on the Pasteur Institute. Much of what emerged was less than flattering to the Pasteur's American counterparts.

The Pasteur director, Dr. Raymond Dedonder, made a long-scheduled appearance in San Francisco before the French-American Chamber of Commerce. Dedonder explained how the French had applied for their patent on the LAV virus in December 1983, while Dr. Gallo had applied for the NCI patent on HTLV-III in early 1984. Dr. Gallo's patent was approved immediately; the Pasteur Institute patent still had not been approved. Without a patent, the Pasteur could not market its blood test in the United States or enjoy the substantial royalties that would accrue from LAV blood tests. The Pasteur would sue, Dedonder warned.

Bit by bit, the story of the fierce scientific warfare between the French and the Americans began to be assembled. The Hudson episode and its attendant publicity rapidly turned into a major embarrassment for American science in general and the federal government in particular.

In Paris, Dr. David Klatzmann of the Pasteur Institute exclaimed that, at last, "we are out of the desert."

Sunday, July 28

AIDS was on the front page of virtually every Sunday morning paper in the United States. Any local angle was pursued with a vengeance, and entertainment sections were crowded with retrospectives on Rock Hudson's career. There was something about Hudson's diagnosis that seemed to strike an archetypal chord in the American consciousness. For decades, Hudson had been among the handful of screen actors who personified wholesome American masculinity; now, in one stroke, he was revealed as both gay and suffering from the affliction of pariahs. Doctors involved in AIDS research called the Hudson announcement the single most important event in the history of the epidemic, and few knowledgeable people argued.

In Los Angeles, a huge crowd turned out for an AIDS Walkathon for the AIDS Project–Los Angeles. The event raised $630,000 in one afternoon, a record for an AIDS fund-raiser, and Los Angeles Mayor Tom Bradley joined a host of movie celebrities praising Hudson's disclosure as a crucial reason for the day's success.

In Washington, Secretary Margaret Heckler abruptly canceled her appearance on "Face the Nation" with Representative Henry Waxman. Acting Assistant Secretary for Health James Mason took Heckler's place, assuring viewers that in recent years, "Money has not in any way incapacitated or slowed us down in moving ahead. . . . We've been working ever since the disease was first identified in 1981, and it is our first priority."

As proof of the administration's commitment, Mason pointed to the increase in AIDS funding announced just that week. Mason didn't mention the threat of the congressional subpoena.

In the suburbs of San Francisco, Rick Walsh grew angrier with each passing day of the Rock Hudson revelations. Big deal, he thought. One guy named Rock Hudson gets AIDS and everybody starts paying attention. When one guy named Gary Walsh died a slow, excruciating death, nobody cared. To the end, Rick knew that his Uncle Gary had believed there might be a reprieve, a cure. But it never came because nobody cared, and now Gary was dead, and thousands more like him were dead. Nobody gave a damn about any of them, just this guy named Rock Hudson. It had never crossed Rick Walsh's mind that politics might have something to do with medicine. Now he knew better.

Monday, July 29
PHILIP BURTON MEMORIAL FEDERAL BUILDING,
SAN FRANCISCO

The Mobilization Against AIDS held a press conference to plead again with Ronald Reagan to say something, anything, about the epidemic, now that he, like the gay men of San Francisco, had a friend who was dying of AIDS. "The president's silence on AIDS is deafening," said the group's director, Paul Boneberg. "Still, he has not said one word about the disease."

A White House press spokesperson said that the president would have no comment on either the press conference or the AIDS epidemic.

Both *Times* and *Newsweek* hit the newsstands with huge stories about Rock Hudson and the AIDS epidemic. Every major news organization in the country was gearing up to do investigative series on the epidemic. As calls flooded the AIDS Activities Office at the Centers for Disease Control, all available staffers were diverted to handling press inquiries. Dr. Harold Jaffe, who had worked on the epidemic since the day Sandra Ford had first alerted the CDC to the mysterious pentamidine orders, wanted to scream into his phone: "Where have you been for the last four years?"

As Don Francis watched the drama unfold, he thought back to one day he had had after beating back the virulent outbreak of Ebola Fever virus in Africa. He and the other scientists from the World Health Organization had thwarted the spread of a horribly deadly disease, risking their lives in the process. When the plane carrying them back to Europe had landed, thousands were waiting on the runway to greet them. The crowds, however, were not on hand for the weary WHO doctors but for a basketball team that had just won an international championship. A bunch of damn athletes, Francis had thought.

To Francis, the Hudson episode was not a celebration of one man's courage but an indictment of our era. A lot of good, decent Americans had perished in this epidemic, but it was the diagnosis of one movie star, who had demonstrated no previous inclination to disclose his plight, that was going to make all the difference.

That afternoon in Atlanta, the CDC released new figures showing that in the past week the number of AIDS cases in the United States had surpassed 12,000. As of that morning, 12,067 Americans were diagnosed with AIDS, of whom 6,079 had died.

In Beijing that day, health authorities reported the first case of AIDS to be detected in the People's Republic of China.

July 30
PARIS

Two minutes before midnight, a chartered Boeing 747 Air France jet, bearing only Rock Hudson and six medical attendants, taxied onto the runway of Orly International Airport. Hudson had wanted to be transferred from the American Hospital to Percy Hospital, where he could undergo HPA-23 treatments, but Dr. Dormant had dissuaded him, informing the actor that he would die soon. Nothing more could be done. When Dormant learned that Hudson had paid $250,000 to rent the jumbo airliner for his return trip, he was dumbstruck. Hudson could have traveled on a commercial jetliner, Dormant knew. The charter was totally unnecessary.

"Two hundred fifty thousand dollars is more than my budget for four years of AIDS research," Dormant groaned.

The plane landed in Los Angeles International Airport at 2:30 A.M. Pacific time. Hundreds of newspeople had gathered for a glimpse of the actor as he was transferred from the plane to a helicopter. Television cameras with telescopic lenses cluttered the airport's rooftops, and photographers jostled for the moment when the world would get the first glimpse of Hudson since his AIDS disclosure. Momentarily, the cameras caught the gaunt form clad in a white hospital gown and covered by a white sheet, as the gurney was wheeled to the helicopter.

In Hawaii, Cleve Jones wanted to put his fist through the television set as he watched the grotesque spectacle of news choppers vying for exclusive footage of the world's newest celebrity AIDS patient. The television stations could afford helicopters to record fifteen seconds of Rock Hudson on a stretcher, but they had never afforded the time to note the passing of the thousands who had gone before him. Cleve recalled the line of pale, anxious faces stretching down the stairs from the one-room office of the KS Foundation on Castro Street in the summer of 1982. All those boys were dead now, and they had died unlamented and unremarked by the media. This is what it took, Cleve thought, some famous closet case to collapse in a hotel lobby.

A few days before, Cleve had heard a new report that scientists had isolated the AIDS virus in the tears of AIDS patients. This discovery and the Hudson spectacle melded into one thought as Cleve watched his television set. "Okay," he said to himself, "I'm not going to cry anymore. I'm going to fight you bastards."

Cleve Jones had come to Hawaii broken and weak. He had found sobriety now and had reclaimed his confidence. He was strong enough to make a difference once again. He would return to Castro Street. It was where he belonged and where he was needed. He would return to Castro Street, and he would not leave again.

◯

From the plate glass windows on the tenth floor of the UCLA Medical Center in Westwood, Michael Gottlieb watched Rock Hudson's helicopter land on the hospital helipad. Bright lights from the television news helicopters overhead bathed the scene in a surreal, even macabre glow. Gottlieb had offered to go to Paris and accompany his patient back to Los Angeles, but Dr. Dormant assured him that Hudson was well in hand. When Gottlieb later examined Hudson, he could tell that the patient was deathly ill, barely cognizant of what was going on around him.

Throughout the night, the medical center continued to be bombarded with media requests on the patient's status. Gottlieb was aware that, as of yet, no physician had confirmed Hudson's diagnosis. The only statement had been Yannou Collart's garbled announcement in Paris. Gottlieb felt he needed to set the record straight if the media siege was ever to lift.

In the morning, he prepared a simple statement and read it to Hudson.

"Sure," Hudson said. "Go ahead."

It was four years, one month, and twenty-five days since Gottlieb's first report on the five unexplained cases of *Pneumocystis carinii* pneumonia had appeared in the *Morbidity and Mortality Weekly Report*. Since then, he had treated 200 AIDS patients, most of whom were dead by now. Gottlieb felt numbed with grief and weariness. After all his years of warnings and pleas, he was aggravated that it had taken this, the diagnosis of a movie star, to awaken the nation. He was troubled by what this said about America and the nation's much-vaunted regard for the sanctity of human life. Nevertheless, Gottlieb could see that Rock Hudson's diagnosis had irrevocably changed everything for the AIDS epidemic. After such a burst of attention, AIDS would never again be relegated to the obscurity to which it had long been assigned.

The UCLA media relations staff informed the news media of an impending announcement, and Gottlieb returned to his dilapidated office to gather his laboratory staff. They had shared the years of frustration and despair, and together they would share the moment that would transform the epidemic.

As he strode to the podium, Gottlieb could see his staff, lined up expectantly in the rear of the crowded auditorium. The chattering of the reporters faded as Gottlieb adjusted the microphone, and there was silence.

Gottlieb paused.

He looked from one side of the auditorium to the other. Gottlieb knew that he needed to be deliberate in every word he spoke. More than anything else, he did not want to sound embarrassed. That, he knew, was what had been the problem all along with this infernal epidemic: It was about sex, and it was about homosexuals. Taken altogether, it had simply embarrassed people—the politicians, the reporters, the scientists. AIDS had embarrassed everyone, he knew, and tens of thousands of Americans would die because of that. It was time for people to stop being embarrassed, Gottlieb decided, if our society was ever to beat this horrible enemy.

In calm, firm tones, Gottlieb began reading from his statement.

"Mr. Hudson is being evaluated and treated for complications of Acquired Immune Deficiency Syndrome."

PART IX

EPILOGUE: AFTER

"It was only possible for me to do it," he said, "because it was necessary. I either had to write the book or be reduced to despair: it was the only means of saving me from nothingness, chaos and suicide. The book was written under this pressure and brought me the expected cure, simply because it was written, irrespective of whether it was good or bad. That was the only thing that counted and while writing it, there was no need to think at all of any reader but myself, or at the most, here and there another close war-comrade, and I most certainly never thought then about the survivors, but always about those who fell in the war. While writing it, I was as if delirious or crazy, surrounded by three or four people with mutilated bodies—that was how the book was produced."

—HERMANN HESSE,
The Journey to the East

58 REUNION

May 31, 1987
WASHINGTON, D.C.

A sticky mugginess hung over Washington the day they arrived. The temperature was trapped in the upper nineties, and the air dense with humidity. Occasionally, lightning flashed and conversation stopped expectantly; thunder lumbered through the heavens, then passed. There was to be no relief.

The heat induced a light nausea among even the most acclimatized natives. For the thousands crowding airport cab stands, shuttle buses, and hotel lobbies that afternoon—the scientists and researchers, public health officials and activists converging on the capital city—the oppression was palpable.

The occasion was the Third International Conference on Acquired Immunodeficiency Syndrome, co-sponsored by the World Health Organization and the U.S. Department of Health and Human Services. Though the conference, a successor to the first international symposium held in Atlanta in 1985, would feature state-of-the-art information on all things AIDS-related, the focus of world attention on this event had less to do with such substance than with the conference's timing. Something had happened in the last two or three months; the epidemic had finally hit home.

Dr. Michael Gottlieb had been correct two years earlier when he stood in that auditorium in Los Angeles and realized that everything would be different for the AIDS epidemic from that day on. It was commonly accepted now, among the people who had understood the threat for many years, that there were two clear phases to the disease in the United States: there was AIDS before Rock Hudson and AIDS after. The fact that a movie star's diagnosis could make such a huge difference was itself a tribute to the power the news media exerted in the latter portion of the twentieth century.

Attention to the epidemic waned only slightly in 1986. There were other celebrity AIDS patients now, but for all the media cachet, the disease remained fundamentally embarrassing. When Broadway's star choreographer-director Michael Bennett fell ill, he maintained he was suffering from heart problems. A spokesman for Perry Ellis insisted the famed clothing designer was dying of sleeping sickness. Lawyer Roy Cohn insisted he had liver cancer, even while he

used his political connections to get on an experimental AIDS treatment protocol at the National Institutes of Health Hospital. Conservative fund-raiser Terry
Dolan claimed he was dying of diabetes. When Liberace was on his deathbed,
a spokesman maintained the painist was suffering the ill effects of a watermelon
diet. As these well-known gay men lied to protect their posthumous public
images, it was the first professional athlete to contract AIDS, former Washington Redskin star Jerry Smith, who calmly stepped forward and told the truth.

Even while such stories gave news organizations fresh angles, there was one
aspect to the epidemic that continued to elude intelligent investigation: the
federal government's role in combating the virus. Congress continued its ritual
of force-feeding AIDS funds to a reluctant Reagan administration. Funding
levels increased dramatically, but within the executive branch of government,
there seemed little excitement about launching anything like a coordinated
attack on the disease. Initiatives for development of a vaccine and effective
treatments puttered along at their usual speed.

Nor had the federal government launched anything resembling a coordinated AIDS prevention program. In late 1985, the CDC had actually stopped
money from being spent on AIDS education when conservatives in the White
House worried that the government should not be in the business of telling
homosexuals how to have sodomy. Even Dr. James Mason was heard complaining that since he had become CDC director, he found himself talking to complete strangers about sexual acts he would not discuss with his wife even in the
privacy of his own home.

Liberal congressional aides struggled to interest reporters in these prosaic
stories of federal sluggishness, but the media was unimpressed. Instead, stories
dealt with celebrity AIDS cases or schoolchildren with AIDS or laboratory
"breakthroughs." Just about every newspaper had also, by now, run a series of
profiles following the life of an AIDS patient. And, of course, there were endless
stories about the "spread of AIDS among heterosexuals." No hint that the
disease might spread to straights, no matter how specious, was too small to put
on page one.

Meanwhile, during most of 1986, anxious health officials within the administration desperately tried to turn the media's attention to the more significant
story: the message that the AIDS challenge still was not being met. At one point,
the Public Health Service held a meeting of its eighty-five top AIDS experts at
the Coolfant Conference Center in Berkeley, West Virginia, to make recommendations on federal AIDS policy. Their stunning projections were covered
by the press—that in five years the cumulative number of AIDS cases in the
United States would be 270,000 and deaths would total 179,000. The recommendations—for massive public education, better coordination of the federal
government's AIDS research and a blue-ribbon commission on AIDS to study
whether enough money was being spent on research and treatment—were
largely ignored.

Four months later, the prestigious Institute of Medicine of the National
Academy of Sciences tried to direct the media's attention to the government's
performance on AIDS with a 390-page report that called the administration's

response to the epidemic "woefully inadequate." The academy report called for a permanent national AIDS commission and the start of coordinated planning, as well as scaling up of AIDS spending to $2 billion annually in research and education. Pointedly, the report also called for "presidential leadership to bring together all elements of society to deal with the problem." Again, congressional aides hoped the blast at the administration might prompt ambitious reporters to investigate the Reagan administration's AIDS efforts. To be sure, every major news organization gave the academy report serious news placement the day after its release, alongside assurances that AIDS was the administration's "number-one health priority." That, however, was the end of any investigation. After a few days, the report faded from the news altogether.

Ultimately, it was a report issued in October 1986 that turned the tale, galvanized the media and allowed AIDS to achieve the critical mass to make it a pivotal social issue in 1987.

Dr. C. Everett Koop had come to President Reagan's attention because of his leading role in the anti-abortion movement. His conservative religious fundamentalism horrified liberal, feminist, and gay leaders who had fiercely opposed his nomination as surgeon general in 1981. The administration prevailed, however, and few in the White House inner circle had any trepidations when Reagan went to the Hubert Humphrey Building the day after his 1986 State of the Union speech and asked Koop to write a report on the AIDS epidemic.

Koop spent much of 1986 interviewing scientists, health officials, and even suspicious gay community leaders. Once the text was prepared, he took the unusual step of having tens of thousands of copies printed—without letting the White House see it in advance. When Koop went public with the report, it was clear why. The "Surgeon General's Report on Acquired Immune Deficiency Syndrome" was a call to arms against the epidemic, complete with marching orders. For one of the first times, the problem of AIDS was addressed in purely public health terms, stripped of politics. AIDS education, Koop wrote, "should start at the earliest grade possible" for children. He bluntly advocated widespread use of condoms. Compulsory identification of virus carriers and any form of quarantine would be useless in fighting the disease, Koop concluded.

The surgeon general's research also had led him to some inescapable conclusions about AIDS antibody testing, which continued to be a controversial issue. Mandatory testing would do little more than frighten away from the public health establishment the people most at risk for AIDS, the people who most needed to be tested, Koop said. He reiterated what health officers had been saying for nearly two years—large-scale testing would not be feasible until people did not have to worry about losing their jobs or insurance policies if they took the test. A push for more testing should be accompanied by guarantees of confidentiality and nondiscrimination, Koop said.

Such safeguards proved an anathema to conservatives, who viewed them as coddling homosexuals. In California, conservative Republican Governor George Deukmejian vetoed anti-discrimination legislation for people with

AIDS or the AIDS virus, not once but twice in 1986 alone. Koop, however, saw such laws as tools with which the epidemic could be fought.

The report proved an immediate media sensation. The calls for sex education and condom use at last gave journalists something titillating on which to hang their stories. This wasn't some tedious call for a blue-ribbon commission or bureaucratic coordination, this was about rubbers and sex education. At last, there was also a sensible explanation about why compulsory AIDS testing wasn't such a good idea. Uncorrupted by the language of AIDSpeak, Koop was able to talk in a way that made sense; at last, there was a public health official who sounded like a public health official. Not only that, he was able to utter words like "gay" without visibly flinching.

Koop's impact was due to archetypal juxtaposition. It took a square-jawed, heterosexually perceived actor like Rock Hudson to make AIDS something people could talk about. It took an ultra-conservative fundamentalist who looked like an Old Testament prophet to credibly call for all of America to take the epidemic seriously at last.

Unwittingly, the Reagan administration had produced a certifiable AIDS hero. From one corner of the country to the other, AIDS researchers, public health experts, and even the most militant of gay leaders hailed the surgeon general. Koop quickly became so in demand for speeches that he was called a "scientific Bruce Springsteen."

In the broader historical sense, Koop's role in the epidemic was a bit more ambiguous. After all, the surgeon general had managed to maintain a complete silence on the epidemic for over five years. By the time he spoke out, 27,000 Americans already were dead or dying of the disease; Koop's interest was historic for its impact, not its timeliness. There was no denying, however, that the report proved a watershed event in the history of the epidemic, and conservatives were stunned.

Anti-feminist leader Phyllis Schlafly decreed that the sex-ed recommendations represented little more than a call to institute grammar school sodomy classes. Anti-abortion groups went about the business of withdrawing their previous awards to Koop. President Reagan observed his ritualistic silence, though the PHS officials who had approved the report's printing without White House clearance quickly found themselves exiled to bureaucratic Siberia.

In the early weeks of 1987, conservatives retaliated with a call for AIDS testing, lots of it. The call for massive, even compulsory, AIDS testing carried a homophobic tenor; this was AIDSpeak with a new accent. Public health officials who opposed such testing, conservatives intimated, were patsies for homosexual militants. It was, of course, an ironic argument. Despite the early gay politicization of AIDS issues, it was also true just about anything done to fight AIDS for many years—whether in AIDS education or in lobbying for research—had come solely from the gay community. The new conservative concern in the epidemic belied the fact that conservatives had been entirely indifferent to the threat of the spreading pestilence. To be sure, the gay community's own obstructionism to early public health efforts, particularly on issues like bathhouses, had fueled the public conception that gays would flout the public health for their own interests. And public health officials hadn't helped by framing issues politically themselves. The public was used to hearing health officials sound like politicians, so it didn't sound jarring when politicians started talking like they were health officials.

The testing issue allowed conservatives to seize the AIDS issue as their own with rhetoric implicitly arguing that those thoughtless homosexuals were so awful that they should be forced to submit to testing, to protect all the good people who weren't infected with the virus. Public opinion polls showed most Americans favored massive AIDS testing, perhaps because most people were confident they wouldn't test positive for the virus and would not have to suffer the consequences of forced testing policies. With such popular support, conservative political theorists already were talking about what a good issue AIDS would be for Republicans in the next presidential election.

Meanwhile, the rest of the world was awakening to the AIDS threat. While the disease had been reported in 51 countries in January 1986, by the spring of 1987 there were 113 countries, on every continent except Antarctica, reporting over 51,000 cases. Ultimately, WHO warned, the planet could expect 3 million AIDS cases internationally by 1991.

European countries rushed to provide nationwide educational efforts. English authorities launched a huge campaign of billboards, newspaper advertisements, and television commercials on AIDS education, hammering on one theme: "Don't die of ignorance." Indeed, by early 1987, the only major Western industrialized nation that had not launched a coordinated education campaign was the United States.

The various American controversies over AIDS education and antibody testing continued through the spring. As the international AIDS conference approached, pressure mounted on the Reagan administration. Though Reagan had at last uttered the word AIDS, he still had not given an address on the six-year-old epidemic. By now, his silence was thunderous. Even the hard-bitten White House press corps, which had never considered AIDS a serious issue, clamored for quotes. In his barnstorming for greater AIDS awareness, Dr. Koop met ever more frequently with embarrassing questions about why President Reagan refused to meet with him.

By the beginning of May, public attention forced the Senate, which had been far less active on AIDS issues than the House of Representatives, to pass unanimously a resolution calling on Reagan to appoint a national AIDS commission. The resolution, drafted by Senate Republican leader Senator Robert Dole, drew a remarkable array of Republican and Democratic co-sponsors.

Conservatives were no less anxious for Reagan to take a stand. Education Secretary William Bennett, a leading spokesman for conservatives on AIDS issues, was strident in his calls for mandatory testing and increasingly vocal in his criticism of Koop. Conservative opinion leaders and newspaper columnists joined the chorus; some called for Koop's resignation. Increasingly, all sides wanted to know where the president stood on AIDS.

As the AIDS conference approached, Reagan announced he would accede to the Senate's wishes and appoint an eleven-member presidential commission to advise him on the epidemic, and he would address an AIDS fund-raising dinner on the eve of the conference. By late May, it became clear that this would be more than just another scientific gathering. Here, at the hub of power in the United States, the science, the politics and the people of the AIDS epidemic would come together; these days would be remembered as the prologue to the future course of AIDS in America. The week would be one of those rare times when the past, the present and future converged. And everybody seemed to understand that as they trekked to their Washington hotel rooms on that cloudy, muggy Sunday afternoon.

THAT NIGHT
GEORGETOWN

Just a few days from now would mark the sixth anniversary of the publication of Michael Gottlieb's article on the mysterious cases of *Pneumocystis carinii* pneumonia in five Los Angeles gay men. Six years ago, Gottlieb had been an eager young immunologist in his first months at UCLA. Now, he was co-chair of a foundation hosting a dinner at which the President and First Lady were guests of honor. On Gottlieb's arm was a famous movie star, and senators and congressmen crowded the restaurant, enjoying cocktails and hors d'oeuvres. AIDS had become so respectable, Gottlieb could scarcely believe it.

Gottlieb knew that much of the success of both the evening and the foundation was the work of his escort, actress Elizabeth Taylor. Taylor's interest in AIDS had been building before it became a fashionable Hollywood cause, back when Gottlieb was discussing his plans for a national AIDS fund-raising group with Dr. Mathilde Krim of the AIDS Medical Foundation in New York City. In the last months of his life, Gottlieb's most famous patient, Rock Hudson, had launched the American Foundation for AIDS Research, or AmFAR, with a $250,000 contribution, and Taylor agreed to become the group's national chair, giving the epidemic the star quality it had long lacked.

As Gottlieb walked with Taylor through the restaurant, many people at the dinner whispered to each other about the circumstances of Gottlieb's recent departure from UCLA. Even though Gottlieb's expertise as one of the world's leading AIDS clinicians had helped secure a $10.2 million federal grant for the institution, he remained something of a persona non grata in Westwood. Yes, he was one of the most published and celebrated researchers at UCLA, but that did little more than inspire jealousy among senior academicians who had never considered AIDS to be legitimate research. If he were truly dedicated to research, they reasoned, why was he running around with movie stars, raising money and indulging in the tainted world of politics?

Gottlieb understood, of course, that much of his colleagues' antipathy dated back to 1983, when he and Dr. Marcus Conant had gone over the heads of University of California administrators to secure an emergency legislative appropriation for AIDS research. Conant had suffered a similar academic exile at UCSF and had largely limited his recent AIDS activities to his private practice.

By early 1987, Gottlieb realized the breach of academic politics had destroyed his university career as well. In just six months, Gottlieb, who remained a mere assistant professor, was turned down for tenure three times. There was also talk that the envious academicians thwarting his tenure would also effectively black-ball any move he might try to make to any other university research center.

Gottlieb couldn't help but recall a conversation he had had with Marc Conant in April 1982, after they had appeared at the first congressional hearing on AIDS to plead for more funding and more concern. At that time, the pair thought that once people realized how serious the threat was, they would be cast as villains for not being more strident in their warnings. Now, both Gottlieb and Conant found themselves undone, not because people believed they hadn't cared enough, but because they cared too much. A few weeks before the conference, Gottlieb left his position at UCLA and opened a private practice of immunology in Santa Monica.

◯

The night's main event was scheduled before dinner, outside, in a huge tent that had been properly secured by Secret Service agents for President Reagan's speech. As people filtered from the restaurant to the tent, their master of ceremonies was on hand to greet them. Easily recognizable by his shock of silver hair, Dr. Mervyn Silverman, former director of the San Francisco Department of Public Health, was now the president of AmFAR. Of all the early AIDS figures who had left an ambiguous legacy, it was Silverman who had taken the most redeeming course in recent years.

After his resignation as health director, he had quickly been tapped by a number of national medical groups to articulate the public health perspective on AIDS issues. During the LaRouche AIDS initiative in California, which called for mandatory AIDS testing, his mediagenic demeanor provided anti-hysteric forces with their most reasoned spokesman. As antibody testing emerged as a potent and divisive issue around the nation in 1987, it was Silverman who patiently explained the public health point of view. In the previous days, he had worked with Reagan speech writers on early drafts of that night's presidential address. It was a long way from painful meetings with sexual liberationists who worried that the city's safe-sex warnings sounded too "anti-sexual." Silverman had been a man of good intentions when AIDS policy was determined by the people of good intentions. Though he had sometimes bum-bled, he was also a visible reminder in these less hospitable times that the people of good intentions would ultimately do far less harm to the cause of public health than the people of bad intentions.

◯

While Dr. Silverman greeted colleagues and chatted with movie stars at the front of the tent, Dr. Paul Volberding took a seat near the back, away from the crowd. The first heat of the summer reminded him of the epidemic's first appearance. For Volberding, that day had been July 1, 1981, his first day on the job at San Francisco General Hospital, when the man whom he was replacing had pointed into an examining room and said, "There's the next great disease waiting for you." It had been an uncannily prescient introduction to Volberding's first Kaposi's sarcoma patient; his subsequent six years of AIDS reesarch had made him one of the world's leading AIDS clinicians. Today, he had suffered a typically hectic schedule, awaking early for an appearance on "Meet the Press." He also had been chosen as one of nine members on a committee organizing an International AIDS Society. A week of speeches, meetings, and interviews lay ahead. In a few days, he would announce that San Francisco had been chosen as site of the 1990 international AIDS conference.

The band struck the fanfare from "Hail to the Chief," and everybody rose as the president and Mrs. Reagan walked into the tent.

As Silverman gave his opening remarks, Volberding marveled at how far the epidemic had come—to the forefront of American life. Where would it go in another six years? Volberding couldn't comprehend what it would be like. He certainly understood the projections of cases, and he had some grasp of what it would mean for his hospital and his clinic. But he truly couldn't comprehend what it meant in a larger sense—what it meant for the nation, for the world, for history. He was too involved to allow himself to get frightened; yet, he knew that if he weren't so involved, he would be very frightened.

$$\bigcirc$$

The crowd cheered loudly, even pointedly, and stood when Elizabeth Taylor presented a special award to the surgeon general. After Koop delivered his brief remarks, glancing toward the president when he endorsed "voluntary" testing with guarantees of confidentiality and nondiscrimination, Dr. Silverman introduced Dr. Gottlieb, who was about to hand out the first of two scientific awards for AIDS research.

A restrained but courteous applause greeted Dr. Robert Gallo when he walked to the podium to accept his award from Gottlieb. Gallo, of course, gave a nod to the French for their contributions to AIDS research and talked about how international cooperation was necessary among scientists to overcome the epidemic. In the tent, however, significant glances darted quickly among the gathered scientists. The events of the past two years of bitter feuding between French and American scientists was hardly a tribute to international cooperation.

The Pasteur Institute's lawsuit against the National Cancer Institute, filed in late 1985, had threatened to bring their ugly dispute to trial in federal court. Though the suit asked only for a share of the royalties that the NCI had accrued from its AIDS blood test patent, the scientific community understood that the French were really suing for the full recognition that had been denied them. To be sure, the Rock Hudson affair had brought worldwide attention to the Pasteur Institute's work in AIDS treatments. And the Pasteur continued to produce world-class AIDS research, most notably with the discovery of a second AIDS-like virus in late 1986. But they still felt they had been robbed of recognition for their most important achievement, the discovery of the elusive AIDS virus.

The United States government, which had so brazenly transformed Gallo's work into political capital for the Reagan administration, tenaciously held on to the myth that Gallo had discovered the AIDS virus. This meant adhering to Gallo's notion that the virus was a relative of the HTLV family that Gallo also had discovered, and that he had the right to name the virus, as viral discoverers always do. Ultimately, it had taken an international committee to rule that, no, this was not a leukemia virus and, no, Dr. Gallo did not have the right to name it. To smooth ruffled feathers, however, the committee arrived at a compromise name: Human Immunodeficiency virus, or HIV.

Throughout 1986, however, the Pasteur pursued its depositions and Freedom of Information Act requests against the National Cancer Institute. It slowly became obvious to even the most obdurate government lawyers that the lawsuit could prove very embarrassing for the United States government. A pithy memorandum from Dr. Don Francis on the potentials of such a suit warned the administration, "If this litigation gets into open court, all of the less-than-admirable aspects will become public and, I think, hurt science and the Public Health Service. The French clearly found the cause of AIDS first and Dr. Gallo clearly tried to upstage them one year later." On the most central issue of whether HTLV-III was the product of viral pilfering, Francis posed the hypothetical question: Could the prototype isolates of HTLV-III and LAV be identical merely by coincidence? And he answered, "Probably not." However, two years later, at the request of Dr. Gallo, Francis wrote to Gallo, "I do not now, nor ever have, supported the claim that you or anyone in your laboratory 'stole' LAV."

For his part, Gallo dismissed the notion with a wave of his hand. He already was a star in the field of human retrovirology without the discovery of HTLV-III, he said. Of course, he wanted a Nobel Prize and he believed he deserved one, but he would not commit a scientific felony to achieve it.

Facing the possibility of open court hearings, the U.S. government began to reconsider fighting the French. In the early months of 1987, Dr. Jonas Salk shuttled between the warring scientists like an ambassador at large, forging a compromise. Ultimately, the settlement was signed by President Reagan and French President Jacques Chirac in a White House ceremony. It was one of the first times in the history of science that heads of state were called upon to resolve a dispute over a viral discovery.

The settlement accorded each researcher partial credit for various discoveries on the way to isolating HIV. It was from this settlement, and because none of the mainstream press had pursued the controversy in any depth, that the pleasant fiction had arisen that Drs. Robert Gallo and Luc Montagnier were "co-discoverers" of the AIDS virus. To this extent, Gallo had won. Now, moments before the president was to deliver his first speech on the epidemic, Gallo accepted his award for being a "co-discoverer" of HIV.

Dr. Mathilde Krim stepped forward to give a comparable award to Montagnier. Perhaps it was all the memories that jarred the normally unflappable Krim that night. Until that point the ceremony certainly had been polite enough. Krim, however, had spent so many of the past four years fighting for people to care, whether in the New York City Department of Health or in the federal government, that she would not be silent and courteous, not when there was still so much to do.

There were AIDS treatments on the shelf that needed to be tested, for instance, but the drug testing process had been stalled. There was talk that no treatment or vaccine would get quick FDA approval for experimentation unless it was developed by the federal government; among AIDS organizers, NIH had become the acronym for the agency disinterested in treatments that were Not Invented Here. There was no stop the government did not pull out for AZT, a drug the NCI had originally developed. However, there seemed no bit of red tape too minor to delay the release of other treatments. Throughout the country, vast networks of gay men now distributed their own AIDS treatments, some obtained in Mexico, others put together in kitchen laboratories.

The delays and disorder, Krim knew, was due less to malevolence than to incompetence, bureaucratic bumbling, and, most importantly, the lack of any leadership on AIDS within the administration.

Krim told the crowd that she had heard optimistic talk about a vaccine that might come for AIDS, someday, and she had heard of possible treatments, someday.

"But when?" Krim pleaded, as her audience suddenly fell silent.

Outside the tent, where the echo of protesters could be faintly heard, was a candlelight vigil, she noted.

"Thousands of candles, carried by people with AIDS, are flickering in the night, asking the question of us. 'When?' The answer to that question depends on the national will."

Tim Westmoreland sat near the back of the tent, a few rows behind Paul Volberding, waiting for the applause for Dr. Montagnier to die down. President Reagan would speak next.

As counsel to the House Subcommittee on Health and the Environment, Westmoreland had worked on AIDS for longer than just about anyone on Capitol Hill, back in the days when he and Bill Kraus counted themselves lucky if their struggles could get an extra $2 million for AIDS research tacked on to a supplemental appropriations bill. The days of such nickel and diming were past. Only a week earlier Senator Kennedy had introduced legislation calling for nearly $1 billion in AIDS spending for the next year, and it appeared that a figure close to this amount would ultimately be enacted. Money was no longer the key issue, Westmoreland understood. It was leadership.

Westmoreland hoped the president's speech would not focus on testing, but on research and education, the only real ways the epidemic could be fought. Westmoreland and Senate aides had been carefully formulating bipartisan AIDS legislation for this session of Congress. Democrats and moderate Republicans both seemed eager for some compromise, because most leaders understood that AIDS had a dangerous potential if it were overly politicized. It touched too many nerves and engendered too many fears; it was better left to the offices of public health departments. As the old saying went, when war is contemplated, turn to your politicians; when war is declared, turn to your generals. By declaring a national war on AIDS, Westmoreland thought, Reagan could at last give his moral support to the generals of public health and pull the battle away from the politicians and all their calls for mandatory AIDS testing.

"Ladies and gentleman," Dr. Silverman said, "the President of the United States."

Ronald Reagan grinned boyishly and started his first address on AIDS with the words, "Many years ago, when I worked for General Electric Theater . . ."

After a brief reminiscence about GE Theater, the president decided to tell a little joke. It was a story he told often at fund-raising dinners, about a charity committee that goes to the wealthiest man in town to seek a contribution.

"Our book shows that you haven't contributed any money this year," the committee tells the man.

The prosperous businessman asks if the charity committee's book shows that he has an infirm mother and a disabled brother.

"Why no," the committee says. "We didn't know that."

"Well," the man retorts. "I don't give them any money. Why should I give any to you?"

The crowd laughed uncertainly. Tim Westmoreland marveled at how much the joke summed up Reagan's handling of AIDS: He hadn't ascribed much importance or funding priority to any other non-armaments program during his presidency, why should he have given any to AIDS?

"That wasn't a joke," said Westmoreland to the friend sitting next to him. "That was a fable."

In the next twenty minutes, the president laid out his views on AIDS. There was little talk of education and a lot of talk about testing. There was no mention, however, of confidentiality guarantees or civil rights protection for those who tested positive. Reagan's program, of course, would do very little to actually stop the spread of AIDS. Though testing heterosexuals at marriage license bureaus created the illusion of action, very few of these people were infected with the virus and very few lives would be saved. But then saving lives had never been a priority of the Reagan administration. Reagan's speech was not meant to serve the public health; it was a political solution to a political problem. The words created a stance that was politically comfortable for the president and his adherents; it was also a stance that killed people. Already, some said that Ronald Reagan would be remembered in history books for one thing beyond all else: He was the man who had let AIDS rage through America, the leader of the government that when challenged to action had placed politics above the health of the American people.

◯

All afternoon, Larry Kramer had asked himself how he would respond this night to President Reagan's speech. Though Larry remained one of the most outspoken gay activists in the country, he was no longer alone in his rage against the Reagan administration. Even Kramer's sharpest critics could no longer maintain he was wrong, even if his personal style had been off-putting; he had only been ahead of his time. With the success of *The Normal Heart,* Kramer had found his measure of vindication, and another play was beginning to form itself in his imagination. He had even made his peace with Paul Popham, the staid GMHC president with whom he had had so many struggles in the early years. When they talked for the last time, only days before Paul died, Larry apologized for their fights, and Paul just said, "Keep fighting."

Though mellower, Kramer still felt compelled to make some protest when Reagan spoke. Other gay advocates present that night agreed, but no protest had been organized. Dr. Krim had passed word that she and other AIDS researchers would walk out if Reagan endorsed mandatory testing, but his speech had artfully dodged such a call. In fact, the speech seemed crafted to touch on all the right themes. There were calls for compassion and understanding, and tributes for the volunteer efforts helping people with AIDS. Reagan even singled out San Francisco's Shanti Project for praise.

As Larry listened, he became aware the president's speech made no mention of the word "gay." There was talk about hemophiliacs who got AIDS, transfusion recipients, and the spouses of intravenous drug abusers, but the G-word was never spoken. And then Reagan turned to the nitty-gritty of testing.

Larry's temper began to rise. There was something so utterly dishonest about discussing almost every aspect of the AIDS epidemic in this address and not mentioning the fact that it was homosexuals who had been killed and homosexuals who had, in fact, done so much of the work in fighting the epidemic for all those years that Reagan had ignored it.

On the night President Reagan finally spoke, Paul Popham was three weeks dead, having gone to his grave profoundly disillusioned with the United States, the country in which he had always believed, the country for which he had fought in Vietnam. This country had turned its back on Popham and his friends and let them die. And now Reagan refused to talk about Paul Popham or any of the gay men who had shown such courage for so many years, as if Popham had played an embarrassing role in the epidemic and not Reagan himself. And when Reagan started talking about testing, as if he were really proposing policies that might at last do something to stop the epidemic, the anger of six years welled up inside Larry Kramer, and he began to jeer.

⬭

By the time President Reagan had delivered his first speech on the epidemic of Acquired Immune Deficiency Syndrome, 36,058 Americans had been diagnosed with the disease; 20,849 had died.

THE NEXT MORNING
WASHINGTON HILTON

When Dr. Dan William remembered the San Francisco Gay Freedom Day Parade on a sunny day in June 1980, he was struck by how naive he had been.

That must have been what it was like in Europe in the 1920s, before the Depression and war, when everyone was so rambunctiously and hedonistically joyous and so oblivious to the future and their own vulnerability.

By mid-1987, 185 of his patients had contracted AIDS. William currently was treating 350 patients who were in some stage of HIV-related illness. If someone had told him seven years ago that he would be treating hundreds of terminally ill patients, he would have dismissed them as crazy. Still, the fact that he had adjusted to the work load and preserved his sanity demonstrated how success-fully people could acclimate to the cruelest realities of the AIDS epidemic. On the practical end, AIDS had become easier to treat as experience made it more predictable and more manageable than in those frightening first years. There was still sadness at the relentlessness of the disease, but today, there also was reason for hope.

This was the assessment of many of the doctors and scientists gathering on the concourse level of the Washington Hilton early that morning for the first day of the AIDS conference. There was sadness and there was hope.

All the old-timers had returned. There was Dr. Alvin Friedman-Kien, the dermatologist who had first realized that a handful of Kaposi's sarcoma cases was part of a broader epidemic, and Dr. Linda Laubenstein, the researcher who had seen New York's first two KS cases in 1979, only to be told that she should try to find a French-Canadian airline steward named Gaetan, because he had those funny spots too. Dr. Marcus Conant bustled through the crowd. Dr. Willy Rozenbaum walked toward the opening session with his Parisian colleagues Drs. Jean-Claude Chermann and Francoise Barre. And the veterans of the early CDC work were there too: Dale Lawrence, Bill Darrow, and Harold Jaffe were all still working on various epidemiological projects, and Jim Curran was still the head of CDC AIDS work. AIDS was like middle age, Curran often said now. It wasn't an experience anyone looked forward too, but there was no way to avoid it either. Dr. Mary Guinan, who had conducted so many of the first interviews with AIDS patients in the frustrating summer of 1981, had advanced to be an assistant CDC director. Still, she had come to the conference that day toting more AIDS research, never convinced that people were taking the epi-demic seriously enough.

While the first AIDS conference in 1985 was marked by shock at the dimen-sions of the unfolding problem and the 1986 conference in Paris was note-worthy for its gloom, this conference seemed cautiously optimistic. By now, the substance of the new science to be presented at the conference was well known. It was a mixture of bad news and good news, and since any news that was not horrible had been so rare for so long in this epidemic, there was at least some relief to be found among the hundreds of studies announced that day.

The most important good news was spelled AZT, the first treatment to interfere with the life cycle of the AIDS virus and extend the lives of patients. It was a primitive drug at best and had many harmful side effects. But it worked. It indicated that more sophisticated treatments could be found as well to lengthen life, even if there was no cure. While doctors currently estimated that an HIV-infected person had a life expectancy of only seven years after infection, five of which were spent incubating the disease, some experts privately predicted that within five years, they would be able to ensure a 20-to-25-year longevity after infection.

Though obstacles remained for a vaccine, they no longer seemed as insurmountable as they had two years before. One French researcher had already vaccinated himself with a prototype that was being tested on Zairians. Several other experimental vaccines were in refrigerators, going through the languorous process of FDA approval. Indeed, the problem with getting the federal government to wage an all-out campaign for an AIDS vaccine convinced some scientists that the most formidable barriers were not technological but bureaucratic. In this area too, however, there was reason to hope.

Hope was important now in large part because of the bad news presented at the conference, the news about the virulence of HIV. The ongoing survey of the 6,700 San Francisco gay men who had participated in the hepatitis B vaccine in the late 1970s provided the most stunning bad news of the week. Of 63 men infected with HIV for at least six years, 30 percent had developed AIDS while another 48 percent had ARC. Only 22 percent had no symptoms of disease. Moreover, the numbers of people falling ill seemed to rise dramatically once the subjects were infected with the virus for more than five years. Rather than declining, the proportions of people getting AIDS seemed to be skyrocketing.

The men suffering ARC had no pretty future to look forward to either, according to another study conducted by Dr. Donald Abrams, assistant director of the San Francisco General Hospital AIDS Clinic. Abrams had begun to follow patients with swollen lymph nodes in 1981, optimistically believing that lymphadenopathy would prove to be a protective response to infection with the AIDS virus, one that would keep a patient from getting AIDS. In the first years of his study, Abrams's hypothesis seemed to bear this out. Now he saw that once their lymph nodes had been swollen for more than three years, they started getting AIDS. In fact, Abrams now figured that half of his patients would have AIDS within five years of the onset of lymphadenopathy, and so far there was no reason to believe this number would not, in time, reach nearly 100 percent.

With the future so clearly laid out, however, the depressing prognosis of HIV-infected people could at least serve the purpose of encouraging more aggressive experimentation with antiviral drugs, since it was clear that hundreds of thousands needed them just in the United States. Already, marketing managers at pharmaceutical corporations were talking eagerly about the "ARC market."

Of course, these projections weren't particularly newsworthy to people familiar with the epidemic. The figures reported at the conference in June of 1987 had already been mapped out on that December day in 1983 when Dale Lawrence realized the average incubation period of the disease was five years, the day he clearly saw the marathons of AIDS runners. AIDS was, once again, merely living up to everyone's worst fears.

⬭

The predictability of all that was happening was one of the aspects of the epidemic that continued to fascinate Don Francis. It had brought him moments of bittersweet vindication. New data on transfusion-associated AIDS cases indicated, for example, that far more Americans were destined to die of AIDS-contaminated transfused blood after the federal government and blood banking industry were fully aware of the problem than before. An estimated 12,000 Americans were infected from transfusions largely administered after the CDC had futilely begged the blood industry for action to prevent spread of the disease. "How many people have to die?" Francis had asked the blood bankers in early 1983. The answer was now clear: thousands would.

On the conference program was a seminar offered for blood bankers about how to defend themselves in blood transfusion lawsuits. The seminar speaker was an attorney for San Francisco's Irwin Memorial Blood Bank, recently the first blood bank to make an out-of-court settlement with the family of a transfusion victim. The Borchelts had been on the way toward probably winning a huge jury award when Irwin decided to settle. In an odd twist, the Borchelt family lawyers had tried to subpoena Don Francis to testify, having heard of his frustration with the blood industry. In the end, the U.S. attorney filed a petition on behalf of the federal government in federal court blocking Francis's appearance; it simply would have been too embarrassing for the government.

If so much of the past had been painfully predictable to Francis, then so was the future. He had come to Washington as a co-author of a paper that plotted the simple course the epidemic would take in the United States. As Francis had long ago realized, you had only to know the transmission routes of hepatitis B to predict the future of AIDS, and that analysis was what Don Francis would present at this conference.

When the panel moderator introduced Francis to deliver his paper, however, she got his name wrong; she apparently had never heard of him before. And in the audience, two staffers from the gay Howard Brown Memorial Clinic in Chicago shuffled their Italian loafers impatiently while Don talked about his fears that AIDS would become an endemic disease among poor inner city neighborhoods where drug addicts spread the virus to their sexual partners. Finally, one of the bored gay staffers whispered loudly to the other, "Who is this pompous guy, talking on so long?"

A lot of people now central to the battle against AIDS had no idea who Don Francis was. Robert Gallo now said that Don Francis was "irrelevant" to AIDS work.

Few doubted that Francis's fall from grace stemmed from his conflicts with Gallo during "the war" between French and American researchers. The fact that Francis had proved so troublesome to bureaucrats, always pleading for more money, had not helped him either. Now, the government scientific establishment was lashing back vindictively. No paper that listed Francis as a presenter was accepted for presentation at the AIDS conference this year. Even a paper on vaccine research that he had written with Dr. Jonas Salk was refused. Francis was only able to make this workshop presentation because the woman who was supposed to give the talk couldn't get to Washington that day.

In his office in Berkeley, Francis had continued to chart AIDS prevention programs for California. He also made regular trips to the University of California campus in Davis, where he was working on an AIDS vaccine with Salk. Yet, he was no longer on the front line, and he was impatient. Before the conference convened, he had been approached by the World Health Organization to consider returning to his old work, fighting disease in Africa. AIDS was spreading rapidly north from the equatorial belt, and someone with Francis's experience on that continent was badly needed.

Francis considered the proposition. It was what he had wanted to do from the start, hold back this disease. To this day, Francis did not feel he had been beaten by AIDS; he had only been beaten by the system, and because of that the disease had won, gaining its foothold throughout the United States. By the day the conference opened in Washington, he knew that he would return to Africa to fight this pestilence. His first assignment was to be in the Sudan. There, away from the governmental politics of budget and the scientific politics of prestige, he had a chance to make a difference.

THAT AFTERNOON
1600 PENNSYLVANIA AVENUE

Large crowds of angry gay people always excited Cleve Jones, and he felt a nostalgic tinge of militant exhilaration as he led the marchers toward the White House, chanting, "History will recall, Reagan did the least of all."

The film of members of the audience jeering President Reagan at last night's fundraising dinner had made all the morning newscasts. Today, Cleve heard that a similar chorus of heckles greeted Vice President George Bush when he gave the opening speech at the AIDS conference and defended the president's newly announced policies for testing. This afternoon, every news organization in the country seemed to have a crew at the White House for the civil disobedience Cleve had spent the past week organizing.

The White House protests had originally been organized by a handful of national gay leaders who wanted to put photographs of themselves being arrested on Pennsylvania Avenue in their next fund-raising brochures. The demonstration, however, came as a wave of frustration was sweeping over the gay community, and organizers from across the country had decided to join the protest. Given his legendary reputation as a media-savvy street activist, Cleve was called in from San Francisco to coordinate the picket line.

As the Washington police prepared to arrest sixty-four gay leaders blockading the White House driveway, they pulled on long rubber gloves. Police had requested full protective suits with face masks, the kind one wears when venturing into a nuclear reactor meltdown, but city officials had persuaded them that rubber gloves would suffice. Cleve watched scores of newspaper reporters and TV cameramen jostling for shots of the protesters and the costumed police, and he marveled at how much things had changed.

He had no doubt that the media's belated involvement in AIDS was responsible for all the concern the epidemic was generating in every quarter of the nation. Virtually every major newspaper in the country now had a full-time AIDS reporter. *The New York Times* was on the verge of announcing that, at long last, it would allow the adjective "gay" to be used when describing homo-sexuals. The *Washington Post,* which had done such a singularly deplorable job in covering federal AIDS policy in years past, had dispatched six reporters to cover the opening of the AIDS conference and its attendant protests.

People were paying attention finally, Cleve saw, but that wasn't all that had changed. The numbers of victims had changed. In San Francisco, tens of thousands, including Cleve, were infected, and more than 3,300 were diagnosed. Even as he plotted his latest militant exploit or planned his 1988 campaign for supervisor, Cleve wondered if he would survive.

Much of what he had once dreamed for would not come to pass; Cleve accepted that now. In years past, Cleve and the other citizens of Castro Street had looked ahead to a time when they had rooted out prejudice against gay people altogether and healed the lives that the prejudice had scarred. They might be old men by then, but they would be able to entertain each other with reminiscences of the old days when they had all believed they could change the world, and know that to a certain extent, they had. Many of those people were dead now, and Cleve accepted that most of his friends would be dead before they reached anything near old age.

What hadn't changed for Cleve was the dream itself; what they had fought for, what Harvey Milk had died for, was fundamentally right, Cleve thought. It had been a fight for acceptance and equality, against ignorance and fear. It was that fight that had brought Cleve to Washington on this day.

The numbers of AIDS cases measured the shame of the nation, he believed. The United States, the one nation with the knowledge, the resources, and the institutions to respond to the epidemic, had failed. And it had failed because of ignorance and fear, prejudice and rejection. The story of the AIDS epidemic was that simple, Cleve felt; it was a story of bigotry and what it could do to a nation.

The legacy of the nation's shame could be read in the faces that Cleve always carried in his memory, the faces of the dead. Cleve could see those faces now as he led the chant at the wrought iron gates of the White House: "Shame. Shame. Shame." Tears streamed down his cheeks as he raised his fist toward the Oval Office. He saw Simon Guzman and Bobbi Campbell, Gary Walsh and Felix Velarde-Munoz. And, of course, he saw Bill Kraus.

KENT: "Is this the promised end?"
EDGAR: "Or image of that horror?"
—*King Lear,* V:iii

"I want my glasses!"

Bill Kraus wanted his glasses; that was all. Why was everybody looking at him so strangely?

"I want my glasses!"

Dennis Seely and a number of other friends eyed Bill warily as they rushed in, not sure of what to say. Bill was sprawled on the floor where he had fallen.

"I want my glasses!" Bill shouted.

All anyone could hear, however, was: "Glubsh nein ubles sesmag."

It was as if Bill was speaking some strange mix of German and gibberish. Somewhere between his brain and his mouth, his words were lost.

"Bill, you're not speaking English," Dennis said.

A sheepish grin crossed Bill's lips.

"Gluck eye bub glenish?" he asked tentatively.

"No," Dennis said. "You're not speaking English. We can't understand anything you're saying."

Bill rolled his eyes upward. From the number of syllables he uttered, Dennis could tell he was saying, "Jesus Christ."

Outside, the day was sunny and the sky was breathtakingly clear, as if painted on a porcelain heaven. It was such clarity that gave the San Francisco gay parades their added magic every June. This was January, however, and without a blanket of warming winter fog, the clear skies brought only a sharp and bitter chill to the air.

It could have been any day in the history of the AIDS epidemic and it could have been any city, because such little dramas were, ultimately, what all the numbers behind the AIDS statistics were about: promising people, who could have contributed much, dying young and dying unnecessarily. As it was, however, the day was January 5, 1986, the city was San Francisco, the person was William James Kraus, and the number he would soon be assigned in the statistics was that of the 887th San Franciscan to die in the AIDS epidemic.

Bill's old friend from the Harvey Milk Gay Democratic Club, Catherine Cusic, knelt down next to Bill on the floor.

"Bill, you need to go to a hospital," she said. "C'mon."

Bill's roommate, Michael Housh, had seen the symptoms of neurological disorder almost from the day Bill had returned from Paris four months earlier. Bill had been barely able to hold a glass of orange juice at the breakfast table because his arm trembled so severely.

"You didn't see that," Bill had commanded on more than one occasion.

In those last months, Bill had rarely ventured from his flat to Castro Street, believing his political enemies, the ones who had branded him a "traitor" and a "fascist," would revel at his misfortune. Bill's friends tried to convince him he was depriving himself of the adulation with which many had come to regard him. Once Bill had been the virtual embodiment of gay political aspirations. When the epidemic struck, there had hardly been an AIDS issue in which he had not been at the center, whether it was for federal funding, public education, gay community responsibility, or wider accessibility of treatments. He had served as the bridge for many gay people making the transition from Before the epidemic to After. He was also the first to articulate a way for gay idealism to survive the ravages of the epidemic, by redefining what the gay community and the gay movement was all about. Though once controversial, Bill's redefinition had largely come to pass. Finally, people were beginning to appreciate his contributions; some called him a hero.

By Christmas, Bill was having a hard time keeping food down and suffering from oppressive diarrhea. He weighed 120 pounds. Headaches pounded his brain like heavy wooden mallets. He resisted friends' urgings that he go to the hospital, insisting that he was suffering from only a touch of stomach flu that would surely pass. His friends had been meeting in the kitchen this cold Sunday afternoon, trying to figure out what to do, when they heard the thud from Bill's bedroom.

Catherine noted that Bill had lost his continence. He had obviously had some sort of seizure, but still it took substantial goading to get him to agree to go to a hospital.

Dr. Marcus Conant quickly ordered a bed for him at the UCSF Medical Center. When it was time to leave, Bill refused to let anyone help him walk. Slowly, he pulled himself from the floor, stood, threw his chest out and started down the stairs.

Outside, in the bitter winter chill, Bill could see his breath. He pulled his coat tightly around him as he left his flat for this last trip out of the Castro neighborhood.

His friends agreed to take shifts and spend twenty-four hours a day with him. Bill's one great love, Kico Govantes, was a frequent hospital visitor. He was now a successful artist, but he remained the emotional foil to Bill's cerebral demeanor, and Bill's friends were afraid he would be too sensitive to man the all-night vigils. Dennis and Harry Britt scheduled themselves for the night shifts, and the anxious waiting began.

Late that first night, as Dennis Seely stretched out on the floor of the hospital room, Bill was speaking normally again.

"Once you guys got power over me, you became fascists," Bill said.

"What are you talking about?"

"I wanted my glasses and you wouldn't give them to me."

"Bill, we couldn't understand what you were saying," Dennis said. "You weren't speaking English."

"Oh," said Bill.

He hadn't remembered that.

⬭

The next day, doctors administered a battery of neurological tests. Bill was lucid about half the time, though it appeared he had lost some use of his cranial nerves. He was seeing double.

"Who is the president?" a doctor asked, trying to judge Bill's presence of mind.

"Kennedy," Bill said.

The doctor looked worried. "I think it's Reagan," he said.

"Please, don't remind me!" Bill groaned. "I'm sick enough already. Don't make it any worse."

The diagnosis: cryptococcal meningitis. Any brain disease was serious, but treatments for cryptococcus were available, the doctors said, and there was no reason to believe that Bill wouldn't pull through. Nevertheless, Bill was in despair over the determination. More than anything else, he was terrified by the thought that the disease might turn on his brain. His intelligence meant more to him than any other quality.

"Are you afraid of dying?" Bill's brother Mike asked.

"I'm more afraid of what happens if I live," Bill said.

⬭

The unseasonably cold weather persisted all week. Sharon Johnson was sitting with Bill on Saturday afternoon when he dozed off. After the previous days' fitfulness, Sharon was relieved to see some serenity return to Bill's face as he slept. He seemed to have made some sort of decision. As Sharon watched him, she remembered where she had seen that expression on Bill before. It had been in Lourdes nearly a year earlier, when Bill had sat transfixed for all those hours on a stone bench in front of the statue of the Virgin Mary. She had never seen Bill so at peace before, and she had not seen him so tranquil since, not until now.

Later, Dennis Seely came to spend the night on the hospital floor. Bill's friends had insisted that the nurses stop coming into the room in the middle of the night to take his temperature. He was never getting a decent night's sleep, they argued, and the nurses finally agreed.

So it was not until 6 A.M. that Dennis woke up, when the nurse came in the next morning.

"Don't wake him," Dennis said.

"I've got to take his temperature," she insisted.

Dennis sat up and stretched, feeling rested. Of all the nights he had spent in Bill's room, it was the first time Bill's loud snoring hadn't kept him up.

Though it was still dark, Dennis could make out the form of the nurse putting the thermometer in Bill's mouth.

Then there was the sound of glass clicking against Bill's teeth as the thermometer fell from his gaping jaw.

"William?" the nurse said. "William?"

"Call him Bill," Dennis said, getting up.

"Bill?"

Dennis walked to the bedside and saw Bill lying motionless, his head tilted so that his curly brown hair lay limp on the pillow.

"I think he's dead," Dennis said.

The nurse was pretty and blond, and as she looked down on her patient, a tone of amazement crept into her voice.

"I'm new," she said. "I've never had anyone die before."

The sheets were tucked neatly around Bill's chin. There had been no final struggle, only a last quiet breath in the night.

"Now I can see," the nurse said softly. "He's dead, but that really isn't *him,* is it?"

The nurse regarded Bill's motionless form, not morbidly but with a genuine fascination, as if she just then were reaching some conclusion about life, about death.

"Oh, I know that's him," she said, a little flustered.

"But that's not *him,*" she said. *"He's* not really dead."

NOTES
ON SOURCES

This book is a work of journalism. There has been no fictionalization. For purposes of narrative flow, I reconstruct scenes, recount conversations and occasionally attribute observations to people with such phrases as "he thought" or "she felt." Such references are drawn from either the research interviews I conducted for the book or from research conducted during my years of covering the AIDS epidemic for the *San Francisco Chronicle*.

Many of the people who play a key role in this book had been sources for many years before the AIDS epidemic appeared. My interviews with Drs. Selma Dritz, Dan William, and David Ostrow, for example, go back to 1976 when I was a reporter for a gay newsmagazine writing about health issues. Similarly, a number of the San Francisco political figures and gay community leaders in the book were also people whom I had interviewed dozens of times in the past decade, both as a television reporter and as the author of a book on San Francisco politics. For purposes of convenience, however, the following notes list only interviews relating to aspects of the AIDS epidemic that are covered within this book. This is not a record of every interview I conducted concerning AIDS in the past five years. Such a list would include more than 900 people.

The interview dates after the names refer both to telephone and personal interviews. In months where I conducted more than one interview with a given source, the number of interviews is indicated in parentheses after the date.

In this particular book, where chronology played such an essential part, I was aided by the fact that scientists routinely keep journals noting specific dates of insights and conversations with other researchers. Medical charts and death certificates also helped provide detail on the AIDS sufferers profiled in the book. Other essential documents and sources are noted when appropriate.

Washington Politics

Congress: Rep. Henry Waxman 7/85, 2/86; Rep. Barbara Boxer 12/83; Rep. Sala Burton 11/84; Michael Housh, aide to Rep. Boxer 2/85, 1/86, 3/86; Susan Steinmetz, staff, Intergovernmental and Human Resources Subcommittee, 2/85, 10/86; Bill Kraus, aide to Reps. Phil & Sala Burton 10/82, 3/83 (3), 4/83, 5/83, 6/83, 10/83, 11/83/, 12/83 (2), 1/84, 2/84 (4), 3/84, 4/84, 10/84, 11/84, 11/85, 6/85, 7/85, 9/85, 10/85 (6), 11/85; Tim Westmoreland, counsel, House Subcommittee on Health and the Environment 2/85, 11/85, 2/86, 6/87; Larry Miike, Office of Technology Assessment 2/86; David Sundwald, counsel, Senate Committee for Labor and Human Resources 2/86; Dan Maldonado, counsel, House Appropriations Subcommittee for Health 2/86; Rep. Ted Weiss 12/83.

Reagan Administration: Dr. Edward Brandt, Assistant Secretary for Health 12/83, 2/85; Surgeon General C. Everett Koop 3/87; Dr. Lowell Harmison, Deputy Assistant Secretary for Health 2/85; Dr. Anthony Fauci, dir. NIAID, 2/85, 9/85, 2/86; Dr. Richard Krause, dir. NIAID 2/86; Dr. James Whitescarver, asst. to dir. NIAID 2/86; Peter Fischinger, asst. dir. National Cancer Institute 2/85; Dr. James Mason, dir. CDC & acting Asst. Sec'y for Health 2/86; Dr. Don Hopkins, asst. dir. CDC 2/86; Dr. Walter Dowdle, director, Center for Infectious Diseases 4/84; Bill Grigg, spokesman, FDA 2/85.

Internal governmental memoranda were obtained under provisions of the Freedom of Information Act. Requests were made in 1983 to Office of Management and Budget, Department of Health & Human Services, Centers for Disease Control, and National Institutes of Health. Requests were made again in 1985 to the same agencies and to the U.S. Department of Defense and U.S. Department of Justice. Further documentation for federal funding decisions came from the "Review of the Public Health Service Response to AIDS" by the Office of Technology Assessment (1985) and from "The Federal Response to AIDS," a report by the Intergovernmental Relations and Human Resources Subcommittee of the House of Representatives Committee on Government Operations (1983).

AIDS Researchers and Physicians

New York: Dr. Mathilde Krim, AIDS Medical Foundation & Memorial Sloan-Kettering Cancer Center 2/85, 1/86; Dr. Arye Rubinstein, Albert Einstein College of Medicine 2/85, 2/86; Dr. Joyce Wallace, St. Vincent's Hospital 2/85; Dr. Michael Lange, St. Luke's-Roosevelt Hospital 2/85, 2/86; Dr. Dan William 1/86, 6/87; Dr. Alvin Friedman-Kien, NYU Hospital 1/86; Dr. Linda Laubenstein 1/86, 6/87; Dr. Larry Mass 1/86; Virginia Lehman, Bellevue Hospital 2/86; Dr. Donna Mildvan, Beth Israel Medical Center 2/86; Dr. Stuart Nicholls 2/86.

The account of the February 1985 AIDS conference sponsored by AIDS Medical Foundation was taken from a videotaped recording of the conference provided by American Foundation for AIDS Research. The name of the AIDS-stricken child at Jacobi Hospital was changed to Diana to protect her confidentiality; this was the only name alteration in the book.

San Francisco: Dr. Marcus Conant, University of California at San Francisco 4/82, 4/83, 10/83, 2/84, 3/84, 6/84, 8/84, 10/84, 11/84, 12/84, 3/85, 4/85, 8/85, 10/85, 12/85, 1/86, 7/86, 9/86 (2), 10/86; Dr. Paul Volberding, dir. San Francisco General Hospital AIDS Clinic 3/84, 8/84, 1/85, 2/85, 1/86, 2/86, 3/86, 12/86, 6/87; Dr. Constance Wofsy, assoc. dir. SFGH AIDS Clinic 5/83, 1/85; Dr. Donald Abrams, asst. dir. SFGH AIDS Clinic 10/83, 2/85, 5/85, 7/85, 8/85, 9/85, 10/85, 1/86, 1/87; Dr. Andrew Moss, epidemiologist, SFGH AIDS Clinic 3/83, 7/83, 2/84, 7/84, 11/84, 3/85; Dr. Jay Levy, UCSF Center for Human Tumor Virus Research 8/84, 3/85, 7/86; Dr. Mort Cowan, UCSF 7/86; Dr. Michael Gorman, epidemiologist 3/83; Dr. James Groundwater, dermatologist 11/83, 1/86, 2/86; Dr. Robert Bolan 3/83, 5/86; Peter Arno, UCSF Institute of Health Policy Studies 8/85; Dr. Edward Shaw, polio expert 10/85; Dr. Warren Winkelstein, professor of epidemiology, UC Berkeley 10/83, 11/84, 10/85, 5/87; David Lyman, San Francisco's Men's Study 8/84; Cliff Morrison, AIDS Coordinator, SFGH 10/83, 1/84, 3/84, 11/84, 5/86; Bill Barrick, RN, SFGH AIDS Ward 10/83; Cathy Juristo, RN, SFGH AIDS Ward 10/83; Bill Nelson, RN, SFGH AIDS Ward 11/84; Alyson Moed, RN, SFGH AIDS Ward 11/84; Paul O'Malley, SF City Clinic hepatitis study 3/86; John S. James, editor, *AIDS Treatment News* 3/87; Dr. Samuel Stegman, dermatologist 4/83; Dr. Arthur Ammann, UCSF 8/83; Dr. Dan Stites, UCSF 8/83; Dr. Cornelius Hopper, special asst. to UC pres. 8/83; Dr. Rudi Schmid, dean of UCSF school of medicine 8/83; Dr. James Wiley, SF Men's Study 10/84.

Centers for Disease Control, Atlanta: Dr. Don Francis, laboratory coordinator, AIDS Task Force 8/85, 10/85 (4), 11/85 (2), 1/86, 5/86; Dr. James Curran, dir. AIDS Task Force 6/83, 10/83, 12/83, 2/84, 4/84, 8/84, 12/84, 2/85, 4/85, 4/86, 2/87; Dr. V.S. Kalyanaraman 4/86; Dr. Bruce Evatt 3/86, 4/86; Don Berreth 4/84; Bill Darrow 4/86, 2/87; Dr. Harold Jaffe 4/82, 4/84, 11/84, 2/85, 2/86; Dr. Mary Guinan 4/84, 4/86; Dr. Dale Lawrence 4/86 (2), 2/87; Ward Cates 4/86; Dr. Paul Weisner 4/86; Dr. James Allen 2/85, 4/86, 2/87; Dr. Meade Morgan 1/86; Dr. Richard Selik 3/83, 12/83; Sandra Ford 4/84; Mary Cumberland 4/84; Dr. Thomas Spira 4/84; David Cross 4/84; Dr. Russ Havlak, Center for Prevention Services 1/86.

National Institutes of Health, Bethesda: Dr. Bill Blattner, NCI 2/86; Dr. Samuel Broder, clinical dir. NCI 2/86; Dr. James Goedert, NCI 2/86; Dr. Robert Biggar, NCI 2/86; Dr. Harry Haverkos, NIAID (previously with CDC) 3/84, 2/86; Dr. Robert Gallo, NCI Division of Tumor Cell Biology 4/86.

Los Angeles: Dr. Joel Weisman 3/86; Dr. Michael Gottlieb, UCLA 3/86, 9/86; Dr. David Auerbach UCLA 3/86; Dr. Wayne Shandera 5/86.

Miami: Drs. Mark Whiteside and Caroline MacLeod, Miami Institute of Tropical Medicine 4/85.

Paris: Dr. Luc Montagnier, Pasteur Institute 9/84, 12/85; Dr. Jean-Claude Chermann, Pasteur 9/84, 2/85, 6/87; Dr. Willy Rozenbaum, Pitie-Salpetriere Hospital 9/84, 12/85, 6/87; Dr. Francoise Brun-Vezinet, Claude-Bernard

Hospital & Pasteur 12/85; Dr. Francoise Barre, Pasteur 12/85; Dr. Jacques Leibowitch, Rene Descartes University 9/84, 12/85; Dr. David Klatzmann, Pitie-Salpetriere & Pasteur 12/85; Dr. Jean-Baptiste Brunet, World Health Organization 12/85; Michael Pollack, sociologist 12/85; Dr. Didier Seux, Pitie-Salpetriere 12/85.

Brussels: Dr. Nathan Clumeck, University of Brussels 11/85.

Kinshasa, Zaire: Dr. Z. Lurhama, Clinique Universitaires 11/85.

Boston: Dr. Myron Essex, Harvard School of Public Health 2/86.

Chicago: Dr. David Ostrow 10/83, 4/85, 11/85.

Copenhagen: Dr. Bo Hoffman, Rigshospitalet 12/85; Dr. Viggo Faber, Rigshospitalet 12/85; Dr. Ib Bygbjerg, Rigshospitalet 12/85; Dr. Jan Gerstof, State Serum Institute 12/85. Other friends of Dr. Grethe Rask were interviewed, though they asked not to be identified.

City, County, and State Officials

New York City: Dr. David Sencer, Commissioner of Health 2/85; Kevin Cahill, NYC Board of Health 2/85; Mel Rosen, director New York State AIDS Institute 2/85, 2/86.

San Francisco: Mayor Dianne Feinstein 10/82, 5/83, 10/83, 3/84, 4/84, 5/84, 6/84; Dr. Mervyn Silverman, director, Department of Public Health 5/83, 6/83, 10/83, 1/84, 2/84. 3/84, 5/84, 6/84, 10/84, 11/84, 1/85, 2/85, 3/85, 4/85, 8/85, 3/86, 6/87; Dr. Selma Dritz, asst. dir. SF DPH Bureau of Communicable Disease Control 4/82, 3/83, 4/83, 5/83, 6/83, 7/83, 10/83, 11/83, 2/84, 1/86; Bill Cunningham, AIDS coordinator 9/83; William Petty, health inspector 10/84; City Attorney George Agnost 3/84; Deputy City Attorney Victoria Hobel 11/83; Deputy City Attorney Phil Ward 10/84; Dr. Dean Echenberg, dir. Bureau of Communicable Disease Control 7/84, 8/84, 11/84, 3/85, 4/85, 8/85; Board of Supervisors President Wendy Nelder 6/83, 9/83, 5/84, 10/84; Supervisor Richard Hongisto 3/84; Supervisor Bill Maher 9/83; Supervisor Harry Britt 6/83, 9/83, 2/84, 5/84, 6/84, 10/84; Supervisor Carol Ruth Silver 6/83; Dr. Steve Morin, CA DHS AIDS Task Force 1/84, 2/84, 6/85; Bruce Decker, CA AIDS Advisory Committee 9/85, 8/86; Dana Van Gorder, aide to Supervisor Harry Britt 3/83, 5/83, 6/83, 8/83, 9/83, 11/83, 2/84, 3/84, 4/84, 5/84, 6/84, 8/84, 12/84, 7/86; Assembly Speaker Willie Brown 8/83; Assemblyman Art Agnos 3/85, 4/85, 6/86, 7/86; Dr. Robert Benjamin, Alameda County Bureau of Comm. Diseases 8/85.

Sacramento: Dr. Ken Kizer, dir., Calif. Dept. of Health Services 3/85, 7/85, 7/86, 2/87; Dr. James Chin, dir. infectious diseases, Calif. Dept. of Health

Services 8/85; Dr. Robert Anderson, Calif. DHS Office of AIDS 11/84, 6/86, 7/86, 5/87; Stan Hadden, aide to Sen. Pres. David Roberti 8/86.

The Gay Community, People With AIDS, AIDS Service Organizations and Related Interviews

Los Angeles: James Kepner, AIDS History Project, International Gay & Lesbian Archives 3/86; John Mortimer, AIDS Project Los Angeles 9/86; Paul Van Ness, exec. dir. APLA 9/86; Bill Meisenheimer, exec. dir. APLA 9/85.

New York City: Virginia Apuzzo, dir. National Lesbian/Gay Task Force 1/86; Charles Ortleb, publisher, *New York Native* 2/85, 2/86; Rodger McFarlane, executive director Gay Men's Health Crisis 8/84, 2/85, 2/86; Larry Kramer, organizer GMHC 2/85, 1/86 (3), 4/86; Paul Popham, pres. GMHC 2/86, 4/86; Enno Poersch, GMHC board member 4/86; Richard Dunne, exec. dir. GMHC 2/86, 5/86; David Nimmons 2/86; Terry Biern, American Foundation for AIDS Research 2/85, 2/86; Jeff Richardson 2/85, 2/86; Dr. Stephen Caiazza, pres. NY Physicians for Human Rights, 2/85, 10/85, 1/86.

San Francisco: Cleve Jones 8/82, 10/82, 3/83 (2), 5/83, 3/84, 4/84 (2), 12/84, 9/85, 1/86, 6/86; Catherine Cusic, Harvey Milk Gay Democratic Club 6/83, 6/85, 12/85; Jack McCarty and Victor Amburgy, hostages 7/85; Gary Walsh, PWA, 5/83, 6/83, 7/83, 8/83, 12/83, 1/84; Rick and Angie Walsh, 10/85; Lu Chaikin, 9/85, 10/85 (2); Matt Krieger 5/83, 9/86, 11/86; Joseph Brewer, 11/84, 10/85 (2), 11/85; Larry Bush, journalist and aide to Assemblyman Art Agnos 4/84, 10/84, 11/84, 1/85, 2/85, 3/85, 6/85, 7/85; Paul Lorch, editor, *Bay Area Reporter* 4/84; Konstantin Berlandt 5/83, 6/84; Allen White, *Bay Area Reporter* 7/84; Pat Norman 3/83, 6/86, 7/86, 8/86; Sharon Johnson 1/87; Dennis Seely 1/87; Bill Jones, proprietor, Sutro Bathhouse 6/83, 6/84; Randy Stallings, pres. Alice B. Toklas Democratic Club 3/83; Martin Cox, People With AIDS 5/83, 10/83, 11/83, 10/84; Paul Castro, PWA 6/83; Bob White, PWA in Paris for HPA-23 9/85, 11/85; Wayne Friday, pres. Tavern Guild 6/83, 12/86; Andrew Small, PWA 6/83; Lawrence Wilson, Alice B. Toklas Democratic Club 6/83; Russ Alley, businessman 6/83; Silvana Strangis 1/85; Anthony Ford 1/85; Louis Gaspar, proprietor, Hothouse 7/83; Steve Folstad, exec. dir. Pacific Center for Human Growth 4/83; Leon McKusick, psychologist 4/83, 10/83, 2/84; Karl Stewart, leather columnist *Bay Area Reporter* 4/83; Mark Feldman, PWA 5/83; Hal Slate, proprietor, The Cauldron 5/83; Gloria Rodriguez, PWA mother 10/83; Gary Ebert, Shanti volunteer 11/84; Bob Owen, proprietor, Academy sex club 10/84; Roberta Achtenberg, Lesbian Rights Project 10/84; John Wahl, Committee to Preserve Our Sexual & Civil Liberties 1/85; Deotis McMather, PWA 10/83; Bruce Schneider 10/83; Nick DiLorea, PWA 10/83; Dale Bentley, proprietor, Club Baths 3/84; Bill Morse, Animals sex club 6/84; Ron Huberman, Harvey Milk Gay Demo Club 11/86; Wayne Friday, *Bay Area Reporter* 11/86; Gwenn Craig, Harvey Milk Gay Democratic Club 12/86; Dick Pabich 11/86; Ken Maley 12/86; Larry Littlejohn 3/84, 4/84, 12/86; Jocelynn Nielsen 1/87; Carole

Migden, pres. Harvey Milk Gay Demo. Club 4/84, 11/86; Sal Accardi, Northern California Bathhouse Owner Assn. 3/84, 5/84; Jim Foster, former pres. Alice B. Toklas Demo. Club, 2/85; Mike Kraus 1/86, 3/86; Mary Kraus Whitesell 1/86; John Graham & Larry Benson, friends of Ken Horne 2/86; Enrique Govantes 3/86; Bobbi Campbell 4/82; Ron Carey 4/82; Tom Simpson, Lambda Funeral Guild, 3/85; Dean Sandmire, Mobilization Against AIDS 9/85; Sam Puckett, SF AIDS Foundation 6/84; Larry Bye, Research & Decisions, Corp. 10/84; Tristano Palermo, social services dir. SF AIDS Foundation 11/84, 1/85; Ed Power, projects dir. SF AIDS Foundation 5/83, 10/83; Jim Geary, exec. dir. Shanti Project 4/82; Sam Pichotto, Operation Concern 10/83. Richard Rector, SF People With AIDS 10/85; Dan Turner, People With AIDS 6/83, 1/86; Kenn Purnell, KS Foundation 2/86; *Op. cit.* Kraus.

Washington: Jeff Levi, National Gay & Lesbian Task Force 4/85, 8/85, 2/86; Garry MacDonald, Federation of AIDS-Related Organizations 8/85; Don Michaels, publisher, *Blade* 2/86; Vic Basile, Human Rights Campaign Fund 2/86.

Minneapolis: City Councilman Brian Coyle 4/84; State Senator Allan Spear 4/84; State Rep. Karen Clark 4/84.

Boston: City Councilman David Scoundras, 4/84.

Vancouver, British Columbia: Kevin Brown, PWA 3/86, Bob Tivey, AIDS Vancouver 3/86. Two friends of Gaetan Dugas consented to interviews only on the condition that their names not be used in the book.

The chronology of Rock Hudson's last days in Paris was drawn from contemporary news accounts, interviews, and the two biographies of the actor, *Rock Hudson: His Story* and *Idol—Rock Hudson: The True Story of an American Film Hero.*

Counts on the number of media stories about AIDS in major newspapers and periodicals were based on a NEXIS analysis of AIDS coverage commissioned by the Centers for Disease Control.

Excerpts from Matthew Krieger's journal were taken directly from his diary and are used with his permission.

Statistics on patterns of gay migration to San Francisco in the late 1970s and early 1980s are taken from the 1984 demographic study of the San Francisco gay community conducted by Research & Decisions Corporation and commissioned by the San Francisco AIDS Foundation.

Historical information on San Francisco's gay community is drawn largely from research for *The Mayor of Castro Street: The Life & Times of Harvey Milk.*

Meteorological data used in this book was provided by Steve Newman of the Earth Environment Service in San Francisco.

Blood Industry

Dr. Joseph Bove 3/86; Dr. John Klok, Pacific Presbyterian Cancer Research Center 8/84; Brian McDonough, president, Irwin Memorial Blood Bank 3/85,

4/85, 3/86; Dr. Herb Perkins, med. dir. Irwin 8/84; Gerry Sohle, Los Angeles Red Cross Blood Services 8/84; Dr. Robert Huitt, exec. dir. Council for Community Blood Centers 8/84; Dr. Edgar Engleman, Stanford Medical Center Blood Bank 8/84, 10/85; Ruth Cordell, lab. mgr. Irwin 3/85; Ray Price, sales rep., Abbott Labs 3/85; Dr. J. Lawrence Naiman, dir. blood services, Santa Clara Red Cross 3/85; Robert and Cathy Borchelt 3/86; Borchelt family attorneys James Waite and Sarah Jane Burgess 3/86. *Op. cit.* Dritz, Evatt, Lawrence, Curran, Francis, Jaffe, Westmoreland and Brandt.

Account of January 1983 policy meeting from interviews with participants as well as contemporary press releases and news accounts, most notably those of Philadelphia *Inquirer, New York Native* and "The Truth About AIDS." General information and blood industry also was drawn from "Blood Policy & Technology," a report from the Office of Technology Assessment (1985).

INDEX